# THE WASHINGTON MANUAL™ OF PEDIATRICS

# THE WASHINGTON MANUAL™ OF PEDIATRICS

*Editors*

## Susan M. Dusenbery, MD
Clinical Instructor of Pediatrics
Washington University School of Medicine
St. Louis Children's Hospital
St. Louis, Missouri

## Andrew J. White, MD
Assistant Professor and Program Director of Pediatrics
Washington University School of Medicine
St. Louis Children's Hospital
St. Louis, Missouri

Wolters Kluwer | Lippincott Williams & Wilkins
Health

Philadelphia • Baltimore • New York • London
Buenos Aires • Hong Kong • Sydney • Tokyo

*Acquisitions Editor:* Sonya Seigafuse
*Managing Editor:* Kerry Barrett
*Project Manager:* Bridgett Dougherty
*Marketing Manager:* Lisa Parry
*Manufacturing Manager:* Bengamin Rivera
*Design Coordinator:* Stephen Druding
*Cover Designer:* Stephen Druding
*Production Service:* Aptara, Inc.

© 2009 by Department of Pediatrics, Washington University on behalf of the School of Medicine

Printed in China

**Library of Congress Cataloging-in-Publication Data**

The Washington manual of pediatrics / editors, Susan M. Dusenbery, Andrew White.
   p. ; cm.
  Includes bibliographical references and index.
  ISBN 13: 978-0-7817-8576-1 (pbk. : alk. paper)
  ISBN 10: 0-7817-8576-6 (pbk. : alk. paper)
  1. Pediatrics—Handbooks, manuals, etc. I. Dusenbery, Susan M.
II. White, Andrew, 1964 Mar. 17 III. Title: Manual of pediatrics.
  [DNLM: 1. Pediatrics—Handbooks. WS 39 W319 2010]
  RJ48.W327 2010
  618.92—dc22

                   2009000200

The Washington Manual™ is an intent-to-use mark belonging to Washington University in St. Louis to which international legal protection applies. The mark is used in this publication by LWW under license from Washington University.

Care has been taken to confirm the accuracy of the information present and to describe generally accepted practices. However, the authors, editors, and publisher are not responsible for errors or omissions or for any consequences from application of the information in this book and make no warranty, expressed or implied, with respect to the currency, completeness, or accuracy of the contents of the publication. Application of this information in a particular situation remains the professional responsibility of the practitioner; the clinical treatments described and recommended may not be considered absolute and universal recommendations.

The authors, editors, and publisher have exerted every effort to ensure that drug selection and dosage set forth in this text are in accordance with current recommendations and practice at the time of publication. However, in view of ongoing research, changes in government regulations, and the constant flow of information relating to drug therapy and drug reactions, the reader is urged to check the package insert for each drug for any change in indications and dosage and for added warnings and precautions. This is particularly important when the recommended agent is a new or infrequently employed drug.

Some drugs and medical devices presented in this publication have Food and Drug Administration (FDA) clearance for limited use in restricted research settings. It is the responsibility of health care providers to ascertain the FDA status of each drug or device planned for use in their clinical practice.

To purchase additional copies of this book, call our customer service department at **(800) 638-3030** or fax orders to **(301) 223-2320**. International customers should call **(301) 223-2300**.

Visit Lippincott Williams & Wilkins on the Internet: http://www.lww.com. Lippincott Williams & Wilkins customer service representatives are available from 8:30 am to 6:00 pm, EST.

10 9 8 7 6 5 4 3 2 1

*This book is dedicated to my mother, Hyon Dusenbery; my husband, Daniel Bohl; and my daughters Abigail and Katherine Bohl.*

*—Susan Dusenbery*

# TABLE OF CONTENTS

**Ana Maria Arbelaez, MD**
Assistant Professor
Department of Pediatric Endocrinology
Washington University School of Medicine
St. Louis, Missouri

**Leonard B. Bacharier, MD**
Associate Professor
Department of Pediatrics
Washington University School of Medicine
Clinical Director
Division of Pediatric Allergy, Immunology,
   and Pulmonary Medicine
St. Louis Children's Hospital
St. Louis, Missouri

**Susan J. Bayliss, MD**
Professor
Departments of Medicine (Dermatology)
   and Pediatrics
Washington University School of Medicine
Director
Department of Pediatric Dermatology
St. Louis Children's Hospital
St. Louis, Missouri

**Anne Beck, MD**
Associate Professor
Department of Pediatrics
Washington University School of Medicine
Director of Dialysis Unit
Department of Pediatric Nephrology
St. Louis Children's Hospital
St. Louis, Missouri

**Avraham Beigelman, MD**
Fellow
Department of Pediatrics
Division of Allergy and Pulmonary
   Medicine
Washington University School of Medicine
St. Louis Children's Hospital
St. Louis, Missouri

**William E. Bennett, Jr., MD**
Clinical Fellow
Department of Pediatrics
Washington University School of Medicine
St. Louis Children's Hospital
St. Louis, Missouri

**Anne E. Borgmeyer, MSN, RN, CPNP, AE-C**
Pediatric Nurse Practitioner
Department of Nursing Administration
St. Louis Children's Hospital
St. Louis, Missouri

**Kristina N. Bryowsky, PharmD, BCPS**
Team Leader
Pharmacy
SSM St. Clare Health Center
Fenton, Missouri

**Douglas W. Carlson, MD**
Associate Professor
Department of Pediatrics
Washington University School of
   Medicine
Chief
Department of Pediatrics
Division of Hospital Medicine
St. Louis Children's Hospital
St. Louis, Missouri

**Li Ern Chen, MD**
Fellow
Department of Pediatric Surgery
Medical College of Wisconsin
Children's Hospital of Wisconsin
Milwaukee, Wisconsin

**Jennifer W. Cole, MD**
Associate Professor
Department of Anesthesiology
Washington University School of
   Medicine
Director of Ambulatory Procedure Center
   and Sedation Services
Department of Anesthesiology
St. Louis Children's Hospital
St. Louis, Missouri

**Megan A. Cooper, MD, PhD**
Fellow, Pediatric Rheumatology
Department of Pediatrics
Washington University School of
   Medicine
St. Louis Children's Hospital
St. Louis, Missouri

**Nathan P. Dean, MD**
Assistant Professor
Department of Pediatrics
Children's National Medical Center
Washington, DC

**Karen DeMuth, MD**
Instructor
Department of Pediatrics
Washington University School of Medicine
St. Louis, Missouri

**Marcella M. Donaruma-Kwoh, MD**
Assistant Professor
Department of Pediatrics
Baylor College of Medicine
Department of Pediatric Emergency
   Medicine
Texas Children's Hospital
Houston, Texas

**Susan M. Dusenbery, MD**
Clinical Instructor of Pediatrics
Washington University School of Medicine
St. Louis Children's Hospital
St. Louis, Missouri

**Elyra D. Figueroa, MD**
Fellow
Department of Pediatric Allergy and
   Immunology
Washington University School of Medicine
St. Louis, Missouri

**Stephanie A. Fritz, MD, MSCI**
Instructor
Department of Pediatrics
Washington University School of Medicine
Attending Physician
Department of Pediatrics
St. Louis Children's Hospital
St. Louis, Missouri

**Christina A. Gurnett, MD, PhD**
Assistant Professor
Department of Neurology
Washington University School of Medicine
St. Louis, Missouri

**Patti M. Gyr, MSN, RN, CPNP, AEC**
Pediatric Nurse Practitioner
Department of Nursing Administration
St. Louis Children's Hospital
St. Louis, Missouri

**Caroline C. Horner, MD**
Instructor
Department of Pediatrics
Washington University School of Medicine
St. Louis, Missouri

**David A. Hunstad, MD**
Assistant Professor
Department of Pediatrics
Washington University School of Medicine
Attending Physician
Department of Pediatrics
St. Louis Children's Hospital
St. Louis, Missouri

**Mark C. Johnson, MD**
Associate Professor
Department of Pediatrics
Washington University School of Medicine
St. Louis Children's Hospital
St. Louis, Missouri

**James P. Keating, MD, MSc**
Director, Division of Diagnostic Medicine
W. McKim O. Marriot Professor
Department of Pediatrics
Washington University School of Medicine
St. Louis, Missouri

**Robert M. Kennedy, MD**
Professor
Department of Pediatrics
Washington University School of Medicine
Attending Physician
Department of Emergency Services
St. Louis Children's Hospital
St. Louis, Missouri

**Lila C. Kertz, MSN, RN, CPNP**
Pediatric Nurse Practitioner
Department of Pediatrics
Division of Allergy and Pulmonary
   Medicine
St. Louis Children's Hospital
St. Louis, Missouri

**Nikoleta S. Kolovos, MD**
Assistant Professor
Department of Pediatrics
Washington University School of Medicine
Medical Director
Pediatric Intensive Care Unit
St. Louis Children's Hospital
St. Louis, Missouri

**Keith A. Kronemer, MD**
Assistant Professor
Mallinckrodt Institute of Radiology
Washington University School of
  Medicine
Radiologist
Department of Radiology
St. Louis Children's Hospital
St. Louis, Missouri

**Amit Malhotra, MD**
Associate Residency Director
Department of Pediatrics
The Permanente Medical Group
Attending Neurologist
Department of Pediatrics
Division of Neurology
Kaiser Permanente Medical Center
  Oakland
Oakland, California

**Amit Mathur, MBBS, MD**
Associate Professor of Pediatrics
Department of Pediatrics/Newborn
  Medicine
Washington University School of
  Medicine
Associate Medical Director Neonatal ICU
Department of Pediatrics/Newborn
  Medicine
St. Louis Children's Hospital
St. Louis, Missouri

**William H. McAlister, MD**
Professor of Radiology and Pediatrics
Department of Radiology
Washington University School of
  Medicine
Radiologist
Department of Pediatric Radiology
St. Louis Children's Hospital
St. Louis, Missouri

**Tracy L. McGregor, MD**
Instructor
Department of Pediatrics
Vanderbilt University
Nashville, Tennessee

**Kara Sternhell Nunley, MD**
Chief Resident
Department of Dermatology
Washington University School of
  Medicine
Barnes Jewish Hospital
St. Louis, Missouri

**Kathryn L. Plax, MD**
Assistant Professor
Department of Pediatrics
Washington University School of Medicine
Director, Adolescent Center
Department of Pediatrics
St. Louis Children's Hospital
St. Louis, Missouri

**Aarati Rao, MD**
Assistant Professor
Department of Pediatrics
University of South Alabama
Department of Pediatrics: Hematology
  Oncology
USA Children's and Women's Hospital
Mobile, Alabama

**Tyler E. Reimschisel, MD**
Assistant Professor of Pediatrics and
  Neurology
Department of Pediatrics
Vanderbilt University
Nashville, Tennessee

**Edward K. Rhee, MD, FACC**
Director, Arrhythmia Services
Eller Congenital Heart Center
St. Joseph's Hospital and Medical Center
Phoenix, Arizona

**Katherine Rivera-Spoljaric, MD**
Instructor
Department of Pediatrics
Washington University School of Medicine
St. Louis, Missouri

**Stacie P. Shepherd, MD, PhD**
Associate Medical Director
Department P4MD
Abbott Laboratories
Abbott Park, Illinois

**Eli Silver, MD**
Instructor
Department of Pediatrics
Washington University School of Medicine
St. Louis, Missouri

**Sweety Srivastava, MD**
Attending Staff Physician
Department of Pediatrics
Hurley Medical Center
Attending Physician
Department of Pediatrics
Hamilton Community Health Network
Flint, Michigan

**Lynne M. Strauser Sterni, MD**
Instructor
Department of Pediatrics
Washington University School of Medicine
Pediatric Hospitalist
Department of Hospital Medicine
St. Louis Children's Hospital
St. Louis, Missouri

**Sthorn Thatayatikom, MD, MSc**
Former Allergy and Immunology Fellow
Department of Pediatrics
Washington University School of Medicine
St. Louis, Missouri
Allergist
Asthma and Allergy Center
Pikesville, Kentucky

**Sarah Tycast, MD**
Instructor
Department of Pediatrics
Washington University School of Medicine
Instructor, Adolescent Medicine
Department of Pediatrics
St. Louis Children's Hospital
St. Louis, Missouri

**Akshaya J. Vachharajani, MD, MRCP (UK)**
Assistant Professor
Department of Pediatrics
Washington University School of Medicine
Department of Pediatrics/Newborn Medicine
St. Louis Children's Hospital
St. Louis, Missouri

**Arpita Kalla Vyas, MB, ChB**
Fellow
Department of Pediatric Endocrinology
Washington University School of Medicine
St. Louis, Missouri

**Brad W. Warner, MD**
Apolline Blair/St. Louis Children's Hospital Professor of Surgery
Director, Division of Pediatric Surgery
Washington University School of Medicine
Surgeon-in-Chief
Department of Pediatric Surgery
St. Louis Children's Hospital
St. Louis, Missouri

**Andrew J. White, MD**
Assistant Professor
Department of Pediatrics
Washington University School of Medicine
Program Director
Department of Pediatrics
St. Louis Children's Hospital
St. Louis, Missouri

**David B. Wilson, MD, PhD**
Associate Professor
Department of Pediatrics
Washington University School of Medicine
St. Louis, Missouri

The first edition of *The Washington Manual™ of Pediatrics* was created from *The Washington Manual™ Pediatric Survival Guide* to provide concise and quickly accessible information to interns, residents, and medical students while they care for children on call, in a critical care setting, in the emergency unit, and in subspecialty outpatient clinics. For this reason, this manual does not contain a complete description of each pediatric subspecialty or an extensive description of the pathophysiology of the diseases discussed. However, it does provide established approaches to the diagnosis and treatment of common inpatient pediatric problems. In addition, it supplies evidence-based medicine references where they are available for the described management approaches.

The authors of the manual were interns, residents, chief residents, subspecialty fellows, and junior and senior faculty at St. Louis Children's Hospital. It has been a pleasure to work with these many talented, enthusiastic, and caring physicians to provide a manual for house officers and medical students. I would like to thank all of the authors that contributed to this manual as well as Dr. Ana Maria Arbelaez and Dr. Tami Garmany, who wrote *The Washington Manual™ Pediatric Survival Guide*. I would also like to thank Dr. Jamie Sutherell, Dr. Jeffrey Bednarksi, and Dr. Jennifer York for their assistance with the creation of *The Washington Manual™ of Pediatrics*, and Dr. Kimberly Quayle for the DKA emergency room management card included with this manual, and Andrew J. White.

*Susan M. Dusenbery*

■ Learning to care for children is best done through experience; however, there are common concerns encountered with every child.

■ This chapter addresses common concerns that are seen during an inpatient hospital stay or a visit to the emergency department.

# FEEDING

## General Principles

### *Infants*

■ Breast milk

  ■ The American Academy of Pediatrics (AAP) recommends breastfeeding for the first 12 months of life (exclusively for the first 6 months).

  ■ Breastfed infants initially nurse 5 minutes on each breast every 1–3 hours and gradually work up to 10–15 minutes on each breast. At 1 month of age, most infants sleep for up to 5 hours, which is the longest time period they will go without needing to be fed.

  ■ Adequate nutrition can be assessed by an infant's history of weight gain. Although infants may lose up to 10% of their birth weight in the first week of life, they have regained that weight by the second week and gained 2–3 lb by the fourth week of life. Birth weight is generally doubled by 4 months of age and tripled by 1 year. Infants gain about 1 oz in weight per day.

  ■ The AAP recommends that 200 IU of vitamin D per day be introduced to the diet of breastfed infants within the first 2 months of age, and it may be wise to start at birth.

■ Formula

  ■ If a family chooses to provide formula as the primary source of nutrition to their infant, the recommended amount is 100 kcal/kg/day. In newborns, this is 2–3 oz every 3–4 hours, and it increases to 4 oz every 3–4 hours at 1 month of age.

  ■ There are many brands and varieties of formula.

    • For a more complete description, refer to Chapter 2, Nutritional Problems.

    • It is most important that if powdered formula is used, family members are following the instructions for making it accurately.

  ■ At 12 months of age, infants should be receiving at least 16 oz of formula a day. At this time, children can be transitioned from breast milk or formula to whole milk containing calcium and vitamin D. Earlier transitioning to whole milk is associated with the development of iron deficiency anemia.

■ Solids

  ■ Single-grain cereal is added to an infant's diet at 4–6 months of age. Initially it is added to breast milk or formula and spoon-fed to the infant. Once a child is able to eat cereal from a spoon, typically at 6 months of age, additional solid foods can be added.

  ■ "Orange" pureed vegetables, such as carrots, sweet potatoes, and butternut squash, are often an infant's first vegetables. Each vegetable is introduced alone over a 3-day period so that it is possible to watch for an allergic reaction. After 3 days, another vegetable can be added.

- "Green" pureed vegetables, such as peas and green beans, can then be introduced.
- Once an infant is able to enjoy vegetables, pureed fruits can be given. Fruits are often started later than vegetables because of the belief that vegetables are less palatable after an infant learns to like the taste of fruit.
- Lastly, pureed meats are added to an infant's diet at approximately 8 months of age.
  - At 8 months of age, most children are beginning to use their pincer grasp to reach finger food.
  - By 12 months of age, most children are eating soft food that the rest of the family is eating as well. This includes 4–5 oz of protein, a half cup of cereal or grain, a half a slice of bread, and one to two pieces of fruit and/or vegetables.

### Toddlers

- Feeding a child in the second year of life is modeled around three meals, with food as described above. The amount increases as a child's weight and energy needs increase.
- By 12–15 months of age, toddlers start to drink on their own out of a "sippy cup" and eventually a regular cup by 2–3 years of age.
- Children in this age group are difficult to feed because of their newfound ability to make choices and declare their independence.

### Children

- As children become 4–5 years of age, they begin to use utensils well and have developed table manners. They continue to eat three meals a day, with possibly one to two snacks.
- Meals should include protein, dairy products, carbohydrates, and fruits and vegetables.
- A multivitamin should be provided if the child's diet is deficient in vitamin D, calcium, or iron or if it is not well balanced with fruits, vegetables, and a source of iron.

## Diagnosis: Common Difficulties

### Food Allergy

- Clinical presentation
- Often urticarial rash
- Also spitting up, vomiting, diarrhea, bloody stools, and breathing difficulties
- History
  - Detailed dietary history, including dates that foods were introduced, types of formula, cereal, and solid food
  - Dates that the rash was noticed and what helps the rash
  - Stooling history, particularly any history of blood in stools
- Physical examination
  - Head, ears, eyes, nose, throat: possible periorbital or perioral swelling
  - Skin: hives or dry scaly rash (eczema)
  - Respiratory: possible tachypnea, wheezing
  - Gastrointestinal: possible guaiac-positive stools (questionable significance)
- Treatment (for further information, refer to Chapter 11, Allergic Diseases)
  - Standard treatments for an allergic reaction that causes swelling or difficulty breathing include removing the offending allergen and giving diphenhydramine (Benadryl), steroids, and subcutaneous epinephrine.
  - If only a rash is noted, discontinue the food that initiated the rash.
  - Milk protein allergies may present before solids are introduced. Differentiate symptoms of a milk protein allergy from lactose intolerance. Cow's milk-based formulas can be switched to soy-based formulas if a cow's milk protein allergy is suspected.

### Spitting Up

- Definition: liquids that are "burped" or "spit-up" out of mouth after feedings, up to 1 year of age
- History and physical examination
  - Parents describe that the infant was picked up following a feeding and some milk or curds or mucus came out of the mouth. The milk did not come out forcefully. No crying is associated with the event.

- There is no history of weight loss.
- Physical examination is within normal limits.
- Treatment
  - Reassurance. Ensure that the infant has been consistently gaining weight.
  - To decrease spitting up:
    - Place the infant at a 30-degree angle after feedings.
    - Use smaller and more frequent feedings.
  - Unlike vomiting from gastroenteritis, hydration status is not a concern in spitting up.
  - Forceful or projectile vomiting that appears at 4–6 weeks of age and is associated with weight loss, which is concerning for pyloric stenosis. This is evaluated with abdominal ultrasound or upper endoscopy; an examination finding of a palpable olive, felt during contraction; and treated with pyloromyotomy.
  - See Chapter 15, Gastroenterologic Diseases for further information on vomiting.

### Slow Weight Gain
- Clinical presentation: wasted appearance, poor growth
- History
  - Dietary and social history, as well as history of weight loss and gain, are critical. Watch the child eat during the history and examination.
  - Any other medical problems or medications must be understood.
  - Family history is also important because many genetic conditions are associated with poor weight gain.
- Physical examination
  - Obtain weight, height, and head circumference values and percentiles.
  - Many other features can be found on examination, depending on the cause of the weight loss.
- Laboratory studies
  - Newborn screen, complete blood count (CBC) with differential, electrolytes, sweat test, antitissue transglutaminase, and immunoglobulin A for celiac disease (if gluten has been introduced to the diet).
  - Additional tests can include repeating free thyroxine, thyroid-stimulating hormone, fat-soluble vitamins, urine organic acids, and serum amino acids.
- Treatment
  - Refer to Chapter 2, Nutritional Problems for further information.
  - If an infant is breastfed, the mother can pump and then provide breast milk to her child in a bottle to be able to quantify the amount of milk the child is receiving.
  - If weight loss is significant, children are admitted, weighed daily, and the amount of food consumed is calculated carefully. Formulas may change during a hospital stay if it is suspected that the child is not able to absorb nutrients from his or her current formula.

### "Picky" Eating
- Typically, these are children 2–3 years of age who eat only certain types of food.
- History
  - Ask about diet. For example, the "white diet" consists of rice, pasta, crackers, cheese, and milk.
  - Parents describe struggling with the child at meal time and may state that they make separate meals for the child.
- Physical examination and laboratory studies
  - Examination is usually within normal limits.
  - Testing may involve a CBC for iron deficiency anemia.
- Treatment. Recommend that caregivers:
  - Provide a variety of foods at each meal in all of the basic food groups.
  - Do not pressure the child to eat any particular food.
  - Do not make a separate meal for the child. Sometimes "picky" eating is a toddler's means of self-expression and independence.

■ If the child is not receiving meat, fruit, and vegetables, or if the CBC indicates that the child has iron deficiency, then provide a daily chewable multivitamin containing iron.

## Iron Deficiency

■ Epidemiology
  ■ This may occur throughout infancy, childhood, and adolescence.
    • Full-term infants have adequate iron stores until 6 months of age; premature infants have adequate iron stores until 2–3 months of age.
    • Children 9–18 months of age are at the highest risk for iron deficiency anemia because of a rapid rate of growth and inadequate dietary iron.
    • During adolescence, it may be seen in girls once they begin their menstrual cycles, particularly when bleeding is heavy.
  ■ Hemoglobin levels <10 g/dL have been associated with developmental delay and behavior difficulties.

■ Clinical presentation
  ■ Lethargy and decreased activity
  ■ Tachycardia and tachypnea if anemia is severe

■ History
  ■ During infancy, history may reveal that the infant received regular cow's milk or goat's milk as a substitute for breast milk or formula, was preterm or low birth weight, received a formula that was not fortified with iron, drank more than 24 oz of whole milk after 12 months of age, or was breast-fed and did not have an additional iron source after 6 months of age.
  ■ Toddlers may be "picky" eaters, as described above, who do not receive enough iron-containing foods. This may apply to children and adolescents.
  ■ There may be a history of lead exposure.
  ■ There may be a history of blood loss in the stool or urine.
  ■ If the patient is an adolescent female, obtain a history about the length of menstrual cycles, how many days between periods, and the number of pads or tampons used.

■ Physical examination
  ■ Vital signs may show tachycardia.
  ■ A child may appear pale, particularly on the mucosal membranes, conjunctiva, and nail beds.
  ■ A systolic flow murmur may be present.

■ Laboratory studies and imaging
  ■ A CBC with smear is necessary. The hemoglobin and hematocrit are low, and platelets may be high. The smear shows microcytic, hypochromic red blood cells. Confirm that the smear does not show schistocytes, which suggest hemolysis. The red cell distribution width is often the first laboratory test to rise in iron deficiency.
  ■ Iron studies, such as a total iron binding capacity (TIBC), transferrin saturation, iron level, and ferritin level, can be obtained to confirm the anemia is iron deficiency, but these are generally not necessary in most clinical scenarios.
  ■ All iron studies are low in iron deficiency except the TIBC, which is high. The ferritin level may be normal if there is a concurrent illness because ferritin is also an acute phase reactant.
  ■ A chest radiograph may be obtained in severe anemia to look for cardiomegaly.
  ■ If there is any history of lead exposure, consider sending a serum lead level.

■ Treatment
  ■ In infants and toddlers, treat with iron drops: 6 mg/kg/day of elemental iron.
  ■ In school-age children, treat with iron tablets: 60 mg/day.
  ■ In adolescents, treat with iron tablets: 60–120 mg/day.
  ■ In all children, continue iron supplement daily for 1 month and recheck the CBC.
  ■ If the hemoglobin has increased by 1 g/dL or the hematocrit by 3%, then the diagnosis of iron deficiency is confirmed. Continue iron supplementation for 2 months and recheck the CBC in 6 months.

- If the hemoglobin is unchanged, further evaluation of anemia must be considered. See Chapter 17, Hematology and Oncology for further details.
- Consider giving a packed red blood cell transfusion if the hemoglobin is ≤4–5 g/dL or symptoms, such as with respiratory distress or acute bleeding, are present. Blood transfusions in severe anemia can precipitate or worsen heart failure. Therefore, they should be done slowly and with close monitoring.
- Other interventions for iron deficiency anemia include:
  - Stop feeding regular cow's milk or goat's milk if younger than 1 year of age.
  - Introduce iron-containing food to the child's diet.
  - Decrease milk consumption if >24 oz/day in a child older than 12 months of age.
  - If serum lead level is elevated, take the child from the home until source is known and removed. See "Lead Poisoning" section of this chapter for further details.
- Refer an adolescent with history of heavy menstrual cycles to obstetrician/gynecologist for evaluation of menorrhagia.

# LEAD POISONING

## Epidemiology

- The normal lead level is zero.
- Elevated lead levels (even <10 µg/dL) have been shown to affect IQ and behavior in children.
- Between 1976 and 1980, the median lead level for children 1 to 5 years of age was 15 µg/dL, and in 1999, it was 1.9 µg/dL. The decreases in median levels were because of removal of lead from gasoline, removal of lead paint from homes, and the removal of lead-based solder from food-containing tin cans.

## Clinical Presentation

- The child may be asymptomatic.
- He or she may have headaches, abdominal pain, constipation, and lethargy.
- He or she may present with seizures, encephalopathy, and coma.

## History

- There may be a history of living in a home built before 1978.
- The home may have chipping paint.
- The home may have been recently renovated.
- There may have been a history of pica (eating soil or paint chips).
- Hobbies of either the child or other family members may include pottery, fishing, or hunting.
- There may be a history of elevated lead levels in the child or his or her family members. Obtain a history of imported pottery or food, particularly canned food.

## Physical Examination

- The child may show developmental delay, particularly language delay.
- Mental status changes or seizures may be present.
- Lead poisoning is associated with short stature.

## Laboratory Studies

- A CBC may show microcytic, hypochromic anemia.
- Basophilic stippling may be seen on a smear.
- A serum lead level is necessary.

## Treatment

- Additional information about treatment is provided in detail in Chapter 17, Hematology and Oncology.

- No treatment is necessary for lead levels <10 µg/dL.
- If the lead level is between 10 and 20 µg/dL, the level should be rechecked. An environmental evaluation for the source of lead should be performed for levels >10 µg/dL.
- Lead levels between 20 and 44 µg/dL can be treated with oral succimer to decrease the lead level. However, there is no evidence that succimer treatment improves cognitive or behavioral outcome at this level.
- Lead levels >44 µg/dL are treated with oral succimer or parenteral Ca EDTA if oral therapy is not tolerated.
- Lead levels >70 µg/dL are treated with parenteral Ca EDTA.

## SLEEPING

### General Principles

- All infants should be placed on their backs to sleep to decrease the risk of sudden infant death syndrome (SIDS). Side sleeping is not sufficient.
- The risk of SIDS is also decreased by removing blankets and toys from the infant's crib, by having parents refrain from or quit smoking, and by not sleeping with the infant.
- It is expected that infants younger than 4 months of age may not sleep through the night because of their feeding schedule.
- After 4 months of age, infants may continue to wake up because of the establishment of a routine.
- Toddlers often wake up in the middle of the night because of night terrors and nightmares.

### Diagnosis: Common Difficulties

*Not Sleeping Through the Night (Infants)*
- Infant begins crying in the middle of the night.
- The condition may be because of hunger, but consider infection and teething.
- Physical examination and laboratory studies
  - Look for fever, acute otitis media, signs of an upper respiratory tract infection, or teeth breaking through the gum line.
  - No laboratory studies are necessary, unless the history or physical examination suggests illness.
- Treatment
  - If the patient is otherwise healthy, have the parents continue to feed the infant every 2–4 hours as described in the "Feeding" section.
  - Between 4 and 6 months of age, the infant can be weaned from a middle-of-the-night feeding regimen.
    - This involves stopping the feedings in the middle of the night for three nights and not picking up the infant when he or she cries. Parents can pat the child or look at him or her from the door, but are encouraged not to pick up the child.
    - The crying should resolve after 3 nights.

*Night Terrors*
- Clinical presentation
  - Children can begin having night terrors at 2 years of age. They present with screaming or crying between the first 1–4 hours of sleep or during the non–rapid eye movement (REM) sleep.
  - The crying can last from 5–30 minutes, and children do not wake up, even if their eyes are open.
  - They typically do not remember the event in the morning.
- Physical examination and laboratory studies
  - Examination: within normal limits
  - Laboratory tests: none

- Treatment
  - Tell parents not to attempt to wake the child during the night terror.
  - Tell them to watch to ensure that the child does not fall off the bed or hurt himself or herself in any way.
  - Ensure that the child has a regular sleeping routine.

### *Nightmares*
- Clinical presentation
  - Children can begin having nightmares at the same age they begin having night terrors.
  - Nightmares occur during REM sleep and therefore later in the night than night terrors.
  - Children can remember nightmares, unlike night terrors.

- Physical examination and laboratory studies
  - Examination: within normal limits
  - Laboratory tests: none

- Treatment
  - Tell parents to ensure that the child has a regular sleep routine.
  - Tell them to avoid scary or horror movies before bed.

## COLIC

### General Principles

- Colic is defined as "intermittent unexplained excessive crying" multiple times per day, 4 days/week for a week or more in an infant between 1 and 4 months of age.
- Each episode lasts 30 minutes to 2 hours, and the infant cries for a total of about 3 hours or more per day. Colic usually occurs in the evenings or is worse in the evenings.
- This is a diagnosis of exclusion. There are multiple unproven theories about the cause of colic, including an increased need for being held and cow's milk whey protein intolerance.

### *Diagnosis*

### *Clinical Presentation*
- Inconsolable crying in a child 1–4 months of age, without fever, lethargy, or any other symptoms
- Taking formula well and gaining weight appropriately

### *Physical Examination and Laboratory Studies*
- The examination is within normal limits.
- No laboratory tests are necessary.

### *Treatment*
- Studies have evaluated the effectiveness of several interventions for colic. Interventions with a modestly statistically significant improvement included a hypoallergenic diet (diet free of milk, egg, wheat, and nut products) for a breastfeeding mother, soy formula in formula-fed infants, and reduced stimulation of the infant.
- Simethicone drops, car ride stimulators, and holding infants more frequently did not show a statistical difference in colic.

## STOOLING

### General Principles

- Breastfed infants have loose, yellow seedy stools that occur frequently. Initially, this may occur after every episode of nursing. Formula-fed infants have firmer stools less often than breastfed infants, perhaps only once every 3 days. The color of the stool may normally vary between yellow and green.

- Once children begin to eat solid food, their stools become firmer.
- Children with bloody stools should be evaluated by a physician.

## Diagnosis: Common Difficulties

### Constipation

- The definition of constipation is variable, and the normal range of bowel movement frequency is wide, from 1 per week to 8 per day, making the definition of constipation difficult.
- Clinical presentation
    - The stool may be hard and may be accompanied by blood. Children may strain and turn red-faced while stooling, although this may also be normal.
    - Stool leakage (encopresis) may develop in chronic constipation.
- Physical examination and laboratory studies
    - Rectal examination may show fecal impaction or fissures.
    - Abdominal examination is normal, and scybala may be palpated.
    - An abdominal film is not necessary unless there is concern for a diagnosis other than ordinary constipation based on the history and physical examination. If the patient has abdominal distension or other findings that suggest intestinal obstruction, an abdominal film is imperative.
    - Consider Hirschsprung disease in infants who present with constipation. After a careful history and physical examination, a rectal suction biopsy can help confirm the diagnosis.
- Treatment
    - Initially, manage toddlers and children who present with constipation with the addition of more fruits and vegetables to the diet. If the constipation persists, treat these children with an osmotic agent such as polyethylene glycol (MiraLax) until they have a regular stooling pattern.
    - Refer to Chapter 15, Gastroenterologic Diseases for further details on management of difficult constipation.

### Diarrhea

- Clinical presentation: frequent, loose, watery stools, with or without blood, vomiting, or fever
- Physical examination
    - Look for signs of dehydration, dry mucous membranes, sunken eyes, tachycardia, poor skin turgor, poor capillary refill, loss of tears, and a decreased amount of urination (dry diaper).
    - Abdominal examination may show diffuse tenderness but with normal bowel sounds and no abdominal distension. Look for signs of appendicitis, including right lower quadrant pain, guarding, and peritoneal signs.
- Laboratory studies: depends on the clinical scenario
    - A rectal swab for bacteria and virus can be taken if a fresh stool sample is not available.
    - A stool ovum and parasites may be sent if the history suggests a parasitic infection as a possible cause.
    - If the patient has an acute abdomen, a surgical consult is imperative.
    - Signs of dehydration should prompt a BMP.
- Treatment
    - Most diarrhea in children represents viral gastroenteritis and takes 5–10 days to resolve.
    - The most important treatment is hydration with electrolyte-containing fluids. Oral rehydration therapy is preferable to intravenous and should be attempted repeatedly.
        - Infants should continue to receive formula, which can be supplemented with Pedialyte. The type of formula may be changed to a formula without lactose, if the diarrhea persists.

- Refer to Chapter 2, Nutritional Problems for discussion of intractable diarrhea of infancy.
- Refer to Chapter 3, Fluid and Electrolyte Management for further details on treatment of dehydration.
- Refer to Chapter 15, Gastroenterologic Diseases for a further discussion of diarrhea.

# URINATING

## General Principles

- Pediatricians expect infants and toddlers to wet at least three diapers per day, although there are usually more than that. If a child is not wetting at least three diapers per day, that should raise the concern for dehydration.
- Older children who suddenly begin to urinate more frequently should be evaluated for urinary tract infection, diabetes mellitus, or diabetes insipidus.

### Enuresis
- Definition
  - Enuresis in children older than 5 years of age is defined as two bed-wetting episodes per week for 3 consecutive months or distress from bed-wetting episodes.
  - In 5-year-old children, this condition occurs in 7% of boys and 3% of girls. This percentage decreases in 18-year-old men to 1%, and it is very rare in 18-year-old women.
- Clinical presentation and history
  - Patients are older than 5 years of age and present with multiple episodes of wetting the bed at night (nocturnal enuresis) or wetting their pants during the day (diurnal enuresis).
  - It is important to ask if the child was born prematurely, has a nervous system disorder, has ever had surgery to their genital area, or has parents with a history of nocturnal enuresis.
  - The history should also include questions about the frequency and amount of urination during the day and night. In addition, questions about pain with urination, as well as constipation, should be asked.
  - Consider the following causes of diurnal enuresis: micturition deferral, urinary tract infections, diabetes, chemical urethritis, constipation, and giggle incontinence.
- Physical examination and laboratory studies
  - Examination is within normal limits if the diagnosis is nocturnal enuresis.
  - Perform a complete neurologic examination to look for signs of spinal cord dysfunction.
  - Carefully evaluate the abdomen for masses.
  - Perform a urinalysis to look for signs of infection.
- Treatment
  - Begin treatment with behavioral modification, including rewards for staying dry, urinating before bedtime, and waking the child 2–3 hours after sleeping to void. This method is successful 85% of the time.
  - Use of a bed-wetting alarm is less successful.
  - Desmopressin (DDAVP) is second-line treatment for nocturnal enuresis.
  - Both the alarm and DDAVP have a high relapse rate when discontinued.

# VACCINATIONS

- Vaccinations are the most important preventive therapy that pediatricians provide to children.
- There is no scientific evidence to support any association between vaccination and autism.

- The vaccine schedule for children and adolescents, as well as a catch-up schedule, is available on the Centers for Disease Control and Prevention (CDC) Web site and is updated regularly (see Suggested Readings).
- See Appendix A, Child and Adolescent Immunization Guidelines, 2008 for the 2008 immunization schedule.
- Some vaccines are associated with fever, irritability, and rash. Each individual vaccine has a different side-effect profile that parents and physicians should understand before vaccination.
- The contraindications to specific vaccines are also listed on the CDC Web site (see Suggested Readings).

## Suggested Readings

American Academy of Pediatrics Committee on Environmental Health. Lead exposure in children: prevention, detection, and management. Pediatrics, October 2005;116:1036–1046.

Brazelton T, Sparrow J. Feeding the Brazelton way. Cambridge, MA: Da Capo Press, 2004.

Centers for Disease Control and Prevention (CDC). Recommendations to prevent and control iron deficiency in the United States. MMWR Morb Mortal Wkly Rep 1998;47(RR-3); 1–36.

Centers for Disease Control and Prevention (CDC). Recommended immunization schedule for persons aged 0–18 years—United States 2008. MMWR Morb Mortal Wkly Rep January 11, 2008;57(01):Q1–Q4. Date accessed 3/3/08.

Garrison MM, Christakis DA. A systematic review of treatments for infant colic. Pediatrics 2000;106;184–190.

Guide to contraindications of vaccinations. Available at: http://www.cdc.gov/vaccines/recs/vac-admin/contraindications.htm. Date accessed 3/3/08.

Kliegman RM, et al. Nelson Textbook of Pediatrics, 18th Ed. Philadelphia: WB Saunders, 2007.

Sears W, et al. The Baby Sleep Book. New York: Little, Brown and Company, 2005.

Thiedke C. Nocturnal enuresis. Am Fam Physician April 1, 2003;67(7).

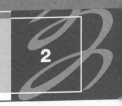

# 2

# NUTRITIONAL PROBLEMS
*William E. Bennett, Jr. and James P. Keating*

## COMMON INFANT ENTERAL NUTRITION

Although breast milk should be the first choice for infant nourishment, there are many infant formulas that provide adequate nutrition. It is common practice to switch formulas in infants with difficulty gaining weight, frequent physiologic reflux, or other feeding difficulties. Specialized formulas are frequently much more expensive than standard formulas, and thoughtful advice should be given to parents, especially those with limited resources (Table 2-1).

## INTRACTABLE DIARRHEA OF INFANCY

### General Principles

- Also called postenteritis enteropathy, intractable diarrhea of infancy (IDI) is a prolonged diarrhea caused by the loss of enterocytes and thus absorptive capacity.
- It occurs initially because of infection, but as malabsorption worsens, resultant malnutrition prevents regrowth of mucosa.
- It is a severe problem in the developing world.

### Diagnosis

- Clinical evidence: diarrhea persisting beyond course of infectious illness and despite appropriate formula choice
- Absence of other factors that may cause chronic diarrhea: parasitic infection, pancreatic insufficiency, or congenital small bowel mucosal defect

### Treatment

- Begin with lactose-free, sucrose-free protein hydrolysate (e.g., Pregestimil) or chemically defined formula (e.g., Neocate).
- If diarrhea continues despite this change, stop feeds and institute total parenteral nutrition (TPN) for 2–4 weeks to allow mucosal rehabilitation.
- Institute bowel rest for 2–4 weeks.
- Restart feeds with lactose-free, sucrose-free formula.
- If diarrhea persists, pursue congenital causes of diarrhea, such as congenital small bowel mucosal defects, autoimmune enteropathy, and vasoactive intestinal polypeptide (VIP) secreting tumors.

## SLOW WEIGHT GAIN

### General Principles

- "Failure to thrive" is also a common term for slow weight gain in infants.
- The most common cause is inadequate intake because of psychosocial causes.
- Other causes should be investigated based on specific clinical characteristics.

| TABLE 2-1 | Common Infant Enteral Nutrition | | | |
|---|---|---|---|---|
| Formula | Carbohydrate | Protein | Fat | Clinical use |
| Breast milk | Lactose | Milk whey protein | Vegetable oils, others | Infant nutrition |
| Enfamil Similac | Corn syrup and lactose | Cow milk whey protein | Vegetable oils, others | Standard formula |
| Isomil | Corn syrup and sucrose | Soy protein isolate | Vegetable oils, others | Cow's milk protein intolerance |
| ProSobee | Corn syrup | Soy protein isolate | Vegetable oils, others | Cow's milk protein intolerance, galactosemia |
| Alimentum Nutramigen | Corn syrup | Casein hydrolysate | Vegetable oils, others | Fat/protein malabsorption, cholestasis |
| Pregestimil | Corn syrup, dextrose | Casein hydrolysate | Vegetable oils, others | Fat/protein malabsorption, cholestasis |
| EleCare Neocate | Corn syrup | Amino acids | Vegetable oils, others | Severe cow's milk protein intolerance or multiple food allergies |
| Nutren Jr. PediaSure | Sucrose, maltodextrin | Milk protein | Vegetable oils, others | Standard formula (children >1 year of age) |
| Peptamen | Corn syrup, maltodextrin | Hydrolyzed milk protein | 60% medium-chain triglycerides | Malabsorption (children >1 year of age) |

## Diagnosis

- Obtain record of growth for both length and weight to establish associations that may be causal.
- Take a focused social history and family psychological history with special attention to high-risk situations:
  - Multiple caregivers
  - Adolescent or developmentally delayed mothers
  - Inadequate formula availability (e.g., poverty)
  - Incorrect formula preparation
  - Postpartum depression
  - Abuse
- Observe infant feeding, both by parents or other caregivers, preferably in the home environment.
- Period of observation with frequent weights and reassessments is necessary.
- For further investigations, use various clues (not a comprehensive list):
  - Dysmorphic features, microcephaly, and so on: congenital anomalies
  - Prematurity
  - Intrauterine growth retardation: growth restriction that may delay later growth up to 2 years
  - Poor suck: neurologic disorder, cleft palate, premature reflexes
  - Signs of abuse/neglect

■ Diarrhea: cystic fibrosis, chronic infection
■ Respiratory symptoms: cystic fibrosis

## Treatment

■ Address remediable social factors; education for psychosocial growth failure.
■ Address disease-based causes individually (see previous discussion).

## VITAMIN DEFICIENCY PEARLS

The varied presentations of specific vitamin deficiencies can be nonspecific and broad. Table 2-2 summarizes common findings in children with specific vitamin deficiencies.

## WARNING ABOUT OVERESTIMATES OF CALORIC NEED

■ Pediatricians should resist the urge to treat all chronically or seriously ill children with more calories.
  ■ Recent evidence suggests that high caloric intake in critically ill patients is not only ineffective, it may actually be harmful.
  ■ A thoughtful, conservative approach to choosing caloric targets should take activity into consideration and appreciate the wide range of normal intake.

| TABLE 2-2 | Clinical Signs of Vitamin Deficiency |
| --- | --- |
| **Vitamin/Mineral** | **Clinical pearls** |
| A | • Bitot spots (corneal haziness/edema) <br> • Nyctalopia (night blindness) <br> • Follicular hyperkeratosis <br> • Bulging fontanelle |
| B₁ (thiamine) | • Cardiac failure ("wet beriberi") <br> • Ophthalmoplegia |
| B₂ (riboflavin) <br> B₆ (pyridoxine) | • Cheilosis/cheilitis <br> • Glossitis <br> • Infantile spasms |
| B₁₂ | • Megaloblastic anemia <br> • Neuropathy |
| C | • Pain on weight bearing <br> • Skeletal x-ray abnormalities <br> • Purpura |
| D | • Increased alkaline phosphatase <br> • Hypocalcemia <br> • Bowed legs/knocked knees |
| E | • Hyporeflexia (in children older than 5) <br> • Ataxia |
| K | • Coagulopathy <br> • Elevated prothrombin time |
| Folate <br> Iron <br> Niacin | • Megaloblastic anemia <br> • Microcytic anemia <br> • Crusted rash <br> • Photosensitive dermatitis |
| Zinc | • Acral rash |

- Also of concern is the increasingly common practice of providing calorically concentrated formulas to children with growth problems or chronic disease.
  - Although concentrated formulas are widely used in populations of children with difficulty handling liquid volume (such as preterm infants), their use in other populations does not have a strong evidence base.

- TPN represents another potential for inadvertently inappropriate calories. TPN allows adults to give plentiful calories easily, although more calories and more weight gain do not mean better health. In fact, children receiving TPN frequently are given extra calories with the aim of improving their health, but are instead saddled with the complications of the methods used to deliver the extra calories.

## Suggested Readings

https://secure.peds.wustl.edu/apps/tpn/calculator.html
The link above is a useful nutrition calculator. Its primary function is to produce TPN order sheets at St. Louis Children's Hospital, but it is also a good general guide for the optimum fluid and calorie requirements for children receiving all types of nutrition.

Avery GB, Villavicencio O, Lilly JR, et al. Intractable diarrhea in early infancy. Pediatrics 1968 Apr;41(4):712–722.

Bryk J, Zenati M, Forsythe R, Peitzman A, et al. Effect of calorically dense enteral nutrition formulas on outcome in critically ill trauma and surgical patients. J Parenter Enteral Nutr 2008 Jan-Feb;32(1):6(11.

Kleinman R, ed. American Academy of Pediatrics' Pediatric Nutrition Handbook. 5th Ed. Elk Grove Village, Ill: American Academy of Pediatrics, 2004.

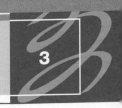

# 3

# FLUID AND ELECTROLYTE MANAGEMENT
### Susan M. Dusenbery and James P. Keating

- This chapter serves as a quick reference for fluid and electrolyte abnormalities in children, focusing on definitions, differential diagnosis, and common presentations.
- Basic approaches to treatment are addressed below.

## FLUID MAINTENANCE

- Calculation of maintenance intravenous fluid (IVF); the IVF in mL/hr is calculated by multiplying the body surface area by 1,500 and dividing by 24, or:

$$\text{IVF } [1.5 \text{ L/m}^2/\text{day}] = \text{Body surface area} \times 1,500 \text{ mL}/24 = [\text{mL/hr}]$$

  - Body surface area (Hosteller formula) = $\sqrt{([\text{Height (cm)} \times \text{Weight (kg)}]/3,600)}$. The body surface area is calculated by multiplying the length in centimeters by the weight in kilograms, dividing by 3,600, and then taking the square root.
  - Alternatively, the nomogram in Figure 3-1 may be used to estimate body surface area even if only the weight is known and it is assumed that the child is of normal height and weight. A 3-kg child is 0.2 m$^2$, a 10-kg child is 0.5 m$^2$, and a 30-kg child is 1 m$^2$.
- Estimated maintenance needs (1,500 mL/m$^2$/day) are calculated by adding the 500 mL/m$^2$/day [insensible water losses (ISWL)], the 500 mL/m$^2$/day [to allow excretion of the renal solute load with normal diet], and the 500 mL/m$^2$/day [to provide for patients with increased ISWL or decreased renal concentrating ability].
- This is usually provided as a solution containing 5% dextrose and 40 mEq/L of sodium.
- ISWLs can be much higher (100–200 mL/kg/day) in extremely low-birth-weight infants.

## ISOTONIC DEHYDRATION AND HYPOVOLEMIA

- This is usually a result of acute diarrhea and vomiting, with losses in excess of retained intake.
- Assessment of degree of dehydration and hypovolemia is marked by the following physical findings: listlessness; lethargy; doughy skin; sunken eyes; sunken fontanel; thready, weak, pulse; capillary refill of >2 seconds; absent tears; and dry mucous membranes.
- Mild dehydration is ≤5% weight loss.
  - Oral rehydration therapy (ORT): 60 mL/kg of oral rehydration solution (e.g., Pedialyte) over 4 hours
    - Give small frequent amounts (5–10 mL [1–2 teaspoons]) every 1–2 minutes to give total volume of oral rehydration solution calculated over 4 hours. Patient is to continue breastfeeding as tolerated.
    - Reassess the patient hourly.
    - Serum electrolytes are not necessary for mild and moderate dehydration (see Suggested Readings).
- Moderate dehydration is 6%–9% weight loss.
  - Attempt ORT with 100 mL/kg of oral rehydration solution over 4 hours; begin with small frequent amounts as stated above and advance as tolerated.
  - Again, patient may continue breastfeeding as tolerated.

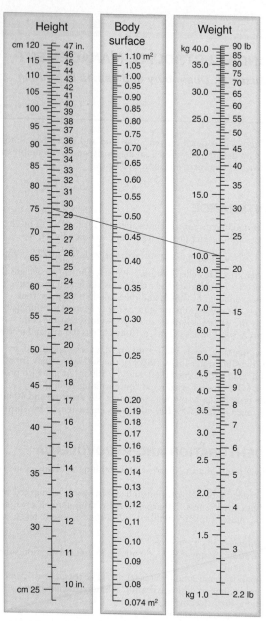

**Figure 3-1.** Body surface area nomogram. The surface area for calculating intravenous fluid rates can be obtained in two ways with this figure. If you know the height and weight, you can draw a line between them in the figure to determine surface area. This figure shows an example where a line is drawn between the height (75 cm at the 50th percentile) and the weight (10 kg [22 lb]), allowing you to determine that the surface area is 0.48 m³. If only the weight is known, the same surface area can be obtained using the line for children of normal height and weight (i.e., 22 lb [10 kg] results in a surface area of 0.49 m³). Modified from Briars GL and Bailey BJ. Surface area estimation: pocket calculator v nomogram. Arch Dis Child 70:246–247, 1994.

- If ORT fails, then begin intravenous (IV) treatment with 40 mL/kg of normal saline over 1 hour, and then begin $D5_{1/2}NS$ at 1.5 × maintenance for up to 60 minutes while continuing to attempt an oral challenge.
- Severe dehydration is ≥10% weight loss and is life threatening.
  - Notify your attending physician immediately.
  - Obtain serum electrolytes and glucose.
  - If there is an electrolyte abnormality, refer to appropriate section in this chapter for further management.
  - Treat glucose that is <60 mg/dL.
  - Recognize that patients with severe dehydration show signs of poor perfusion and shock.
  - Give rapid IV hydration of 20 mL/kg normal saline over 20–30 minutes.
  - Give repeat normal saline boluses over 20 minutes repeatedly to improve perfusion.
- Discharge criteria
  - Absent dehydration symptoms and/or return to base weight
  - Minimal vomiting
  - Taking fluids by mouth
- Admission criteria
  - Continuing tachycardia
  - Protracted vomiting
  - No or minimal urine output

As a general rule, pharmacologic agents should not be used to treat acute diarrhea.

 # ELECTROLYTE ABNORMALITIES

## HYPERNATREMIA

### Definition and Etiology

- Hypernatremia is defined as a serum sodium >150 mEq/L.
- The causes of excess water loss resulting in hypernatremia include:
  - Insensible losses
  - Gastrointestinal (GI) loss: infectious diarrhea (rotavirus). Fecal losses contain more water than sodium (fecal analysis: 35–60 mEq Na/L).
  - Less commonly renal concentrating defects: obstructive uropathy and diabetes insipidus (DI)
- Using skimmed cow's milk (high solute), either boiled or nonboiled, to treat diarrhea of infancy has been shown to result in hypernatremic dehydration.

### Clinical Presentation and Physical Examination

- Hypernatremia most commonly presents with jitteriness (which can be mistaken for seizures) and lethargy.
- Findings of dehydration may be lessened relative to the degree of dehydration because of relative preservation of extracellular fluid.

### Treatment

- Phase I
  - Replace water orally or intravenously.
  - If treating intravenously, begin with isotonic saline to restore systemic perfusion. Use 20 mL/kg over 30 minutes repeatedly until hypovolemia is corrected. (There may be an initial elevation in sodium of 5–8 mEq/L after initial treatment because of a physiologic adjustment period. No intervention should be performed in response to this transient elevation.)

■ The targeted rate of lowering the plasma sodium is 12–15 mEq/L/day. (Fluid administration rates will be lower than with isotonic dehydration to avoid complications.)
■ Phase II
    ■ Begin IV fluids of 5% dextrose quarter normal (40 mEq/L sodium) solution at 2–2.5 L/m$^2$/day.
    ■ Measure sodium serum every 4–6 hours. If correction is too slow, increase the rate of IV fluids. If correction is too fast, decrease the rate of IV fluids.

## Case

■ HPI: A 6-month-old male infant with watery diarrhea at home for the past 5 days and vomiting for 1 day presents with intermittent lethargy and irritability.
    ■ He has also not had any wet diapers for the past 24 hours.
    ■ He has nursed poorly.
■ PE
    ■ Vital signs are temperature 102°F, respiratory rate 40 breaths/min, O$_2$ saturation 95%, and heart rate 190 beats/min.
    ■ He is crying without tears.
    ■ He has increased muscle tone in all extremities.
■ Therapy
    ■ Phase I
        • During placement of an IV line, a set of electrolytes is obtained.
        • After administration of an isotonic saline bolus at 20 mL/kg, the initial serum sodium returns as 185 mEq/L. Another saline bolus of 20 mL/kg is given to complete the restoration of perfusion.
    ■ Phase II
        • D5$_{1/4}$NS + 20 mEq/L KCl was then started at 2 L/m$^2$/day.

# HYPONATREMIA (WATER INTOXICATION)

## Definitions

■ Hyponatremia is defined as a serum sodium of <135 mEq/L.
■ Water intoxication is defined as an "acute neurologic disturbance that results from rapid, excessive water intake." The associated rapid decrease in sodium can result in lethargy, seizures, coma, and death.

## Epidemiology and Etiology

■ Forty percent of children in children's hospitals have a serum sodium of <135 mEq/L as a result of chronic illness. They are asymptomatic and do not require special intervention.
■ Causes of water intoxication include excessive parenteral or enteral water administration by medical personnel, excessive oral ingestion of water in an infant, repeated immersion, and excessive voluntary oral ingestion of water.
■ During a review of 34 patients with water intoxication at St. Louis Children's Hospital between January 1975 and July 1990, investigators found that excessive water was usually ingested with a bottle. There were multiple reasons given for giving the infants excessive water, including "ran out of formula, gave water for diarrhea, and gave water for irritability or fussiness."

## Clinical Presentation and Physical Examination

■ Clinical presentation: 3- to 6-month-old infant who presents with apnea or seizures
■ Physical examination
    ■ Careful neurologic examination, including evaluating mental status
    ■ Low body temperature despite warm summer environment

## Treatment

- Central pontine myelinolysis occurs from rapid correction of chronic hyponatremia. The recommended rate of serum sodium increase in patients with chronic hyponatremia is 0.5 mEq/L. This rate is inappropriate for the treatment of water intoxication because it is a symptomatic acute hyponatremia.
- For water intoxication, the serum sodium should be increased at a minimum of 1 mEq/L/hr up to a recommended increase of 2–3 mEq/L/hr.
- The clinician treating the patient must decide whether isotonic (normal saline) or hypertonic (3% saline) will be used to increase the patient's serum sodium. Previous data support using 3% saline if the patient has not had a spontaneous water diuresis at the time of evaluation and treatment.
- Before giving parenteral sodium, it is necessary to calculate the patient's sodium deficit:

$$\text{Total body water (TBW)} = 0.7 \times \text{weight}$$

$$\text{Sodium deficit} = (140 - \text{serum sodium}) \times \text{TBW}$$

## Case

- HPI: A 4-month-old female infant presents with seizures.
- PE
    - The infant is shaking in all extremities.
    - The airway is intact.
- Therapy
    - Diazepam (Diastat) was initially given to stop the seizure. The seizure continued while an IV line was placed and lorazepam (Ativan) was also administered without resolution of the seizure.
    - During placement of an IV, serum glucose and electrolytes are obtained. Glucose is 100 mg/dL, but serum sodium is 115 mEq/L.
    - Isotonic saline infusion had been initiated before knowing the patient's serum sodium. When the serum sodium returned, a 3% saline infusion is started and the correction is set at a rate of 2 mEq/L/hr until the seizures stop. The correction rate is then reduced to 10–12 mEq/L for the first 24 hours following presentation with isotonic saline.
- Resolution: On further questioning, the parents reported that they stopped putting formula in their daughter's bottle and replaced it with tap water because of the hot weather. This resulted in the water intoxication.

# HYPERKALEMIA

## Definition and Etiology

- Hyperkalemia is defined as a serum potassium >6 mEq/L.
- It is commonly caused by increased intake, cellular breakdown, or decreased output.

## Clinical Presentation and Physical Examination

- Symptoms: usually none; can present with cardiac arrest
- Physical examination: irregular heartbeat and decreased or lost pulses

## Differential Diagnosis

- Increased potassium intake from oral or IV supplementation
- Cellular breakdown from trauma, surgery, burns, and chemotherapy
- Decreased urinary potassium excretion caused by renal failure or hypoaldosteronism from nonsteroidal anti-inflammatory drugs, cyclosporine, primary adrenal insufficiency, or congenital adrenal hyperplasia
- Hemolyzed sample; need to check with laboratory for falsely elevated potassium levels

## Treatment

- Check that the test sample is not hemolyzed and redraw a venous potassium level, remove potassium containing fluids/supplements, and check an electrocardiogram (ECG).
- Monitor the patient with telemetry.
- If the patient has symptomatic hyperkalemia, treat with calcium, glucose, insulin, $\beta_2$-adrenergic agonists, and diuretics. Consider dialysis if the hyperkalemia is life threatening.

## Case

- HPI: A 2-week-old, full-term, previously healthy male infant with a 1-day history of vomiting and decreased oral intake presents with increased sleepiness.
  - The parents report that their son had been eating well before his 1 day of vomiting but not gaining weight. They describe the vomiting as projectile, nonbilious, and nonbloody.
  - The infant had been afebrile without upper respiratory symptoms, diarrhea, or rash.
  - The parents became concerned today when their son would not wake up sufficiently to nurse.
- PE
  - The infant is minimally responsive.
  - Vital signs show that he is afebrile and tachycardic, and with a blood pressure measured by Doppler of 50 mm Hg.
  - The anterior fontanel is sunken, lungs are clear, abdomen is soft without masses or distension, femoral pulses are weak, and extremities are cool.
  - Increased pigmentation was evident in the patient's diaper area when his femoral pulses were palpated.
- Therapy
  - The patient is intubated because of poor respiratory effort, and an IV is placed for fluid resuscitation. During IV placement, electrolytes and other laboratory tests are obtained and sent.
  - During the patient's second 40 mL/kg normal saline bolus, the electrolytes returned with a serum sodium of 120 mEq/L, potassium of 6.5 mEq/L, $CO_2$ of 8 mEq/L, blood urea nitrogen of 50 mg/dL, and creatinine of 0.7 mg/dL.
  - An ECG is obtained because of the patient's elevated potassium; it does not show peaked t waves. If abnormalities had been seen on the ECG, calcium should be given.
  - A dose of IV hydrocortisone is given, resulting in significant improvement in blood pressure and perfusion.
- Resolution: The patient is subsequently diagnosed with 21-hydroxylase deficiency.

# HYPOKALEMIA

## Definition and Etiology

- Hypokalemia is defined as a serum potassium <3.5 mEq/L.
- It is a result of potassium losses in excess of replacement. Potassium can be lost through the GI tract as well as the kidneys.

## Clinical Presentation and Physical Examination

- Symptoms: constipation, fatigue, muscle weakness, and paralysis
- Physical examination
  - Check for possible irregular heartbeat.
  - Evaluate for signs of muscle weakness/paralysis.

## Differential Diagnosis

- Decreased intake as a result of low dietary intake or IV fluids without potassium
- Increased GI losses from vomiting, nasogastric suction, or diarrhea

- Increased urinary losses because of loop and thiazide diuretics
- Mineralocorticoid excess
- Liddle syndrome (autosomal dominant with increased sodium resorption)
- Bartter or Gitelman syndromes
- Amphotericin
- Hypomagnesemia

## Treatment

- Administer oral or IV potassium supplements.
- Correct hypomagnesemia.
- Stop diuretics and amphotericin if possible.

## Case

- HPI: A 6-week-old female infant presents to the emergency department with persistent nonbilious, nonbloody vomiting. A full-term infant, she has been healthy, eating well, and gaining weight.
    - She began vomiting 1 week ago; in the past 2 days, she has vomited after every episode of nursing.
    - Her parents have taken her to their pediatrician. At their pediatrician's office, it was noted that the infant had not gained weight since her 1-month checkup.
- PE
    - Infant is alert but fussy and attempting to "root" on the pediatrician's hand.
    - The fontanel is sunken, and the skin turgor is poor.
    - An abdominal ultrasound reveals pyloric stenosis.
- Therapy and Resolution
    - Electrolytes reveal a potassium of 2.8 mEq/L, chloride of 95 mEq/L, and $CO_2$ of 30 mEq/L.
    - She is admitted for fluid hydration and electrolyte correction before a pyloromyotomy.

# HYPERCALCEMIA

## Definition and Etiology

- Hypercalcemia is defined as a calcium concentration >10.6 mg/dL (total) and 5.6 mg/dL (ionized).
- The physiologic actions of calcium are dependent on the ionized form.

## Clinical Presentation and Physical Examination

- Symptoms: nausea and vomiting, constipation, abdominal pain, mental status changes, and lethargy
- Physical examination: possible bradycardia, proximal muscle weakness, increased reflexes, and abnormal mental status

## Differential Diagnosis

- Hyperparathyroidism
    - Primary neonatal
    - Secondary as a response to maternal hypocalcemia
    - Primary as part of multiple endocrine neoplasia (MEN) 1 or MEN 2A syndrome
    - Secondary as a response to a parathyroid adenoma
        - Immobility
        - Iatrogenic causes: thiazide diuretics, theophylline, lithium, total parenteral nutrition, excess vitamin D, excess vitamin A, milk alkali

- Cancer: lymphoma, leukemia, Ewing sarcoma, rhabdomyosarcoma, neuroblastoma, Langerhans cell histiocytosis
- Addison disease
- Williams syndrome
- Granulomatous diseases (tuberculosis and sarcoidosis)
- Familial hypocalciuric hypercalcemia

## Treatment

- Treat underlying cause.
- Can acutely treat with isotonic fluids intravenously and a loop diuretic.
- Possibly use a bisphosphonate.
- For severe hypercalcemia with renal failure, use dialysis if necessary.

## Case

- HPI: A 10-year-old previously healthy boy presents to his pediatrician for evaluation of acute abdominal pain. His mother reports that her son has not been himself lately. He has not wanted to spend time with friends or go to school.
  - He says that he does not have the strength to ride his bike or play soccer with friends anymore.
  - Today he has been nauseated, with one episode of emesis and abdominal pain that began at 2 PM.
  - He denies fevers, weight loss, diarrhea or constipation, or rashes. He does report dysuria.
- PE: The boy is in moderate distress from pain.
  - The examination is unremarkable except for left-sided costovertebral angle tenderness.
  - A urinalysis (UA), serum electrolytes, and an abdominal flat plate are obtained.
    - The UA shows an elevated specific gravity and blood.
    - The serum electrolytes are normal, except for calcium of 14.5 mg/dL.
    - The abdominal flat plate shows an opacity in the renal collecting system consistent with a stone.
- Therapy
  - The boy is admitted to the hospital.
  - At the hospital, he receives IVF hydration with normal saline and intermittent doses of morphine for pain control. The parathyroid hormone (PTH) level is elevated.
  - Furosemide is added following hydration until the total calcium is below 14 mg/dL.
  - An ECG shows a short QT interval and a prolonged PR interval.
- Resolution: The boy is diagnosed with MEN type 1 syndrome.

# HYPOCALCEMIA

## Definition

- Hypocalcemia is defined as a concentration <8.8 mg/dL (total calcium) and 4.0 mg/dL (ionized calcium).
- The total calcium concentration drops 0.8 mg/dL for every 1 g/dL drop in serum albumin.

## Clinical Presentation and Physical Examination

- Symptoms: irritability, mental status changes, seizures, muscle weakness/spasm, numbness and tingling, loss of hair, and difficulty breathing
- Physical examination

- Alopecia
- Wheezing or stridor with respiratory distress
- Chvostek sign (tapping anterior to the ear causes contraction of ipsilateral facial muscle)
- Trousseau sign (placing blood pressure cuff on arm and inflating above systolic blood pressure for a few minutes causes flexion of the hand at the wrist)

## Differential Diagnosis

- Hypoparathyroidism
  - Congenital (DiGeorge syndrome, APECED, Kearns-Sayre syndrome)
  - Surgical
  - Autoimmune
  - Secondary to elevated maternal calcium
- Pseudohypoparathyroidism
- Rickets (borderline normal to low calcium levels)
  - Vitamin D deficiency
  - Rarely because of inadequate calcium and phosphorus intake
- Iatrogenic causes
  - Aminoglycosides, loop diuretics
  - Short bowel syndrome
  - Intestinal bypass
- Abnormalities of minerals
  - Hypomagnesemia
  - Wilson disease (excess copper)
  - Hyperphosphatemia
- Sequestration of calcium
  - Pancreatitis
  - Rhabdomyolysis
  - Hypoalbuminemia (causes pseudohypocalcemia)

## Treatment

- Correct underlying cause if possible.
- If patient is asymptomatic, give oral calcium and vitamin D supplements.
- If symptomatic, give calcium intravenously.
- Correct hypomagnesemia.

## Case

- HPI: A 3-month-old male infant presents with difficulty breathing.
  - His mother reports that he is an otherwise healthy full-term infant. He has not had a fever or upper respiratory symptoms.
  - Today when she picked him up from day care, he was breathing faster than usual. She said he was also "wheezing." The day care facility reports that his breathing worsened over the course of the day, and he was not taking his bottle well.
- PE: The infant is lying in the mother's arms in mild respiratory distress.
  - He is afebrile, with a respiratory rate of 40 breaths/min, a heart rate of 140 beats/min, an $O_2$ saturation of 95% on room air.
  - The examination is remarkable only for stridor, subcostal and supracostal retraction, and a clear chest, with good aeration bilaterally.
- Therapy
  - The infant is given multiple treatments of racemic epinephrine and a single dose of oral dexamethasone. He shows minimal improvement.
  - An IV is placed for IVF hydration, and electrolytes are sent. Total calcium returns at 5 mg/dL. Additional laboratory tests include an elevated phosphorous level and an undetectable PTH level. Calcium gluconate is added to the IVF.

- An ECG shows a prolonged QT interval. He is admitted for telemetry.
- Oral calcium and vitamin D supplements are necessary.

- Resolution: After the diagnosis of hypoparathyroidism, the infant is placed on long-term treatment with calcium and vitamin D.

# HYPERPHOSPHATEMIA

## Definition and Etiology

- Hyperphosphatemia is defined as a phosphorus value of >7 mg/dL in infants and 4.5 mg/dL in adolescents and adults.
- This condition used to be common during the newborn period when infants were fed cow's milk.
  - It is usually not seen beyond the newborn period unless the individual has kidney disease.
  - However, large amounts of phosphorus from either oral laxatives or enemas can cause hyperphosphatemia and hypocalcemia at any age.

## Clinical Presentation and Physical Examination

- Symptoms: usually from the condition that is causing the elevated phosphorus. Symptoms of hypocalcemia can also occur.
- Physical examination: possible physical findings consistent with hypocalcemia

## Differential Diagnosis

- Rhabdomyolysis
- Hyperparathyroidism
- Hypocalcemia
- Phosphate-containing enema or laxative
- Tumor lysis syndrome
- Excess phosphorus-containing formula in the newborn period
- Renal failure

## Treatment

- For acute treatment, give IV hydration and a loop diuretic.
- Treat the underlying cause.
- Consider dialysis, which may be necessary.

## Case

- HPI: A previously healthy 3-month-old male infant presents to the emergency department with a 24-hour history of fever, lethargy, and respiratory distress.
- PE:
  - The patient has a temperature of 40°C, heart rate of 203 beats/min, respiratory rate of 70 breaths/min, blood pressure of 100/40 mm Hg, $O_2$ saturation on room air of 80%, which increased to 100% with supplemental oxygen.
  - He is lethargic with intermittent muscle spasms.
- Therapy
  - The infant is given normal saline and antibiotics.
  - A complete blood count, electrolytes, blood culture, urine culture, and CSF culture are obtained. The electrolytes show a sodium level of 155 mEq/L, creatinine of 0.9 mg/dL, calcium of 5.1 mg/dL, and a phosphorus of 38 mg/dL.
  - The child receives calcium gluconate and calcium chloride intravenously as well as fluid hydration.
    - As the calcium level normalizes, the muscle spasms and respiratory distress resolve.

- The phosphorus level decreases to within the normal range within the first day of presentation with isotonic fluid hydration.

■ Resolution: On further questioning, the parents reveal that they were giving an over-the-counter oral laxative to the infant; this caused this child's severe hyperphosphatemia.

## HYPOPHOSPHATEMIA

### Definition

■ Hypophosphatemia is defined as a phosphorus value of <2.5 mg/dL.
■ Phosphorus is important because it is a component of ATP, which the body requires for survival. Hypophosphatemia can lead to a renal tubular acidosis and rickets.

### Clinical Presentation and Physical Examination

■ Symptoms: lethargy, ileus, myalgia, weakness
■ Physical examination: small stature, frontal bossing, enlarged wrists, bowing of legs

### Differential Diagnosis

■ Diuretics
■ Hypoparathyroidism
■ Diabetic ketoacidosis
■ Fanconi syndrome
■ Refeeding syndrome
■ Inadequate dietary intake
■ Excess aluminum ingestion

### Treatment

■ For acute treatment, give oral or IV phosphorus.
■ Treat the underlying cause.

### Case

■ HPI: A 3-month-old female infant presents to the GI clinic with poor weight gain and diarrhea.
  ■ She has been exclusively breastfed and taking 4–5 oz of breast milk every 3–4 hours.
  ■ At 3 weeks of age, she was diagnosed with gastroesophageal reflux, and rice cereal was added to breast milk.
  ■ At 10 weeks of age, her spit-ups were considered worse, and she was started on a proton pump inhibitor.
  ■ Since 13 weeks of age, she has had watery diarrhea.
■ PE:
  ■ Weight: 3.87 kg (fifth percentile)
  ■ Frontal bossing with craniotabes and no other abnormalities
■ Therapy
  ■ Serum electrolytes and a phosphorus level are obtained. Calcium was 10.5 mg/dL, and phosphorus was 1.4 mg/dL. PTH and 1, 25 vitamin D levels were normal; 25 vitamin D level was 9 ng/mL (just below normal range).
  ■ The infant receives phosphorus, calcium, and vitamin D supplementation.
  ■ A bone survey shows diffuse osteopenia with physis widening and metaphysis fraying, consistent with rickets.
■ Resolution: The infant is diagnosed with rickets. On further questioning, the parents describe giving the infant large quantities of an aluminum-containing antacid for reflux, which was determined to be the cause of her hypophosphatemia and rickets.

## Suggested Readings

Bhatia J. Fluid and electrolyte management in very low birth weight neonate. J Perinatol 2006;26:S19–S21.

Briars GL, Bailey BJ. Surface area estimation: pocket calculator v nomogram. Arch Dis Child 1994;70:246–247.

Domico MB, et al. Severe hyperphosphatemia and hypocalcemic tetany after oral laxative administration in a 3-month-old infant. Pediatrics 2006;118:e1580–e1583.

Finberg L. Water and Electrolytes in Pediatrics, Physiology, Pathophysiology and Treatment. 2nd Ed. Philadelphia: WB Saunders Company, 1993.

Fomon SJ. Nutrition of Normal Infants. St. Louis: Mosby, 1993.

Lentner C. Geigy scientific tables. Basle, Switzerland: Ciba-Geigy, Limited. 1981;8(1): 226–227.

Owen GM, et al. Concentrations of calcium and inorganic phosphorus in serum of normal infants receiving various feedings. Pediatrics March 1963;31:495–498.

Rose BD. Clinical Physiology of Acid Base and Electrolyte Disorders. 5th Ed. New York: McGraw Hill, 2001.

Santosham M, et al. Oral rehydration therapy and dietary therapy for acute childhood diarrhoea. Pediatr Rev March 1987;8(9):273–278.

Teach SJ, Yates EW, Feld LG. Laboratory predictors of fluid deficit in acutely dehydrated children. Clin Pediatr (Phila) 1997;36:395–400.

Zitelli BJ. Atlas of Pediatric Physical Diagnosis. 5th Ed. St. Louis: Mosby, 2007.

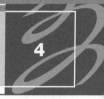

$\mathcal{R}$emember, emergency department visits are stressful for both children and their parents. When it is a busy day, conditions can become chaotic, and patients and their parents can become impatient and restless. To improve this situation, adhere to the following:

- Introduce yourself to the parents and the child, and explain your role in the emergency department assessment.
- Wash your hands when you come into the room, and again when you leave.
- If emergent treatment is needed, obtain a brief history relevant to the problem so as to institute prompt and appropriate therapy. A more detailed history can be obtained after your initial intervention.
- Always think anticipation (if possible), airway, breathing, and circulation (AABC).
- Perform the auscultation portion of the examination first (lungs, heart, and abdomen) and the more invasive parts at the end (ears and throat). If possible, keep toddlers on a parent's lap (or very close by) during the physical examination. You may use the parents' help during the examination (e.g., let a parent position the stethoscope in the chest).
- Keep the parents informed about their child's clinical progress. Explain what to expect in the course of illness and what they need to look for to prompt reevaluation.
- Any time you go into a room and find a patient in distress or one you are uncomfortable managing, let your attending or senior resident know immediately.

## CARDIOPULMONARY RESUSCITATION

- Identify the cause early. Past medical history and history of present illness may affect therapy.
- Patients who received delayed resuscitation or who present in asystole have a poor prognosis.

### Etiology

- Most common causes:
  - Traumatic: motor vehicle crashes, burns, child abuse, firearms
  - Pulmonary: foreign body aspiration, smoke inhalation, near drowning, respiratory failure
  - Infectious: sepsis, meningitis
  - Central nervous system: head trauma, seizures
  - Cardiac: congenital heart disease, myocarditis
  - Others: sudden infant death syndrome (SIDS), poisoning, suicide, dehydration, congenital anomalies
- In most patients, hypoxia from respiratory failure causes bradycardia, followed by cardiac arrest.

### Treatment (basic life support; Table 4-1)

- Focus on hard, rapid compressions with minimal pauses.
- The goal is to optimize cardiac output and sustain tissue oxygen delivery (mainly to the heart and brain).

| TABLE 4-1 | Basic Techniques of Pediatric Life Support | | |
|---|---|---|---|
| Maneuver | Child 1–8 yr | Infant <1 yr | Newborn |
| **Airway** | Head-tilt–chin lift. If trauma is present, use jaw thrust | Head-tilt–chin lift. If trauma is present, use jaw thrust | Head-tilt–chin lift. |
| **Breathing** | | | |
| *-Initial* | 2 breaths at 1–1.5 sec/breath | 2 breaths at 1–1.5 sec/breath | 2 breaths at 1–1.5 sec/breath |
| *-Subsequent* | ~20 breaths/min | ~20 breaths/min | ~30–60 breaths/min |
| *-Foreign Body Aspiration* | Heimlich maneuver | Back blows and chest thrusts | |
| **Circulation** | | | |
| *-Pulse check* | Carotid | Carotid, brachial or femoral | Brachial or femoral |
| *-Compressions* | Lower half of sternum | | |
| *landmark* | Heel of one hand | One finger width below mammary line | One finger width below mammary line |
| *method* | 1–1.5 in or one third to one half depth of chest | Two thumbs encircled hands | Two thumbs encircled hands |
| *depth rate* | 100/min | 0.5–1 in or one third to one half depth of chest ≥100/min | 0.5–1 in or one third depth of chest 120/min |
| *compression/ ventilation ratio* | 15:2 (two rescuers) pause for ventilation until trachea is intubated | 15:2 (two rescuers) pause for ventilation until trachea is intubated | 3:1 for intubated newborn (two rescuers) |

American Heart Association, Guidelines CPR ECC 2006. Handbook of Emergency Cardiovascular Care. Field JM, Hazinski MF, and Gilmore D, eds.

## COMA

- History: trauma, ingestion, infection, fasting, diabetes, drug use, seizure
- Physical examination: heart rate, blood pressure, respiratory pattern, temperature, pupillary size and response, rash, abnormal posturing, focal neurologic signs
- Laboratory studies
  - Dextrostick, complete blood count, electrolytes, transaminases, ammonia, lactate, toxicology screen, blood gas, blood culture
  - In infants: plasma amino acids and urine organic acids
- Treatment
  - Use airway, breathing, circulation (ABC) and oxygen.
  - Consider naloxone. Flumazenil is appropriate for benzodiazepine overdose, but seizures may result. Thiamine is mainly used in an adult setting.
  - If infection suspected, start antibiotics.
  - Consider head computed tomography (CT).

## TRAUMA

- Trauma is the most common cause of death in children beyond the first months of life.
  - Motor vehicle crashes are the most common cause of death in children older than 1 year of age.
  - Homicide as a result of child abuse is the most common cause of death in children younger than 1 year of age.

■ Drowning ranks second among unintentional trauma deaths, with peaks in preschool and late teen years.

## Primary Management of the Polytraumatized Patient (ABCs)

■ **A**irway
  ■ Immobilize cervical spine.
  ■ Inspect for foreign objects or loose teeth in mouth.
  ■ Intubate if necessary.

■ **B**reathing
  ■ Administer supplemental oxygen if airway is patent.
  ■ Consider orogastric tube to decompress stomach.
  ■ Inspect chest for open wounds and/or pneumothorax.

■ **C**irculation
  ■ Apply direct pressure with sterile gauze to bleeding wounds.
  ■ Realize that heart rate and capillary refill are the best indicator of circulatory status in children (hypotension occurs late; maintained blood pressure should never be considered "reassuring" in a trauma setting).
  ■ Insert an intravenous (IV) catheter with two large-bore IV lines.
  ■ Insert an intraosseous needle (if <8 years of age) or a femoral venous line if IV access delayed
  ■ Administer a rapid infusion of warmed lactated Ringer or normal saline at 20 mL/kg for up to three boluses. If patient remains unstable, give colloid and/or blood products and obtain emergent surgical evaluation (if not done so already).

■ Disability. Determine the following:
  ■ Level of consciousness (alert/responding to verbal stimuli/responding to pain/unresponsive)
  ■ Pupil equality and responsiveness to light
  ■ Muscle tone (unilateral/bilateral flaccidity)

## Secondary Survey

■ Remove all clothing and perform a thorough head-to-toe evaluation.
  ■ Head-ear-eyes-nose-throat: scalp/skull injury, periorbital ecchymosis (think orbital fracture), pinna ecchymosis or hemotympanum (think basilar skull fracture), cerebrospinal fluid (CSF) leak from nose or ears, pupil size, corneal reflex, hyphema, cervical spine tenderness or deformity, trachea midline
  ■ Chest/abdomen/pelvis: clavicular deformity or tenderness, breath sounds, heart tones, rib tenderness or deformity, chest wall symmetry, subcutaneous emphysema, abdominal tenderness or distension, bloody orogastric aspirates, palpate spleen for tenderness, pelvic instability
  ■ Genitourinary: rectal tone, blood in stool, blood at urethral meatus
  ■ Back: step-off along spinal column, tenderness along spine
  ■ Extremities: deformity or point tenderness, neurovascular examination (mainly for compartment syndrome, spinal shock; 4 Ps: forearm **p**ain with passive movement of fingers/toes, **p**aresthesia, **p**allor, **p**ulselessness)
  ■ Skin: capillary refill, lacerations, abrasions, contusions
  ■ Neurologic: mental status, Glasgow coma scale, muscle tone, purposeful movement of extremities, intact sensation

## Laboratory Studies and Imaging

■ Order the following laboratory tests:
  ■ Hemoglobin and hematocrit (baseline)
  ■ Transaminases
  ■ Type and cross
  ■ Amylase/lipase
  ■ Urinalysis

- Consider a toxicology screen and a urine pregnancy test.
- Obtain the following radiographs:
  - Plain films: cervical spine, chest, pelvis, any extremity with pain or deformity
  - CT: low suspicion to obtain head or abdomen CT
- Consider an echocardiogram if there is poor cardiac output despite volume administration and/or distended veins in a patient with penetrating trauma.

## Prevention

- Motor vehicle
  - <20 lb: infant seat in rear seat facing backwards
  - >20 lb: toddler seat in rear seat facing forward
  - <13 years: ride in the backseat
  - Until age 8, 80 lb, and 57 inches: booster seat and seat belt with shoulder straps
- Bicycle: **always** wear a helmet.

## Head Trauma

- Concussion: immediate and transient alteration of consciousness, vision, and equilibrium
  - A functional injury, a concussion typically results in the rapid onset of neurologic impairment, which then resolves spontaneously.
  - It may or may not involve loss of consciousness and is typically associated with normal imaging studies.
- Epidural hematoma: located between dura and skull
  - Natural history includes a loss of consciousness followed by a lucid interval. If not treated, it results in rapid deterioration.
  - Lens-shaped opacity on CT
  - Eighty-five percent of patients have a skull fracture, most often overlying the middle meningeal artery.
  - Infants are at especially high risk. They take longer to show lethargy because open sutures separate to accommodate mass effect of expanding hematoma.
- Subdural hematoma: located under dura and over the brain, often associated with cerebral contusion and cerebral edema
  - Typically there is no lucid interval; this is a serious brain injury.
  - Crescent-shaped opacity on CT
- Contusion: associated with skull fractures; focal symptoms are present at site of injury or at contrecoup site.

### Diagnosis and Treatment

- Infants (<12 months)
  - Alert: if scalp hematoma present, consider skull films. If fracture is present, perform head CT to evaluate for intracranial bleeding.
  - Not alert: head CT
- Minor head trauma with no loss of consciousness
  - Thorough history and physical examination, including a neurologic examination
  - Observation in clinic, office, emergency department, or home
  - CT and magnetic resonance imaging (MRI): not recommended
- Minor head trauma with brief (<1 minute) loss of consciousness
  - History and physical examination, including a neurologic examination
  - Observation or head CT. (Skull radiographs and MRI are not recommended.)
- If you discharge the patient, be certain that the parents understand warning signs and symptoms. The indicators for seeking medical attention are persistent headache, persistent vomiting up to 6 to 8 hours after injury, drowsiness, weakness, blurry or double vision, or ataxia. Instruct to wake child at 4-hour intervals during the night. Irritability or change in behavior, neck pain, seizures, fever, and watery discharge from the nose or ears are also problematic and warrant return to the emergency department for repeat medical evaluation.
- For more information about the evaluation and management of concussion, see Table 4-2.

| TABLE 4-2 | Evaluation and Management of Concussion |
|-----------|------------------------------------------|

**Features**

| Cognitive features | Symptoms | Signs |
|--------------------|----------|-------|
| Loss of consciousness | Headache | Loss of consciousness or impaired |
| | Double vision | consciousness |
| Confusion | Dizziness | Ataxia |
| Amnesia | Nausea | Vomiting |
| Disoriented to time/ | Sleepiness/sleep | Slurred speech |
| date/place | disturbance | Personality changes |

**Assessment**
- A full neurologic assessment is mandatory in an assessment of head trauma. This includes a cervical spine evaluation.
- Imaging is typically only necessary when you suspect structural injury (i.e., the history of the mechanism of injury or the physical findings make you concerned for skull fracture, cervical spine injury, intracranial bleeding)

**Management:** "So when can I get back into the game?"
- **Rest** is the cornerstone of management. This means rest until all symptoms—including feelings of being dazed, dizzy, sleepy, and headache—have vanished. The risk of dangerous second impact syndrome may be reduced in this way (repeated injury predisposing the already injured brain to manifest a more deleterious—even fatal—response after a second concussive event).
- In addition, the athlete must be protected from the situation in which decreased alertness, coordination, or responsiveness could predispose him or her to further injury of any sort. **This is the critical and mandatory phase of treatment for concussive injury.**
- **Return to play** should occur in a controlled and stepwise fashion. Light aerobic activity may progress to sport-specific training, noncontact training, medical reevaluation, then progression to full contact training and then competitive play. **This process should involve the minimum of 1 full week of recovery time after injury.**

## Neck Injury

- Always rule out a fracture or dislocation!

### Diagnosis and Treatment
- Immobilization of neck
- May clear cervical spine without radiographs if:
  - The patient is alert and responds to commands.
  - There is no midline neck pain on palpation.
  - The neurologic examination is normal.
  - There is no major distracting injury (e.g., long bone fracture).

- Obtain radiographs of the cervical spine (anteroposterior, lateral, and open mouth views) if the patient complains of neck pain or is unresponsive.
  - If the films or examination are abnormal and the patient can cooperate, consider flexion-extension views to evaluate ligament injury or obtain a cervical spine CT.
  - If there are symptoms of spinal cord injury, obtain a noncontrast MRI to rule out spinal cord hematoma, edema, and stenosis.
  - If the patient is unresponsive, consider obtaining a cervical spine CT.

- Patients can return to play when they have a full, pain-free range of motion, normal strength and sensation, and normal lordosis of the cervical spine.

## BURNS

- The character of a burn may change over the first few days after the injury. Keep this in mind when deciding whether to admit and when discussing prognosis.
- Classification: burn severity
  - First-degree/superficial: involve epidermis only; painful and erythematous

- Second-degree/partial thickness: involve epidermis and dermis, sparing dermal appendages. Superficial second-degree burns are blistered and painful. Deep second-degree burns may be white and painless; they may require grafting.
- Third-degree/full thickness: leathery and painless; they require grafting.
- Electrical burns often involve tissues in excess of the superficial skin damage. High voltage may cause rhabdomyolysis. This is more typical of industrial, not household, current.

## Diagnosis and Treatment

- Use caution regarding inhalation with burns from a fire in enclosed space, facial burns, singed nares, carbonaceous material in nares or mouth, cough, hoarseness, shortness of breath, or wheezing. Airway edema and obstruction may be imminent; intubate early if in doubt.
- If a chemical burn, wash away remaining chemicals on the patient.
- Order laboratory studies as indicated by patient status; consider carbon monoxide level for victims entrapped in enclosed space with flames or smoke.
- Airway
  - Consider the possibility of airway decline secondary to swelling, if there is inhalational injury.
  - If airway stable, give humidified 100% $O_2$.
  - Pulse oximetry is not accurate if the carbon monoxide level is significant; obtain $PaO_2$ from blood gas measurement.
- Breathing: Monitor closely for signs of distress.
- Circulation
  - Give 20 mL/kg of lactated Ringer or normal saline if body surface area (BSA) is >10% in infants or >15% in children.
  - If hypotensive, manage according to trauma principles first. Maintain at least 1 mL/kg/hr urine output.
- Fluid management
  - Use Parkland formula (first 24 hours):

$$4 \text{ mL/kg} \times \% \text{ BSA burned} + \text{maintenance fluids}$$

**OR**

$$5,000 \text{ mL/m}^2 \text{ BSA burned} + 2,000 \text{ mL/m}^2 \text{ BSA/24 hours}$$

  - Administer half of this total over the first 8 hours and then the remaining over the next 16 hours
- GI: Consider nasogastric tube, begin $H_2$ blocker for stress ulcer (Curling ulcer) prophylaxis.
- GU: Monitor urine output with Foley catheter if >15% BSA burn.
- Ophthalmology: If eye injury is suspected, consult ophthalmology.
- Analgesia: Use IV, not subcutaneous or oral, route for medications.
- Admission guidelines: consider inpatient burn management for:
  - Burns >10% BSA in infants or >15% in children (Figure 4-1)
  - Electrical or chemical burns
  - Burns that involve the face, hands, feet, perineum, or joints
  - Inhalation injury
  - Children with unsafe environment at home or uncertain follow-up
  - Underlying medical condition

## LACERATIONS (TABLE 4-3)

- Most lacerations, including those on fingers and toes, can be anesthetized with topical gels, such as lidocaine (4%) plus epinephrine (1:1,000) plus tetracaine (0.5%) [LET], to reduce patient anxiety. If additional local anesthesia is needed, lidocaine or lidocaine

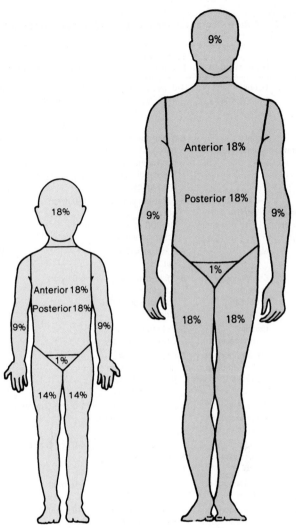

**Figure 4-1.** Rule of nines for child (left) and adult (right). The surface area of the palm and fingers is approximately 1% BSA in a child. The palm is approximately 1% of BSA in an older child/teen. (Adapted from Scherer JC. Introductory medical-surgical nursing, 4th Ed. Philadelphia: Lippincott, 1986:687)

with epinephrine should be buffered 1:10 with standard 8.4% sodium bicarbonate and injected slowly using a 30-gauge needle to minimize injection pain.
■ Many superficial hand and foot lacerations <~2 cm in length heal well with simple bandaging.

## POISONING

■ Ingestions in toddlers typically do not cause symptoms because of the small amounts actually ingested. However, clinicians must be prepared for the rare significant poisoning.

| TABLE 4-3 | Suture Characteristics for Lacerations in Various Locations | | | |
|-----------|-------------|-------------|-------------|----------|
| Location | Deep sutures | Skin sutures (absorbable)* | Skin sutures (nonabsorbable) | Duration (days) |
| Scalp | Usually unnecessary | 4-0 chromic gut or 4-0 Vicryl RAPIDE | Absorbable preferred May consider staples | Until absorbed 7–10 |
| Face (no tension) | Usually unnecessary | 6-0 fast-absorbing gut plus tissue adhesive and/or tissue-adhesive Steri-strips[†] | 6-0 nylon | 3–5 |
| Face (with tension; e.g., chin or eyebrow) | 5-0 Monocryl or Vicryl | 6-0 fast-absorbing gut or 5-0 Vicryl RAPIDE plus tissue adhesive | 6-0 nylon | 5–7 until absorbed |
| Eyelid | None | 6-0 fast-absorbing gut | – | Until absorbed |
| Ear | 5-0 Monocryl or Vicryl in cartilage | 6-0 fast-absorbing gut plus tissue adhesive and Steri-strips[†] | 6-0 nylon | |
| Oral mucosa | Usually unnecessary | 5-0 chromic gut if closure necessary | – | |
| Vermilion border | 5-0 Monocryl or Vicryl in deep dermis | 6-0 fast-absorbing gut on cutaneous portion; 5-0 chromic gut on vermilion | – | |
| Trunk and Extremities | 4-0 or 5-0 Monocryl or Vicryl | 4-0 or 5-0 chromic gut or Vicryl RAPIDE | 4-0 or 5-0 nylon | 7 (10–14 if over a joint) |
| Palm of Hand[‡] | Usually unnecessary | 4-0 chromic gut No tissue adhesive No Steri-strips | 4-0 or 5-0 nylon | 7 |
| Dorsum of Hand | 5-0 Monocryl or Vicryl | 5-0 chromic gut or Vicryl RAPIDE | 5-0 nylon | 7 |
| Sole of foot | 4-0 Monocryl or Vicryl | 4-0 chromic gut or Vicryl RAPIDE plus tissue adhesive and Steri-strips[†] | 4-0 nylon | 7–10 |

*Absorbable sutures are generally preferred because they avoid the need for a second medical visit for suture removal, which causes marked distress in many young children.
[†]*Note:* Steri-strips should be placed under the tissue adhesive—perpendicular to the cut—to provide support.
[‡]Most palm, finger, and foot lacerations do **not** need suturing. Approximate wound edges with bandage and keep dry and clean for 3–7 days.

The history is typically absent or incomplete because these children lack effective verbal and cognitive skills and the symptomatic child may have an altered mental status.

- Careful observation alone is usually indicated for the asymptomatic toddler found playing with or mouthing pills. If the child is seen within an hour of suspected ingestion, oral charcoal may be considered but should not be forced. Administration of syrup of ipecac or gastric lavage is no longer recommended. Supportive care is the cornerstone of treatment.
- Do not waste time if the child is symptomatic.
- Perform initial resuscitation and stabilization.
  - ABCs
  - Dextrostick
  - IV access
  - If comatose, give bolus of 0.5g/kg (2mL/kg $D_{25}W$) glucose followed by naloxone IV.

- Obtain history, perform a physical examination, and gather as much exact information of substance ingested as you can to assess its toxicity.
- Obtain an electrocardiogram and laboratory evaluation to help identify the toxic agent or underlying disease.
- Order a basal metabolic profile to measure bicarbonate and assess kidney function. If possible, obtain a blood sample for future testing.
- Determine specific serum levels of the agent.
- Treatment
  - Provide symptomatic treatment (for seizures, arrhythmia, or shock).
  - Give special care to toddlers for ingestion of oral hypoglycemics.
  - Realize that most treatment is supportive; antidotes are rare.

- Be aware that elimination of poison occurs from GI tract, skin, and eyes.
- Discuss with a poison control center or toxicology service.
- See Chapter 5, Poisonings for more information.

## BITES

- Contact a poison control center for advice on venomous bites. Tetanus prophylaxis is advisable (Table 4-4). Antihistamines may help treat minor local symptoms.

### Human

- Most common organisms: anaerobes, *Staphylococcus aureus*, and streptococci
- Treatment
  - Use **copious** irrigation and débridement.
  - Leave unsutured. **No tissue adhesive should be used to treat this mechanism of injury!**

| TABLE 4-4 | Tetanus Prophylaxis | |
|---|---|---|
| **Clinical scenario** | **Clean wound** | **Tetanus prone** |
| Fully immunized and <5 yr since last booster | None | None |
| Fully immunized and 5–10 yr since last booster | None | Td |
| Fully immunized and >10 yr since last booster | Td | Td |
| Incompletely immunized or unknown | Td | Td and tetanus immunoglobulin |
| Td = tetanus and diphtheria toxoid | | |

- If located on the face, consider delayed primary closure (clean, cover, close in 4 days).
- If cosmetically significant, clean thoroughly, close, and inspect in 2 to 3 days for evidence of infection.
- Administer tetanus prophylaxis if necessary.
- Consider antibiotic prophylaxis in hand or foot bites (amoxicillin-clavulanic acid or clindamycin).
- Ensure urgent surgical exploration for joint involvement.

## Mammal

- Most common organisms: anaerobes, *S. aureus*, group A streptococci, *Pasteurella multocida*
- Determine circumstances of the attack and the state of health of the animal.
- Treatment: same as for human bites
- Contact local health department to assess local risk of rabies.
    - Cat bite: more like a puncture wound and so more difficult to irrigate
    - Dog bite: think of this as a crush-type injury; will result in more infection-prone, devitalized tissue
    - Bat bite: most commonly arises in the presence of a dead bat and uncertain circumstances of an actual "bite." Rabies prophylaxis is recommended if any possibility of a bat bite exists (e.g., when a bat is discovered in a child's room). Children sleep heavily and may not awaken from the presence of a small bat in their room, and a bat bite can be superficial and not easily noticed.

## Hymenoptera (Bees, Wasps, and Ants)

- A bite from any member of this family may result in fatal anaphylaxis.
- Lesions are immediately painful with a burning sensation, and rapidly progress to an intense erythematous wheal.
- Inspect wound for any persistent foreign body (i.e., stinger). Do not use tweezers to extract a stinger; this risks compression of the venom sack and further injection into the wound site. Use a plastic credit card edge, or something equally dull to scrape it off.
- Tetanus prophylaxis is unnecessary.
- Antihistamines such as diphenhydramine are typically recommended for first-line therapy to reduce swelling and itching. A mild analgesic may also be prescribed.
- If the lesion is extensive and disabling, then a systemic steroid such as prednisone may be given.
- The features of **anaphylaxis** from an insect sting are the same as those from anaphylaxis from any other cause: flushing, angioedema, and generalized urticaria, followed by airway compromise, hypotension, and shock. Symptoms commonly present within 10–20 minutes of the sting, but reactions as long as 72 hours later have been reported.
    - For treatment, give subcutaneous epinephrine (1:1,000) as soon as possible (formulation of 1 mg/mL, 0.01 mL/kg of body weight subcutaneously, maximum dose 0.3–0.5 mL). Aerosolized epinephrine is **not** an equivalent therapeutic measure, although it may be administered in conjunction with subcutaneous therapy.
    - After administration of epinephrine, proceed with appropriate supportive measures.
    - Patients with known anaphylactic reaction should carry injectable epinephrine with them.

## Spiders

- Brown recluse
    - This spider is endemic in the midwestern and southeastern United States.
    - The vast majority of bites result in mild reactions, with local vesicle, redness, and swelling. The actual bite is typically painless.
    - In severe cases, local tissue and vascular damage can occur with systemic reactions, such as disseminated intravascular coagulation, hemolysis, arthralgias, fever, urticaria, and vomiting.
    - Treatment is supportive. Steroid and dapsone use are controversial. No antivenin is available.

- Black widow
  - This spider produces a neurotoxin that causes pain, muscle cramps, and rigid abdomen rapidly after envenomation.
  - A bite can also cause ascending motor paralysis, seizures, shock, and fever.
  - Treatment is supportive. Give diazepam and calcium gluconate for muscle spasms and narcotics for pain. Antivenin is available for patients who are not allergic to horse serum.

# PROCEDURAL SEDATION IN CHILDREN

- Indications and strategies for procedural sedation should be individualized in every patient. If procedural pain can be effectively managed with local anesthesia and/or oral analgesia, many children do not require sedation. For young children, allowing the parent to participate, for example, suturing while the toddler sits in the parent's lap or provides distraction, greatly reduces the child's anxiety and the need for sedation.
- For urgent and emergent procedures, the risks and benefits of sedation should be carefully considered, and the lightest effective sedation should be used. The risk of vomiting correlates poorly with the length of fasting in children sedated in the emergency department. The risk of pulmonary aspiration is unknown but rare.
- Inhaled nitrous oxide can provide mild to moderate anxiolysis and analgesia without the need for a frightening intravenous catheter. When 50% nitrous oxide is combined with oral oxycodone and injection of lidocaine into the fracture site, forearm fracture reduction may be well tolerated, although many patients remain verbally responsive. Increasing experience with ketamine-based deep sedation suggests that the risks of pulmonary aspiration are low when diligent direct patient observation and immediate airway clearing (e.g., turning patient to side to clear oropharynx) are used.
- For additional information about sedation, see Chapter 24, Sedation.

## Suggested Readings

American Academy of Pediatrics, Committee on Quality Improvement: the management of minor closed head injury in children. Pediatrics 1999;104–1415.

American Heart Association, Subcommittee on Pediatric Resuscitation: Pediatric Basic and Advance Life Support 1994–1997.

Fleisher GR. The management of bite wounds. N Engl J Med 1999;340:138–140.

Guzzetta P, Randolph J. Burns in children. Pediatr Rev 1983;4:271.

Kennedy RM, Luhmann JD. The "ouchless emergency department": getting closer: advances in decreasing distress during painful procedures in the emergency department. Pediatr Clin North Am 1999;46(6):1215–1247.

Kissick J, Johnston KM. Return to play after concussion: principles and practice. Clin J Sport Med 2005;15:426–431.

Luhmann JD, Kennedy RM, Porter FL, et al. A randomized clinical trial of continuous flow nitrous oxide and midazolam for sedation of young children during laceration repair. Ann Emerg Med 2001;37:20–27.

Luhmann JD, Schootman M, Luhmann S, et al. A randomized comparison of nitrous oxide plus hematoma block versus ketamine plus midazolam for emergency department forearm fracture reduction in children. Pediatrics 2006;118(4):e1–e9.

McAllister JD, Gnauck KA. Rapid sequence intubation of the pediatric patient: fundamentals of practice. Pediatr Clin North Am 1999;46(6):1249–1284.

McGuigan, ME. Poisoning in children and adolescents. Pediatr Rev 1993;14:411–422.

Quinn J, Cummings S, Callahan M, et al. Suturing versus conservative management of lacerations of the hand: randomized controlled trial. BMJ 2002;325:299–301.

Steen CJ, Janniger CK, Schutzer SE, et al. Insect sting reactions to bees, wasps, and ants. Int J Derm 2005;44:91–94.

White NJ, Kim MK, Brousseau DC, et al. The anesthetic effectiveness of lidocaine-adrenaline-epinephrine gel on finger lacerations. PEC 2004;20(12):812–815.

Wiley JF, II. Difficult diagnoses in toxicology. Poisons not detected by the comprehensive drug screen. Pediatr Clin North Am 1991;38(3):725–737.

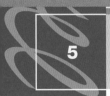

# POISONINGS
## 5
### *Marcella M. Donaruma-Kwoh*

- When you are faced with a patient whom you think has been a victim of poisoning, whether accidental or intentional, remember to think ahead!
    - It is important to consider the need for toxicologic testing early in the clinical evaluation.
    - This is a simpler task when faced with a patient who presents with a classic toxidrome (remember "mad as a hatter, dry as a bone"), but it is equally important when faced with a child who simply presents with a diagnostic dilemma.
- **When drawing blood during the acute phase of illness, always secure extra samples when clinically possible.** Collect whatever samples you deem necessary in the context of the patient's signs and symptoms; blood and urine (and occasionally vomit or feces) may be helpful.
- Include poisoning in the differential diagnosis.
- **Poison control centers** can be an excellent source of information (telephone **1-800-222-1222**).
- For a discussion of emergency management and the general approach to initial management and stabilization of a poisoning victim, see Chapter 4, Emergencies.

## Classification (Age)

### *Infants*
- Based on their limited developmental capabilities, accidental ingestions are rare in children younger than 12 months of age.
- Consider misuse of medication (administering medication prescribed for another household member to an infant).
- Consider inappropriate dosing (concentration or measurement error) of prescription or over-the-counter medicine.

### *Toddlers*
- Toddlers have a potentially deadly developmental combination of independent mobility, evolving manual dexterity, and impulsivity.
- In recent data from poison control centers, >50% of all poisoned children were younger than 3 years of age.
- Male predominance

### *School-Aged Children*
- Evaluate with increased caution; children in this age group with normal developmental achievement **do not** typically ingest toxic substances unless the toxin is improperly stored (e.g., antifreeze stored in a soda container).

### *Adolescents*
- Second most common age range of pediatric poisoning victims
- Female predominance
- Intentional poisonings are more commonly recognized in this age group.
    - Suicide attempts
    - Recreational ingestion for amusement/altered perception/intoxication leading to unintentional overdose
    - More severe clinical effects of toxin
    - Higher associated morbidity and mortality with intentional poisonings in all age ranges (i.e., suicide attempts or deliberate poisonings)

# DIAGNOSIS

## History

- None (i.e., "found down")
    - The number one chief complaint of poisoning victims is **altered mental status.**
    - Secure the available timeline of progression of symptoms.
        - Presence of a prodrome
        - Symptoms that a stressed caretaker may have tried to "treat"

- Recent introduction of new compound into the environment
    - This is particularly appropriate to toddlers (e.g., the household car's brake fluid was just changed and the container left accessible in the driveway).
    - Holidays may increase availability of alcohol-containing beverages within a child's reach.

- New caretaker
    - Possible diminished level of alertness to child's activity
    - New household members, such as elderly relatives taking prescription medications that may be accidentally stored within the arm's reach of a small child

- Home environment
    - More than 90% of poisonings occur in the home (Centers for Disease Control and Prevention, 2006). Cosmetics, cleaning products, and over-the-counter products (e.g., analgesics, topical agents, antihistamines, vitamins, and cough and cold preparations) are among the most frequently encountered poisons in accidental ingestions.
    - Prescription medications are available to all household members. **Child-resistant caps are not childproof.** Anticipatory guidance must include keeping all prescription and over-the-counter medications, as well as potentially toxic products, in their original containers, as well as securing these products with the use of a lock or latch.
    - A repeat visit with a chief complaint of ingestion is a concern. Affected patients are likely to be **chemically abused children.** One of the following is true:
        - The home environment is unsafe and endangering (e.g., methamphetamine "lab").
        - Caretakers practice neglectful supervision.
        - The child was intentionally administered a toxic substance. See section on Child Abuse by Poisoning.
    - Plants
        - Common backyard plants of concern are listed in Table 5-1.
        - Mushrooms are also common sources of alarm in pediatric ingestions.
            - Mushrooms from backyards are unlikely to be poisonous as opposed to those found in woody areas.
            - Mushrooms with pale or white undersides should be regarded with suspicion.
    - Hobbies may lead to exposure to hydrocarbons, heavy metals, or foreign body aspiration/ingestion.
    - Often, child protective services can help in assessing the home environment to confirm the details in the history by conducting a home inspection.
        - Helps assist parents with childproofing and instruction in appropriate supervision
        - May help provide a safe alternative environment
        - Recent life change/emotional upset. This may prompt a suicidal gesture with available household products/medications.

## Clinical Presentation

- Prescription medication ingestion (Table 5-2)
- Nonprescription substance ingestion/exposure (Table 5-3)

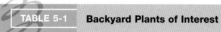

| TABLE 5-1 | Backyard Plants of Interest | | | |
|---|---|---|---|---|

| Plant | Appearance | Toxin | Poisonous parts | Symptoms |
|---|---|---|---|---|
| Deadly nightshade (*Atropa belladonna*) | Cream-colored, bell-shaped, violet-tipped flowers with shiny black berries | Alkaloids (hyoscyamine; atropine is a derivative) | All parts; berry is most commonly ingested | Anticholinergic Mydriasis, dry mouth, urinary retention, agitation, ataxia, seizures |
| Jimson weed (*Datura stramonium*) | Broad, serrated leaves, spiny seed pod that led to nickname "thorn apple" | Alkaloids (hyoscyamine, scopolamine) | All parts; leaves and seeds are most commonly ingested | Anticholinergic Mydriasis, dry mouth, urinary retention, agitation, delirium, ataxia, seizures |
| Mistletoe (*Viscum album*) | Found on deciduous trees, waxy white berries | Alkaloids (tyramine) | All parts **except** the berry | Nausea/ vomiting/ diarrhea, mydriasis, bradycardia, muscle weakness |
| Rhubarb (*Rheum officinale* or *R. palmatum*) | Magenta stalk (like celery), fades to greenish white at tip, large broad leaves | Oxalates, Cyanogenic glycosides | Leaves | Nausea/ vomiting/ diarrhea, hypocalcemia because of chelation by oxalates |
| Wisteria (*West sinensis* or *W. floribunda*) | Woody climbing vines with dangling clusters of white or violet flowers | Cyanogenic glycosides | Seeds (large quantities must be eaten for toxic effect) | Nausea/ vomiting/ diarrhea |
| Woody nightshade (*Solanum dulcamara*) "Bittersweet" | 5-petal purple flower with yellow center, green berries turn bright shiny red | Alkaloids (solanine) Cyanogenic glycosides | All parts; particularly the unripe berries | Nausea/ vomiting, ataxia, drowsiness, seizures |
| Yew (*Taxus*) | Evergreen with flat narrow leaves, matte red berries | Alkaloids (solanine) | All parts except the berries | Nausea/ vomiting, bradycardia, mydriasis, seizures, oropharyngeal irritation |

| TABLE 5-2 | Common Findings and Management Approach in Prescription Drug Ingestion | | |
|---|---|---|---|
| **Poison** | **Signs and symptoms** | **Antidote/ Treatment** | **Comments** |
| Atropine/ antihistamines/ anticholinergics | Dry mouth, mydriasis, tachycardia, hyperthermia | Physostigmine 0.02– 0.06 mg/kg IV | Can produce seizures or bradycardia Requires telemetry |
| Benzodiazepines | Miosis, respiratory depression | Flumazenil 0.2 mg IV bolus, then 0.2 mg/ min up to max 3 mg | Administration of flumazenil can precipitate seizures in habituated patients. |
| β-blockers | Bradycardia, hypotension, hypoglycemia | Glucagon, 0.05 mg/ kg bolus, then 0.07 mg/kg. Continuous infusion of dextrose- containing fluids | Requires telemetry |
| Barbiturates and anticonvulsants | Slurred speech, hypothermia, nystagmus, ataxia, CNS depression | Charcoal, urine alkalinization | — |
| Calcium channel blockers | Hypotension, arrhythmias, hyperglycemia possible | Calcium chloride 10–25 mg/kg; not to exceed 1 g slow IV bolus May repeat dosing q 10–20 minutes up to 3 doses | Requires telemetry |
| Digitalis | Arrhythmia, hypotension, hyperkalemia | Fab fragments; 80 mg inactivates 1 mg of digoxin | Requires telemetry |
| Insulin | Sweating, dizziness, pallor, syncope, seizure, coma | Continuous infusion of dextrose- containing fluids | Frequent blood glucose checks are warranted to reach appropriate glucose infusion rate and avoid iatrogenic hyperglycemia |
| Iron | Nausea, bloody diarrhea, abdominal pain, shock, agitation/delirium (later stages of intoxication) coma, leukocytosis, metabolic acidosis | Desferoxamine: 40– 90 mg/kg IM q8h or if shock or coma 15 mg/kg/hr × 8 hr; hemodialysis if iron level >180 μmol/L or anuric | Toxic dose 20– 60 mg/kg iron High toxic dose > 60 mg/kg Lethal dose 200–300 mg/kg |
| Narcotics/clonidine | Miosis, hypotension, hypothermia, respiratory depression, coma | Naloxone 0.1 mg/kg IV | Half-life of naloxone is less than that of clonidine or given narcotic; repeat dosing may be necessary |

*(continued)*

| TABLE 5-2 | Common Findings and Management Approach in Prescription Drug Ingestion (Continued) | | |
|---|---|---|---|
| Poison | Signs and symptoms | Antidote/ Treatment | Comments |
| | | | If clonidine is suspected substance, telemetry is required |
| Phenothiazines (such as haloperidol, chlorpromazine, many others) | Fever, agitation, weakness, hypotension, arrhythmia, extrapyramidal reaction | Diphenhydramine 1–2 mg/kg/dose (max 50 mg) | — |
| Oral hypoglycemics | Lethargy, coma seizures, severe hypoglycemia | Continuous infusion of dextrose-containing fluids; octreotide 1 µg/kg SC q12h | Hypoglycemia may be resistant to IV dextrose; frequent monitoring of blood glucose necessary |

## Laboratory Studies

### Blood Glucose and Serum Electrolytes

- Sodium
  - Salt loading resulting in hypernatremia may be distinguished from hypernatremic dehydration by a measurement of the patient's fractional excretion of sodium ($FE_{Na}$). A child who has a high-sodium burden is expected to have a high $FE_{Na}$ (>2%) as the body attempts to achieve equilibrium. Conversely, a child with hypernatremia as a result of dehydration still has an avid renal response of water resorption, facilitated by sodium resorption; therefore the $FE_{Na}$ should be low (<1%).
  - $FE_{Na}$ equation:

$$[Urine_{Na} \times Plasma_{creatinine} / Plasma_{Na} \times Urine_{creatinine}] \times 100$$

- Bicarbonate
  - MUDPILES (**m**ethanol, **u**remia, **D**KA, **p**araldehyde, **i**ron/INH, **l**actic acid, **e**thanol/ethylene glycol, **s**alicylates) remains a useful, if not comprehensive, mnemonic to begin analysis of anion gap metabolic acidoses in ingestion cases: methanol, metformin, phenformin, iron, isoniazid, ibuprofen, ethylene glycol, and salicylates.
  - CAT (**c**arbon monoxide, **c**yanide, **c**affeine, **a**lbuterol, **t**oluene, **t**heophylline) can cover a large remainder of offending substances. These agents may also lead to an anion gap metabolic acidosis, either as the primary anions themselves, or via induction of increased lactic acid production.

### Blood Gas

- Arterial blood gas analysis is useful in assessing acid-base status in a more detailed fashion than an isolated bicarbonate value.
- Remember, a patient with methemoglobinemia (from ingestion of sulfonamide, mothballs, quinine, nitrates, and nitrites) sufficient to produce cyanosis may have a normal $PaO_2$ and calculated oxygen saturation, although pulse oximetry may be slightly low.
  - Methemoglobinemia of >30% is treated with methylene blue 1–2 mg/kg IV administered over several minutes. Repeat dosing may be necessary.

**TABLE 5-3**   **Common Findings and Management Approach in Nonprescription Substance Ingestion or Exposure**

| Poison | Signs and symptoms | Antidote/ Treatment | Comments |
|---|---|---|---|
| Acetaminophen | Toxic dose >150 mg/kg Nausea, vomiting, lethargy, >24 hr: liver damage, jaundice, encephalopathy, >7 day renal failure | N-Acetylcysteine 140 mg/kg initial dose, followed by 17 doses of 70 mg/kg q4 hr Activated charcoal if <4 hr. | See toxicity nomogram and treatment algorithm (Figures 5-1 and 5-2) Check level 4 hr postingestion Follow liver damage by checking blood glucose and coagulation parameters Only oral dosing route for N-acetylcysteine is Food and Drug Administration-approved, unless brand name Acetadote is ordered for parenteral use; **know your pharmacy policy!** |
| Alkaline corrosives | Dysphagia, oral and esophageal burns | **Do not give emetic or gastric lavage.** If eye or skin contact: rinse with water. | Esophagoscopy 3–5 days after ingestion. Esophageal stricture occurs in 15% |
| Carbon monoxide | Headache, obtundation, cerebral edema (sluggish pupillary reflex) | Delivery of supplemental oxygen | Pulse oximetry and arterial blood gas analysis may be normal |
| Ethanol (also present in perfume, aftershave, mouthwash) | Slurred speech, delirium, nausea, vomiting, hypoglycemia, hypothermia, ataxia, respiratory depression, coma | Airway management Dextrose-containing IV fluids Supportive care (warming) (Give thiamine 100 mg IV/IM in **chronic abuse cases** to avoid neurologic injury) | Younger children with smaller glycogen stores more likely to present with low blood sugar. In teens, remember to check for pregnancy, recreational drug use, coexisting trauma |
| Ethylene glycol | Tachypnea (compensatory for metabolic acidosis), obtundation, renal failure with oxalate crystal deposition and acute tubular necrosis, death | Ethanol drip (competitor for alcohol dehydrogenase) controversial Fomepizole (inhibitor of alcohol dehydrogenase) trials in adults are | Fluorescein in ethylene-glycol based antifreeze may be present in urine/vomitus, and will glow under Wood lamp, if ingestion recent |

*(continued)*

| TABLE 5-3 | Common Findings and Management Approach in Nonprescription Substance Ingestion or Exposure *(Continued)* |

| Poison | Signs and symptoms | Antidote/ Treatment | Comments |
|--------|--------------------|--------------------|----------|
| | | occurring in United States at the time of this writing. **Check your hospital's policy.** Dialysis may assist in removing the toxic alcohol and its metabolites. | |
| Hydrocarbons | Inhalation/aspiration can lead to respiratory distress and failure, sometimes delayed up to 12–24 hr after exposure | Supportive care Steroids controversial without evidence-based medicine support | Remember that symptoms of respiratory distress may be delayed |
| Ipecac | Repeated emesis | Cessation of administration of emetic | Chronic ipecac use/abuse has been shown to lead to skeletal muscle weakness and cardiomyopathy |
| Laxatives (typically magnesium-containing) | Diarrhea, skin breakdown with chemical dermatitis mimicking burns, electrolyte imbalances/ arrhythmias rare | Cessation of laxative administration | |
| Salicylate | Emesis, pyrexia, tinnitus, coma, hyperventilation, seizures, bleeding, metabolic acidosis, and respiratory alkalosis | Gastric emptying if <1 hr activated charcoal Urine alkalinization (keep pH: 7.5–8) Hemodialysis if renal failure, pulmonary edema, salicylate level >100 mg/dL, CNS changes | Toxic dose >150 mg/kg Lethal dose >500 mg/kg Obtain level at admission and at 6 hr postingestion |
| Salt | Altered mental status, seizures (typically in hyponatremia rather than hypernatremia), cerebral edema, coma | Careful adjustment of serum osmolarity over time. For necessary elaboration, see Chapter 3, Fluid and Electrolyte Management. | Often because of misconceptions of infant feeding (i.e., giving free water PO, as enema, or mixing dilute formula) or because of inappropriate discipline (forced ingestion of salt load). **Parental education and child safety are paramount.** |

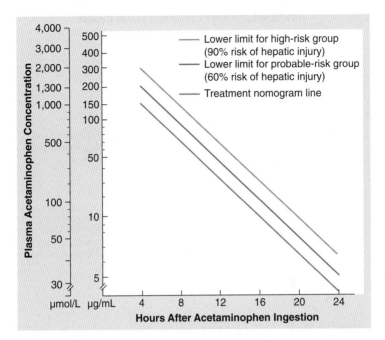

**Figure 5-1.** Nomogram showing plasma or serum acetaminophen concentration versus time post-acetaminophen ingestion.

**CAUTIONS FOR USE OF THIS CHART:**

1. The time coordinates refer to time post ingestion.
2. Serum levels drawn before 4 hours may not represent peak levels.
3. The graph should be used only in relation to a single acute ingestion.

■ **Methylene blue is contraindicated in patients with glucose-6-phosphate deficiency because of its antioxidant qualities;** patients with glucose-6-phosphate dehydrogenase (G6PD) deficiency may not have sufficient NADPH to reduce it. Use in patients with G6PD deficiency may result in severe hemolysis.

■ Carbon monoxide intoxication may also have normal values on arterial blood gas and pulse oximetry, although carbon monoxide inhalation does not produce cyanosis.

*Institutional Drug Screen*
■ Urine and serum "comprehensive" drug screens are not completely comprehensive for drugs of abuse.
■ It is imperative to know your hospital's routine urine and serum drug screening panel.
■ In some drug classes, a common metabolite is the compound that is assayed; this can miss some members of that family.
   ▪ Benzodiazepines: neither lorazepam (Ativan) nor alprazolam (Xanax) have the downstream metabolite of oxazepam. Thus, these ingestions have a falsely negative routine urine drug screen.
   ▪ Synthetic opiates (e.g., hydrocodone, oxycodone, methadone, and fentanyl) as well as "designer drugs" (e.g., fentanyl/sufentanil)
   ▪ Illicit recreational substances: lysergic acid diethylamide (LSD), gamma hydroxybutyric acid (GHB), flunitrazepam (Rohypnol), and ketamine, which are often abused as well as used in chemically assisted sexual assaults. These drugs are not commonly included in routine urine assays and often need to be ordered by name. Check with your chemistry section of laboratory medicine for proper processing.

## ACETAMINOPHEN POISONING FLOW CHART

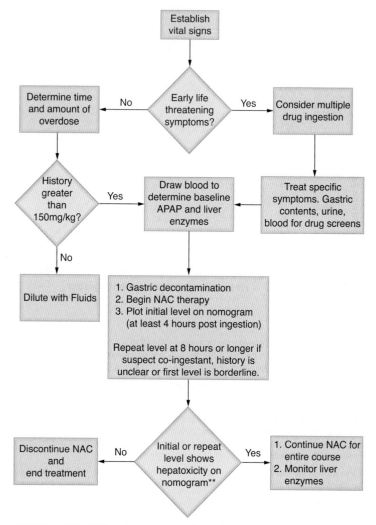

** In late presentation APAP overdoses an acetaminophen level may be meaningless. if there is clinical evidence of liver toxicity the patient should receive a full course of NAC. NAC may be useful even when liver failure has ensued.

**Figure 5-2.** Treatment algorithm for acetaminophen poisoning.

## Specific Laboratory Studies

### *Intentionally Induced Hypoglycemia*
- C-peptide and insulin level
  - Blood for these samples must be drawn concomitantly, and at the time the patient is experiencing hypoglycemia.
  - C-peptide is a subunit of insulin that is cleaved from insulin inside pancreatic islet cells.
  - If insulin level is high, and C-peptide is simultaneously low, one may deduce that the insulin was not manufactured by the patient's pancreas.

- Note that **these values can only be interpreted if drawn before the initiation of glucose therapy.** Levels obtained after therapy is begun may be confused by the patient's own pancreatic response to the glucose bolus.
- Oral hypoglycemic panel
  - Serum assays that measure for members of the sulfonylurea class of drugs, as well as some meglitinides, are available in some laboratory facilities.

### Carboxyhemoglobin

- A good rule of thumb is that symptoms typically begin around a measured carboxyhemoglobin of 10%. This may vary in adolescent patients who are chronic smokers; their levels may approach 10% at baseline.
  - In very young infants, fetal hemoglobin may be read as carboxyhemoglobin.

### Specific Drug Levels

- Emetine (metabolite of ipecac)
  - Level may be assessed in urine or serum specimen if specifically ordered.
  - Best window for collection is within 3 hours of emesis because of the high volume of distribution for drug.
- Specific quantitative drug assays
  - Antiepileptic medications, antihypertensive medications, and anticoagulants are all commonly encountered substances in pediatric ingestion cases. Many of these drug levels are of the send-out category to a specific institution(s) in the nation.
  - **If such an ingestion is considered and the assay for a blood level is sought, it is imperative that the child is not allowed to return to a potentially harmful home environment until the results are known or an alternative diagnosis is made!**

## Other Useful Diagnostic Studies

### Electrocardiography

- Tachyarrhythmias
  - **Tricyclic antidepressants** and **antipsychotic medications** may present as sinus tachycardias, but prolongation of the QT and/or QRS intervals may foretell potentially fatal ventricular arrhythmias.
  - **Digoxin** acts to slow conduction at the sinoatrial and atrioventricular (AV) nodes, and speeds conduction in between, leading most commonly to atrial tachycardias or junctional tachycardias, with or without AV block.
- Bradyarrhythmias
  - β-**blockers** and **calcium channel blockers** typically demonstrate AV block of varying degrees.
- T-wave inversion
  - **Ipecac** in chronic users or at toxic levels may result in T-wave inversion on all leads as well as prolongation of the QT interval.

### Radiography

- Radiopaque foreign bodies that have been ingested or aspirated by the child may be visualized on chest or abdominal films.
- Iron (ferrous sulfate) or enteric-coated tablets may be seen in the gastrointestinal tract.
- A negative radiograph does not rule out ingestion/aspiration.

## TREATMENT

### Elimination of Ingested Poisons

- Activated charcoal may be considered if <1 hour after ingestion; the dose is 0.5–1g/kg (30–50 g). This may be repeated 3–4 times in the first 24 hours.

- Agents absorbed by activated charcoal: atropine, barbiturates, chlorpromazine, cocaine, colchicine, digitalis, amphetamines, morphine, phenytoin, salicylates, theophylline, and tricyclic antidepressants
- Agents not absorbed by activated charcoal: iron
- Methods of secondary elimination
  - Increased transit time (cathartics): magnesium citrate and sorbitol, polyethylene glycol
  - Forced diuresis: use with caution; some poisons enhance pulmonary edema.
  - Alkalinization: for TCA, barbiturates, salicylates, and isoniazid. Administer $NaHCO_3$ and follow urine pH.
  - Acidification: for amphetamines, quinine, fenfluramine, and phencyclidine. Administer ascorbic acid and follow pH.
  - Hemodialysis, hemofiltration, or peritoneal dialysis: methanol, lithium, ethylene glycol, and salicylates

## Antidotes/Therapy for Prescription Medication Ingestion (see Table 5-2)

## Antidotes/Therapy for Nonprescription Substance Ingestion/Exposure (see Table 5-3)

# CHILD ABUSE BY POISONING

- Pediatric condition falsification (PCF) was formerly known as Münchausen syndrome by proxy. The term "Münchausen's" is no longer favored; it is not an appropriate diagnosis for the pediatric patient because it implies a diagnosis of the caretaker.
- PCF is a situation that involves pathologic health care–seeking behavior by a caretaker on behalf of the child, in which the caretaker (often the mother) fabricates, induces, or exaggerates signs and symptoms of illness leading to the perception of an ill child when presented to medical personnel
- The creation of these circumstances may lead to incorrect diagnoses, unnecessary medications, diagnostic interventions, and surgical procedures.
- Evaluation and treatment in such cases require the involvement of a multidisciplinary team familiar with the dynamics of PCF.
- Open confrontation with the suspected caretaker should be avoided until agreed on by the institutional multidisciplinary team.
- In the interest of the child's safety, do not hesitate to keep the child under close inpatient supervision (1:1 nursing, 1:1 sitter) should intentional administration of a harmful substance be suspected (i.e., covert administration of subcutaneous insulin, the willful contamination of a wound or catheter with feces, or any other type of harmful act with the result of inducing ill health).
- The intentional killing of a child by poison is not necessarily synonymous with PCF. Typically, it lacks the repetitive health care–seeking and health care–shopping behaviors characteristic of PCF, although it is no less puzzling.

*Diagnosis*
- To make the diagnosis of intentional poisoning, consider it in the differential diagnosis. This is difficult; pediatricians are trained to take a history from the caretakers and use it to guide patient evaluation and management.
- Ask detailed questions regarding the home environment, caretakers, timeline, access to substances, and attempted interventions before seeking medical care.
  - Typically, in accidental poisoning, <2 hours elapse between the time of ingestion and the time of seeking medical care.
  - Often, parents realize their error and may be fearful of losing their child "to the system" based on their lapse in supervision, and so they fabricate a history and make diagnosis and treatment more challenging.

■ Conduct a developmental assessment of the child, whether based on physical examination (sometimes complicated by altered mental status) or by history; this can be key in validating the mechanism of access to the substances (e.g., a 3-month-old child could not pick up a pill and coordinate its transfer to his mouth, but an 11-month-old child could).

■ **Ask about past medical history of ingestion.** In a 1989 study (Litovitz), there was a trend noted among "repeaters" with a diagnosis of ingestion:

  ■ Children with a history of drug ingestion were 1.49 times more likely to ingest another drug; with household product ingestion, 1.24 times more likely to "repeat"; and with plant ingestion, 2.00 times more likely to "repeat."

  ■ Disturbingly, 12% of the entire group of "repeaters" was younger than 1 year of age. This raises alarming issues based on an infant's limited developmental capabilities; surely a large percentage of these repeaters were victims of child abuse by poisoning.

  ■ Although these numbers may be indicative of deliberate poisoning or neglectful supervision, either scenario is a danger to the child's safety and well-being and is worthy of intervention.

■ In nonverbal or preverbal children who are suspected poisoning victims, a skeletal survey is a reliable screening tool for other abusive injury—when used in conjunction with a thorough history and physical examination.

■ Do not be afraid to ask for help if you have the concern that your patient could have been a poisoning victim. Senior residents, chief residents, social workers, attendings, child abuse team members, and child protective services workers all want to work to treat and protect the patient rather than point a finger at a guilty party.

### Suggested Readings

Diagnostic imaging of child abuse. Pediatrics, 2000;105(6):1345–1348.

Ayoub CC, Alexander R. Definitional issues in Münchausen by proxy. APSAC Advisor 1998;11(1):7–10.

Ayoub CC, Alexander R, et al. Position paper: definitional issues in Münchausen by proxy. Child Maltreatment 2002;7(2):105–110.

Bays J, Feldman KW. Child Abuse by Poisoning. 2nd Ed. In: Block RM, Ludwig S, eds. Child Abuse: Medical Diagnosis and Treatment. vol 1, Philadelphia: Lippincott Williams & Wilkins, 2001:405–441.

Black J, Zenel J. Child abuse by intentional iron poisoning presenting as shock and persistent acidosis. Pediatrics 2003;111:197–199.

Coulthard MG, Haycock GB. Distinguishing between salt poisoning and hypernatraemic dehydration in children. BMJ 2003;326(7381):157–160.

Garrettson LK, et al. Physical change, time of day, and child characteristics as factors in poison injury. Vet Hum Toxicol 1990;32(2):139–141.

Hoffman RJ, Nelson L. Rational use of toxicology testing in children. Curr Opinion Pediatr 2001;13:183–186.

Litovitz TL, et al. 2000 annual report of the American Association of Poison Control Centers toxic exposure surveillance system. Am J Emerg Med 2001;19(5):337–395.

Litovitz TL, et al. Recurrent poisonings among paediatric poisoning victims. Med Toxicol Adverse Drug Exp 1989;4(5):381–386.

Maxwell JC. Party drugs: properties, prevalence, patterns, and problems. Subst Use Misuse 2005;40(9–10):1203–1240.

Meadow R. ABC of child abuse. Poisoning. BMJ 1989;298(6685):1445–1446.

Megarbane B, Borron SW, Baud FJ. Current recommendations for treatment of severe alcoholic poisonings. Intensive Care Med 2005;31(2):189–195.

Paschall RT. The Chemically Abused Child. In Giardino AP, ed. Child Maltreatment, vol 1, 2nd Ed. St. Louis: GW Medical Publishing, 2005.

Riordan M, Rylance G, Berry K. Poisoning in children 5: rare and dangerous poisons. Arch Dis Child 2002;87(5):407–410.

Riordan M, Rylance G, Berry K. Poisoning in children 4: household products, plants, and mushrooms. Arch Dis Child 2002;87(5):403–406.

Riordan M, Rylance G, Berry K. Poisoning in children 3: common medicines. Arch Dis Child 2002;87(5):400–402.

Riordan M, Rylance G, Berry K. Poisoning in children 2: painkillers. Arch Dis Child 2002;87(5):397–399.

Riordan M, Rylance G, Berry K. Poisoning in children 1: general management. Arch Dis Child 2002;87(5):392–396.

Russell AB, Hardin J, Grand W, et al. Poisonous plants of North Carolina; Russell AB, ed. North Carolina State University, 1997.

Shannon M. Ingestion of toxic substances by children. N Engl J Med 2000;342(3):186–191.

Shnaps Y, et al. The chemically abused child. Pediatrics 1981;68(1):119–121.

Scharman EJ, et al. Single dose pharmacokinetics of syrup of ipecac. Ther Drug Monit 2000;22(5):566–573.

Schneider D, Perez A, Knilamus TE, et al. Clinical and pathological aspects of cardiomyopathy from ipecac administration in Münchausen's syndrome by proxy. Pediatrics 1996;97(6 Pt 1):902–906.

Stevens M, Nesom G. Plant guide, U.S.D.O. Agriculture, Editor. 2003, National Plant Data Center: 1–6. Available at: http://npdc.usda.gov/publication/index.html.

Wiseman HM, et al. Accidental poisoning in childhood: a multicentre survey. 2. The role of packaging in accidents involving medications. Hum Toxicol 1987;6(4):303–314.

Wright R, Lewander WJ, Woolf AD. Methemoglobinemia: etiology, pharmacology, and clinical management. Ann of Emerg Med 2004;34(5):646–656.

Yamamoto LG, Wiebe RA, Matthews WJ, Jr. Toxic exposures and ingestions in Honolulu: I. A prospective pediatric ED cohort; II. A prospective poison center cohort. Pediatr Emerg Care 1991;7(3):141–148.

Marcella M. Donaruma-Kwoh and Robert M. Kennedy

# DEVELOPMENTAL HIP DYSPLASIA

## Definition and Etiology

- In this spectrum of abnormalities, the femoral head and acetabulum are misaligned or have abnormal development.
- Etiology may involve mechanical (abnormal in utero positioning), primary acetabular dysplasia, or ligamentous laxity.

## Epidemiology

- Risk factors include breech presentation, oligohydramnios, female sex, postnatal positioning, white ethnicity, and family history. (However, the majority of affected children do not have identifiable risk factors.)
- The left hip is more likely to be affected than the right.
- Associated conditions include torticollis, clubfoot (metatarsus adductus), scoliosis, plagiocephaly, and low-set ears.

## Diagnostic Tests

- Ortolani and Barlow maneuvers (up to 12 weeks of age) (Figure 6-1)
  - Asymmetry of gluteal and thigh folds
  - Leg-length discrepancy. Allis and Galeazzi signs also may be present on physical examination (see Figure 6-1).
  - Limited abduction in older child (>3 months of age)
- Ultrasound is useful. Up to 90% of newborns with mild dysplasia present on ultrasound resolve spontaneously between 6 weeks and 6 months.

## American Academy of Pediatrics' (AAP) Recommendations

- Serial clinical examinations at well-child checkups
- Hip imaging in breech female infants (general imaging is **not** recommended as a screening tool for all infants)
  - Ultrasound of the hips at birth up to 4 months
  - Anteroposterior (AP) radiographs of the hips after 3–4 months
- Optional imaging in breech male infants, or in girls with a positive family history

## Treatment

- Management occurs in tandem with a pediatric orthopedic surgeon.
- Risks associated with intervention are not inconsequential, particularly avascular necrosis of the femoral head.
- Treatment method by age:
  - 0–6 months:
    - Pavlik harness and hip spica cast
    - Triple diapering is not recommended.

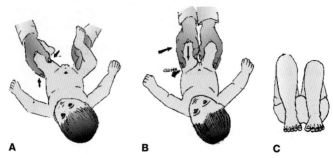

**Figure 6-1. A.** Ortolani maneuver (hip is dislocated). **B.** Barlow maneuver (hip is dislocatable). **C.** Allis or Galeazzi sign (leg-length discrepancy).

- 6–18 months:
  - Traction for 3 weeks followed by attempt at closed reduction and spica cast
  - Open reduction if necessary
- Older than 18 months
  - Open reduction and osteotomy

## TODDLERS WITH ACUTE SKELETAL SYMPTOMS

- Children in this age group, in particular, can be difficult to assess because of the combination of their mobility (allowing them to come to harm) out of proportion to their verbal skills (inhibiting the collection of a medical history).

### Complaint: "He Isn't Using That Arm"

- Consider **nursemaid's elbow** in the context of an absent history of fall or trauma that would increase your suspicion for fracture (see "Fractures" section).
- This is radial head luxation in a child who is younger than 5 years of age. It may be secondary to excessive axial traction in an extended elbow.
- Note that radial head/neck fractures may mimic nursemaid's elbow! History is very important!
- The child usually hangs the arm with the elbow slightly flexed and the hand pronated, and he or she is unwilling to supinate or pronate the wrist. There is slight tenderness over the radial head or wrist.
- Radiographs are unnecessary if reduction is successful; if obtained, films are normal and positioning for lateral view often results in reduction.
- Reduction is performed by quickly and fully supinating or pronating the wrist, followed by flexion of the elbow; a "pop" is felt over the radial head at the elbow.
- The patient will start to use that arm normally within 5–10 minutes.

### Complaint: "She Wouldn't Walk This Morning"

- The following diagnoses lead the differential diagnosis of a toddler with either a limp or refusal to bear weight.

### Septic Joint

- This diagnosis is an orthopedic emergency. Children with septic arthritis are usual febrile and systemically ill, although this is less consistent in the neonatal population, who may simply be irritable and demonstrate a "pseudoparalysis" of the affected extremity.
- The joint is often red, hot, and swollen, although less frequently in the hip. These patients strongly resist examination for range of motion of the affected joint (most commonly the hip) and frequently refuse to bear weight.

- Erythrocyte sedimentation rate (ESR) is sensitive (but not specific) when elevated. White blood cell (WBC) count is elevated in about 50% of these patients.
- Plain radiographs may show subtle signs of joint effusion, such as widening of the joint space, soft tissue swelling, obliteration of normal fat planes, or osteomyelitis.
- The definitive diagnosis is made in microscopic examination of synovial fluid obtained through **arthrocentesis.**

## Osteomyelitis

- Osteomyelitis occurs most commonly in patients younger than 5 years of age, and it has a predilection for the long bones of the leg, although any bone may be affected.
- Hematogenous seeding is the most common pathway of infection, and the metaphyses of long bones are highly vascular, providing an ideal environment.
- The patient is usually febrile. In contrast to the child with a septic joint, point tenderness is present; however, the child allows range of motion evaluation of the affected extremity. Redness and swelling may overlie the area of tenderness but are not consistently present.
- Standard assessment includes C-reactive protein, ESR, blood culture, and complete blood count (CBC; although an elevated WBC count is often surprisingly absent).
- Standard plain films may not display destructive changes to bone in the first 10–14 days of illness. Bone scanning or magnetic resonance imaging (MRI) can offer more information.
    - Although an MRI is more sensitive, it more often requires sedation in this age group to obtain a satisfactory study. MRI is also helpful in detailing abscesses in need of surgical drainage.
    - Bone scan may be more helpful in looking for multifocal disease.

## Toxic Synovitis

Also known as transient synovitis, this entity is a diagnosis of exclusion, with its evil twin of septic arthritis ruled out in the following fashion:
- Typically, these children have a nontoxic appearance and are afebrile, although they resist range-of-motion assessment and weight-bearing.
- Normal ESR and normal CBC are required to make the diagnosis.
- Radiographs are recommended to rule out other possible diagnoses. Ultrasound is also frequently performed to confirm the presence of an effusion.
- These patients may be followed clinically and may be conservatively managed with nonsteroidal anti-inflammatory drugs (NSAIDs). The prognosis is excellent, although a small percentage of cases recur.

## Toddler Fracture (see discussion below)

# FRACTURES

Evaluation of any patient with suspected fracture: **5 Ps**
    **P**oint tenderness
    **P**ulse distally
    **P**allor
    **P**aresthesia distally
    **P**aralysis distally
- Fractures in infants younger than 18 months of age or with an unclear mechanism of injury should lead to a suspicion of nonaccidental trauma.
- Fractures can be classified using the Salter-Harris system (Table 6-1).

## General Management

- Keep patients nil per os (NPO) in case of need for surgery or sedation.
- Cover open wounds with a sterile dressing.

| TABLE 6-1 | Types of Salter-Harris Fractures |

| | I | II | III | IV | V |
|---|---|---|---|---|---|
| Diagnosis/ Associated Conditions | Difficult to diagnose if not displaced; rarely associated with growth disturbance | Most common type; growth disturbance rare | High risk of growth disturbance and posttraumatic arthritis | High risk of growth disturbance | Difficult to diagnose; usually diagnosed when growth disturbance manifested |
| Treatment | Immobilization for 10–14 days | Closed reduction with 3–6 weeks of cast placement | May require open reduction and fixation if displaced | May require open reduction and internal fixation | Anticipatory guidance about possible asymmetric healing and growth |
| Appearance | | | | | |
| | I | II | III | IV | V |

- **Remember** that early pain management involves splinting and oxycodone 0.2 mg/kg.
- Open fractures require tetanus prophylaxis, antibiotics, immediate débridement, and surgery.
- Angulation in plane of motion may not need reduction if angle is <10°–20° and growth plates are open.
- Open reduction is indicated in failed closed reduction, displaced intraarticular fractures, unstable fractures, or open fractures.
- After placement of a **cast**, it is very important to pay close attention to signs and symptoms of compartment syndrome (Figure 6-2), which include the following:
  - Pain with passive motion of the fingers
  - Marked swelling
  - Cyanosis or pallor of the extremity distal to the cast

## Clavicular Fracture

- This frequently occurs in newborns because of difficult deliveries.
- It may occur in older children as a result of falling on an outstretched arm or shoulder.
- Treatment
  - Sling or swathe to bind the arm to the trunk for few days to 3 weeks. Union occurs at 2–4 weeks.
  - Surgery only in cases of open fracture or neurovascular injury

## Colles Fracture

- This fracture of the distal radius with displacement results in classic dinner fork deformity of the wrist.
- It occurs secondary to falling with the pronated hand outstretched and the wrist dorsiflexed.
- Treatment: Buckle fractures of the distal radius or ulna are treated with a:
  - Splint or short-arm cast if pain on supination/pronation is minimal
  - Long-arm cast if displacement has occurred or cortices are broken

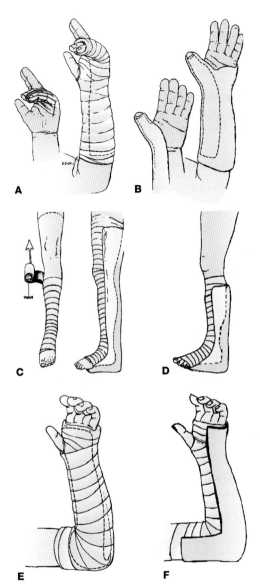

**Figure 6-2.** Casts appropriate for various fractures. **A.** Boxer's fracture. **B.** Scaphoid and thumb fracture. **C.** Knee injury and/or spiral fracture. **D.** Ankle sprain; foot, ankle, or distal fibula fracture. **E.** Distal radius and wrist fracture. **F.** Elbow and wrist injury.

## Boxer Fracture

- This is fracture of the fifth metacarpal with apical dorsal angulation.
- Treatment
  - Reduction usually unnecessary and unstable
  - Splinting with an ulnar gutter splint (see Figure 6-2)

## Scaphoid Fracture

- Characteristics include snuffbox tenderness or pain on supination with resistance.
- This is the most common carpal bone fracture.

- It has a high risk of malunion or avascular necrosis.
- Radiographs may be normal; request scaphoid views.
- Treatment
  - Splint or cast if pain is significant
  - Repeat radiographs in 2–3 weeks

## Slipped Capital Femoral Epiphysis (SCFE)

- SCFE is displacement with external rotation of the femoral head relative to the femoral neck at the epiphyseal plate. Think of this as a Class I Salter-Harris fracture (see Table 6-1).
- The male:female ratio is 3:1.
- SCFE is more frequent in pubertal African-American and obese children, as well as in those with endocrinopathies.
- Between 25% and 50% of cases are eventually bilateral.
- Onset is usually insidious.
- A limp is present with lack of internal rotation and limited abduction and flexion of the hip.
- Pain may be referred to the knee.
- Obtain AP and frog-leg radiographs.
- Treatment
  - No weight bearing and surgical pinning
  - Orthopedic consult

## Osgood-Schlatter Disease

- This painful chronic stress fracture of the tibial tuberosity occurs as a result of a vigorous quadriceps pull in a growing child.
- Symptoms may persist for 1–2 or more years and resolve as tibial epiphyses close.
- Diagnosis is by point tenderness at the tibial tubercle (i.e., insertion of patellar tendon).
- Radiography shows enlargement of the tibial tubercle, but this is unnecessary if the presentation is classic.
- Treatment
  - Rest
  - Knee immobilizer and crutches if pain is severe
  - Quadriceps and hamstring stretching
  - NSAIDs

## Ligament Injuries of the Knee (Table 6-2)

### Toddler Fracture

- This oblique nondisplaced fracture of the distal tibia in a child 9 months to 3 years of age occurs because of low energy forces.
- The child presents with antalgic gait and refusal to bear weight. There is often minimal tenderness to palpation but severe pain with internal or external rotation of the ankle.
- These fractures are usually spiral and nondisplaced.
- Radiographs may not be revealing; order an oblique view of the tibia if necessary.
- Treatment
  - Cast for 3 weeks

## Ankle Sprains

- These injuries occur due to inversion during plantar flexion.
- Talofibular ligament disruption is most common.
- Patients present with pain anterior to the lateral malleolus swelling and ecchymosis.
- Imaging
  - Ankle radiographs. To make a decision about ordering these, follow the **Ottawa Ankle Rules.** If the pain is near the malleoli and *either:*

| TABLE 6-2 | Injuries to Ligaments of the Knee | | |
| --- | --- | --- | --- |
| Ligament | Injury | Physical examination | Management |
| Medial collateral | Twisting or lateral blow to the knee | Joint effusion and limitation of motion, pain over ligament | Ice, elevation, NSAIDs, no weight bearing, orthopedic consult once swelling improved |
| Anterior cruciate | Hyperextension with foot planted | Anterior drawer test after pain resolved, hemarthrosis, and avulsion fracture acutely | Crutches, knee immobilizer, refer for orthopedic consult |
| Posterior cruciate | Direct blow to tibia while knee is flexed | Posterior knee tenderness and small effusion | Ice, elevation, NSAIDs, no weight bearing, orthopedic consult once swelling improved |

- The patient is unable to bear weight immediately after the injury and at the time of assessment (four steps) *or*
- Bone tenderness is present at the posterior edge or tip of either malleolus
- Foot radiographs should be obtained if pain is present in the midfoot and *either:*
  - The patient is unable to bear weight *or*
  - Bone tenderness is present over the navicular base or the base of fifth metatarsal
  - Normal radiographs. It is difficult to exclude a Salter-Harris I fracture.

- Treatment
  - Grade I: elastic wrap or air cast, ice, elevation, NSAIDs, and weight bearing as tolerated
  - Grade II and III: cast or posterior splint for 3 weeks
  - If there is suspicion of Salter-Harris I: cast or splint, elevation, and orthopedic consult in 1 week
  - **RICE** (treatment mnemonic for sprains)
    **R**est: Ambulation allowed if it is not painful and does not result in swelling.
    **I**ce: With the skin protected by cloth, ice area for 15–20 minutes every 2 hours for the first 48 hours after injury.
    **C**ompression: Use Ace wrap or air cast.
    **E**levation: Keep elevated as often as possible. The child may need a note for school.

# PARENTAL CONCERNS

## Legg-Calve-Perthes Disease

- This disorder involves idiopathic avascular necrosis of the femoral head.
- The disease occurs more frequently in males who are 4–8 years of age.
- Patients present with limp, referred knee pain, and limited hip internal rotation and abduction.
- Diagnosis is made by radiographs—AP and frog-leg views of the hips.
- All patients must be referred for orthopedic evaluation.

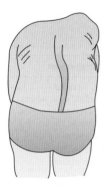 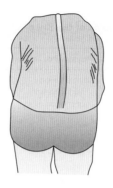

**Figure 6-3.** Scoliosis. **A.** Deformity. **B.** Normal spine.

## Scoliosis

- This disorder involves structural lateral and axial rotation of the spine.
- Between 2% and 3% of the population has scoliosis (curvature ≥10°).
- The condition affects females more commonly than males.
- Classification depends on magnitude, location, direction, and etiology. Eighty percent of cases are idiopathic, occurring in adolescence (during growth spurts), but causes may be congenital or neuromuscular.
- Curve progression is more likely in patients with curves equal to or >30° to 40° or in younger patients.
- Screening should begin at 6–7 years of age.
- The incidence of backache, except in patients with thoracolumbar curvature, is no greater than in the general population. Pulmonary function is abnormal in patients with severe (≥90°) thoracic curves.
- In the physical examination, evaluate body asymmetry (hips, shoulders, scapulae, spine) when looking from behind (Figure 6-3). Leg-length differences are most apparent when palpating the iliac crest.
- Forward bend test: with hands together posterior ribs prominent on convex side; a scoliometer reading of 5°–7° correlates with a curve of 15°–20°.
- Treatment
  - Referral for the patients with:
    - Angle of trunk rotation >6°
    - Vertebral angulation >20°–25°
  - Therapeutic methods
  - Bracing: skeletally immature patient with curve 25°–40°
  - Surgery: curves ≥45°

## In-toeing

- This is characteristic of three conditions (Table 6-3).
- On examination, determine the foot progression angle, range of internal and external hip rotation, thigh-foot angle, and degree of metatarsus varus.

## Out-toeing

- Almost all children have out-toeing because of external femoral torsion. This usually self-corrects when patients start to roll over and bear weight.

## Bow Legs (Genu Varum)

- Differential diagnosis
  - Physiologic varus (corrects by 2 years of age)
  - Rickets

| TABLE 6-3 | Types of In-toeing | | |
|---|---|---|---|
| **Condition (incidence)** | **History** | **Physical Examination** | **Therapy** |
| Metatarsus adductus (5%–10%) | Diagnosis as newborn, associated with hip dysplasia Common to have positive family history | Forefoot in varus, C-shaped | Flexible: observe 3–9 mo Rigid: refer for casting. If >2 yr: surgery |
| Internal tibial torsion (5%–10%) | Diagnosis at 1.5–4 yr More frequent when sitting or sleeping on feet with feet turned in | Abnormal thigh-foot angle (normal: 0°–20° at birth; 20° by age 2–3; 0°–40° adults) | Growth corrects the majority of cases by 3–4 yr. Refer to specialist if no improvement over first year of walking. Surgery if severe >8–10 yr |
| Femoral anteversion (80%–90%) | Diagnosis at 3–8 yr | Femoral neck rotated anteriorly from femoral shaft Internal rotation > external rotation up to 90° | Discourage sitting in "W" position. Usually resolves by 8–12 years old. Surgery if: internal rotation ≥80°, external rotation ≤15°, severe gait disturbance persists >8 yr |

- Familial bowlegs
- Traumatic growth disturbance
- Blount disease. This nontraumatic growth disturbance of the medial epiphysis of the tibia often results in progressive bowlegs. It is more common in African-American children.
    - Infantile: occurs in early walkers and in obese patients; those who are 1–2 years of age; bilateral in 50%–75% of patients
    - Adolescent: associated with obesity; more often requires surgical intervention than bracing; may result in early arthritis as a result of uneven wear on cartilage
- Diagnosis is made by radiograph of the knee and lower leg; characteristic changes are apparent in the proximal tibial epiphysis, growth plate, and metaphysis.

## Knock Knees (Genu Valgum)

- This condition is first noticed around 2–3 years of age, progresses for 1–2 years, and spontaneously corrects at 3–4 years of age.
- Differential diagnosis
    - Physiologic valgus
    - Rickets
    - Other bony dysplasias

# CONCERNS RELATING TO NONACCIDENTAL TRAUMA

- Although there is no such thing as "pathognomonic" in this nonphysiologic process, certain kinds of fractures are highly specific for inflicted injury.
- When considering a pediatric patient who is younger than 3 years of age and nonverbal, the following fractures should raise your suspicion for child abuse, along with a nonexistent, implausible, or frequently changing history of present illness.

## Rib Fractures

- Rib fractures may be present posteriorly, laterally, or anteriorly along the rib shaft.
  - Posterior rib fractures are most often associated with anteroposterior-directed thoracic compression, creating strain along the posterior rib arcs.
  - Lateral and anterior rib fractures may also occur after such squeezing, and they are also more often vulnerable after a direct impact.
- Look closely at the ribs above and below the known fracture because a direct blow often fractures several ribs simultaneously.
- If you need more information about the ribs, order oblique chest views.

## Classic Metaphyseal Lesions ("Corner Fractures" or "Bucket Handle Fractures")

- Think of these as avulsion fractures at the growth plate, in which either a crescent (bucket handle) or fragment (corner) of bone is torn from the zone of provisional calcification and contained by the periosteum.
- These are most often present after a whiplash-type force has been applied to the bone.

## Multiple Fractures

- A patient who is younger than 3 years of age and presents without a plausible mechanism of injury needs a complete skeletal survey to evaluate for the presence of additional fractures.
- Should multiple fractures be present and unaccounted for in the history of present illness, a reasonable suspicion for nonaccidental trauma exists. Varying ages of fracture are also concerning for repeated inflicted injury over time.

## Complex Skull Fractures

- These skull fractures contain more than one line of fracture, sometimes described as a stellate pattern, and they may be accompanied by displacement or diastasis.
- Most accidental injuries are the results of falls onto a flat surface with resultant linear fractures over the convexity of the skull. The presence of a complex skull fracture implies a greater level of force applied to the skull than is usually expected in a short fall onto a flat surface (i.e., off a bed or couch onto the floor).

### Suggested Readings

American Academy of Pediatrics. Clinical practice guidelines: early detection of developmental dysplasia of the hip. Pediatrics 2000;105:896–905

Baronciani D, et al. Screening for developmental dysplasia of the hip: from theory to practice. Pediatrics 1997;99(2):e5.

Beaty JH, Kasser JR, eds. Fractures in Children, vol 3, 6th Ed. Philadelphia: Lippincott-Raven, 2005.

Connolly LP, Connolly SA. Skeletal scintigraphy in the multimodality assessment of young children with acute skeletal symptoms. Clin Nucl Med 2003;28(9):746–754.

Craig C, Goldberg M. Foot and leg problems. Pediatr Rev 1993;14:395.

Kleinman PK. Diagnostic Imaging of Child Abuse. 2nd Ed. St. Louis: Mosby, 1998.

Marsh J. Screening for scoliosis. Pediatr Rev 1993;14:297.

Plint AC, et al. Validation of the Ottawa ankle rules in children with ankle injuries. Acad Emerg Med 1999;6:1005.

US Preventive Services Task Force. Screening for developmental dysplasia of the hip: recommendation statement. Pediatrics 2006;117:898–902.

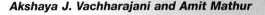
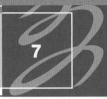

# NEWBORN MEDICINE
## Akshaya J. Vachharajani and Amit Mathur

**7**

## APPROACH TO THE NEONATE IN RESPIRATORY DISTRESS

- You are looking at a newborn infant in respiratory distress.
    - Assessment and appropriate treatment of this neonate should be the immediate goal.
    - Determination of the underlying causes should be the secondary goal.
- The algorithm in Figure 7-1 summarizes the approach to the infant in respiratory distress.

### History

- Is the neonate term or preterm?
- Are there any risk factors for sepsis in maternal history?
- Was meconium noted at delivery?

### Physical Examination

- Note color and oxygen saturations, capillary refill, pulse volume, and blood pressure.
- Measure vital signs; these are vital in diagnosing the severity of the respiratory distress and also indicate the urgency of the situation.

### Etiology

- Signs of respiratory distress such as flaring of alae nasi, chest wall retractions, and grunting point to a respiratory etiology.
- An inspiratory stridor indicates upper airway obstruction.
- An inspiratory stridor with poor cry suggests vocal cord paralysis.
- Tachypnea (respiratory rate >60 breaths/min) without chest wall retractions is a good clue to an underlying cardiac etiology or metabolic acidosis (sepsis, shock, inborn error of metabolism). For more information about cardiac causes, see Figure 7-2.

### Laboratory Studies and Imaging

- A chest radiograph to differentiate parenchymal (hyaline membrane disease, pneumonia, meconium aspiration, fluid in the minor fissure) from pleural (effusion, pneumothorax) or chest wall causes (diaphragmatic hernia) of respiratory distress
- A capillary blood gas to follow pH and $CO_2$
- A complete blood count (CBC) and differential white blood cell count further strengthen or rule out an infectious etiology for the distress. A blood culture is the gold standard for diagnosing or ruling out sepsis, although it can be false-negative in 30% of cases for a variety of reasons (common causes: inadequate blood sample and pretreatment with antibiotics).

### Treatment

- Guidelines for intubation/surfactant therapy
    - Some indications for endotracheal intubation and mechanical ventilation of an infant include apnea, poor oxygen saturation despite supplemental oxygen either by nasal cannula or continuous positive airway pressure, severe respiratory distress with anterior chest wall retracting to the spine, or poor capillary refill or color.

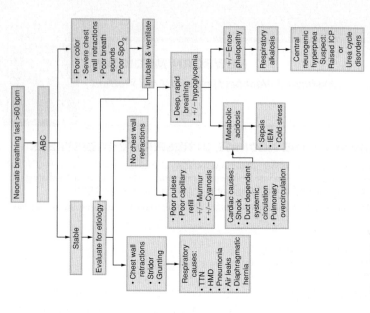

Figure 7-2. Algorithm to use when cardiac disorder should be suspected in a neonate. Look at relevant sections and algorithms for further information about the symptoms and signs mentioned here.

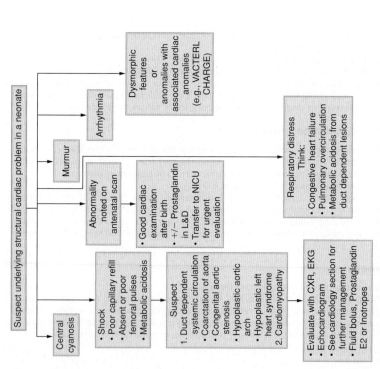

Figure 7-1. Approach to respiratory distress in a neonate. *ABC*, airway, breathing, circulation; *TTN*, transient tachypnea of the newborn; *HMD*, hyaline membrane disease; *IEM*, inborn error of metabolism; *ICP*, intracranial pressure.

| TABLE 7-1 | Endotracheal Tube Size in Neonates | |
|---|---|---|
| Tube size (internal diameter in mm) | Weight (g) | Gestational age (wk) |
| 2.5 | <1,000 | <28 |
| 3 | 1,000–2,000 | 28–34 |
| 3.5 | 2,000–3,000 | 34–38 |
| 3.5–4 | >3,000 | >38 |

- Prophylactic surfactant therapy through an endotracheal tube is given to infants who are <28 weeks estimated gestational age.
- See Tables 7-1 and 7-2 for further information about endotracheal intubation in neonates.
- Ongoing fluid management
  - Maintaining fluid and electrolyte balance with 80 mL/kg/day of maintenance fluids (50 mL/kg/day of starter total parenteral nutrition plus 30 mL/kg/day of $D_{10}W$) is a good prescription for the first 24 hours after birth.
  - Subsequently, the gestational age, urine output, daily weight, and serum electrolytes help guide the amount and type of maintenance fluids including the commencement of enteral feeds.

## Special Considerations: Pulmonary Hypertension

- Term and late preterm infants with respiratory distress (especially small for gestational age and meconium-stained liquor) are at a risk of developing pulmonary hypertension. Their size and gestation may delay aggressive intervention (intubation, mechanical ventilation). They could develop pulmonary hypertension (because unlike preterm infants, they have well-developed media in their pulmonary arteries that respond to hypoxia with vasoconstriction).
- The first sign of trouble is poor handling and desaturation, especially with handling. Preductal and postductal saturation differential of >10 (differential cyanosis, pink hands, blue feet) indicates right-to-left shunting across the patent ductus arteriosus. Absence of this sign does not preclude shunting and the right-to-left shunting may be across the foramen ovale.
- It is advisable to maintain oxygen saturation >95% in term infants until their disease process is identified and pulmonary hypertension is ruled out.

| TABLE 7-2 | Endotracheal Tubes and Depth of Insertion in Neonates[*] |
|---|---|
| Weight (g) | Depth of insertion (cm from upper lip) |
| 1 | 7 |
| 2 | 8 |
| 3 | 9 |
| 4 | 10 |
| *Rule of thumb: Weight + 6 = depth of insertion. | |

## APPROACH TO THE NEONATE WITH A HEART MURMUR

- I hear a murmur today! You have missed it (did you examine the infant?), and the nurse hears it.
- A murmur may or may not indicate heart disease.
- Examine the infant.
  - Use the fifth sign (pulse oximetry) for its diagnostic value.
  - Measure blood pressure on all four limbs.
  - Look at chest radiograph and electrocardiogram (ECG) if possible.
  - Perform a hyperoxia test if necessary.
  - The composite information can be used for a diagnosis.

### Differential Diagnosis

- Does this neonate have heart disease?
  - A neonate who has any of the characteristics in the flow chart above should be suspected to have heart disease.
  - If a term or preterm neonate looks well and has a normal examination, then think of the following:
    - Innocent murmur. In a term infant who is on room air, has a pulse oximetry >95%, is feeding well, looks well, and has a normal examination except the murmur, the murmur is very unlikely to represent a cardiac emergency requiring an urgent echocardiogram and consult. A majority of such murmurs are innocent and need only monitoring and clinical follow up.
    - Tricuspid regurgitation from physiologic pulmonary hypertension.
    - Hemodynamically insignificant patent ductus arteriosus (PDA) that is closing. Repeat examinations confirm the disappearance of the murmur.
- Is the neonate in shock or congestive heart failure?
  - Poor capillary refill, poor pulse volume, tachycardia, low blood pressure, and metabolic acidosis suggest shock. Remember the definition of compensated and hypotensive shock from PALS (compensated shock is shock without hypotension and hypotensive shock is shock with hypotension). Use it clinically.
  - Tachycardia, tachypnea or respiratory distress, hepatomegaly, or cardiomegaly on chest radiograph suggests congestive heart failure.

### Etiology

- Is the heart disease cyanotic or acyanotic? The differential diagnosis is extensive, and the diagnosis is difficult. Use the algorithm presented in Figure 7-3 for guidance.
  - A hyperoxia test is useful, and making a diagnosis of pulmonary hypertension versus cyanotic heart disease is critical. If the $SpO_2$ is >95% on room air or supplemental oxygen, it is unlikely that the neonate needs a hyperoxia test.
  - Pulmonary hypertension is best diagnosed based on clinical circumstances. The presence of the murmur of tricuspid regurgitation is a small piece of information that is not diagnostic. Red flags for pulmonary hypertension are in Figures 7-3 and 7-4.
    - A term infant with meconium-stained liquor at birth with low pulse oximetry and hazy lung parenchyma with high $PCO_2$ and low $PO_2$ and differential cyanosis probably has pulmonary hypertension from meconium aspiration syndrome. If the infant has a normal $PCO_2$ and a low pulse oximetry, cyanotic heart disease may be suspected in this same infant because the normal or low $PCO_2$ points against significant lung disease. The hyperoxia test may not be diagnostic in this situation. A very low $PaO_2$ can be obtained on the hyperoxia test in both severe pulmonary hypertension and cyanotic heart disease.
  - The information from pulse oximetry, outlined in Figure 7-4, may be useful in diagnosing congenital heart disease.
  - A big infant (term) with hazy lungs and low $PaO_2$ should make the clinician suspicious for total anomalous pulmonary venous return (TAPVR) with obstructed veins. Big infants do not commonly have hyaline membrane disease, and making a diagnosis

of pulmonary hypertension in these infants and starting nitric oxide can be lethal if they have the TAPVR; the nitric oxide will cause pulmonary edema and worsen the prognosis. It is imperative to consider nitric oxide therapy very carefully. An echocardiogram should be obtained as soon as possible.

■ The etiology is not as important as recognizing the physiologic situation, instituting the treatment (prostaglandin or after load reducing agents), and calling for urgent cardiology evaluation.

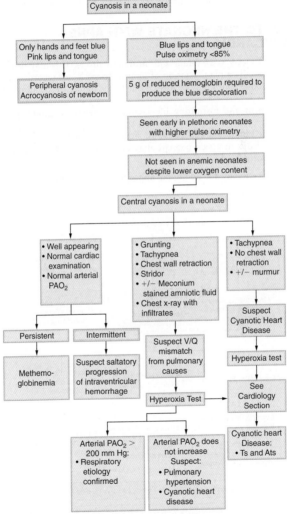

**Figure 7-3.** Differential diagnosis of cyanosis in a neonate. *Ts,* tetralogy of Fallot, transposition of great vessels, total anomalous pulmonary venous return, truncus arteriosus. *Ats,* Pulmonary atresia, tricuspid atresia. Hyperoxia test can be performed by delivering 100% oxygen (use oxygen analyzer in the hood) with Oxy-hood or intubating and ventilating a neonate. (Adapted from Park MK. Pediatric Cardiology for Practitioners, 5th Ed. Philadelphia: Mosby Elsevier, 2008.)

## Clinical Diagnoses

- Certain heart murmurs are **common** in certain clinical scenarios.
  - Murmur in a big infant of a diabetic mother or a neonate on chronic steroid therapy: Think of cardiomyopathy.
  - Murmur in a neonate with trisomy 21: Think of atrioventricular canal defect.
  - Murmur in a preterm neonate: Think of PDA.
  - Murmur in a preterm neonate with a cataract: Think of PDA and rubella syndrome.
  - Murmur in a neonate with an arrhythmia: Think of the Ebstein anomaly, especially if the mother received lithium while pregnant.
- For further details on murmurs, please see Chapter 12, Cardiac Concerns.

## APPROACH TO THE NEONATE WITH APNEA AND BRADYCARDIA

- You are called to look at an infant with heart rate drops. This may be the only evident sign, but it is usually a manifestation of apnea. Apnea is not recorded if one is not observant; obstructive apnea may be missed due to the nature of the monitors used in clinical practice.
- Urgent assessment and instituting life-saving interventions should be the immediate goal.
  - Examine the infant first and assess for signs of well-being or sepsis.
  - Heart rate drops in a sick neonate may demand **urgent therapeutic interventions** such as endotracheal intubation.
- Think about the etiology and additional appropriate intervention after initial stabilization.

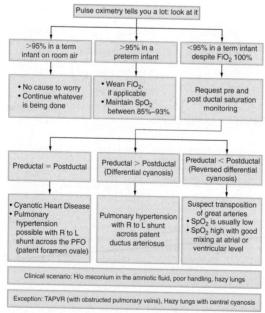

**Figure 7-4.** Diagnostic use of pulse oximetry. *TAPVR,* Total anomalous pulmonary venous return. (Adapted from Koppel RI, Druschel CM, Carter T, et al. Effectiveness of pulse oximetry screening for congenital heart disease in asymptomatic newborns. Pediatrics 2003 Mar;111(3):451–455.)

## Differential Diagnosis

■ Events are recent in onset and the neonate is ill appearing.

  ▦ Sepsis. Management includes a CBC, blood culture, chest radiograph (pneumonia) or obstructive series (necrotizing enterocolitis), lumbar puncture, and commencement of antibiotics. Lumbar puncture is considered mandatory in a neonate with heart rate drops because this may be the only symptom of meningitis. Up to 30% of meningitis cases can exist with a negative blood culture.

  ▦ Respiratory distress. Management includes increasing respiratory support such as administering continuous positive airway pressure (CPAP), which should be administered before ordering a capillary gas analysis. A capillary gas analysis may reveal normal pH and $CO_2$ because minute ventilation is maintained by increasing the respiratory rate. Waiting to institute CPAP until the capillary gas results are abnormal may lead to alveolar atelectasis that may not respond to CPAP. Mechanical ventilation through endotracheal intubation may then be required.

■ Events are recent in onset and the neonate is well appearing.

  ▦ Sepsis. Indications for septic workup include a history of temperature instability, feeding intolerance, abdominal distension, and lethargy. See previous discussion for management.

  ▦ PDA. Evaluate pulse volume, pulse pressure, and precordial pulsations. PDA can occur with or without a murmur.

  ▦ Blocked ectopic atrial beat. This is a common cause of heart rate drop in preterm infants and is self-limiting. It does not necessarily cause hemodynamic compromise and warrants an ECG.

  ▦ Obstructive apnea from incoordinated suck and swallow, if associated with recently introduced oral feeds or noticed while the infant is feeding from a bottle

  ▦ Incorrect position of a feeding tube. Check with chest radiograph.

  ▦ Eye examination for retinopathy of prematurity. This is a common cause of heart rate drop as a result of the vagal stimulation from eyeball compression during the examination (these infants could also have tachycardia from anticholinergic effects of cyclopentolate drops for the eye examination).

  ▦ Vagus nerve induced. In a ventilated infant where the airway is patent (endotracheal tube), it is unlikely to be obstructive in origin and more likely to be central. Consider vagus nerve–induced bradycardia from increased intracranial pressure or more commonly a low-lying endotracheal tube irritating the carina.

  ▦ Not ready for weaning. In an infant who is being weaned from ventilator support, heart rate drops and apnea indicate that it is necessary to think twice about extubating the infant or weaning the current support irrespective of blood gas analysis. It may also be a clue to starting or adjusting the dose of caffeine before extubating or stopping CPAP.

  ▦ Intraventricular hemorrhage (IVH). Consider if it is the first 24 hours of life in an extremely premature infant (<26 weeks gestation), especially if there is a rapid hemoglobin drop. An ultrasound of the head would be diagnostic. IVH is most likely to occur in the first week of life, and hence ultrasound of the head after the first week of life (in response to apnea and bradycardia) is less likely to be fruitful.

  ▦ Hydrocephalus. Consider if an infant with known IVH has an increasing occipitofrontal circumference, bulging fontanel, and increasing frequency of heart rate drops. Weekly ultrasounds should be considered.

■ Events are not new in onset and the neonate has a history of heart rate drops.

  • If the infant is well, then spending time on eliciting history is worth the time and trouble.

  • Always talk to the nurse, examine the charts, and examine the infant before jumping to conclusions.

  ▦ Benign. The event is more significant if it is associated with cessation of breathing and/or color change, or it lasts >20 seconds. Transient, self-resolving heart rate drops may not be significant and may not deserve embarking on an expensive and unnecessary diagnostic expedition. Heart rate in the 80–100 beats/min range in a

term infant who is sleeping is probably not pathologic. The infant may have had heart rate drops in the past and may need only weight-appropriate dose adjustments of caffeine.
- Seizures. These should be considered in all neonates with no good explanation for apnea. Heart rate increases with subtle seizures. Think of seizures if apnea is associated with abnormal eye or limb movements.

- Apnea of prematurity. This is a diagnosis of exclusion and hence mentioned at the end. It is due to immaturity of the respiratory center. It could be central or obstructive but usually is mixed in etiology. Once a diagnosis is made, loading with caffeine citrate followed by maintenance dosing may be useful in ameliorating the problem.

# APPROACH TO THE NEONATE WITH AN UNACCEPTABLE BLOOD GAS ANALYSIS RESULT

- An infant on a ventilator has a "bad" gas result showing respiratory acidosis.
- Do not guess the next change to be made on the ventilator and do not ask supervisors or colleagues what should be done. Examine the infant.
- Determine whether this is an emergency.
  - Consider it an emergency if the infant's color is poor, heart rate is dropping, and the chest is not expanding well.
  - Ask for a chest radiograph and continue examining the infant.

## Imaging

- A chest radiograph helps in making a diagnosis and deciding on treatment in some but not all situations.
  - For example, unless the patient ventilator asynchrony is observed, it will never be corrected, and patent ductus arteriosus can be better diagnosed clinically than by radiography.
  - The gold standard for diagnosing patent ductus arteriosus is an echocardiogram.
- A malpositioned endotracheal tube, atelectasis versus pneumonia, and air leak syndrome can all be diagnosed on a chest radiograph, and appropriate therapy can be instituted.

## Etiology and Treatment

- Problem: DOPE
  - DOPE mnemonic from PALS is useful.
    D: **D**isplacement of endotracheal tube. If the chest wall is not expanding well with ventilator breaths, auscultate the chest for breath sounds. Are they present? A gold standard test to check for endotracheal intubation is to use the $CO_2$ detector (if the Pedicap turns yellow, the tube is in the trachea; if the indicator is purple, the tube is not in the trachea).
    O: **O**bstruction. Can you pass a suction catheter through the endotracheal tube?
    P: **P**neumothorax. Are breath sounds unequal (atelectasis or pneumothorax)? Transillumination with fiberoptic light and observing for the "halo" around the light source may diagnose pneumothorax in a premature neonate (false-negative and false-positive results possible).
    E: **E**quipment malfunction. Disconnecting the infant from the ventilator and mechanical bagging with a flow-regulated breathing bag can help determine the adequate pressure required to move the chest wall (if higher than the current peak inspiratory pressure, then the lung compliance has worsened). If the chest wall moves with the current inspiratory pressure, then there is an equipment malfunction.
  - Treatment involves fixing the identified problem.

- Problem: possible asynchrony
  - Does the neonate exhale when the ventilator delivers its breath? Does it appear that there is a see-saw movement of the chest and abdomen? This indicates patient ventilator asynchrony. This is uncommon with synchronized intermittent mandatory ventilation available on modern ventilators.
  - Treatment (in pressure ventilation)
    - Increasing the ventilator rate or providing pressure support for breaths initiated by the neonate can improve the ventilation without switching the mode of ventilation (if the ventilator allows this mode)
    - Switching to assist mode of ventilation so that each breath is ventilator supported can also be tried (this is a poor mode for weaning support)
    - Sedating the infant so that he or she does not "fight" the ventilator. It is very important to prevent this phenomenon in large-term infants to prevent pneumothorax.
- Problem: changing (worsening) lung compliance
  - Observe the respiratory therapist's note or talk to one and note whether the tidal volume delivered by the ventilator is decreasing over a period of time; this indicates a worsening lung compliance.
    - Check the position of endotracheal tube (is it at the same level where it was originally taped? Has it slipped in or out?).
    - Do you hear a murmur or feel bounding peripheral pulses (is the ductus arteriosus patent and causing decreased compliance)?
    - Is there temperature instability? Has the character of endotracheal secretions changed (such as an increased amount of secretions or a change in secretion color to yellow)? If these secretion changes are seen, this indicates that the patient may have pneumonia which would worsen lung compliance.
    - Is the infant on the ventilator for a long time and developing chronic lung disease?
  - In volume control mode of ventilation, suspect all the above possibilities if you note increasing pressure generated by the ventilator to deliver the same volume.
- *Sometimes it is good to think outside the box*
  - Is the blood gas result unacceptable because of an extrapulmonary cause?
    - Is the abdomen distended (necrotizing enterocolitis, intestinal obstruction)? Is the abdominal distension compromising the tidal volume of the lung? This is seen in infants with unrepaired abdominal wall defects who are being treated with a Silastic pouch (silo), and the contents of the silo are progressively reduced into the abdominal cavity.
  - Does the infant have sufficient ventilatory drive?
    - Is he or she too sedated?
    - Does the ventilator rate need to be increased? (In nurses' parlance: the infant is "riding the vent.")
  - Is the endotracheal tube very old? Think of changing it even if there are protests; a blocked endotracheal tube can cause respiratory acidosis.

## APPROACH TO THE NEONATE WITH PREGAVAGE ASPIRATE

- Always examine the infant with pregavage aspirate (PGA) rather than trying to locate his or her last CBC or blood culture!
- Immediate examination and assessment for necrotizing enterocolitis should be the primary goal.

### Diagnosis and Treatment

#### Necrotizing Enterocolitis

- Assess for signs of necrotizing enterocolitis and ascertain whether the neonate looks well or ill. In an ill-appearing infant, the possibility of necrotizing enterocolitis is high.
- Stop enteral feeds, decompress the stomach with continuous nasogastric suction (to prevent emesis and aspiration as well as respiratory compromise), evaluate for sepsis (CBC,

blood, urine, and possibly cerebrospinal fluid culture), and evaluate for pneumatosis intestinalis radiologically.

- Start broad-spectrum antibiotics (vancomycin and gentamicin). Clindamycin is reserved for intestinal perforation by some but preferred routinely by others.
- Consider surgery. Intestinal perforation is an absolute indication, whereas progressive thrombocytopenia and metabolic acidosis are relative indications. The neonate should hence be monitored very closely with frequent clinical examination, complete blood counts, electrolytes, blood gases, and abdominal radiographs (anteroposterior and lateral decubitus films) for these parameters.
- Consider mechanical ventilation and analgesia, which are important adjuncts to the successful management. Consider inotropic support.

### Intestinal Obstruction

- Assess for signs of intestinal obstruction and ascertain whether the neonate looks well or ill. A well-looking infant with bilious or green PGA should prompt evaluation for intestinal obstruction. A patent anus and absence of obstructed inguinal hernias rule out two common causes of intestinal obstruction (**imperforate anus and obstructed inguinal hernia**).
- Mainstays of treatment: stop enteral feeds, nasogastric (Replogle tube) decompression of stomach, and administer parenteral fluid or nutrition
- Radiologic investigations, such as plain abdominal radiograph and contrast studies: confirm the diagnosis and help delineate the cause

### Incorrectly Placed Feeding Tube

- The tip of the tube may be in the duodenum and is a common benign cause of these PGAs.
- Passage of meconium does not rule out intestinal obstruction, and hence an abdominal obstructive series is helpful.
- Nonbilious, partially digested PGAs are the bane of existence for the house staff, especially in the middle of the night.

### Intestinal Dysmotility

- Assess for normal physical examination. Radiologic examination should also be normal. Preterm infants have **intestinal dysmotility** that improves over time.
- Treat the underlying condition as warranted.
    - As a rule of thumb, if the PGA is nonbilious and the infant is well-looking, it would be prudent to continue enteral feeds if the volume of PGA is ≤50% of the total volume fed.
    - Consider reducing volume of gavage feeds.
    - Consider reducing the osmotic load of the enteral feeds by stopping breast milk fortification or reduce caloric density of feeds (reduce from 24 cal/oz to 22 cal/oz). However, there is no evidence to support this practice.

## APPROACH TO THE NEONATE WITH POOR FEEDING

### Clinical Presentation and Physical Examination

- A term infant does not feed by mouth.
- Examine the infant. Is he or she ill or well appearing?

### Diagnosis and Treatment

- In an **ill-appearing** infant, evaluate for sepsis, respiratory distress, and congestive heart failure. Appropriate evaluation depending on signs and symptoms would be then indicated.
- In a **well-appearing** infant, consider whether he or she is (has):
    - Borderline preterm? Telltale signs include thin red skin, poorly developed breast tissue, undescended testes or poorly developed scrotal rugae (prominent labia minora), and few creases on the anterior third of the feet. A detailed Ballard score would also be helpful.

- Not feeding because he or she has never fed so far or may be very young (only a few hours old) and not learned how to feed. Tincture of time is all that may be required.
- Very sleepy from just being a normal infant or from maternal magnesium sulphate or narcotics? Cold? Hypoglycemic? All these are easily reversible and require observation.
- Anatomical barriers to feeding (cleft palate, small chin)?
- Topical infection (oral thrush)? Tongue tie is not a cause of poor feeding.
- Any dysmorphic features (trisomy 21) or respiratory distress? Is the infant neurologically normal?
- Floppy? The floppy infant who feeds poorly should raise suspicions of Prader-Willi syndrome. Abnormal neurologic examination in association with poor feeding is commonly seen in hypoxic ischemic encephalopathy; trisomy (dysmorphic features and hypotonia); Prader-Willi syndrome (undescended testes and dysmorphic features); and many muscle disorders, of which myotonic dystrophy is easy to diagnose by examining the mother. See Figure 7-5 for more information.
- Withdrawing from maternal narcotic drug abuse? In this case, the infant is more likely to suck vigorously and not gain weight rather than not suck at all.

- Recall that feeding is a team effort; the "team" consists of the infant and the mother (if breastfed) and the infant and the caregiver (if bottlefed).
  - Maternal reasons for poor feeding include inexperience, anxiety, engorged breasts, or fissure of the nipple.
  - Caregiver (e.g., mother, father, nurse) reasons include inexperience; feeding varies from "good" (finishes a bottle in <20 minutes) to "poor"!

## APPROACH TO A NEONATE WITH HYPOGLYCEMIA

- A blood glucose <40 mg/dL may be hazardous in neonates.
  - The threshold for collecting critical samples varies among physicians.
  - Most infants are asymptomatic when diagnosed with low blood glucose because of the monitoring protocols in most nurseries.
- Always confirm a blood glucose obtained by bedside monitoring methods with urgent laboratory glucose estimation. Also measure insulin thyroxine, growth hormone, cortisol, lactate, and pyruvate.
- Treatment is important because low blood glucose is one of the risk factors for adverse neurodevelopmental outcomes. Therapeutic maneuvers take precedence over diagnostic maneuvers and in reality are performed in parallel to each other (Figure 7-6).
- See Chapter 14, Endocrine Diseases for details.

## APPROACH TO THE NEONATE WHO HAS NOT PASSED URINE

- Do not panic; undocumented urine void in labor and delivery or in the nursery is the most common cause of lack of urine output in the first 24 hours after birth.

### Definition: Oliguria Urine Output <1 mL/kg/hr

### Etiology

- Prerenal
  - If the infant looks well, is hemodynamically stable, has normal genitalia, and no abdominal mass, then the most important cause is inadequate intake, especially if he or she is breastfed. Hence, this infant needs to be monitored closely for feeding and urine output.
  - Prerenal causes of oliguria have a very good prognosis and hence should be identified early (hemorrhage, hypovolemia, sepsis, shock) and treated appropriately.

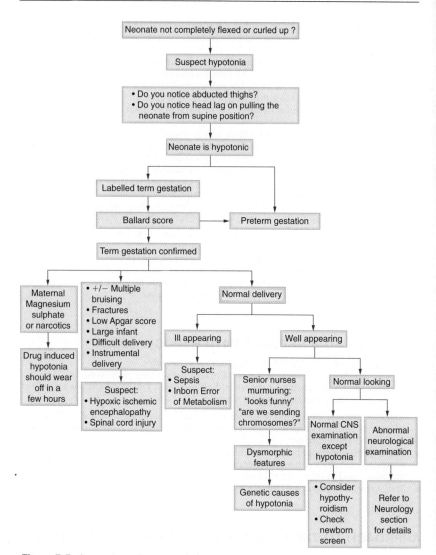

**Figure 7-5.** Approach to a floppy neonate.

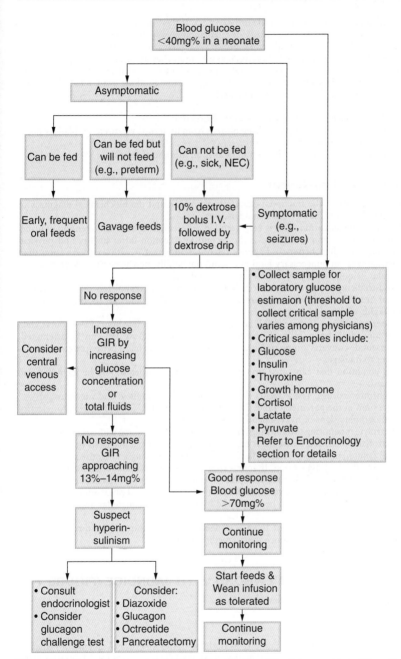

**Figure 7-6.** Approach to a neonate with hypoglycemia. Target blood glucose values differs with different authors; generally >70 mg% are acceptable. *GIR,* glucose infusion rate; *NEC,* necrotizing enterocolitis.

- Renal: anatomic anomalies of the urinary tract. If there are antenatal indicators of urinary tract anomalies (family history of renal anomalies, pelvic dilatation, or another renal anomaly on ultrasound scan), physical stigmata of underlying renal problems (preauricular pits, wrinkled abdominal skin), anomalies associated with renal malformations (e.g., tracheoesophageal fistula and VACTERL association), it may be worthwhile to get a baseline electrolyte and serum creatinine along with renal ultrasound while monitoring intake and output closely.
- Postrenal
  - A palpable bladder suggests urethral obstruction.
  - Palpable kidneys suggest hydronephrosis from ureteropelvic, ureteral, bladder neck, or urethral obstruction.
  - Retention of urine may be seen in infants on morphine/sedation.

## Diagnosis and Treatment

- For details about the fractional excretion of sodium and the biochemical diagnosis of renal failure, see Chapter 22, Renal Diseases.
- Urinary catheterization. This is very useful in differentiating between retention of urine, oliguria, and anuria and hence is the second intervention (after history and physical examination). It is better to diagnose retention and treat it with catheterization than treating with an unnecessary fluid bolus and potentially increasing the risk of intraventricular hemorrhage in very small premature infants.
- Fluid challenge. Lack of urine on catheterization may not completely differentiate prerenal from intrinsic renal failure and hence a fluid challenge (normal saline 10 mL/kg/dose) should be attempted.
- Diuretic challenge. If there is still no urinary output after a few hours (2–4 hours), then a second fluid bolus followed by furosemide (1 mg/kg/dose IV) can be attempted. Furosemide converts anuric to oliguric renal failure, which has a better prognosis and is easier to manage.
- Any condition that can cause prerenal failure. The disorder should be identified and treated.
- Nephrotoxic drugs. These agents should be stopped (gentamicin and vancomycin).
- Potassium in the parenteral fluid. This should be removed, and monitoring for electrocardiographic signs of hyperkalemia should be aggressive.
- Electrolyte monitoring. Monitoring phosphorus and calcium along with serum and urinary electrolytes, urea, and creatinine is helpful in further defining a diagnosis (prerenal versus renal failure), tailoring parenteral fluid composition, and giving a prognosis to the family.
- Ongoing fluids and nutrition. If anuria is present, then fluid intake should be restricted to 400 mL/kg/m$^2$ body surface area plus the ongoing urine output, if any; protein intake should be minimum to prevent catabolism (1 gm/kg/day); and potassium intake should be zero. Catabolism should be minimized by providing adequate fat and carbohydrate calories.
- Dialysis. This is indicated if there is congestive heart failure or life-threatening electrolyte abnormalities not amenable to medical treatment.

## APPROACH TO THE NEWBORN WITH JAUNDICE (FIGURE 7-7)

- Examine the infant and review the history.

### Epidemiology

- Identify the risk factors for jaundice as outlined in the American Academy of Pediatrics (AAP) guidelines on jaundice. Note that these guidelines are only for infants at a gestational age of ≥35 weeks, not for preterm infants at a gestational age of <35 weeks.
- Emphasis should be on identifying risk factors for hemolysis and ruling out hemolysis in all infants with jaundice. Rapidly rising bilirubin and falling hemoglobin is a good indicator of hemolysis. Risk factors for kernicterus should be identified.

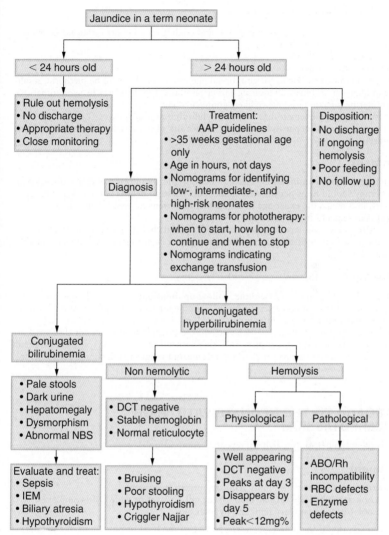

**Figure 7-7.** Approach to a term neonate with jaundice. *DCT,* Direct Coombs test; *IEM,* inborn error of metabolism.

## History and Physical Examination

- Note adequacy of feeding, passing stools, and voiding (risk factors for increased entero-hepatic circulation of bilirubin).
- Examine for the following:
- Well-being (no sepsis)
- Growth parameters. (Small for gestational-age infants are likely to be plethoric, resulting in higher bilirubin and requiring earlier phototherapy. This may be symptomatic of intrauterine infection and hence likely conjugated jaundice.)
- Bruising and cephalhematomas (increasing bilirubin production)
- Pallor, edema, and hepatosplenomegaly (indicators of hemolysis and congestive heart failure)

## Treatment

- Commencement, continuation, discontinuation, and monitoring effectiveness of phototherapy should be as per the AAP guidelines. These guidelines are based on the age in hours, and hence the exact age in hours should be remembered when deciding on the treatment (e.g., 17 hours, not day 1).
- Breastfed babies who are jaundiced present a special challenge. Mothers should not be discouraged from breastfeeding, and support from a lactational consultant (if available) should be sought.

## Follow-Up

- Monitoring clinically with/without follow-up bilirubin after discharge should be arranged within 48 hours after discharge from the hospital. Breastfed infants are at the highest risk of getting readmitted with dehydration and increased bilirubin levels.
- Follow-up arrangements after discharge and the possible time frame for discharge are important. If discharge takes place over the weekend or on holidays, it means difficult home health arrangements for checking feeding and weight trends, home phototherapy, and bilirubin estimation.


# APPROACH TO THE NEONATE WITH "HIGH" SERUM POTASSIUM

- Was the sample hemolyzed? If so, repeat a venous sample.

## Treatment

- Identify hemodynamic instability requiring urgent treatment.
    - Look at the bedside cardiac monitor for tall T waves or wide QRS complexes.
    - Look for poor capillary refill and hypotension.
- If you see any of the above, then irrespective of the level of potassium, the neonate is symptomatic and hence needs emergency treatment.
- Evaluate for causes of hyperkalemia after emergency treatment. Some of the common causes are excess potassium in total parenteral nutrition (TPN) or intravenous (IV) fluids, poor urine output, bruising, hemolysis, or metabolic acidosis.

### Emergency Treatment

- IV fluids with potassium should be stopped immediately while awaiting calcium gluconate administration.
- IV 10% calcium gluconate is best because it is has a directly opposite effect on the myocardium. Potassium stops the heart in diastole, and calcium counteracts this with its positive inotropic effect. It is long lasting and very effective.
- Sodium bicarbonate is also useful because it causes metabolic alkalosis and shifts potassium intracellularly, reducing serum potassium. A 2 mL/kg/dose of 4.5% sodium bicarbonate should be used.

### Nonemergency Treatment

- Emergency measures may not be required even if serum K levels are 5.5–6.5 mEq/L in preterm infants if
  - There is no cardiac arrhythmia.
  - Urine output is adequate (>1 mL/kg/hr).
  - Potassium supplementation in the parenteral fluid is adequate (2–3 mEq/kg/day).
  - Blood pH is not acidotic.

- It may be prudent to watch clinically and monitor serial potassium levels and urine output.
- Reducing potassium in the parenteral fluid is also an option.
- If serum potassium is >7.5 mEq/L, even without cardiac arrhythmia, removing potassium from parenteral fluid, increasing glucose infusion rate (to increase endogenous insulin, which will then shift potassium intracellularly) with or without insulin drip, and adding calcium to the parenteral fluid either all at once or sequentially is a reasonable option.
- It is necessary to continue monitoring for hemodynamic compromise.
- Inducing respiratory alkalosis by increasing ventilator support (especially minute ventilation by increasing the rate of ventilation). This is a simple way of treating hyperkalemia if IV access is not established.
- Continuous nebulizations with albuterol ($\beta_2$-receptor agonist) cause transcellular shift of potassium and reduce potassium.
- Lack of IV access is usually not an issue because hyperkalemia is seen in "micropreemies" (nonhemolytic hyperkalemia caused by bruising, poor urine output because of high antidiuretic hormone level, poor renal cortical blood flow, and low glomerular filtration rate) in the first few days of life when most neonates have umbilical lines.

## APPROACH TO THE NEONATE WITH "HIGH" BLOOD PRESSURE

- Hypertension is defined as blood pressure in the >95th percentile on Zubrow nomograms based on postconceptual age.
- Ideal conditions to measure blood pressure in an infant are:
  - 90 minutes after a feed
  - Sleeping or quiet for 15 minutes
  - In prone position

- Before ordering a battery of tests, check for the conditions under which blood pressure was measured as above.
- A correct-sized cuff should be used; the cuff should cover two thirds the length of the arm and 75% of the limb circumference. Blood pressure should be measured in the arms rather than the legs (where it is normally higher).
- A single measurement is not diagnostic, and three successive readings at 2-minute intervals should be made before deciding on "hypertension."
- Rule of thumb: systolic blood pressure >100 mm Hg in a term infant a few weeks old should be treated.

### Etiology

- Agitation and inadequate pain control are two common explanations for high blood pressure recorded.
- Caffeine, theophylline, and corticosteroids are common medications implicated.
- Excessive parenteral fluid and sodium administration over the past few days are two important causes that can be missed unless TPN prescriptions are scrutinized closely.

### History

- History of umbilical arterial lines is a common predisposing factor for renovascular hypertension.

- Stigmas of renal disease (as outlined previously) should increase suspicions of intrinsic renal disease (vesicoureteric reflux, multicystic dysplastic kidney, horseshoe kidney).
- An infant with chronic lung disease often has hypertension from multiple etiologies.
- Endocrine disorders are not seen commonly in neonates (except Cushing syndrome with steroid therapy, and neonatal hyperthyroidism, which is rare).

## Physical Examination

- Check for unequal pulses and blood pressure in arms and legs (coarctation of aorta).
- Palpate for ballotable renal mass and auscultate for renal bruit on either side of the umbilicus (renovascular causes are the most common causes of hypertension). Infants of diabetic mothers can present with gross hematuria. These infants should be evaluated for hypertension and palpable renal mass(es), which are indicative of renal vein thrombosis.

## Laboratory Studies and Imaging

- Laboratory evaluation involves:
  - Urine examination (macroscopy, microscopy, and culture; infection is still the most common cause of renovascular hypertension)
  - Renal measures such as blood urea nitrogen, serum creatinine, and electrolytes
  - Renal ultrasound for anatomical anomalies
  - Doppler studies for vascular anomalies
  - Echocardiogram for coarctation of aorta
  - Ratio of renin to aldosterone levels
- The ratio of renin to aldosterone is recommended to distinguish primary from secondary hyperaldosteronism, but turnaround time for results is too long and interpreting the results in small "preemies" may not be very helpful clinically. If no cause is found in the initial screening tests, then it is hoped that the subspecialties would have become involved a while ago. Urinary levels of vanillylmandelic acid to diagnose pheochromocytoma are not required routinely.

## Treatment

- Treatment depends on the cause, but symptomatic drug therapy is beyond the scope of this discussion.
- Angiotensin-converting enzyme inhibitors such as enalapril are preferred.

# NUTRITIONAL REQUIREMENTS OF NEONATES

- Breast milk is the preferred source of nutrition whenever possible.

## Calories

- Parenterally fed premature neonates require 90–100 kcal/kg/day to promote sustained growth.
- Enterally fed neonates require 120 kcal/kg/day.
- Factors that may increase caloric demand include thermal stress, increased metabolic rate (e.g., hyperthyroid state, postoperative recovery), and increased fecal losses (malabsorption).
- Maintenance fluid requirements for both term and preterm infants by the end of the first week are about 150 mL/kg/day. Human breast milk and formulas for mature, term infants provide 20 kcal/oz, whereas formulas for premature infants provide either 20 or 24 kcal/oz. At full maintenance fluid intake, the term infant takes in 100 kcal/kg/day with breast milk or term formula and a preterm infant takes in 120 kcal/kg/day with the preterm 24 kcal/oz formula.

## Proteins

■ Adequate protein intake is estimated to be approximately 2.5 g/kg/day in term and 3.5–4.0 g/kg/day in preterm infants (approximately 10%–15% of caloric intake). Parenterally, TrophAmine is used as a source of amino acids.

## Fats

■ Approximately 40%–45% of caloric intake should come from fat.
■ Premature infants are unable to digest long-chain fatty acid in formula (lack of bile salts).
■ Premature formulas use medium-chain fatty acids as a predominant source of fat. Parenterally, Intralipid 20% is used to provide fat calories. Infusion is initiated at 0.5 g/kg/day and gradually increased to 3 g/kg/day.

## Carbohydrates

■ Approximately 40%–45% of caloric intake comes from carbohydrates. Parenterally, dextrose is used as a carbohydrate source. Usual starting glucose infusion rates are 6–8 mg/kg/min. This is gradually advanced to deliver more calories, to a maximum of 10–12 mg/kg/min.
■ Lactose is the predominant carbohydrate in breast milk and formula, and it is well absorbed in premature infants.

## Strategies for Providing Nutrition

■ In premature infants who are unstable after admission to the nursery, start an infusion of "starter total parenteral nutrition," or "starter TPN." This TrophAmine solution provides 2.5 g/kg/day of protein when infused at 50 mL/kg/day.
■ To make up maintenance fluid requirements, $D_{10}W$ is "piggybacked" to the TPN at 30 mL/kg/day. Regular TPN with adjustment of fluid intake is commenced on day of life no. 1 with 2.5 g/kg/day of protein, 0.5 g/kg/day of Intralipid, and $D_{12.5}W$ ± electrolytes depending on weight loss, electrolytes, and urine output.
■ For administration, a central catheter is preferred (umbilical artery catheter, central umbilical venous catheter, peripherally inserted central catheter). In peripherally placed lines, to avoid injury to vessels, the maximum allowed concentration of dextrose is 12.5%. All central catheters have 500 U of heparin per liter.
■ "Trophic feeds" (up to 20 mL/kg/day) are usually started by gavage feeds on day of life nos. 2–4, depending on the infant's clinical condition and the availability of breast milk. The volume of initiating and the rate of advancement of feeds depends on the infant's birth weight and tolerance of feeds. The goal is to achieve full enteral nutrition by 10–14 days of life. Breast milk is preferred and is fortified with human milk fortifier once intake reaches 100 mL/kg/day.

## Nutrition Monitoring

■ Parameters used to track growth are daily weights, weekly lengths, and occipitofrontal circumference.
  ■ Iron supplements are started at 3 weeks of life at 2–4 mg/kg/day.
  ■ Premature infants need higher amounts of calories, protein, calcium, phosphate, iron, and sodium intake compared with their term counterparts.
■ Infants at high risk for metabolic bone disease (<30 weeks gestation, prolonged TPN, diuretics, steroids) should have ionized calcium, phosphorus, and alkaline phosphatase levels monitored at 3 weeks and every 2 weeks thereafter.
■ Infants on prolonged TPN should have the following laboratory tests every 2 weeks: serum electrolytes including calcium, magnesium, albumin, alkaline phosphatase, and phosphate.

*Expected Weight Gain*
- Term infants: 20–30 gm/day for the first 3 months, 15–20 gm/day for the next 3 months, and 10–15 g/day for the next 6 months. These infants will double their birth weight in 5 months, triple it in 1 year, and quadruple it in 2 years.
- Preterm infants: 15 gm/kg/day

*Expected Increase in Head Circumference*
- Term infants: 2 cm/mo for first 3 months, 1 cm/mo for the next 3 months, and 0.5 cm/mo for the next 6 months
- Preterm infants: 0.5 cm/wk

# RETINOPATHY OF PREMATURITY

- Retinopathy of prematurity (ROP) is a disorder of the developing retinal vasculature that occurs with interruption of the forming retinal vessels. Constriction and obliteration of the advancing capillary bed are followed by neovascularization of the retina, which can extend into the vitreous (Figure 7-8).
- The incidence varies inversely with gestational age.
- The most serious and feared complication of ROP is retinal detachment and associated loss of vision that may occur in 6%–8% of infants.
- Disease occurs when vessels posterior to the ridge become dilated and tortuous.

## Classification (Table 7-3)

## Screening

- Who should be screened?
  - Infants with a birth weight of <1,500 g or ≤32 weeks gestational age **and** selected infants between 1,500–2,000 g or >32 weeks gestation with an unstable neonatal course (as defined by the neonatologist). Pupils are dilated using cyclopentolate and phenylephrine.
  - Pacifiers and oral sucrose is recommended for comfort during the examination.
- When should screening take place?
  - ROP is not detected before 31 weeks corrected gestational age.
  - Infants born at 22–27 weeks gestational age should be screened when at 31 weeks of age.
  - Infants born at 28–32 weeks gestational age should be screened at 4 weeks of age.

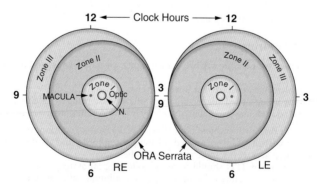

**Figure 7-8.** Schema of the right and left eye showing the zones and clock hours used in the description of retinopathy of prematurity.

| TABLE 7-3 | International Classification of Retinopathy of Prematurity |
|---|---|

| Stage | Description |
|---|---|
| 1 | A line of demarcation develops from the vascularized region of the retina and the avascular zone. |
| 2 | The line becomes a ridge that protrudes into the vitreous; there is histologic evidence of an atrioventricular shunt. |
| 3 | Extraretinal vascular proliferation occurs with the ridge; neovascular tufts can be found posterior to the ridge. |
| 4 | Scarring and fibrosis can occur when the neovascularization extends into the vitreous; this can cause traction on the retina, leading to retinal detachment. |
| 5 | Total retinal detachment |

## Treatment

- Laser photocoagulation is aimed at the avascular part to reduce the production of the growth factors responsible for exuberant vascular growth. There are well-defined criteria to identify infants needing laser therapy.
- Other therapeutic options include cryotherapy and scleral banding/vitrectomy for later stages.

### Suggested Readings

AAP. Clinical practice guideline: management of hyperbilirubinemia in the newborn infant 35 or more weeks of gestation. Pediatrics 114(1):297–316.

American Academy of Pediatrics. Neonatal resuscitation. Chapter 5, pp 1–34.

Cornblath M, Hawdon JM, Williams A, et al. Controversies regarding definition of neonatal hypoglycemia: suggested operational thresholds. Pediatrics 2000;105:1141–1145.

Ewer AK, Yu VY. Effect of fortifying breast milk on gastric emptying. Arch Dis Child Fetal Neonatal Ed Jan 1996;74(1):F60–2.

Faix RG, Polley TZ, Grasela TH. A randomized, controlled trial of parenteral clindamycin in neonatal necrotizing enterocolitis. J Pediatr Feb 1988;112(2):271–277.

Lucas A, Morley R, Cole TJ. Adverse neurodevelopmental outcome of moderate hypoglycemia. Br Med J 1988;297:1304–1308.

McClure RJ, Newell SJ. Gastric emptying in pre-term infants: the effect of breast milk fortifier. Acta Paediatr Sep 1996;85(9):1112–1115.

Nwanko MU, Lorenz JM, Gardiner JC. A standard protocol for blood pressure measurement in the newborn. Pediatrics 1997;99:e10.

Policy Statement: American Academy of Pediatrics: Screening examination of premature infants for retinopathy of prematurity. Pediatrics 2006;117:572–576.

Zubrow AB, Hulman S, Kushner H, et al. Determinants of blood pressure in infants admitted to neonatal intensive care units: a prospective multicenter study. J Perinatol 1995; 15:470–479.

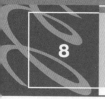

# 8 CRITICAL CARE
## Nathan P. Dean and Nikoleta S. Kolovos

## ACUTE RESPIRATORY FAILURE

- This is the inability of the respiratory system to provide adequate oxygen to meet the body's metabolic requirements and/or to excrete the carbon dioxide produced by the body.

### Causes of Hypoxemic and Hypercapnic Respiratory Failure

*Alveolar Hypoventilation*
- Definition: inadequate minute ventilation resulting in the buildup of $CO_2$ and drop in alveolar $PO_2$
- Etiology: impaired respiratory drive (narcotics, coma, status epilepticus), upper airway obstruction, impaired peripheral nervous system function (Guillain-Barré syndrome, botulism), respiratory muscle fatigue (muscular dystrophy, excessive work of breathing)
- Physical examination findings: apnea, hypopnea, suprasternal retractions, stridor, muscular weakness, encephalopathy
- Treatment
  - Supplemental oxygen may improve mild cases.
  - Invasive mechanical ventilation may be necessary in moderate to severe cases.
  - Proper airway position or placement of an oral or nasal airway device may resolve an upper airway obstruction.
  - Helium:oxygen (Heliox) mixtures may reduce turbulent flow and overcome increased resistance caused by partial airway obstruction.

*Ventilation/Perfusion Mismatch*
- Definitions
  - One extreme is perfused alveoli without ventilation (or dead space ventilation).
  - Other extreme is ventilated alveoli that are not perfused.
- Etiology
  - Dead space: asthma, acute respiratory distress syndrome (ARDS), bronchopulmonary dysplasia (BPD), atelectasis, mucous plugging, pneumothorax
  - Perfusion abnormalities: pulmonary embolus (absence of $CO_2$ retention)
- Physical examination findings: retractions, tachypnea, wheezing, crackles, nasal flaring, prolonged expiration. A massive pulmonary embolus may result in cardiovascular collapse.
- Treatment
  - Supplemental oxygen often overcomes hypoxemia.
  - Treatment of the underlying disorder improves hypercapnia, although severe cases may require invasive mechanical ventilation.

### Causes of Hypoxemic-Only Respiratory Failure

- Diffusion abnormalities: diffusion of oxygen into the bloodstream depends on the following:
  - Thickness of the alveolar wall
  - Area available for gas exchange
  - Partial pressure difference between the two sides.

■ Any disruption can result in impaired diffusion and hypoxia. $CO_2$ readily diffuses across the alveolar surface, and thus its elimination is not affected by these changes.
■ Causes: pulmonary fibrosis
■ Treatment
    ■ Increase the area available for gas exchange with continuous positive airway pressure (CPAP) or positive end-expiratory pressure (PEEP) by mechanical ventilation.
    ■ Increase the partial pressure difference with supplemental $O_2$.

## Shunt

■ Definition: occurs when mixed venous blood directly bypasses the pulmonary capillary-alveolar interface and mixes with oxygenated blood coming into the heart from the pulmonary vein
■ Etiology: right-to-left shunting cardiac lesions (e.g., hypoplastic left heart, truncus arteriosus)
■ Physical examination: from cyanotic only (no distress) to signs of cardiogenic shock (diminished pulses and perfusion, respiratory distress, hepatomegaly)
■ Treatment
    ■ Administration of oxygen has no effect on arterial $P_{O_2}$ and saturation. Patients will require correction or palliation of their lesion.
    ■ Prostaglandin $E_1$ may be required in neonates with a patent ductus arteriosus to promote a more balanced mixing between the right and left heart circulations.

# INTUBATION

## General Principles

### Major Indications
■ Respiratory failure
■ Cardiovascular dysfunction: to decrease systemic or myocardial oxygen consumption by decreasing the work of breathing
■ Clinical condition requiring controlled ventilation (intracranial hypertension, surgical, or intensive care unit [ICU] procedure)
■ Upper airway disease requiring intubation
■ Altered sensorium with absent protective airway reflexes

### Preparation
■ Before intubation, have the following available: oxygen, suction and catheters, ventilation bag, mask, laryngoscope with appropriate blade, endotracheal tube of the expected size as well as one larger and smaller, stylet, end-tidal $CO_2$ detector, pulse oximetry, secure intravenous (IV) access.
■ Consider pharmacotherapy (Table 8-1). Sedatives and neuromuscular blocking agents are used to aid in the visualization of the airway and for patient comfort.

### Signs of a Difficult Airway
■ Consider the presence of an anesthesiologist if the patient has micrognathia, facial clefts, midface hypoplasia, maxillary protrusion, facial asymmetry, small mouth, short neck, limited cervical spine mobility, upper airway bleeding, edema, or foreign bodies.

## Bag-Mask Ventilation

### Basics
■ It is reasonable to assume that acutely ill or traumatically injured patients have full stomachs; therefore, application of bag-mask ventilation along with cricoid pressure is recommended.
■ A properly fitting mask is essential; it may be necessary to use an oral airway to adequately ventilate the patient.

| TABLE 8-1 | Selection of Medications for Intubation | | | |
|---|---|---|---|---|
| **Class** | **Dose** | **Time of onset** | **Advantages** | **Disadvantages** |
| **Sedatives** | | | | |
| Thiopental | 3–5 mg/kg | 30–60 sec | Short-acting barbiturate. Decreases cerebral oxygen consumption and decreases cerebral blood flow | Potent myocardial depressant and venodilator |
| Etomidate | 0.2 mg/kg | 30–60 sec | Short-acting anesthetic, potent respiratory depressant, can decrease cerebral blood flow | Perhaps adrenal insufficiency |
| Midazolam | 0.1–0.3 mg/kg | 1–5 min (peak effect at 5 min) | Benzodiazepine that produces sedation and amnesia. Best when combined with narcotic | No pain relief, mild myocardial depressant |
| Fentanyl | 1–3 mg/kg | Almost immediate | Narcotic used in combination with a benzodiazepine to relieve pain associated with laryngoscopy | Bradycardia and chest wall rigidity if given rapidly in large doses |
| Ketamine | 1–2 mg/kg | 30 sec | Nonnarcotic analgesic and anesthetic, increases systemic blood pressure and cardiac output, acts as a bronchodilator | May be complicated by severe laryngospasms; increases cerebral blood flow and intracranial hypertension, causes increased salivation; emergence can be complicated by delirium and hallucinations |
| **Neuromuscular blocking agents** | | | | |
| Vecuronium | 0.1 mg/kg | 1–3 min | No hemodynamic effects, metabolized in the liver, lasts 30–60 min | Less ideal agent in patients with full stomach because of time of onset |

| TABLE 8-1 | Selection of Medications for Intubation *(Continued)* | | | |
|---|---|---|---|---|
| **Class** | **Dose** | **Time of onset** | **Advantages** | **Disadvantages** |
| Rocuronium | 1 mg/kg | 30–60 sec | No hemodynamic effects, metabolized in the liver, lasts 15–30 min | Less ideal agent in patients with full stomach because of time of onset |
| Pancuronium | 0.15 mg/kg | 2–3 min | Excreted in the kidneys, lasts 45–60 min | Less ideal agent in patients with full stomach because of time of onset. Causes short-lived tachycardia |
| Succinylcholine | 1 mg/kg | 30–60 sec | Rapid onset of action an ideal for emergent intubation of patients with full stomachs Depolarizing agent, lasts 5–10 min | May increase intracranial pressure; may see hyperkalemia in patients with crush injuries, spinal cord injuries, or neuromuscular disease; may trigger malignant hyperthermia |
| Atracurium/ cis-atracurium | 0.4–0.5 mg/kg | 1–4 min | Metabolized by plasma esterases and Hofmann degradation; can be useful in patients with hepatic and/or renal failure | Atracurium causes histamine release |

- Two people may be needed to perform this task, one to position the patient properly and the other to operate the bag.
- If you cannot ventilate a patient with a bag and mask, do not give neuromuscular blockade.

### Ventilating Bags
- Self-inflating bags: easier to use; however, they continue to fill even when disconnected from an oxygen source.
- Anesthesia bags: require an ideal mask seal to fill; however, they have no inspiratory valves and allow for spontaneous respiration.

### Selection of Laryngoscopy Blade and Endotracheal Tubes
- Tube types
  - Miller: straight blade with slightly curved tip, which allows for visualization of the larynx without lifting the epiglottis. It is particularly helpful in younger children and infants with a floppy epiglottis.

- Macintosh: curved blade, requires lifting of the epiglottis for visualization of the larynx. It provides more room to assist passing cuffed endotracheal tubes.
- Cole formula: rough guide for determining the appropriate sized endotracheal tube
  - Tube size = Age(yr)/4 + 4
  - Not as reliable for infants. Term infants should be intubated with a 3.0- to 3.5-mm endotracheal tube.
  - The appropriate sized tube should pass easily, allow an air leak at pressures of 15–30 cm $H_2O$, but fit well enough to allow delivery of adequate tidal volumes
  - Children with trisomy 21 require a 0.5–1 mm tube size smaller than expected for age
- Cuffed versus noncuffed endotracheal tubes
  - The narrowest point of the airway in the young child is the subglottis, allowing for a snug fit without the presence of a cuff, whereas the narrowest point in the adult larynx is at the vocal cords, and a cuffed tube is required to prevent an air leak at low pressures.
  - Traditionally, uncuffed endotracheal tubes are used in children <8 years of age.
  - More recently, the use of cuffed endotracheal tubes in children >1 yr and even <1 yr has been advocated, and demonstrated no increased risk of postextubation stridor. Patients may require a tube 0.5 mm smaller than estimated by the Cole formula (see Duracher and Newth suggested readings).

### After Intubation

- When the vocal cords are visualized, the endotracheal tube should be observed to pass through the vocal cords.
- Position should be confirmed with end-tidal $CO_2$ detection, symmetrical chest wall rise, and equal auscultation over both chest walls.
- Carefully note the depth of tube intubation; a quick rule of thumb is 3 times the size of the endotracheal tube (i.e., a 4-mm tube should be inserted to the 12-cm mark).
- Obtain a chest radiograph to confirm position.

## MECHANICAL VENTILATION

- Mechanical ventilation uses positive pressure to move gas into the lungs. Although modern ventilators offer several different modes, the goal is to select a strategy that maintains oxygenation and ventilation, is comfortable to the patient, and causes minimal trauma to the lung.
- A primary objective is avoiding iatrogenic ventilator-induced lung injury or other complications such a pneumothorax, cardiovascular compromise, or respiratory muscle atrophy.

### General Principles

- Two basic principles guide ventilator management:
  - The major determinants of oxygenation are alveolar lung volume and fraction of inspired oxygen ($FiO_2$). Alveolar lung volume is affected primarily by measures that affect mean airway pressure, such as PEEP, inspiratory time, and peak airway pressure, and less so by tidal volume and respiratory rate.
  - The major determinant of the elimination of $CO_2$ is minute ventilation. Minute ventilation is determined primarily by the respiratory frequency and the tidal volume.
- In all modes of conventional mechanical ventilation, a regulated gas flow generates pressure (airway pressure) that moves a volume (tidal volume) of gas into the lung. The modes differ by parameter(s): flow, pressure, or volume. These are set by the clinician. Table 8-2 summarizes the differences in modes of ventilation.
  - The most common modes of ventilation are those in which the clinician sets either the tidal volume (volume control) or the peak airway pressure (pressure control). For most patients, volume control modes are comfortable and provide adequate gas exchange with minimal risk of injury to the lung.

| TABLE 8-2 | Volume Control Versus Pressure Control Ventilation | |
|---|---|---|
| **Mode** | **Volume control** | **Pressure control** |
| Clinician set parameter | Tidal volume | Peak inspiratory pressure |
| Variable parameter | Peak inspiratory pressure | Tidal volume |
| Mean airway pressure | Lower for given tidal volume, inspiratory time, and peak airway pressure | Higher for given tidal volume, inspiratory time and peak airway pressure |
| Other parameters to set | Rate, PEEP, inspiratory time, $Fio_2$ | Rate, PEEP, inspiratory time, $Fio_2$ |
| Flow pattern | Constant inspiratory flow | Decelerating inspiratory flow |
| Advantages | Guaranteed tidal volume and minute ventilation | Peak airway pressure is limited. |
| | Changes in respiratory system compliance easily detected (peak inspiratory pressure increases) | Decelerating flow pattern can decrease peak airway pressure and increase mean airway pressure, decreasing risk of further lung injury. |
| Disadvantages | Peak airway and alveolar pressures may vary excessively. Continuous flow may be low enough to cause patient discomfort, asynchrony and increased work of breathing | Tidal volume varies with changes in compliance and may be too high or too low. Changes in respiratory system compliance are not as easily detected. |

PEEP, positive end-expiratory pressure.

- For patients with conditions that decrease lung compliance such as severe pneumonia or ARDS, pressure control modes may be safer by limiting the high airway pressures that may be necessary in these conditions.
- For patients with large leaks around the endotracheal or tracheostomy tube, pressure control modes can compensate for the volume lost via the leak.

■ Most ventilators allow setting both a tidal volume and an airway pressure limit (e.g., pressure-regulated volume control).
   - Most ventilators allow ventilation to be synchronized to respiratory effort in the spontaneously breathing patient to increase patient comfort.
   - Patient effort is sensed either as initiation of inspiratory flow (flow triggering) or as a reduction in the airway pressure (pressure triggering).
■ In addition to controlling the volume or pressure delivered, the clinician can adjust the timing and pattern of the ventilator-delivered breaths. This is described as mandatory, assisted, or supported ventilation.

### Mandatory (Controlled) Ventilation (volume- or pressure-controlled)
■ The machine provides a set number of breaths with the set tidal volume or pressure limit. Inspiratory time is fixed.
■ This mode is useful for patients with limited and/or absent respiratory drive (e.g., patients who are apneic from sedation, anesthesia, central nervous system (CNS) injury, drug overdose, neuromuscular blockade), or for patients whose respiratory drives need to be suppressed.

- Intermittent mandatory ventilation (IMV) allows spontaneous breathing between ventilator breaths delivered at a fixed interval.
- Synchronous IMV (SIMV) refers to IMV breaths that are synchronized with the patient's breathing effort. If the ventilator does not sense patient effort, a mandatory IMV breath is delivered. If the patient makes respiratory effort between SIMV breaths, spontaneous breathing is allowed.

### Assisted Ventilation (volume- or pressure-controlled)
- In patients with spontaneous respiratory effort, assist modes deliver ventilator breaths with a set volume or pressure and with a fixed inspiratory time whenever the ventilator senses patient effort. One drawback is that the inspiratory time is fixed; this may be uncomfortable for the spontaneously breathing patient.
- In assist control mode, the machine provides a preset tidal volume or pressure in response to patient-initiated breaths. It also delivers the mechanical tidal volume at a preset frequency if the patient fails to initiate a breath within a preselected time. Patients with weak respiratory effort have complete, maximal support. This allows patient-ventilator synchrony but can lead to hyperventilation and respiratory alkalosis.

### Supported Ventilation
- Frequency and inspiratory time of ventilator breaths are regulated by patient effort. Support modes can only be used for patients with adequate respiratory drive.
- Pressure support ventilation (PSV) is a commonly used mode of supported ventilation in which the ventilator gives an inspiratory flow of gas, with a decelerating flow pattern whenever the patient triggers a breath, to a preset pressure limit. Patient effort regulates the respiratory cycle. The tidal volume is determined by the patient's effort, preset pressure limit, and respiratory system compliance. PSV may decrease inspiratory work caused by endotracheal tube impedance.
- PSV may be combined with SIMV modes of ventilation whereby the spontaneous patient breaths are supplemented with pressure support. These modes may used in weaning the patient from mechanical ventilation.
- Volume support ventilation adjusts pressure support to attain a selected tidal volume; this may also be useful in separation from mechanical ventilation.

### CPAP
- In this method of respiratory support, a constant level of pressure is maintained in the circuit while the patient breathes spontaneously.
  - Patients must have an adequate respiratory drive.
  - CPAP improves gas exchange and decreases respiratory effort by helping maintain end expiratory lung volume.
- CPAP is used noninvasively for patients with upper airway obstruction or a tendency for airway collapse. It may also be used during weaning from mechanical ventilation before extubation.

### Pressure-Regulated Volume Control (PRVC)
- Newer ventilators combine the advantages of a guaranteed tidal volume (such as volume control) with a decelerating inspiratory flow pattern to limit airway pressure (such as pressure control). This strategy may minimize risks for ventilator-induced lung injury and maximize patient comfort.
- Mechanical ventilation in PRVC modes can be provided in a SIMV mode or an assist-control mode with a set inspiratory time and minimum rate.
  - If patient effort decreases, tidal volume is augmented by increasing gas flow (within preset limits) to maintain minute ventilation.
  - A potential disadvantage is that an unnatural respiratory pattern of slow, large breaths may occur.

### High-Frequency Oscillatory Ventilation (HFOV)
- HFOV allows the use of lower tidal volumes and avoidance of barotrauma (avoids alveolar shear injury) by using supraphysiologic ventilatory frequencies (900–3600 cycles

per minute) with low tidal volumes (less than or equal to physiologic dead space in conventional ventilation).
■ It is used in patients with severe hypoxia or hypercapnia despite maximal (or toxic) settings via a conventional ventilator ($FiO_2$ >60% and $SaO_2$ <88%, peak airway pressures >40 cm $H_2O$).

## Setting Ventilator Parameters

■ Tidal volume
  ▪ The average resting tidal volume for a spontaneously breathing nonintubated person is 5–7 mL/kg. To account for volume lost in the ventilator circuit and lack of natural sigh breaths (which expand the lung bases and maintain functional residual capacity), a larger tidal volume of 10 mL/kg is selected. The goal is to achieve a net delivered tidal volume of 6–8 mL/kg. An adequate tidal volume produces an adequate chest rise. For patients with diffuse lung injury, smaller tidal volumes (4–6 mL/kg) may be associated with a decreased risk of further lung injury.
  ▪ Volume lost in the circuit can be estimated by subtracting the PEEP from the peak airway pressure. That number is multiplied by 1.5 for children using a pediatric circuit (>12 mo of age) or by 1 for children using an infant circuit (<12 mo). This number is the approximate volume lost as a result of the compliance of the tubing.
    • The smaller the patient, the more significant this volume loss becomes, and close attention must be paid to infants being supported in volume modes of ventilation.
  ▪ Some newer ventilator models are capable of calculating volume lost breath to breath, in the circuit, and autocorrect the volume administered, providing a more accurate indication of the amount of tidal volume received by the patient.
  ▪ Permissive hypercapnia: Often an elevated $PCO_2$ is tolerated to achieve lower tidal volumes or lower peak airway pressures to minimize ventilator-associated lung injury.
■ Rate: A physiologic norm for age is selected and then adjusted according to assessment of $PaCO_2$.
■ Inspiratory time
  ▪ A physiologic, age-specific time is selected, resulting in an average inspiratory:expiratory ratio of 1:2.
  ▪ Reasonable starting points are 0.4–0.5 seconds for infants, 0.6–0.8 seconds for younger children, and 0.8–1.2 seconds for adolescents and adults.
■ $FiO_2$
  ▪ This is determined by clinical circumstances.
  ▪ Attempts should be made to keep it below nontoxic levels, usually <60%.
■ PEEP
  ▪ A value of 3–5 cm $H_2O$ is usually sufficient for most patients. Higher levels may be needed for patients with impaired lung compliance.
  ▪ Increases are made in 1- to 2-cm $H_2O$ increments, with careful attention to the hemodynamic effects excessive PEEP may have by decreasing venous return.
  ▪ Avoid overdistension of the lung caused by excessive PEEP.
■ HFOV settings
  ▪ ΔP (or amplitude)
    • This influences ventilation.
    • It is set so that the oscillation or "jiggle" of the patient goes to the lower groin.
  ▪ Mean airway pressure (MAP, or pulmonary artery wedge pressure)
    • This influences oxygenation.
    • It is set 3–5 cm $H_2O$ higher than the MAP on the conventional ventilator.
    • It is increased by 1–2 points until adequate oxygenation is achieved.
  ▪ Frequency (hertz)
    • This influences the tidal volume; the lower the value, the larger the tidal volume.
    • Typically it is set at 6–12, with larger patients requiring a lower hertz.
  ▪ Weaning to conventional ventilation, which typically occurs when a MAP of <20 cm $H_2O$ is achieved

## Assessment of Mechanical Ventilation

- Clinical assessment of aeration, chest wall movement, and work of breathing are essential. Do not fall into the trap of thinking that increased work of breathing is caused by lack of sedation. Often, it is a sign that a patient's respiratory needs are not being met. This could be true despite a "normal" blood gas.
- Blood gas analysis is often used to assess adequacy of mechanical ventilation.
  - Arterial blood gas (ABG) is the most reliable indicator.
  - In patients without arterial access, capillary blood gases are a good estimate of the patient's pH and $PaCO_2$ but do not accurately reflect a patient's $PaO_2$. Mixed venous blood gases (those coming from a central line) can be used as well.
  - The $PCO_2$ of a venous blood gas is typically 5 mm Hg higher than the arterial $PCO_2$.
  - Peripheral venous gases are unreliable and should not be used.
- End-tidal $CO_2$
  - This is measured at the end of the endotracheal tube and typically is a few mm Hg lower than a patient's true $PaCO_2$. Proper square wave form should be seen to assess the accuracy of the measurement.
  - Patients with extensive dead space ventilation (BPD, asthma) may have a larger discrepancy between their end-tidal $CO_2$ measurement and the true $PaCO_2$.

## Noninvasive Mechanical Ventilation

- Definition: application of positive pressure ventilation without the use of an endotracheal tube or tracheostomy but rather a tight-fitting facial or nasal mask
- Indications: static or slowly progressive neuromuscular disease, central hypoventilation, chronic respiratory failure, chronic obstructive lung disease, severe asthma attacks
- Advantages: avoidance of artificial airway, greater acceptance by parents, decreased need for sedation
- Disadvantages: requires degree of patient cooperation, may not be suitable for small children, does not aid airway protection
- Biphasic positive airway pressure (BIPAP): supplies pressurized air during inspiration (inspiratory positive airway pressure [IPAP]) and expiratory positive airway pressure (EPAP)
  - Requires a tightly fitting mask
  - Breaths triggered by detection of change in airflow generated by the patient
  - IPAP settings start at 8–10 cm $H_2O$ and can be titrated up based on patient compliance and improved work of breathing.
  - EPAP settings start at 4 cm $H_2O$ and are titrated up to improve oxygen saturations.
  - Can be used to administer EPAP alone (CPAP)
  - Can set up back-up rate for patients with hypoventilation

# SHOCK

- Shock is a clinical syndrome that is caused by inadequate tissue perfusion, which ultimately leads to deranged homeostatic mechanisms and irreversible cellular damage. It is a clinical diagnosis and should not be judged on the basis of blood pressure alone.
- Because circulatory function depends on blood volume, vascular tone, and cardiac function, all shock states result from abnormalities in one or more of these factors.

## Classification

- Shock has been classified in many ways and any classification must allow for overlaps. In other words, any given patient in shock, regardless of initial etiology, may have pathophysiologic characteristics of different types of shock at different time periods in the illness (Table 8-3).
- Eventually, irreversible stage of shock may develop where there are abnormalities of multiple organ systems.

| TABLE 8-3 | Classification of Shock | | | |
|---|---|---|---|---|
| **Types of shock** | **Hypovolemic** | **Distributive** | **Cardiogenic** | **Septic** |
| **Etiology** | Dehydration<br>Gastroenteritis<br>Deprivation<br>Heat stroke<br>Burns<br>Hemorrhage<br>Major abdominal surgery/third spacing | Anaphylaxis<br>Neurogenic<br>Drug toxicity<br>Septic | Congenital<br>Ischemic<br>Traumatic<br>Cardiomyopathy<br>Drug toxicity<br>Tamponade | Bacterial<br>Fungal<br>Viral<br>Protozoan |
| **Pathophysiology** | Decreased intravascular volume → decreased venous return → decreased myocardial preload | Vasomotor tone abnormalities → maldistribution of circulatory volume → peripheral pooling and vascular shunting → hypotension | Pump failure Inadequate Cardiac output | Invasive organism → cytokine release → impaired endothelial, cellular function → circulatory derangements Direct tissue damage |
| **Diagnosis** History and physical examination are of utmost importance | Early<br>Compensated<br>Cool extremities<br>Tachycardia<br>Normal blood pressure<br>Increased systemic vascular resistance (SVR)<br>Decreased-perfusion urine<br>Cardiac output filling pressure (or normal filling pressure)<br>Uncompensated hypotension<br>Altered sensorium<br>Anuria<br>Cardiac and respiratory failure | Decreased cardiac output<br>Profound hypotension<br>Anaphylaxis → other manifestations<br>Spinal shock → accompanying bradycardia | Poor perfusion<br>Pulmonary edema<br>Hepatomegaly<br>Cardiomegaly<br>Abnormal heart sounds<br>Increased systemic vascular resistance | Tachypnea<br>Tachycardia<br>Fever or hypothermia<br>Hyperdynamic circulation followed by hypoperfusion<br>Altered central nervous system function<br>Oliguria<br>Lactic acidemia<br>Impaired organ function<br>Hypoxemia<br>Renal failure<br>Evidence of infection |
| **Initial Treatment** | Volume repletion | Volume repletion<br>Pressors | Fluid restriction<br>Pressors<br>Diuretics ± afterload reducer | Volume repletion<br>Pressors<br>Antimicrobials |

## Monitoring

- A high index of suspicion and knowledge of conditions predisposing to shock are important in the early recognition of shock.
- Assessment of decreased tissue perfusion, changes in body temperature, capillary refill, impaired urine output, tachycardia, tachypnea, decreased pulse pressure and peripheral pulse characteristics, and mental status changes should be noted.
- Laboratory investigations should include serum electrolytes, ionized calcium, blood cell counts, and type and screen. ABG analyses, lactate, and mixed venous oxygen saturation can add further information about adequacy of tissue perfusion and cardiovascular performance.
- Continuous cardiopulmonary monitoring, pulse oximetry, temperature, and blood pressure measurements are essential.
  - Intra-arterial catheters can be used for ABG analysis and continuous blood pressure monitoring.
  - Invasive venous and pulmonary arterial monitoring should be considered for determination of cardiac output, volume status, and systemic vascular resistance (SVR) to better guide management.
- Consider placement of a Foley catheter. Urine output of <1 mL/kg/hr suggests renal hypoperfusion.

## Treatment

- Management of shock is aimed at optimizing perfusion of critical vascular beds.
- Treatment of the underlying cause is mandatory (e.g., cessation of hemorrhage, antibiotic therapy).
- Fluid resuscitation. Give 20 mL/kg of isotonic crystalloids (normal saline, lactated Ringer) with assessment between boluses. Colloids and blood products may be necessary. Fluid must be used cautiously if cardiogenic shock is suspected.
  - Patients with septic shock may need repeat fluid boluses every 5–10 minutes and as much as 80 mL/kg of fluid to correct their shock state.
  - Severe metabolic acidosis may be treated with 1–2 mEq/kg sodium bicarbonate IV. Sodium bicarbonate should be given cautiously to patients with impaired ventilation because increased intracellular acidosis may occur.
  - Use of pressor agents, such as dopamine, dobutamine, epinephrine (cold shock), and norepinephrine (warm shock), may be required to improve myocardial function and support blood pressure (Table 8-4).
  - Afterload reduction with milrinone or nitroprusside to improve myocardial performance may be indicated for patients with severe cardiac dysfunction.
  - Dysfunction in other organ systems, such as renal, gastrointestinal, hematologic (coagulation), and CNS, must be identified and treated, if possible.
  - Corticosteroids should be considered in patients who fail to respond to vasopressor therapy and are at risk for adrenal insufficiency (history of CNS abnormality, chronic steroid use, purpura fulminans, or hyperpigmentation). Hydrocortisone doses of 1–2 mg/kg for stress coverage to 50 mg/kg for shock have been recommended. Also, consider drawing a random cortisol level before giving hydrocortisone.
  - In cases of catecholamine refractory shock, consider pericardial effusions, pneumothorax, hypoadrenalism, hypothyroidism, ongoing blood loss, intra-abdominal catastrophe, necrotic tissue, and other problems.
  - Consider Swan-Ganz catheterization for assessment of volume status and systemic vascular resistance if hemodynamic status remains ambiguous by clinical assessment.

# INCREASED INTRACRANIAL PRESSURE

- Increased intracranial pressure (ICP) is a common sequelae of a variety of CNS insults, including trauma, infections, ischemic injury, and metabolic disease.

| TABLE 8-4 | Inotropic and Afterload-Reducing Medications | | | | |
|---|---|---|---|---|---|
| Medication | Dopamine | Epinephrine | Norepinephrine | Dobutamine | Milrinone |
| Indication | First-line agent for warm and cold septic shock, cardiogenic shock, distributive shock | Cold septic shock, cardiogenic shock | Warm septic shock, distributive shock | Cardiogenic shock | Cardiac dysfunction, but stable blood pressure |
| Mechanism of action | Low doses: increase renal and splanchnic blood flow, and contractility  Higher doses: increase heart rate and systemic vascular resistance (SVR) | Increased heart rate, SVR, and contractility | Increased SVR | Increased contractility | Decreased SVR, Increased contractility |
| Dosage | 2–20 μg/ kg/min | 0.01–1 μg/ kg/min | 0.01–1 μg/kg/ min | 5–20 μg/ kg/min | 0.5–1 μg/kg/ min |

- Therapy directed at decreasing ICP has only been shown to improve outcome for traumatic brain injury, but may benefit other carefully selected patients.
- ICP results from the interaction of the brain, intracranial blood volume, cerebral spinal fluid (CSF), and anything else contributing to intracranial volume, such as tumors, hematomas, abscesses, or other mass lesions.
- If the volume of one component of the intracranial vault increases, the volume of the other components, usually blood or CSF, must be reduced to maintain normal ICP.
  - Once the capacity for this mechanism fails, ICP increases.
  - If the pressure is sufficiently high, movement of the brain or brainstem across the tentorium or through the base of the skull can occur. This is defined as herniation and can lead to irreversible damage of the brain or brainstem and death.

## Cerebral Perfusion Pressure and Cerebral Autoregulation

- The brain depends on a constant blood supply to provide oxygen and metabolic substrates. Cerebral perfusion pressure (CPP) needs to be maintained to protect the integrity of the brain cells.
- CPP is used as a measure of the adequacy of cerebral blood flow in the injured brain. It is defined by the equation: CPP = MAP – ICP.
  - Current adult data suggest that maintaining a CPP >70 mm Hg may be associated with improved neurologic outcome.
  - The optimal CPP in children is not known, but a goal of keeping CPP >50 mm Hg is reasonable based on available evidence (see Downward suggested reading).

- Autoregulation refers to the brain's ability to maintain cerebral blood flow (CBF) despite fluctuations in MAP. Under normal circumstances, CBF is well maintained for MAP ranging from 60–150 mm Hg. Above and below this range, it varies with blood pressure.
- At low blood pressures, the CBF may be inadequate and ischemia occurs.
- In the injured brain, autoregulation may be compromised or completely lost. In these circumstances, CBF may vary directly with blood pressure, leading to cerebral ischemia at lower pressures or excessive blood flow at normal to high blood pressures.
- A major factor in autoregulation is the brain's response to changes in arterial $O_2$ and $CO_2$ levels. Hypoxia is a potent cerebral vasodilator and hypocapnia a potent vasoconstrictor. Although other aspects of autoregulation may be lost, these responses are usually preserved in the injured brain.

## ICP Monitoring

- Maintaining CPP requires monitoring of ICP. This is usually done by either a fiberoptic pressure monitor in the brain parenchyma, subdural, or epidural space, or by an intraventricular catheter (ventriculostomy). The latter offers the advantage of the therapeutic removal of CSF.
- Monitor-associated complications are rare but include infection, hemorrhage, seizures, and inaccurate readings.
- Indications for ICP monitoring
  - Glasgow Coma Score ≤8 after traumatic brain injury
  - Abnormal head computed tomograph (mass lesion, contusions, cerebral edema, compression of the basal cisterns)
  - Neurologic examination obscured by sedation or neuromuscular blockade
- Presence of an open fontanel and/or sutures does not negate the utility of ICP monitoring

## Airway Management

- Having a secure airway in patients with elevated ICP is critical to prevent secondary damage from hypoxia and hypercapnia.
- Stimulation of the oropharynx or larynx produces a vagally mediated reflex increase in ICP. Therefore, endotracheal intubation in patients at risk for elevated ICP must include measures to blunt this response. This is most commonly done with the use of sedatives and nondepolarizing neuromuscular blocking agents and also administering either sodium thiopental or lidocaine (1 mg/kg IV), which directly inhibits the ICP response.
  - Drugs that increase cerebral blood flow, such as ketamine and succinylcholine, must be avoided.
  - Hypoxia must be avoided so preoxygenation before intubation is essential.

## Treatment (Children)

- The primary goal in caring for patients with elevated ICP is prevention of secondary brain injury. This is achieved by maintaining adequate supply of oxygen and nutrients to the injured brain and avoiding further insults such as ischemia or excessive metabolic demands (e.g., seizures, hyperthermia).
- Therapy is directed at maintaining CPP by ensuring that blood pressure (MAP) is adequate and keeping ICP as low as possible.
- If necessary, additional fluid boluses or vasopressor medications may be needed to maintain MAP.
- Surgery. Surgical evacuation of mass lesions may be necessary. However, surgical management is often not sufficient, because there is often significant residual brain edema leading to elevated ICP.
- Nonoperative methods. This approach is directed at decreasing ICP by minimizing cerebral metabolism (which increases cerebral blood volume [CBV]) and controlling excessive CBF while maintaining CPP to ensure adequate delivery of oxygen and metabolic substrates to the brain cells.

■ Temperature control. Increased metabolic demand from fever can increase CBV and ICP and damage brain cells. A cooling mattress and rectal acetaminophen can be used to maintain normothermia. Shivering can be controlled by muscle paralysis.

■ Head at 30°. This position facilitates venous drainage to help decrease CBV.

■ Seizure control. Seizures greatly increase cerebral metabolism and blood flow and must be aggressively treated. Prophylaxis with fosphenytoin or phenobarbital for 7 days should be considered for patients at high risk for early posttraumatic seizures (penetrating brain injury, intracranial hematomas, and depressed skull fractures). For acute seizure control, the following agents may be used: lorazepam 0.1– 0.2 mg/kg IV repeated at 5 minutes, fosphenytoin 10 mg/kg IV repeated if necessary in 30 minutes (up to 30 mg/kg), and phenobarbital 10 mg/kg IV repeated every 15–30 minutes until the seizure resolves. Prophylaxis with antiepileptics has no effect on the occurrence of late posttraumatic seizures.

■ Fluid management. Overhydration must be avoided. Isotonic fluids such as lactated Ringer or normal saline must be used. Hyponatremia and hypotonic fluid must be avoided. Hyperglycemia should be avoided and glucose-containing IV fluids in the first 24 hours are not recommended, with the exception of young infants. Serum glucose levels must be monitored closely.

■ Sedation. Decreasing brain metabolism and agitation with sedatives can be very effective in helping control elevated ICP. Benzodiazepines with or without opiates are commonly used. A short-acting barbiturate such as sodium thiopental may be effective for sedation before noxious procedures, such as endotracheal tube suctioning or moving the patient. A nondepolarizing neuromuscular blocking agent may be added to prevent coughing or ventilator dyssynchrony because these are associated with increased ICP.

■ CSF removal. Use of intraventricular catheters to remove CSF is often beneficial for ICP control. In patients with severe edema and very small ventricles, CSF removal may be of little benefit.

■ Osmotic agents and diuretics:
  • Mannitol, given at doses of 0.25–1 g/kg, is the most commonly used osmotic agent to control ICP. It may be given as intermittent doses for acute ICP elevations or scheduled every 4 to 6 hours.
    ◦ High doses of mannitol are associated with renal toxicity. To avoid renal toxicity, serum osmolality is measured periodically. This is compared with the serum osmolality calculated from a basic metabolic profile (BMP).
    ◦ One's serum osmolality is determined by sodium, blood urea nitrogen, glucose, and osmolar substances, such as mannitol and ethylene glycol. It can be calculated using the equation $1.86 \times (Na+K) + (BUN/2.8) + (Glucose/18) + 10$.
    ◦ Osmolar gap: A difference of 20 mOsm/L between the serum osmolality measured in the laboratory and the calculated serum osmolality is thought to represent a safe level of mannitol (see Diringer and Gondim suggested readings).
    ◦ Because a brisk diuresis can ensue, close monitoring of intravascular volume is important.
  • Hypertonic saline (3%) given in boluses of 3 mL/kg followed by an infusion of 1–2 mL/kg/hr titrated to a serum osmolarity of 360 mOsm/L can be used to control elevated ICP (this corresponds to a serum sodium <160 mmol/L). Multiple boluses may be needed to achieve goal serum osmolarity.

■ Hyperventilation
  • Hyperventilation leads to hypocapnia and cerebral vasoconstriction, resulting in decreased CBV and ICP. $PaCO_2$ levels should be maintained between 35 and 40 mm Hg to prevent excessive cerebral circulation.
  • Prophylactic hyperventilation ($PaCO_2$ between 30–35 mm Hg) should be avoided; however, it may be considered in cases of refractory intracranial hypertension after having maximized pharmacologic measures.
  • Transient aggressive hyperventilation may be used for acute control of increased ICP that is unresponsive to other measures (sedation, hyperosmolar therapy).

- Chronic hyperventilation ($Pco_2$ in the 20–30 mm Hg range) can cause further cerebral ischemia if continued for long periods.
- CBF, jugular venous saturations, or brain tissue oxygenation monitoring are suggested to ensure adequate CBF, especially if hyperventilation is needed.
- Barbiturate coma
  - This decreases cerebral blood flow by decreasing cerebral metabolism.
  - It can be considered for patients with ICP refractory to maximal medical and surgical therapy.
    - A pentobarbital loading dose of 5–10 mg/kg over 1 hour followed by continuous infusions of 1–5 mg/kg/hr with dose titration to clinical effect is an initial starting point.
    - High-dose barbiturate therapy commonly produces hypotension, and additional fluid boluses or vasopressor therapy is often necessary.
    - Should the patient progress to herniation, the first brain death examination must be delayed until the pentobarbital has cleared the patient (see later discussion).
- Steroid therapy. This is currently indicated only for vasogenic edema caused by tumors.

# DEATH ON THE BASIS OF NEUROLOGIC CRITERIA (BRAIN DEATH)

## Definition

- Brain death is irreversible damage to the brain, including the brainstem, resulting from a known disease that can result in brain death. Life support is futile and should occur only for organ donation.
- The diagnosis of brain death cannot be made in the presence of conditions that may be responsible for the clinical absence of detectable brainstem functions. These include:
  - Shock
  - Severe electrolyte, acid-base, or endocrine abnormalities
  - Severe hypothermia (core temperature of 32°C or lower)
  - Hypotension
  - Drug intoxication (e.g., barbiturate coma), poisoning, or neuromuscular blockade
- These abnormalities must be corrected before making a diagnosis of brain death. Most hospitals have policies regarding the diagnosis of brain death, and these should be consulted before any final determination.

## Physical Examination

- In most instances, physical examination criteria are sufficient to make the diagnosis of brain death. However, confirmatory tests may be necessary in very young children (<1 year of age).
- The examination must be performed by two physicians, the attending and either a neurologist or a neurosurgeon.
- Two examinations are necessary. The recommended duration between the first and second examinations varies depending on the age of the patient.
  - Infants 1 week to 2 months of age: up to 48 hours
  - Infants up to 1 year of age: 24 hours
  - All other patients: 12 hours
- There is an absence of motor response to painful stimuli, although rudimentary spinal cord reflexes such as triple flexion of the legs with painful stimuli may be present.
- There is an absence of brainstem reflexes:
  - Dilated pupils (4–6 mm)
  - Lack of pupillary response to bright light
  - No oculocephalic movement to rapid turning of head (absent doll's eyes reflex)
  - Absent cold caloric response (i.e., no eye movement toward stimulus in response to irrigation of tympanum with ice water)

- Absent corneal reflex when touched lightly with cotton swab or gauze
- Absent cough response
- Absent gag reflex
- An apnea test is necessary.
  - After preoxygenation with 100% oxygen for 5–10 minutes, the patient is taken off the ventilator.
  - Oxygen is provided via a small catheter placed in the endotracheal tube or by some other means of continuous gas flow.
  - The average increase in arterial PaCO$_2$ is 3 mm Hg per minute and is monitored every 5 minutes.
  - The patient is observed for any sign of respiratory effort as the PaCO$_2$ increases.
  - A positive test is the absence of spontaneous respiratory effort despite a rise in PaCO$_2$ of 60 mm Hg or a value 20 mm Hg above baseline.
  - Patients with severe cardiopulmonary instability may not be able to complete an apnea test and confirmatory tests are recommended to make the diagnosis of brain death.

## Imaging

- Confirmatory tests are optional in adults but recommended in very young children. These provide evidence of lack of CBF or neuronal activity (electroencephalography [EEG]), both indicative of loss of cellular function.
  - Cerebral angiography may document nonfilling of intracranial arteries at the entry to the skull.
  - EEG shows absent electrical activity.
  - Transcranial Doppler ultrasonography shows lack of diastolic flow and very small systolic peaks in early systole.
  - Cerebral scintigraphy with technetium may demonstrate absence of intracerebral uptake of the tracer, indicative of lack of CBF.

# POSTOPERATIVE CARE OF PATIENTS AFTER CARDIAC SURGERY

- Successful postoperative management of cardiac patients can be achieved by the following:
  - Knowledge of preoperative anatomic diagnosis and pathophysiologic effects of the defect
  - Understanding operative details and potential complications
  - Careful postoperative ICU management

## Preoperative Details

- The ICU team should be familiar with the salient historical details of the patient scheduled for surgery even before the patient is taken to the operative room. This includes:
  - Prenatal course and gestational age, if pertinent age and weight of the patient
  - Anatomic details of the lesion
  - Pathophysiologic effects before surgery
  - General health of the patient
  - Noncardiac medical and surgical history
  - Results of any diagnostic procedures (echocardiogram, magnetic resonance imaging, cardiac catheterization) and radiographic studies

## Operative Details

- Details of the operation, including anesthetics used and the duration of cardiopulmonary bypass, aortic cross clamp, and circulatory arrest, should be noted.
  - Cardiopulmonary bypass
    - Catheters are placed in both venae cava to drain blood from the patient, which is then passed through an oxygenator and warmer and returned to the patient via the ascending aorta.

- This results in a nonphysiologic and nonpulsatile blood flow, triggers the inflammatory cascade similar to septic shock, and impairs platelet function.

- Aortic cross-clamp time
  - A clamp is placed on the aorta, preventing blood flow into the coronary arteries.
  - It reflects the actual ischemic time for the heart and lungs.
- Circulatory arrest
  - The patient's entire blood volume is drained into the bypass circuit.
  - Thus, the patient is not perfused (including the brain) during this time.
- Expect greater systemic inflammatory response and end organ dysfunction with longer ischemic/artificial perfusion times.

- Details about the surgical approach, ease of coming off bypass, intraoperative complications—such as arrhythmias, bleeding, or air embolism—are important to know.
- A transesophageal echocardiogram is usually obtained in the operating room to evaluate for residual defects.

## ICU Management: The First Several Hours

- Stabilize the patient after transport from the operating room.
  - Verify placement of the endotracheal tube via auscultation and chest radiography.
  - Note the patient's hemodynamic status (palpate central and peripheral pulses, nail bed capillary refill, extremity temperature, skin color, heart rate).
  - Obtain baseline laboratory tests (ABG, lactate, mixed venous saturations, serum electrolytes, ionized calcium, complete blood count, prothrombin time/partial thromboplastin time).
  - Confirm sinus rhythm.
  - Observe tracing and values of all transduced lines (may include some or all of the following: radial/femoral artery, right atrium, left atrium, central venous pressure).
- Provide respiratory support as necessary. After cardiac surgery, patients who are intubated are normally weaned off the ventilator as tolerated. There are some instances when certain ventilatory strategies may need to be used instead.
  - If the pulmonary vascular resistance is high, the patient may require sedation and neuromuscular blockade for 24–72 hours to prevent pulmonary hypertensive crises. Hyperventilation, high inspired oxygen, and, in some instances, nitric oxide may be used to facilitate pulmonary blood flow.
  - If there is excessive blood flow, such as in a patient with residual intracardiac shunt, hypoventilation and low inspired oxygen may be necessary.
  - In operations, such as the Fontan and Glenn procedures, the patient is extubated as soon as possible, because elevated mean airway pressure can cause diminished pulmonary blood flow.

## ICU Management: Overnight

- Postoperative bleeding. Watch for too much output (>3 mL/kg/hr) or too little output (<1 mL/kg/hr) from chest tubes.
  - Too much output may indicate the presence of coagulopathy that fresh frozen plasma needs correcting; consider platelets (recent cardiac bypass impairs platelet function), frozen plasma (if PT/PTT is prolonged), cryoprecipitate (if fibrinogen is low), protamine (if heparin from the pump circuit has not been fully reversed), or recombinant factor VII (if large volumes of blood products are needed). Alternatively, bleeding from large vessels may require chest reexploration and surgical ligation.
  - Too little output may be followed by cardiac tamponade. Tamponade is manifested by a decrease in blood pressure, elevation in heart rate, and elevation in CVP. This should be brought to the immediate attention of the surgeon; the patient may require exploration of their chest.
- Arrhythmias
  - Junctional ectopic tachycardia (JET)
    - This is more frequently seen in patients undergoing surgery that involves the ventricular septum (atrioventricular [AV] canal, ventral septal defect, tetralogy of Fallot).

- It often starts low and speeds up; once the rate exceeds the sinoatrial (SA) node, it becomes the dominant pacemaker. It is manifested by more QRS complexes than p waves, or 1:1 RP relationship, with p waves inside QRS and QRS complexes are narrowed.
- It causes atrial-ventricular dyssynchrony, and systolic blood pressure is often depressed by 10–15 mm Hg. This dyssynchrony can be identified by the presence of cannon A waves on the central venous pressure (CVP) tracing.
- Treatment includes slowing the rate with amiodarone boluses (5 mg/kg) infused slowly over 30 minutes and a continuous infusion of 15 mg/kg/day. IV amiodarone can cause hypotension as a result of lingering effects of cardiac bypass and lipid soluble carrier vehicle and thus patients require close monitoring during its administration. JET can be made worse by elevated catecholamines; thus, the use of narcotics and avoidance of inotropes can aid in therapy. Cooling (avoiding excessive hyperthermia) the core is important. Peripheral venodilation and the avoidance of heating lamps allows radiation of heat away from the heart. Ice bags can make things worse by causing peripheral vasoconstriction and more central hyperthermia.
- Once the rate is reduced, the patient can be atrial paced at a rate exceeding the JET rate to achieve atrial-ventricular synchrony and improved blood pressure.
- Atrial pacing at higher rates (>180 beats/min) results in impaired ventricular filling and reduced stroke volume, and thus decreased blood pressure.
- The condition often resolves in 12–24 hours.

■ Complete heart block
- This failure of AV node conduction, similar to JET, is seen in patients undergoing surgery involving the ventricular septum (AV canal).
- The underlying escape rate is slow junctional or ventricular and often insufficient to maintain cardiac output.
- Treatment involves setting the pacemaker to pace the ventricle every time an atrial beat is sensed.
- The condition often resolves in the first several days after the surgery. If it persists >2 weeks, a permanent pacemaker will need to be placed.

■ Supraventricular tachycardia
- This condition can be confused with JET.
- It often occurs as a rapid increase in rate versus the slow rate increase of JET.
- If the patient is hemodynamically stable, vagal maneuvers may be attempted (ice to the face) and adenosine can be given.
- If the patient is hemodynamically unstable, synchronized cardioversion should be attempted or the patient may be overdrive atrially paced at a rapid rhythm (>300 beats/min) for several seconds.
- If the patient fails to convert with adenosine, atrial flutter or ectopic atrial tachycardia should be considered. These conditions require rapid overdrive pacing or DC cardioversion.

■ Low cardiac output syndrome: typically reaches its nadir 6–12 hours after the surgery (see Parr and Wernovsky suggested readings)
  ■ Factors that can contribute to low cardiac output: residual or unrecognized structural defects, continuation of perioperative ventricular dysfunction, reperfusion injury/effects of bypass, type of surgical procedure (i.e., ventriculotomy), complication of surgery (compromised coronary arteries during a transposition of the great vessels repair), arrhythmia, pulmonary hypertension, and infection
  ■ Manifestations: decreased mental status, core hyperthermia, cold/mottled extremities, tachycardia, narrowed pulse pressure, hypotension, decreased mixed venous saturations, increased lactic acidosis, increased cardiac size, and pulmonary edema on chest radiograph
  ■ Treatment: Evaluation of CVP, right atrial (RA), and left atrial (LA) pressures, as well as physical examination, can help guide therapy.
    - Low filling pressures (low CVP, RA, or LA pressures) indicate hypovolemia and should be treated with gentle 5 mg/kg boluses of colloids or crystalloids.

- Normal or elevated filling pressures (high CVP, RA, or LA pressures) indicate depressed myocardial function and should be treated with inotropic support (dopamine, epinephrine, milrinone, calcium drips).
- Cool, poorly perfused extremities but stable blood pressure indicate borderline myocardial function and can be treated with afterload reduction (milrinone 0.5–1 µg/kg/min) (see Hoffman suggested reading).
- Should the cardiac output continue to decline, despite interventions, some patients require placement on extracorporeal membrane oxygenation (ECMO) support.
  - Worsening cardiac output can be followed by elevation in serum lactic acid. Should levels climb precipitously, a patient may be placed on ECMO electively (see Trittenwin suggested reading).
  - ECMO should be considered in any patient with refractory hypotension, worsening metabolic acidosis, and/or inotropic requirement of >0.2 µg/kg/min of epinephrine.
  - Support is typically required for 4–5 days.

## ICU Management: The Next Day

- Fluids, diuretics, and nutrition
  - Most postoperative cardiac surgery patients require diuretics after 12–24 hours.
  - Nutrition, either enteral or parenteral, is usually started within 24–72 hours after operation. If the patient requires prolonged mechanical ventilation, nutrition is given through a nasogastric feeding tube or as total parenteral nutrition, if enteral feeding is not indicated.

- Respiratory care
  - Chest tube output should continue to be monitored. It should become clear and serous. Cloudy output could be a sign of damage to the thoracic duct resulting in chylous pleural effusions, which may impair respiration.
  - Occasionally, the phrenic or recurrent laryngeal nerves can be damaged. This can be permanent from direct trauma or temporary from thermal injury caused by hypothermia induced during the surgery.
    - Recurrent laryngeal nerve damage is manifested by stridor and distress after extubation.
    - Phrenic nerve damage is manifested by respiratory distress and paradoxical abdominal wall retractions. Younger infants are more at risk of respiratory failure caused by diaphragmatic paralysis and may require surgical plication of the diaphragm.

# MANAGEMENT OF CHILDREN WITH SINGLE VENTRICLES

- A variety of congenital heart lesions have a common physiology of complete mixing of the systemic and pulmonary venous returns. These lesions are usually associated with atresia of the AV or semilunar valves.
- The result is a single ventricular output that is divided into two parallel circulations: systemic and pulmonary. The relative proportion of flow to these vascular beds is determined by the relative resistances to flow.
- Thus, the single ventricle anatomy can be divided into three broad categories that determine the preoperative management and the surgical treatment.

## Balanced Circulation

- The pulmonary blood flow ($Q_p$) is equal to the systemic blood flow ($Q_s$), and the aortic saturation is about 75%–85%. Intermediate surgery or medical management may not be needed.
- This suggests that the pulmonary vascular resistance (PVR) has not yet dropped to the normal physiologic range.

## Excessive Pulmonary Flow

- The $Q_p$ is greater than $Q_s$. Arterial saturation is higher, reflecting increased pulmonary blood flow, and is expected as PVR falls after birth. If untreated, this may result in congestive heart failure.
- Try to decrease systemic vascular resistance (SVR) so that more blood flows into the systemic circulation. Afterload reduction, such as nitroprusside, milrinone, or oral angiotensin-converting inhibitors may be used. Medications that increase SVR are avoided.
- PVR may be increased by controlled hypoventilation with neuromuscular blockade and with decreased inspired oxygen (blending in nitrogen or carbon dioxide via face mask or tent).
- Increased hematocrit may contribute to increasing PVR by increasing blood viscosity and thus decrease pulmonary shunting.
- Surgical palliation is often necessary once PVR decreases.
- Pulmonary banding is the usual approach. A band is placed around the main pulmonary artery and tightened until oxygen saturation is 75%–85% in the aorta or the gradient across the band is 40–60 mm Hg.
- In hypoplastic left heart syndrome (HLHS), the pulmonary artery is used in the construction of the neoaorta, so banding is not performed.

## Insufficient Pulmonary Blood Flow

- Hypoxemia is present. Oxygen saturation may be 60% or lower. $Q_p$ is less than $Q_s$. The goal of management is to increase pulmonary blood flow.
- Try to increase SVR. Sometimes systemic vasoconstriction agents, such as phenylephrine, may be necessary.
    - PVR may be decreased by increasing supplemental oxygen, hyperventilation, and relative alkalosis.
    - Hypovolemia should be avoided.
    - Direct pulmonary vasodilators, such as nitric oxide and prostacyclin, may be helpful.
- In some cases, pulmonary valve dilation, to increase pulmonary blood flow, or atrial septostomy, to increase mixing at the atrial level, is required.
    - The primary surgical intervention before complete palliation is a systemic-to-pulmonary shunt. A common approach is a modified Blalock-Taussig (BT) shunt, whereby a Gore-Tex tube is anastomosed in an end-to-side fashion to both the subclavian (innominate artery in HLHS) artery and the pulmonary artery.
    - This provides adequate pulmonary blood flow. After successful surgery, oxygen saturation is approximately 75%–85%, indicative of a balanced circulation.

## Treatment

- All patients with single ventricles ultimately undergo similar palliation—systemic to pulmonary venous connections with Norwood, Glenn, and Fontan procedures.
- The ultimate goal is to separate the arterial and venous circulation. This decreases the volume load on the single ventricle that has been pumping blood to both the pulmonary and systemic pulmonary vascular beds.
- If not corrected, this leads to ventricular failure.
- Cardiac catheterization is performed before Glenn and Fontan procedures to evaluate PVR. Both these procedures allow venous blood to flow passively into the pulmonary arteries, and therefore successful outcome is dependent on low PVR and low single ventricle end diastolic pressure.

### Norwood Shunt

- Once pulmonary pressures drop and the patient develops signs of pulmonary overcirculation (oxygen saturations >85%), usually by the first week of life, the patient is taken to the operating room, where the branch pulmonary arteries are removed from the main pulmonary trunk.

■ The main pulmonary trunk is anastomosed to the hypoplastic aorta, creating a neoaorta.

■ Pulmonary blood flow is established with either a Sano shunt or a modified BT shunt.
   • The Sano shunt is a shunt that is surgically created between the right ventricle and the branch pulmonary artery.
   • The goal of the Sano shunt is to avoid diastolic runoff and thus optimize coronary blood flow to a heart that has already been compromised by cardiac bypass and cross-clamping during the repair (see Reemsten and Cua suggested readings).

■ The modified BT shunt is complicated by diastolic runoff, which causes mild coronary artery hypoperfusion.

### Glenn Shunt

■ At about 4–6 months of age, when pulmonary vascular resistance has dropped and the patient begins to outgrow the Sano or BT shunt (manifested by a drop in arterial saturations), the superior vena cava is anastomosed to the pulmonary artery.

■ At this time, the BT shunt or Sano shunt is taken down.

■ If a pulmonary band was previously placed, the surgeon either leaves it alone or removes the band, transects the main pulmonary artery and oversews the pulmonary valve. These patients will still have cyanosis because the inferior vena cava still empties into the heart.

### Fontan Shunt

■ At about 2–3 years of age, the inferior vena cava is anastomosed to the pulmonary artery via either a lateral extracardiac tunnel or a conduit completely excluding the heart.

■ This allows complete separation of the venous and arterial circulations.

■ These patients have near normal saturations. The slight reduction in oxygen saturation occurs because the coronary veins, which contain very unsaturated blood, still empty into the heart.

■ In many patients undergoing Fontan procedures, a small fenestration is placed between the Fontan circuit and the right atrium. This allows a right-to-left shunt at the atrial level to maintain cardiac output in the event that PVR is elevated.

   ■ Blood pressure and cardiac output are maintained while oxygen saturation is decreased.

   ■ Without this "pop off," pulmonary blood flow and subsequently cardiac output decreases, leading to low oxygen saturation and hypotension.

### Suggested Readings

Acute Respiratory Distress Syndrome Network. Ventilation with lower tidal volume as compared with traditional tidal volume for acute lung injury and the acute respiratory distress syndrome. N Engl J Med 2000;342:1301–1308.

Adelson PD, et al. Guidelines for the acute medical management of severe traumatic brain injury in infants, children and adolescents. Pediatr Crit Care Med 2003:4S(3).

Arnold HJ. High-frequency ventilation in the pediatric intensive care unit. Pediatr Crit Care Med 2000;(1)93–99.

Carcillo JA. Clinical practice parameters for hemodynamic support of pediatric and neonatal patients in septic shock. Crit Care Med 2002;30(6):1365–1378.

Cho DY, Wang YC, Chi CS. Decompressive craniotomy for acute shaken/impact syndrome. Pediatr Neurosurg 1995;23:192–198.

Cua CL, Thiagarajan RR, Taeed R, et al. Improved interstage mortality with the modified Norwood procedure: a meta-analysis. Ann Thorac Surg 2005;80:44–49.

Diringer MN, Zazulia AR. Osmotic therapy: fact and fiction. Neurocritical Care 2004; 2:219–234.

Downard C, Hulka F, Mullins RJ, et al. Relationship of cerebral perfusion and survival in pediatric brain injured patients. J Trauma 2000;(49):654–659.

Duracher C, Schmautz E, Martinon C, et al. Evaluation of cuffed tracheal tube size predicted using the Khine formula in children. Pediatr Anesth 2008;18:113–118.

Fuhrman BP, Zimmerman JJ. Pediatric Critical Care, 3rd Ed. Buffalo, NY: Mosby, 2005.

Gondim FAA, Aiyagari V, Shackleford A, et al. Osmolality not predictive of mannitol-induced acute renal insufficiency. J Neurosurg 2005;103:444–447.

Hoffman TM, Wernovsky G, Atz AM, et al. Efficacy and safety of Milrinone in preventing low cardiac output syndrome in infants and children after corrective surgery for congenital heart disease. Circulation 2003;107:996–1002.

Malhotra A. Low tidal-volume ventilation in the acute respiratory distress syndrome. N Engl J Med 2007;357:1113–1120.

Mehta NM, Arnold JH. Mechanical ventilation in children with acute respiratory failure. Curr Opinions Crit Care 2004;10:7–12.

Newth CJ, Rachmann B, Patel N, et al. The use of cuffed vs uncuffed endotracheal tubes in pediatric intensive care. J Pediatr 2004;144:333–337.

Nichols DG, Ackerman AD, Carcillo JA, et al. Roger's Textbook of Pediatric Intensive Care. 4th Ed. Durham, NC: Lippincott Williams & Wilkins, 2008.

Nichols DG, Cameron DE. Critical Heart Disease in Infants and Children. 2nd Ed. Baltimore: Mosby, 2006.

Parr GVS, Blackstone EH, Kirklin JW. Cardiac performance and mortality early after intracardiac surgery in infants and young children. Circulation 1975;51:867–874.

Reemstem BL, Pike NA, Starnes VA. Stage I palliation for hypoplastic left heart syndrome: Norwood versus Sano modification. Curr Opinions Cardiol 2007;22:60–65.

Report of Special Task Force. Guidelines for determination of brain death in children. Ann Neurol 1987;22:616–617.

St. Louis Children's Hospital. Policy on the determination of brain death, 2005.

Trittenwein G, Pansi H, Graf B, et al. Proposed entry criteria for postoperative cardiac extracorporeal membrane oxygenation after pediatric open heart surgery. Artificial Organs 1999;23:1010–1014.

Wernovsky G, Wypij D, Jonas RA, et al. Postoperative course and hemodynamic profile after the arterial switch operation in neonates and infants: a comparison of low-flow cardiopulmonary bypass and circulatory arrest. Circulation 1995;92:2226–2235.

West JB. Respiratory Physiology, the Essentials. 8th Ed. San Diego: Lippincott Williams & Wilkins, 2008.

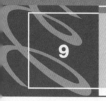

# SURGERY
### Li Ern Chen and Brad W. Warner

- The constellation of pediatric surgical disease is enormous. Of the myriad of congenital and acquired problems that require a pediatric surgeon, the most common are discussed in this chapter, with a focus on diagnosis and presurgical treatment.

# CONGENITAL DISORDERS

## ABDOMINAL WALL DEFECTS

### Definition and Anatomy

- Abdominal wall defects allow herniation of abdominal contents through the abdominal wall.
  - In **omphalocele**, the defect is at the umbilical ring.
  - In **gastroschisis**, the defect is to the right of the umbilicus/umbilical cord.

### Epidemiology

- The incidence of **omphalocele** is 1 in 4,000 births.
- The incidence of **gastroschisis** is 1 in 6,000–10,000 births.
- There is no gender predominance.
- Anomalies associated with the two defects differ.
  - **Omphalocele** is associated with Beckwith-Wiedemann syndrome, pentalogy of Cantrell, cloacal exstrophy, trisomies 13, 18, and 21, Turner syndrome, and Klinefelter syndrome.
  - **Gastroschisis** is primarily associated with jejunoileal atresia but not with an increase in anomalies in other organs.

### Etiology

- **Omphalocele** is thought to occur because of a failure of the intestines to return to the abdomen during gestation.
- **Gastroschisis** is thought to be a defect at the site of involution of the second umbilical vein.

### History and Physical Examination

- Abdominal wall defects are associated with elevated maternal α-fetoprotein levels and can be diagnosed by prenatal ultrasound at 14 weeks gestation.
- In **omphalocele**, the herniated abdominal contents are covered by a membrane. The small and large bowel, the stomach, and sometimes the liver may be visible through the sac.
- In **gastroschisis**, there is no covering membrane; the exposed bowel is thickened, matted together, and may be covered in a fibrin peel. The entire midgut is generally herniated, but other organs, including the stomach or pelvic organs, may also herniate if the defect is large.

### Imaging

- **Prenatal.** Imaging involves thorough ultrasonographic examination to look for other anomalies, fetal echocardiography, and amniocentesis for karyotyping. Cesarean section

and early premature delivery are not indicated unless necessary for other obstetric reasons.
- **Postnatal.** In combination with a detailed physical examination, imaging is directed at identifying other congenital anomalies. Commonly, abdominal ultrasound, cardiac echocardiogram, and other radiographic techniques are used.

## Treatment

### *Postnatal*
- Nasogastric decompression at birth is mandatory.
- An omphalocele membrane should be covered with a sterile saline-soaked gauze and plastic wrap. Herniated bowel in gastroschisis should be treated similarly.
- A heat lamp may be necessary to maintain normothermia.
- Total parenteral nutrition (TPN) is given to patients until defects are repaired.
- Fluid losses can be significant, and fluid status should be monitored closely.
- Antibiotics are indicated in gastroschisis, and in the case of omphalocele membrane rupture.

### *Surgery*
- Primary closure can be performed in infants with small defects where the volume of herniated contents is small.
- Staged closure, using a silo that is placed at the bedside, is used when the intra-abdominal volume at birth is too small to accommodate the extra-abdominal contents.
- Postoperative care in the neonatal intensive care unit (NICU) includes mechanical ventilation and monitoring for abdominal compartment syndrome. Intestinal ileus is expected after closure, and TPN should be continued. Bowel function generally returns more quickly in those with omphalocele than those with gastroschisis.

### *Results and Complications*
- Outcome is largely dependent on gestational age at birth and the presence of other congenital and genetic anomalies.
- Delayed enteral feeding may increase the risk of necrotizing enterocolitis (NEC; see later discussion).
- Long-term complications include gastroesophageal reflux and adhesion-related bowel obstruction.

## CONGENITAL DIAPHRAGMATIC HERNIA

### Definition and Anatomy
- A congenital diaphragmatic hernia (CDH) is a defect in the diaphragm allowing herniation of abdominal contents into the thorax.
- Most cases (80%) are left sided. Rare cases are bilateral.

### Epidemiology
- Incidence is approximately 1 in 2,000–5,000 births.
- The condition is associated with pulmonary hypoplasia and pulmonary hypertension.

### Etiology
- The cause is a defect in diaphragmatic development.
- A genetic cause is not currently known.

### History
- Maternal history of polyhydramnios exists in 80% of cases.
- CDH can be diagnosed on prenatal ultrasound. Prenatal chromosomal analysis should be performed.

## Physical Examination

- Tachypnea, grunting, cyanosis, and decreased breath sounds occur on the affected side.
- A scaphoid abdomen with an asymmetric and distended chest may be seen.
- Hypotension may be present as a result of mediastinal compression and obstruction of venous return to the heart.

## Laboratory Studies and Imaging

- Tests include blood gas analysis as well as preductal and postductal oximetry.
- A chest radiograph showing bowel in the chest and a paucity of bowel gas in the abdomen confirms the diagnosis.
- Cardiac anomalies can occur in up to 25% of infants with CDH; a cardiac echocardiogram is warranted.

## Differential Diagnosis

- Congenital diaphragmatic eventration is a possibility.

## Treatment

- Nitric oxide may be necessary for pulmonary vasodilatation.

### Extracorporeal Membrane Oxygenation (ECMO)

- ECMO may be useful when there is inadequate oxygen delivery in the face of adequate volume resuscitation, circulating hemoglobin, pharmacologic support, and ventilation.
- Infants should generally be >34 weeks gestation, weigh >2,000 g, have no major intracranial hemorrhage, have been on a mechanical ventilator for <14 days, and have no lethal congenital anomalies.

### Surgery

- Surgical closure is not an emergency; rather, it should be performed when the infant is physiologically stable and the pulmonary vascular tone has been maximally optimized.
- Preoperative treatment includes:
  - Nasogastric tube, intravenous fluid, intubation, and mechanical ventilation
  - Ventilation by mask or "bagging" is contraindicated to avoid distension of the bowel.
  - Blood gas analysis, as well as preductal and postductal oximetry, should be monitored serially.

### Results and Complications

- Mortality rates range from 20%–52% (infants with CDH who require ECMO).
- To date, no factors that reliably predict outcome have been identified.
- Pulmonary hypoplasia and pulmonary hypertension are possible.
- Gastroesophageal reflux occurs in 45%–85% of patients.

# ESOPHAGEAL ATRESIA AND TRACHEOESOPHAGEAL FISTULA

## Definition and Anatomy

- Esophageal atresia (EA) is a discontinuity in the esophagus. There may be an associated fistulous connection between the esophagus and the trachea, which is known as a tracheoesophageal fistula (TEF).
- Classification is based on the location of the TEF, if present. Eighty-five percent of patients have a blind-ending upper pouch with a fistula connecting the trachea with the distal esophagus.
  - The fistula can be present in the distal or proximal portion of the esophagus.
  - A fistula can also be present without atresia, resulting in a different clinical presentation.

## Epidemiology and Etiology

- Incidence is approximately 1 in 4,000 live births with a slight male predominance.
- About 50% have an associated congenital syndrome (e.g., VACTERL, trisomies 18 and 21, CHARGE syndrome).
- Abnormal separation of the esophagus and trachea occurs during the fourth week of gestation.

## History

- Maternal polyhydramnios is characteristic.
- Diagnosis can be made by prenatal ultrasound.

## Physical Examination

- A newborn with EA has excessive drooling and episodes of cyanosis or respiratory distress. It is impossible to pass a feeding tube into the infant's stomach.
- A newborn with an isolated TEF swallows normally and does not drool, but may choke and cough while eating.
- A newborn with a distal fistula or an isolated fistula may have a distended abdomen.

## Laboratory Studies and Imaging

- Tests include complete blood count (CBC), electrolyte panel, and type and screen.
- Chest and abdominal radiographs after placement of a catheter into the infant's mouth show catheter location in the esophagus.
  - Air in the stomach suggests a distal or isolated fistula.
  - Patients with a proximal fistula or no fistula at all do not have air in the abdomen.
- Echocardiogram or computed tomography angiogram determines the location of the aortic arch, which is important in operative planning.
- Given the frequent association with other anomalies, an abdominal sonogram and an echocardiogram are also required.

## Treatment: Surgery

- Preoperative treatment includes:
  - Placing the infant in an upright position and placing a nasoesophageal or oroesophageal tube to suction saliva and prevent aspiration and pneumonia. The infant should be nil per os.
  - Providing mechanical ventilation if the infant is in respiratory distress or has a pneumonia. The end of the endotracheal tube must be beyond the fistula. Bag-mask ventilation is contraindicated if a distal fistula is present because it causes abdominal distension.
- The goal of surgery, which is semielective, is to restore esophageal continuity.

*Complications*
- Dysphagia is a common postoperative symptom.
- Gastroesophageal reflux (40%) and recurrent respiratory tract infections from silent aspiration may require fundoplication.
- Late complications include anastomotic stricture and tracheomalacia.

# MALROTATION

## Definition and Anatomy

- Abnormal positioning of the midgut results in a narrow mesenteric base, conferring a risk of life-threatening midgut volvulus, bowel obstruction, and mesenteric vessel occlusion, which is a surgical emergency.
- The ligament of Treitz lies to the right of the midline; there is a narrow mesenteric base and Ladd bands overlying the duodenum.

## Epidemiology and Etiology

- Seventy-five percent of infants present when <1 month of age, and 90% are symptomatic within the first year.
- Malrotation can also present in childhood and adulthood.
- The incidence at autopsy is 0.5%–1%.
- Associated anomalies occur in about 50% of patients and include CDH, abdominal wall defects, tracheoesophageal anomalies, intestinal webs and atresias, anorectal malformations, orthopedic and cardiac anomalies, situs inversus, and asplenia and polysplenia.
- Abnormal rotation and fixation of the small bowel occur during gestation.

## History

- The most common symptoms are bilious vomiting, colicky abdominal pain, and distension.
- If midgut volvulus is present, patients may be lethargic and irritable. Those with chronic midgut volvulus may have a malabsorptive syndrome.
- Children who are not diagnosed in infancy may present with chronic abdominal pain, vomiting, diarrhea, and failure to thrive.
- Occasionally, malrotation is an incidental finding on a radiographic workup for another problem.

## Physical Examination

- Abdominal distension, dehydration, and possibly signs of shock are found.
- Abdominal tenderness and blood on rectal examination are suggestive of bowel ischemia.

## Laboratory Studies and Imaging

- Tests include CBC, electrolyte panel, and type and screen.
- Upper gastrointestinal (GI) contrast study is diagnostic.
- Reversed orientation of superior mesenteric artery and vein can be seen on ultrasonography, which is a good screening tool.
- Small bowel follow-through can be done if the upper GI study is normal but symptoms are consistent with malrotation.

## Surgery

- Preoperative treatment includes nasogastric tube decompression, fluid resuscitation, and correction of electrolyte and acid-base abnormalities. Antibiotic therapy is indicated in patients with midgut volvulus, peritonitis, or sepsis.
- The Ladd procedure involves division of Ladd bands over the duodenum and widening of the mesenteric base, with the bowel left in nonrotation.
  - Emergency surgery is required in cases of malrotation with midgut volvulus. Parents of children with asymptomatic malrotation awaiting surgery should be taught to recognize the signs and symptoms of this emergency.
  - In cases when malrotation is diagnosed without midgut volvulus, the Ladd procedure is performed due to the associated risk of midgut volvulus.

### Complications

- Long-term adhesion-related complications, including bowel obstruction, can occur in about 25% of surgical patients.

# INGUINAL HERNIA

## Definition

- This hernia involves protrusion of intra-abdominal contents (e.g., omentum, bowel, gonad) through a defect in the abdominal wall into the inguinal canal.

## Epidemiology and Etiology

- Most hernias in infants and children are indirect.
- Inguinal hernia repair is the most common surgery performed on children.
- Its incidence in full-term neonates is 3%–5% and as high as 60% in premature infants. The peak incidence is in the first 3 months of life.
- Etiology is a patent processus vaginalis.

## History

- Parents often give a history of intermittent bulging in the groin associated with crying or straining.
- The infant may have irritability and anorexia.

## Physical Examination

- A mass may be present in the groin, and in male infants it may extend into the scrotum.
- Scrotal transillumination can help distinguish between a hernia and a hydrocele.
- A hernia that cannot be reduced is termed incarcerated. If the blood supply is compromised because of incarceration, the hernia is strangulated.

## Imaging

- Ultrasound may be used if diagnosis is equivocal on physical examination.

## Differential Diagnosis

- Hydrocele, testicular torsion, testicular tumor, and lymphadenopathy are possibilities.

## Treatment

*Surgery*
- Infants with an easily reducible hernia should undergo elective outpatient surgical repair within 2 weeks. (Chen LE, Zamakhshary M, Aspelund G, et al. Impact of wait-time on outcomes in infant inguinal hernias. Pediatr Surg Int Online: 16 Dec 2008).
    - The risk of incarceration after difficult manual reduction is significant; if reduction is challenging, the child should be admitted to the hospital and undergo hernia repair within 48–72 hours.
    - An incarcerated or strangulated hernia mandates emergent surgical exploration and repair.
    - Parents of children with an inguinal hernia awaiting surgery should be counseled to recognize the signs and symptoms of incarceration, and they should understand that it is a surgical emergency.
- Primary herniorrhaphy is appropriate. Contralateral exploration is performed in young infants.

*Complications*
- Preoperative complications include incarceration, strangulation, and bowel ischemia necessitating bowel resection.
- Complications associated with elective hernia repair are rare (2%) and include hematoma, wound infection, and gonadal complications.
- The surgical complication rate significantly rises in the setting of incarceration.
- In neonates, repair is associated with up to 8% recurrence. In older infants, the expected recurrence rate is 1%.

# ACQUIRED DISORDERS

## NECROTIZING ENTEROCOLITIS

### Definition and Anatomy

- Necrotizing enterocolitis (NEC) is an acute inflammatory process of the intestines that may progress to necrosis and perforation of intestinal tissue.

- NEC most commonly affects the terminal ileum and right colon but may involve any segment of the GI tract.

## Epidemiology and Etiology

- NEC occurs in 1–3 per 1,000 live births.
- The incidence in the NICU is 2%.
- Etiology is multifactorial. Predisposing factors include prematurity and enteral feeds.

## History

- Classic presentation includes the triad of abdominal distension, bloody stools, and pneumatosis intestinalis.
- The typical infant is 2–3 weeks of age and has been formula fed.

## Physical Examination

- Abdominal examination may be notable for distension, abdominal wall erythema, or a palpable mass (fixed dilated loop of bowel).
- A septic infant may also have tachycardia, hypotension, hypothermia, and signs of poor perfusion.

## Laboratory Studies and Imaging

- Trends in leukocyte and platelet counts, as well as hemoglobin concentration are usefull. Electrolytes and blood gases are also followed.
- Blood cultures may aid in tailoring antibiotic coverage.
- Serial abdominal radiographs (anteroposterior, left lateral decubitus, and lateral) looking for pneumatosis intestinalis, portovenous gas, and pneumoperitoneum are useful. Distended loops of small bowel are commonly seen but can be a nonspecific finding.
- Ultrasonography is useful for detecting pneumatosis intestinalis and portovenous gas.

## Monitoring

- Continuous hemodynamic monitoring is necessary.

## Treatment

### Nonoperative

- Medical management is the treatment of choice for patients with NEC who are neither septic nor have GI hemorrhage. Surgical treatment is required if pneumoperitoneum develops.
- Nonoperative management consists of antibiotics, fluid resuscitation, nasogastric or orogastric decompression, and stopping enteral feeds. Vasopressor support may be appropriate. Parenteral nutrition is also initiated.

### Surgery

- Exploratory laparotomy, resection of necrotic or perforated bowel, and ostomy creation are the mainstay of surgical intervention. More recently, primary peritoneal drainage has been shown to be an alternative treatment with equivalent outcome.
- Preoperative interventions include fluid resuscitation, and correction of electrolytes, anemia, and coagulopathy. Cross-matched blood products must be available for surgery.
- In infants who are gaining weight and are no longer critically ill, reversal of enterostomy is timed at 8 weeks after the initial operation.
- Survival in infants requiring surgical treatment is 70%–80%.

### Complications

- Recurrent NEC occurs in 4%–6% of infants.
- Intestinal stricture is the most common complication.
- Short bowel syndrome and intestinal malabsorption can result depending on the amount of bowel resected.

# INFANTILE HYPERTROPHIC PYLORIC STENOSIS

## Definition

- Infantile hypertrophic pyloric stenosis (IHPS) is narrowing of the pyloric canal caused by circular muscular hypertrophy.

## Epidemiology and Etiology

- Incidence is 2–3 per 1,000 live births.
- The male:female ratio is 4:1.
- Siblings of patients with IHPS are 15 times more likely to develop IHPS than those with no family history.
- The cause is unknown.

## History and Physical Examination

- The classic presentation includes nonbilious vomiting that occurs most commonly in weeks of life 2 through 8. Initially, the infant may regurgitate feeds, but this generally progresses to a characteristic projectile nonbilious emesis.
- An olive-sized pyloric mass may be palpable. The abdomen is soft and nontender.
- Poor skin turgor and a sunken fontanel accompany dehydration.

## Laboratory Studies and Imaging

- An electrolyte panel may reveal a hypochloremic, metabolic alkalosis from vomiting.
- Blood urea nitrogen and creatinine can indicate severity of dehydration.
- Abdominal ultrasonography is diagnostic. If equivocal, a contrast study can also be obtained.

## Treatment

- IHPS is not a surgical emergency; fluid resuscitation, normalization of electrolytes, and correction of acid-base imbalances must be accomplished before operation.
- A nasogastric tube should be inserted for decompression while awaiting surgery.
- Open and laparoscopic pyloromyotomy are acceptable.

### *Results and Complications*

- Feeding is initiated after surgery, and infants are usually discharged home on postoperative day 1 or 2.
- Perforation, wound infection, or dehiscence may complicate pyloromyotomy.

# INTUSSUSCEPTION

## Definition and Classification

- Intussusception involves a segment of the bowel telescoping into a more distal segment.
- Peristalsis causes propulsion of the intussusception into the intussuscipiens, resulting in lymphatic and venous obstruction. Progression of this process leads to bowel wall edema, mucosal bleeding, arterial insufficiency, and eventually bowel necrosis.
- Classification is according to anatomy—ileocolic (most common), ileoileal, or colocolic.

## Epidemiology and Etiology

- Overall incidence is 1%–4%.
- Approximately 95% of cases occur in children <2 years of age; intussusception is the most common cause of intestinal obstruction in this age group.
- Pathologic lead points should be suspected with increasing age. Medical conditions that can create a lead point within the bowel include, but are not limited to, Meckel

diverticulum, intestinal duplication cyst, small bowel lymphoma, polyps, cystic fibrosis, and Henoch-Schönlein purpura.

## History

- The infant or child classically has a history of crying and drawing up their legs during intermittent episodes of abdominal pain. The child may be otherwise asymptomatic between episodes of pain. Most children with intussusception are healthy and well nourished.
- Vomiting (80%) may initially be nonbilious but can become bilious as obstruction progresses. Children with intussusception are often lethargic and may pass bloody stools, known classically as "currant jelly stools."
- Sometimes, a history of recent gastroenteritis or upper respiratory infection is elicited.

## Physical Examination

- Abdominal examination reveals an empty right lower quadrant and a tender "sausage-shaped" mass in the right upper quadrant in 85% of patients. As the process progresses, patients can develop abdominal distension, pain, and peritoneal signs.
- Mucosal bleeding can cause stool to be guaiac positive even in the absence of a history of bloody stool.

## Laboratory Studies and Imaging

- A CBC and electrolyte panel are necessary.
- If the diagnosis is unclear from the history and physical examination, a plain abdominal radiograph may be obtained. If obtained late in the process, the radiograph may show specific distribution of bowel gas and signs of obstruction or perforation.
- Ultrasonography has a sensitivity of 98.5% and 100% specificity.
- An air-contrast enema can be both diagnostic and therapeutic.

## Treatment

### *Nonoperative*

- Hydrostatic reduction of the intussusception with saline or by air enema can be performed by radiologists after notification of a pediatric surgeon. This is contraindicated in patients who have peritonitis or signs of shock.
  - Nonoperative reduction may be complicated by perforation, which is a surgical emergency.
  - Successful reduction is followed by inpatient observation for 24–48 hours.

### *Surgery*

- Operative treatment is indicated in patients with peritonitis or shock.
- Patients with incomplete or unsuccessful reduction, early or multiple recurrences, or a pathologic lead point also require surgical reduction and/or resection.
- Preparation for surgery includes nasogastric tube for decompression, fluid resuscitation, and correction of electrolyte and acid-base abnormalities. Antibiotic therapy is indicated in patients who are septic or have peritoneal signs.
- A population-based study showed that patients necessitating transfer to a teaching hospital were at increased risk for surgical reduction. Patients transferred >1 day after admission were at an even higher risk. This highlights the importance of early recognition and treatment of intussusception.

### *Recurrence*

- After nonoperative reduction, recurrence is 13% in the <2-year age group. A third of these cases occur within 24 hours of reduction.
- After operative reduction, recurrence is infrequent.

## APPENDICITIS

### Definition

- Inflammation of the appendix may progress to necrosis and perforation.

## Epidemiology and Etiology

- Appendicitis is the most common surgical emergency in childhood.
- Peak incidence occurs at 10–12 years of age. The higher rate of perforation in children (30%) compared with adults is attributed to the fact that symptoms are often mistaken for gastroenteritis and to the child's inability to communicate their pain.
- Blockage of the appendiceal orifice causes venous congestion that leads to arterial insufficiency.

## History

- Vague periumbilical pain localizes to the right lower quadrant and is accompanied by nausea, vomiting, anorexia, and fever.
- Diarrhea may also be present.
- Not all symptoms may occur.

## Physical Examination

- Palpation of the abdomen in the right lower quadrant elicits pain. There may be rebound tenderness or guarding.
- Palpation of the left lower quadrant may result in right lower quadrant pain (Rovsing sign).
- Rectal examination results in focal tenderness on the right if the appendix lies in the pelvis.
- If the child is stable and the diagnosis of appendicitis is uncertain, serial abdominal examinations should be performed to monitor the child's clinical trajectory.

## Laboratory Studies

- Patients with appendicitis usually have a low-grade leukocytosis with a neutrophilia.
- Urinalysis should be done to rule out urinary tract infection, which can have a similar clinical presentation.
- If presentation is not classic, liver enzymes, amylase, and lipase levels may be helpful.

## Imaging and Surgical Diagnostic Procedures

- Abdominal ultrasound is a fairly sensitive and specific test for appendicitis.
- Computed tomography (CT) may be useful in some cases but is rarely necessary.
- Diagnostic laparoscopy is especially helpful in teenage girls in whom diagnosis of appendicitis is equivocal.

## Differential Diagnosis

- Conditions to rule out are gastroenteritis, mesenteric adenitis, Crohn disease, urinary tract infection, pyelonephritis, and gynecologic pathology.

## Treatment

- Intravenous antibiotics (e.g., agents that cover aerobic and anaerobic bacteria) are favored in patients with perforated appendicitis with pain for ≥5 days. This should be followed by interval appendectomy in 6 weeks.

### Surgery

- Laparoscopic and open appendectomy are both standard. Recent studies suggest that laparoscopic appendectomy may be associated with a lower wound infection rate and a shorter hospital stay.
- Preoperatively, the patient should be kept nil per os and receive intravenous fluid resuscitation. Antibiotics should be given once diagnosis of appendicitis is made.

### Complications

- Early complications include intra-abdominal abscess and wound infection.
- Late complications include those that are adhesion-related, including bowel obstruction.

# ABDOMINAL TRAUMA

## Definition and Anatomy

- Solid organs commonly injured include the liver, spleen, kidneys, and pancreas.
- Hollow viscus injuries or perforation can occur anywhere along the GI tract.
- Vascular structures may also be injured.
- External landmarks for the boundaries of the abdomen are the nipples superiorly and the pelvis inferiorly.

## Epidemiology and Etiology

- Approximately 50% of all childhood deaths are related to trauma.
- Between 10% and 15% of trauma-related deaths can be attributed to abdominal injury.
- Abdominal injuries are most often caused by blunt trauma.
- Despite careful primary and secondary surveys, injuries are still missed in 2%–50% of children.

## History

- Pertinent history includes the mechanism of injury.
  - Was the mechanism penetrating or blunt?
  - Was the patient restrained?
  - Was the patient thrown on impact?
  - Was there loss of consciousness?

## Physical Examination

- Primary survey for any trauma patient includes evaluating airway, breathing, and circulation (ABCs).
- Secondary survey includes abdominal and rectal examination.
  - On abdominal examination, evaluate for distension and tenderness. Contusion or ecchymosis on the abdominal wall implies significant force to the abdomen.
  - On rectal examination, assess for blood in the stool and rectal tone.
  - Identify wounds that suggest a penetrating injury, looking for entrance and exit wounds.

## Laboratory Studies and Imaging

- Trauma panel (CBC, electrolytes, liver enzymes, amylase, coagulation panel, type and cross-match, urinalysis) is necessary.
- Chest and pelvis radiographs as well as abdominal CT with intravenous contrast are useful.
- Cervical spine series is necessary in patients with significant mechanism of injury.

## Treatment

### Nonoperative

- Patients with a significant mechanism of injury who have no identifiable injury on initial evaluation should undergo serial clinical evaluation with abdominal examination for 24 hours.
- Patients with abdominal injury should receive antibiotic therapy that targets aerobic and anaerobic bacteria.
- Tetanus immunization, if not up to date, is imperative in penetrating trauma. Pain control is also important.

### Surgery

- Surgery is indicated if the patient has peritonitis, uncontrolled abdominal bleeding, pneumoperitoneum, or penetrating abdominal injury.
- Preoperatively, placement of two large-bore intravenous lines, nasogastric decompression, and supplemental oxygen is necessary.

# SOFT TISSUE ABSCESS

## Definition

■ Purulent fluid collects in the skin and subcutaneous tissue.

## Epidemiology and Etiology

■ Methicillin-resistant *Staphylococcus aureus* (MRSA) strains are becoming increasingly prevalent in children with community-acquired staphylococcal infections. The majority of these children have no identifiable risk factors.
■ The cause is violation of the epidermis, with bacterial invasion of the skin and soft tissue.

## History

■ There is often a several-day history of progressive swelling, pain, erythema, and warmth in a localized region of skin.
    ■ There may have been drainage from the wound.
    ■ Fever may be present.
■ It is important to ask about trauma to the skin.
■ Other key elements of the history include previous abscesses, recurrent abscess, and family members with abscesses or with MRSA exposure. There is known community colonization with MRSA in some areas, which makes it valuable to know where the child lives.

## Physical Examination, Laboratory Studies, and Imaging

■ Identify the abscess location, size, induration, fluctuance, drainage, and area of erythema.
■ CBC with differential, and if the lesion is drained, a wound/fluid culture is necessary.
■ Imaging is not usually beneficial.

## Surgical Diagnostic Procedures

■ If it is unclear whether there is a fluid collection to drain, needle aspiration (19-gauge or larger) under local anesthesia can be helpful.
■ If fluid is obtained, aspiration is inadequate and an incision and drainage must be performed.

## Treatment

### Medications

■ Mild cellulitis can be treated with dicloxacillin or cephalexin.
■ If MRSA is suspected, clindamycin or trimethoprim/sulfamethoxazole is recommended.
■ Oral antibiotic therapy is sufficient if the area of infection is small and adequately drained.
■ Systemic signs of infection (fever, leukocytosis) warrant intravenous antibiotics.
■ Notably, the incidence of clindamycin-resistant and trimethoprim/sulfamethoxazole-resistant MRSA is increasing.

### Surgery

■ It may be necessary to use incision and drainage, with twice daily dressing/packing changes, until the wound is healed.
■ Inadequate drainage could result in progressive spread of the infection.

## Referrals

■ A patient with recurrent abscesses should be referred to a specialist in immunology and infectious disease.

## Patient Education

■ Personal hygiene practices should be reviewed with the parent and child.

## Suggested Readings

Bergmeijer JHLJ, Tibboel D, Hazebroek FWJ. Nissen fundoplication in the management of gastroesophageal reflux occurring after repair of esophageal atresia. J Pediatr Surg 2000;35:573–576.

Fujimoto T. Hypertrophic pyloric stenosis. In: Puri P, Hollwarth M, eds. Pediatric Surgery. Heidelberg, Germany: Springer-Verlag, 2000, pp 171–180.

Gahukamble DB, Khamage AS. Early versus delayed repair of reduced incarcerated inguinal hernias in the pediatric population. J Pediatr Surg 1996;31:1218–1220.

Henry MCW, Gollin G, Islam S, et al. Matched analysis of non-operative management vs immediate appendectomy for perforated appendicitis. J Pediatr Surg 2007;42:19–24.

Logan JW, Rice HE, Goldberg RN, et al. Congenital diaphragmatic hernia: a systematic review and summary of best-evidence practice strategies. J Perinatol 2007;Epub July 19:1–15.

Moss RL, Dimmitt RA, Barnhart DC, et al. Laparotomy versus peritoneal drainage for necrotizing enterocolitis and perforation. N Engl J Med 2006;354:2225–2234.

Murphy FL, Sparnon AL. Long-term complications following intestinal malrotation and the Ladd's procedure: a 15 year review. Pediatri Surg Int 2006;22:326–329.

Orzech N, Navarro OM, Langer JC. Is ultrasonography a good screening test for intestinal malrotation? J Pediatr Surg 2006;41:1005–1009.

Owen A, Marven S, Jackson L, et al. Experience of bedside preformed silo staged reduction and closure for gastroschisis. J Pediatri Surg 2006;41:1830–1835.

Somme S, To T, Langer JC. Factors determining the need for operative reduction in children with intussusception: a population based study. J Pediatr Surg 2006;41:1014–1019.

Tirabassi MV, Wadie G, Moriarty KP, et al. Geographic information system localization of community-acquired MRSA soft tissue abscesses. J Pediatr Surg 2005;40:962–966.

Waag K. Intussusception. In: Puri P, Hollwarth M, eds. Pediatric Surgery. Heidelberg, Germany: Springer-Verlag, 2006, pp 313–320.

Yagmurlu A, Vernon A, Barnhart DC, et al. Laparoscopic appendectomy for perforated appendicitis: a comparison with open appendectomy. Surg Endosc 2006;20:1051–1054.

- Adolescence is the time of transition from childhood to adulthood. Typically it begins at 10–14 years of age. It is characterized by rapid physical, cognitive, and emotional growth, as well as sexual development (puberty).
- Adolescents start to develop independence and separation from their parents. Less willing to participate in family activities, many concentrate on peer relationships and challenge parental authority.
- Adolescents are increasingly concerned about their developing body, peer opinion, independence, and sexual exploration.
- Tips for the adolescent clinical interview
  - Interview the adolescent and the parent(s) together and then the adolescent alone.
  - Early in the interview and in front of the parent(s), discuss patient confidentiality. Be sure to say that you will keep your findings and all discussions confidential unless the patient is at risk of hurting himself or herself or others, or someone has hurt the patient.
  - Encourage the adolescent to discuss problems with his or her parents, and encourage parents to create a time in the day to be with their child.
  - The adolescent psychosocial history often includes a **HEADSS** assessment:
    Home dynamics
    Education: school performance
    Activities, Aspirations
    Drugs, Depression,
    Sex, Suicide
  - Offer anticipatory guidance on diet, maturation, sexuality, injury prevention, and good health habits.
  - Other advice includes the following:
    - Before the physical examination, give the adolescent the option of being examined alone or accompanied by the parent. Respect the patient's modesty.
    - When formulating a plan, it is important to reinforce the strengths and achievements of the adolescent both to the patient and to the parent.

## SEXUALLY TRANSMITTED DISEASES

### Definition and Etiology

- Sexually transmitted diseases (STDs) can present as urethritis, vulvovaginitis, cervicitis, genital ulcers or growths, pelvic inflammatory disease (PID), epididymitis, abdominal pain, enteritis or proctitis, hepatitis, arthritis, pharyngitis, rash, or conjunctivitis.

### Diagnosis and Treatment

- Table 10-1 summarizes the characteristics and treatment of the various STDs.
- Adolescents can consent for evaluation and treatment of STDs without parental consent and notification in most states.
- Evaluation should include complete history and physical examination. In females, a pregnancy test, wet prep, assay for *Neisseria gonorrhoeae* and *Chlamydia trachomatis*, *Trichomonas* culture, human immunodeficiency virus (HIV), and rapid plasma reagin (RPR) should be performed. In males, a urine specimen or urethral swab should be taken for diagnosis of infection with *N. gonorrhoeae* and *C. trachomatis*, and HIV and RPR testing should also be completed.

| TABLE 10-1 | Characteristics and Therapy for Sexually Transmitted Diseases | |
|---|---|---|
| **Disease** | **Characteristics** | **Therapy** |
| Gonorrhea | • Caused by *Neisseria gonorrhoeae*<br>• Patients often are coinfected with *Chlamydia*, so treat for both regardless of chlamydia result<br>• Sexual partners should be treated<br>• Screen for syphilis on all patients<br>• May cause mucopurulent cervicitis<br>• **Widespread** resistance to quinolones exists | • **Uncomplicated urogenital, rectal, or pharyngeal:**<br>**Ceftriaxone** 125 mg IM single dose **OR**<br>**Cefixime** 400 mg PO single dose |
| Chlamydia | • Caused by *Chlamydia trachomatis*<br>• Asymptomatic infection is very common among men and women<br>• Sexual partners should be treated<br>• May cause mucopurulent cervicitis<br>• Sexual abuse must be considered in preadolescent children with chlamydia | • **Uncomplicated urogenital:**<br>**Azithromycin** 1 g PO single dose if weight >45 kg or >8 yr **OR**<br>**Doxycycline** 100 mg PO bid for 7 day<br>**Erythromycin base** if <45 kg (50 mg/kg/day divided q.i.d. for 7 day)<br>• **Pregnancy:** erythromycin or amoxicillin |
| Syphilis | • Caused by *Treponema pallidum*<br>• Primary: painless ulcer or chancre<br>• Secondary: rash, mucocutaneous lesions and adenopathy<br>• Early latent syphilis: *within a year of evaluation,* patient has seroconversion or unequivocal symptoms of primary or secondary syphilis, or sex partner with primary, secondary, or early latent syphilis.<br>• All others should be considered to have late latent syphilis.<br>• Tertiary: CNS, cardiac, or ophthalmic lesions, auditory disturbances, gummas<br>• Diagnosis: VDRL or RPR (positive = 4 fold change in titers)<br>  - Cannot compare one to the other—may turn negative after treatment<br>  - Treponemal serologic test to confirm infection (FTA-ABS)—stays positive for a lifetime<br>• Sexual partners should be treated | • **Primary and secondary or early latent:**<br>**Benzathine penicillin G** 50,000 U/kg up to 2.4 million units IM in a single dose (pregnant or not)<br>• **Penicillin allergy:**<br>**Doxycycline** 100 mg PO b.i.d for 14 day **OR**<br>**Tetracycline** 500 mg PO q.i.d. for 14 day<br>• **Late latent:**<br>**Benzathine penicillin G** 2.4 million units IM every week for 3 wk<br>• **Penicillin allergy:**<br>**Doxycycline** 100 mg PO b.i.d. for 28 day **OR**<br>**Tetracycline** 500 mg PO q.i.d. for 28 day<br>• **Tertiary syphilis:**<br>**Benzathine penicillin G** 2.4 million units IM every week for 3 wk<br>• **Neurosyphilis:**<br>**Aqueous crystalline penicillin G** 4 million units IV q4h for 10–14 day followed by |

|  TABLE 10-1 | Characteristics and Therapy for Sexually Transmitted Diseases *(Continued)* | |
|---|---|---|
| Disease | Characteristics | Therapy |
| | | **benzathine penicillin G** 2.4 million units IM every week for 3 wk at the completion of IV therapy. |
| Trichomoniasis | • Caused by *Trichomonas vaginalis*<br>• Malodorous yellow green discharge and irritation but may be asymptomatic<br>• Diagnosis: wet prep and culture<br>• Sexual partners should be treated | **Metronidazole** 2 g PO single dose **OR**<br>**Tinidazole** 2 g PO single dose<br>**If previous treatment fails:**<br>**Metronidazole** 500 mg PO b.i.d. for 7 day |
| Epididymitis | • Usually caused by chlamydia or gonococcus<br>• Epididymal swelling, tenderness, discharge, fever, dysuria | **Ceftriaxone** 250 mg IM single dose **PLUS**<br>**Doxycycline** 100 mg PO b.i.d. for 10 day<br>Follow-up in 72 hr to ensure response to therapy |
| Herpes | • Recurrent, lifelong viral infection<br>• May manifest as painful genital or oral ulcers, cervicitis, proctitis, or be asymptomatic<br>• Pregnant women who acquire infection near time of delivery have a higher risk of perinatal infection (30%–50%)<br>• Use of condoms should be encouraged (↓ transmission if cover lesions)<br>  • May shorten duration of lesions but does not eradicate the virus | **First episode:**<br>**Acyclovir** 400 mg PO t.i.d. for 7–10 day **OR**<br>**Famciclovir** 250 mg PO t.i.d. for 7–10 day **OR**<br>**Valacyclovir** 1 g PO b.i.d. for 7–10 day **OR**<br>**Recurrent episodes:**<br>**Acyclovir** 400 mg PO t.i.d. for 5 day **OR**<br>**Famciclovir** 125 mg PO b.i.d. for 5 day **OR**<br>**Valacyclovir** 500 mg PO b.i.d. for 3 day<br>**Daily suppressive therapy if six recurrences or more per year:**<br>**Acyclovir** 400 mg PO b.i.d. (↓ frequency of recurrences by 75%) |
| Chancroid | • Caused by *Haemophilus ducreyi* and very rare in the United States<br>• One or more painful ulcers and tender suppurative regional lymphadenopathy<br>• All patients should be tested for HIV at time of diagnosis and 3 months after (it is a cofactor for HIV)<br>• Partners must be treated | **Azithromycin** 1 g PO single dose **OR**<br>**Ceftriaxone** 250 mg IM once **OR**<br>**Ciprofloxacin** 500 mg PO b.i.d. for 3 day<br>**Erythromycin** 500 mg PO q.i.d. for 7 day<br>• If treatment is successful, ulcers improve symptomatically in 3 day; |

*(continued)*

| TABLE 10-1 | Characteristics and Therapy for Sexually Transmitted Diseases *(Continued)* | |
|---|---|---|
| **Disease** | **Characteristics** | **Therapy** |
| | | complete healing may require >2 weeks |
| **Genital warts** **Condyloma** **acuminata** | • Caused by human papillomavirus<br>• May manifest as visible genital warts, uterine, cervix, anal, vaginal, urethral, laryngeal warts (types 6, 11)<br>• Associated with cervical dysplasia (types 16, 18, 31, 33, 35)<br>• Condoms reduce but do not eliminate risk of transmission<br>• Patient might remain infectious even though warts are gone<br>• Cervical and anal mucosa warts management should be by expert<br>• Treatment may induce wart-free periods but does not eradicate virus<br>• HPV vaccine now recommended for females at 11–12 years of age | • **External warts:**<br>*Patient administered:*<br>**Podofilox 0.5% topical solution:** b.i.d. for 3 day, then 4 day off; may repeat 4 times this cycle, **OR**<br>**Imiquimod 5% cream:** apply at bedtime 3 × per week then wash off in AM for up to 16 wk<br>*Provider applied:*<br>**Cryotherapy OR**<br>**Podophyllin resin 10%–25% OR**<br>**Trichloroacetic acid OR Surgical or laser removal** |
| **Pediculosis** **pubis** | • Lice or nits on pubic hair<br>• Patients consult because of pruritus or visual nits | **Permethrin 1% cream:** apply for 10 min and rinse<br>**Pyrethrins with piperonyl butoxide:** apply for 10 min and rinse |
| **Scabies** | • Caused by *Sarcoptes scabiei*<br>• In adults may be sexually transmitted but not in children<br>• Pruritus and rash<br>• Treat partners and household contacts, plus household decontamination. | **Permethrin 5% cream:** apply to body from neck down, wash off after 8–14 hr **OR**<br>**Ivermectin** 200 μg/kg PO × 1 then can repeat after 2 wk<br>**Lindane 1% lotion*** |
| **Vaginitis** **Bacterial** **vaginosis** | • Caused by *Gardnerella vaginalis*<br>• Most prevalent cause of pathologic vaginal discharge<br>• Symptoms may include vaginal discharge and odor, vulvar itching, and irritation, although up to 50% are asymptomatic<br>• Partners do not need treatment | **Metronidazole** 500 mg PO b.i.d. for 7 day<br>• Other alternatives:<br>**Clindamycin cream 2%:** 5 g applicator intravaginally for 7 nights<br>**Metronidazole gel 0.75%:** 5 g applicator intravaginally for 5 nights |
| **Candidiasis** | • Symptoms include pruritus, erythema, and white discharge<br>• Partners do not need treatment | **Fluconazole:** 150 mg PO once<br>**Clotrimazole:** 100-mg tablet: 2 intravaginal daily for 3 day or 1 daily for 7 day<br>**Clotrimazole:** 1% cream 5 g intravaginally for 7 nights<br>**Miconazole:** 200 mg vaginal suppository for 3 day |

*Do not use in patients <2 years of age due to neurotoxicity. Only use in cases of treatment failure or if patients cannot tolerate first-line treatments.

- If STD is suspected and followup not certain, treat presumptively for at least gonorrhea and chlamydia.
- Hepatitis C testing should be offered to all HIV-infected patients and patients who abuse intravenous (IV) drugs, or who have partners that do.
- Human papillomavirus (HPV) is a cause of genital warts and cervical cancer. The HPV vaccine (Gardasil) is now approved by the U.S. Food and Drug Administration (FDA) and recommended by the Advisory Committee on Immunization Practices (ACIP) for girls 11–12 years of age; however, it can be given to girls as young as 9 and to women as old as 26. A three-injection series administered over 6 months, the HPV vaccine protects against HPV serotypes 6 and 11 (cause of 90% of genital warts) and 16 and 18 (cause of 70% of cervical cancers). Papanicolaou (Pap) smear screening recommendations still apply because the vaccine does not protect against all types of HPV.
- Condoms, when properly used, can greatly decrease the spread of STDs.
- Initiation of pap smears should occur within 3 years after onset of sexual activity or when the patient is 21 years old. A pelvic exam and pap smear is not required for initiation of birth control.

## Complications

- Long-term sequelae of STDs include infertility, PID, chronic pelvic pain, ectopic pregnancy, cervical dysplasia, and cancer.

# PELVIC INFLAMMATORY DISEASE

## Definition and Etiology

- PID is a spectrum of inflammatory disorders of the upper female genital tract, including endometritis, salpingitis, and oophoritis. Complications may include tubo-ovarian abscess (TOA), perihepatitis, and pelvic peritonitis.
- The most common causal organisms are N. gonorrhoeae and C. trachomatis. Other organisms isolated are Gardnerella vaginalis, Haemophilus influenzae, enteric Gram-negative rods, Streptococcus agalactiae, and Bacteroides fragilis.

## Diagnosis

Lower abdominal pain in a sexually active female with no other identifiable cause and:
- Minimum criteria:
  - Adnexal/uterine tenderness OR
  - Cervical motion tenderness

- Supportive criteria:
  - Oral temperature >101°F (>38.3°C)
  - Abnormal cervical or vaginal discharge
  - Elevated erythrocyte sedimentation rate (ESR) or C-reactive protein
  - Laboratory documentation of N. gonorrhoeae or C. trachomatis infection
  - Presence of white blood cells (WBCs) on saline mount of vaginal secretions

- Definitive criteria:
  - Histopathologic evidence of endometritis on endometrial biopsy
  - Transvaginal sonography or other imaging techniques showing thickened fluid-filled tubes with or without free pelvic fluid or tubo-ovarian complex
  - Laparoscopic abnormalities consistent with PID

- Hospitalization criteria:
  - All pregnant women with suspected PID
  - If surgical emergency such as appendicitis cannot be excluded
  - Inability of patient to follow-up or tolerate outpatient therapy
  - If the patient did not respond clinically to oral antimicrobial therapy
  - If the patient has severe illness, nausea and vomiting, or high fever
  - Patient with TOA

## Treatment

- Parenteral treatment
  - Cefotetan: 2 g IV q12h OR cefoxitin: 2 g IV q6h PLUS
  - Doxycycline: 100 mg IV or PO q12h for 14 day OR
  - Clindamycin: 900 IV q8h PLUS
  - Gentamicin: 2 mg/kg loading dose IV or IM followed by 1.5 mg/kg q8h IV or IM, THEN
  - Continue with doxycycline: 100 mg IV or PO q12h (especially if TOA present) for a total of 14 day.
- Outpatient treatment
  Ceftriaxone: 250 mg IM PLUS
  Doxycycline: 100 mg PO b.i.d. for 14 day
- Metronidazole 500 mg PO b.i.d. may be added for 14 day.
- All sexual partners should be evaluated and treated for gonorrhea and chlamydia infections.

## Follow-Up

- Follow-up examination should be performed within 72 hours to ensure response to therapy.
- Reinforce safer sex practices.

# DYSMENORRHEA

## Definition and Etiology

- Dysmenorrhea is pain with menstruation.
  - Primary: painful menstruation that occurs within 1 or 2 years of menarche; no evidence of organic pelvic disease
    - Cramping usually starts 1–4 hours before menstruation and may last 24 hours, although symptoms may begin 2 days earlier and may last up to 4 days.
    - Episodes typically become less severe with increasing age.
  - Secondary: painful menstruation that appears for the first time or suddenly intensifies in a mature woman.
    - This condition is nearly always a result of a specific pathologic problem, such as endometriosis, chronic PID, benign uterine tumors, or anatomic abnormalities.
- Painful menstruation is caused by release of prostaglandins during menstrual flow.

## Treatment

- Mild symptoms: nonsteroidal anti-inflammatory drugs (NSAIDs) or acetaminophen
- Moderate to severe symptoms: NSAIDs such as ibuprofen 400–600 mg q6–8 h or naproxen 250–500 mg q8–12h. These agents are most effective if given before the onset of menses and continued for 2–3 days after.
- Hormonal contraception, which may be useful if the patient wishes contraception or has pain unresponsive to NSAIDs

# DYSFUNCTIONAL UTERINE BLEEDING

## Definition and Etiology

- Dysfunctional uterine bleeding (DUB) is irregular and/or prolonged vaginal bleeding as a result of endometrial sloughing in the absence of structural pathology.
- DUB is usually a result of anovulation (cycles become ovulatory an average of 20 months after menarche).

## History and Physical Examination

- Take a menstrual, sexual, and endocrine history.
- On physical exam, look for orthostatic blood pressure changes (indicates severe anemia), hirsutism, thyroid changes, galactorrhea, abdominal/pelvic masses, petechiae, and bleeding gums.
- Consider a pelvic examination if the adolescent is sexually active or has a history suggestive of structural pathology.

## Laboratory Studies

- Order a pregnancy test, complete blood count (CBC), and thyroxine ($T_4$)/thyroid-stimulating hormone (TSH).
- Based on the history and physical examination, transaminases, prothrombin time/partial thromboplastin time, platelet function assay, consider von Willebrand factor testing, pelvic ultrasound, gonorrhea/chlamydia testing (if ever sexually active), and luteinizing hormone/follicle-stimulating hormone/testosterone/dehydroepiandrosterone sulfate.

## Diagnosis

- DUB is a diagnosis of exclusion.
- Differential diagnosis: pregnancy, STD, polyp, foreign body (retained tampon, IUD), bleeding diathesis (von Willebrand disease, idiopathic thrombocytopenic purpura, platelet abnormality, clotting factor deficiency), hormonal causes (anovulation, hypothyroidism/hyperthyroidism, polycystic ovarian syndrome, late-onset congenital adrenal hyperplasia, exogenous hormones, such as those in oral contraceptive pills [OCPs], Depo-Provera, Plan B), stress, and excessive exercise

## Treatment

- Treat underlying disorder if present.
- If DUB is the diagnosis, determine that the patient is hemodynamically stable; if so, consider hormonal therapy to stop the bleeding, oral iron supplementation if anemia is present, and NSAIDs if there is accompanying dysmenorrhea.

# CONTRACEPTION

- The goal of contraception in adolescents is a safe and effective method of preventing pregnancy that is both convenient and reversible.
- Table 10-2 summarizes the most common birth control methods available to adolescents.
- **Absolute contraindications to use of estrogen-containing hormonal contraception** include history of thromboembolic disease (myocardial infarction, stroke, pulmonary embolism), pregnancy, breast cancer, exclusive breastfeeding, estrogen-sensitive neoplasias, undiagnosed vaginal bleeding, active viral hepatitis or cirrhosis, major surgery with prolonged immobilization >1 month, symptomatic gallbladder disease, migraine with focal neurologic symptoms, moderate or severe hypertension (systolic blood pressure >160 mm Hg, diastolic blood pressure >100 mm Hg). The World Health Organization guidelines (see Suggested Readings) contain more information.

# EATING DISORDERS

## Definitions and Diagnostic Criteria

- Anorexia nervosa is the pursuit of thinness.
    - Refusal to maintain body weight at or above a minimally normal weight for age and height (e.g., weight loss leading to maintenance of body weight <85% of that expected; or failure to make expected weight gain during period of growth, leading to body weight <85% of that expected)

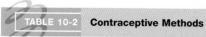

**TABLE 10-2** Contraceptive Methods

| Method | Mechanism of action and characteristics | Failure rate | Adverse effects |
|---|---|---|---|
| **None** | | 85% | |
| **Rhythm method** | Avoidance of coitus during presumed fertile days. Ovulation occurs 14 day before menses. After ovulation, sperm can survive in the vagina 3–4 day and oocytes up to 24 hr. | 6%–38% | |
| **Barrier/chemical** | | | |
| Condom | Mechanical barrier to sperm | 2%–15% | Allergic reaction |
| Diaphragm (placed intravaginally 1–6 hours before intercourse) | Mechanical barrier to sperm | 6%–16% | UTI or vaginal infection |
| Cervical cap (should be used in conjunction with spermicides) | Mechanical barrier to sperm | 16%–32% | Irritation |
| Foam or vaginal tablets | Inactivate sperm; should allow 10–15 min to allow the tablets to dissolve | 15%–29% | Irritation |
| **Intrauterine device** | Inhibits sperm transport and causes direct damage to sperm and ova, affecting fertilization and ovum transport | 0.8% | Dysmenorrhea, PID, uterine perforation (rare) |
| **Combined oral contraceptives** | Suppresses ovulation by inhibiting the gonadotropin cycle, changing the cervical mucus and endometrium | 0.3%–8% | Estrogen-related risk of thromboembolism, hypertension, stroke Irregular bleeding |
| **Birth control patch** | Same mechanism as combined oral contraceptives Releases estrogen and progesterone at controlled rates over 1 wk Changed weekly for 3 wk, then patch-free week for withdrawal bleeding. | <1% | Vaginal spotting, local site reaction (do not put on breasts), less effective if weight >90 kg, detachment, estrogen-related risks |
| **Vaginal ring** | Same mechanism as above Releases estrogen and progesterone at controlled rates over 3 wk, followed by ring-free week for withdrawal bleeding | 0.3% | Must use back-up contraception if out for >3 hr; vaginal spotting, vaginitis, estrogen-related risks |

| TABLE 10-2 | Contraceptive Methods *(Continued)* |

| Method | Mechanism of action and characteristics | Failure rate | Adverse effects |
| --- | --- | --- | --- |
| Medroxypro-gesterone (Depo-Provera) | Inhibits ovulation by inhibiting the midcycle rise of luteinizing hormone; also thickens cervical mucus and causes endometrial thinning | 0.3%–3% | Menstrual irregularities, weight gain, headache |
| Implanon (implantable rod) | Same as above | <1% | Menstrual irregularities, acne, insertion/removal problems |
| Emergency contraception (postcoital) | Plan B (progestin only, may give both pills together as one dose), Ovral 2 pills or Lo Ovral, Triphasil Ovral, Tri-Levlen, Nordette or Levlen 4 pills as soon as possible after unprotected intercourse (within 120 hr) Repeat the dose 12 hr after. | Reduces risk of pregnancy by 89% (Plan B) | Nausea, vomiting (less with progestin-only pills), spotting |

- Intense fear of gaining weight or becoming fat, even though underweight
- Disturbance in the way in which one's body weight or shape is experienced, undue influence of body weight or shape on self-evaluation, or denial of the seriousness of the current low body weight
- In postmenarchal females, amenorrhea (i.e., absence of at least three consecutive menstrual cycles). (A woman is considered to have amenorrhea if her periods occur only following hormone [e.g., estrogen, progesterone] administration.)
- Bulimia nervosa is recurrent episodes of binge eating followed by inappropriate compensatory behaviors.
  - An episode of binge eating characterized by both of the following:
    - Eating, in a discrete period of time (e.g., within any 2-hour period), an amount of food that is definitely larger than most people would eat during a similar period of time and under similar circumstances
    - A sense of lack of control over eating during the episode (e.g., a feeling that one cannot stop eating or control what or how much one is eating)
  - Recurrent inappropriate compensatory behavior to prevent weight gain, such as self-induced vomiting; misuse of laxatives, diuretics, enemas, or other medications; fasting; or excessive exercise
  - Occurrence of both binge eating and inappropriate compensatory behaviors, on average, at least twice a week for 3 months
  - Self-evaluation unduly influenced by body shape and weight
  - The disturbance does not occur exclusively during episodes of anorexia nervosa.

## Epidemiology

- Risk factors:
  - Female sex: 90%–95% of affected individuals
  - Race: >95% Caucasian (this is changing)
  - Athletes: may be gymnasts, ballet dancers, or runners (roles in which thinness is related to success)
  - Age: >80% are adolescents or young adults (third most common chronic illness in adolescents), but younger patients are increasingly more common

## Clinical Presentation

- Anorexia nervosa: amenorrhea, cold hands and feet, constipation, social withdrawal, poor concentration, fainting/dizziness/orthostasis, headaches/lethargy, irritability/depression, and decreased ability to make decisions
- Bulimia nervosa: weight gain, bloating and fullness, guilt/depression/anxiety, and lethargy

## Physical Examination

- Anorexia nervosa: bradycardia, loss of muscle mass, and dry skin/hair loss
- Bulimia nervosa: knuckle calluses, dental enamel erosion, and enlargement of salivary glands

## Laboratory Findings

- Anorexia nervosa: neutropenia/anemia, increased alanine aminotransferase (ALT)/aspartate aminotransferase (AST), decreased serum glucose, prolonged QTc, and electrolyte abnormalities
- Bulimia nervosa: increased serum bicarbonate, decreased potassium, and prolonged QTc or other cardiac arrhythmias

## Treatment

### Therapeutic Guidelines
- Take all concerns seriously.
- Focus on health, not only on weight.
- Follow electrolytes and electrocardiographic (ECG) changes.
- Use team approach, with mental health provider, dietitian, and primary care physician or adolescent medicine specialist.

### Admission Criteria
- Vital sign instability: temperature <36°C (96.8°F), pulse <50 beats/min, on standing a drop in blood pressure of 10 mm Hg or an increase in pulse of 20 beats/min
- Altered mental status or fainting
- Rapid weight loss (>10% in 2 months or >15% overall) or <80% of ideal body weight
- Potassium <3.0 mmol/L, phosphorus <2.0 mg/dL, or dehydration
- Ineffective outpatient management
- Comorbid diagnosis interfering with treatment (i.e., depression, anxiety)
- Unable to eat or drink or uncontrollable binging or purging
- Cardiac arrhythmia or prolonged QTc

## Complications

- Amenorrhea; adequate weight gain should return menses to normal.
- Cardiac conditions: abnormal heart contractility, prolonged QT, and ventricular arrhythmias
- Osteopenia and osteoporosis; weight gain is the most effective method of increasing bone density.
- Refeeding syndrome: greatest risk during first few days of refeeding. Administration of glucose causes extracellular phosphate depletion, which limits the ability of the red blood cell to carry oxygen because of decreased levels of 2,3-diphophosphoglycerate. Phosphate depletion can lead to cardiomyopathy, altered consciousness, hemolytic anemia, and death.
  - Monitor phosphate and other electrolytes at least every 24 hours (magnesium and potassium).
  - Give prophylactic phosphate supplement to prevent phosphorous depletion.

# DEPRESSION

## Definitions

- Major depressive episode
  - Depressed mood or loss of interest for at least 2 weeks
  - Four or more of the following: weight loss/gain, low energy/fatigue, insomnia/hypersomnia, psychomotor retardation/agitation, worthlessness/guilt, poor concentration/indecisiveness, and suicidality
- Dysthymic disorder
  - Irritable or depressed mood for most of the day, most days, for at least 1 year, with significant impairment in functioning
  - Two or more of the following: insomnia/hypersomnia, poor appetite/overeating, low self-esteem, helplessness, low energy/fatigue, and poor concentration/indecisiveness
  - No major depressive episode
- Adjustment disorder with depressed mood
  - Emotional symptoms within 3 months of onset of stressor
  - Distress/impairment in social/occupational/academic functioning
  - Depressed mood, tearfulness, or hopelessness
  - Once stressor has terminated, symptoms persist for no more than 6 months.

## Epidemiology

- The prevalence of major depression in adolescents is estimated at 5%–9% and dysthymic disorder at 3%–8%.
- The female-male ratio in adolescents is 2:1.
- Adolescents may not tell or admit they are depressed.
- Patients feel hopeless, worthless, and helpless.
- School problems, social withdrawal, substance abuse, somatic complaints, and high-risk behaviors should be red flags that a patient may be depressed.
- Risk factors: parental history of affective illness, history of abuse, chronic illness, loss through separation or death, medications, coexisting conditions such as attention-deficit hyperactivity disorder, or mild mental retardation or learning disabilities

## Treatment

- Counseling and medications together have been shown to be effective in treating major depression in adolescents.
- Treat at least for 6 months after initial episode, or 12 months if recurrent episode.
- Selective serotonin reuptake inhibitors (SSRIs), such as fluoxetine, sertraline, paroxetine, fluvoxamine, and citalopram, all show benefit over placebo.
  - Benefits may not be apparent for 4–6 weeks.
  - Response to one SSRI does not predict response to different SSRI.
  - Side effects are few. They may be gastrointestinal (nausea, vomiting, diarrhea, constipation, mouth dryness, appetite change, dyspepsia) or central nervous system–related (headache, nervousness, tremor, insomnia, confusion, fatigue, dizziness, decreased libido).
  - There is an FDA **"black box" warning** for SSRIs. Although overall the evidence shows that antidepressant use in depressed adolescents is beneficial, particularly in conjunction with cognitive behavioral therapy, this warning regarding increased thoughts of suicide may give pediatricians pause in prescribing SSRIs. Principles for treating adolescent depression developed by the Guidelines for Adolescent Depression in Primary Care (GLAD-PC) Working Group, which were published in 2007, were endorsed by the American Academy of Pediatrics. Some of the GLAD-PC recommendations for treatment and ongoing management include the following:
    - Collaboration with a mental health professional is necessary for patients with moderate/severe depression or coexisting psychosis or substance abuse, or if initial treatment is not successful.

- Practitioners should monitor for adverse events during SSRI treatment, with attempts to adhere to the FDA recommendations for follow-up.
- Involvement of the family is necessary in monitoring both response to treatment and adverse events related to medication.
- Regular tracking of outcomes and goals should occur in home, school, and peer settings.
■ Tricyclic antidepressants are not recommended in adolescents.
■ Major cause of failure is nonadherence; relapse rate is as high as 72% after 5 years.

# SUICIDE IN ADOLESCENTS

■ Any patient who talks about suicide should be taken seriously.

## Epidemiology

■ Suicide is the third most common cause of death in adolescents, in whom it represents 12% of all mortality.
■ The rate is four times higher in males, and males outnumber females 6:1 in completed suicides. However, attempts are more frequent in females.
■ Risk factors include: previous suicide attempts, affective disorders, family history or conflict, alcohol and substance abuse, impulsivity, and guns in the home.
■ There is often a precipitating factor and a motivation (gain attention, escape, communicate, express love or anger) in addition to preexisting social isolation.

## Treatment

■ When adolescents feel depressed, ask about their support system. Ask if they ever thought of hurting themselves, and if so, when; how; if they had a plan; if they would do it again; and if they feel the same way now.
■ When patients are suicidal or you are concerned about their safety, you should:
   ▪ Hospitalize.
   ▪ Consider psychiatric consultation.
   ▪ Involve the patient's parents and/or support system.
   ▪ Contract for safety.
   ▪ Consider antidepressant therapy.

# ALCOHOL AND DRUG ABUSE

## Definition and Epidemiology

■ Commonly abused drugs include alcohol, nicotine, marijuana, amphetamine ("speed") and methamphetamine, cocaine, methylenedioxymethamphetamine (MDMA; "ecstasy"), lysergic acid diethylamide (LSD), phencyclidine (PCP), heroin, prescription drugs (oxycodone, Demerol, methylphenidate), "huffing" volatile solvents, and anabolic steroids.
■ More than half of adolescents try an illicit drug before the end of high school.
   ▪ Almost one third of adolescents have used an illicit drug other than marijuana.
   ▪ It is estimated that 80%–90% of adolescents try alcohol by 18 years of age.
■ Drugs are widely present and available, even among older elementary and middle school children.
■ Regular alcohol and drug use; binge drinking; and related injuries, accidents, and physical consequences are problematic and unfortunately, not uncommon.
■ The CRAFFT screening tool for alcohol and drug abuse is for the adolescent age group (two or more "yes" answers is a positive screen).
   C: Have you ever ridden in a CAR driven by someone (including yourself) who was "high" or had been using alcohol or drugs?
   R: Do you ever use alcohol or drugs to RELAX, feel better about yourself, or fit in?

**A:** Do you ever use alcohol or drugs while you are ALONE?
**F:** Do you ever FORGET things that you did while using alcohol or drugs?
**F:** Do your family or FRIENDS ever tell you that you should cut down on your drinking or drug use?
**T:** Have you gotten into TROUBLE while using alcohol or drugs?

■ Contributing factors can include a genetic disposition for alcoholism, parental drug use and role modeling, peer influence, low self-esteem and personality disorders, and depression.

## Treatment

■ Recognize and treat addiction as a disease process.
■ Consider family involvement and support. Resources include Alcoholics Anonymous, National Council on Alcoholism and Drug Abuse, and other local resources for formal drug/alcohol abuse evaluation, counseling, and treatment options.

# CONSENT AND CONFIDENTIALITY

■ These issues are very important when caring for adolescents.
■ Always find out about the laws in your state.

## Definitions

■ Consent is an agreement to medical care (examination, testing, treatment, surgical procedures).
  ▪ Patients have the right to know about their health and treatment options, and the physician should respect their autonomy, rights, preferences (religious, social, cultural, philosophic) and decisions.
  ▪ When obtaining consent it is important to:
    • Provide information (illness, studies, treatments, risks/benefits, options).
    • Assess the patient's understanding.
    • Assess the patient's capacity for decision making.
    • Ensure the patient's freedom to choose.
  ▪ In most situations, a parent or guardian's consent is required for the medical care of a minor. However, there are certain exceptions where adolescents may give consent for their own medical care. Depending on the specific state laws, this may include:
    • An adult 18 years or older (for himself or herself)
    • A minor who is married, on active duty military, or is declared emancipated by the court
    • A parent for a minor child in his/her legal custody (including a minor parent who may consent for himself or herself or for his or her child)
    • Those who present requesting treatment for pregnancy; contraception; sexually transmitted disease testing and/or treatment, including HIV; and drug or substance abuse
■ Confidentiality is the agreement between the patient and the healthcare provider that information will not be shared without explicit permission of the patient.
  ▪ The goals of confidentiality are to protect the patient's privacy, ensure access to healthcare, and encourage open and honest communication.
  ▪ The Health Insurance Portability and Accountability Act (HIPAA) designates parents or guardians of unemancipated minors as "personal representatives" with access to their children's personal health information. This does **not** apply to evaluation and treatment of STDs, pregnancy, contraception, or substance abuse under most state laws. Depending on the state, if a minor seeks evaluation for pregnancy, STD, drug or substance abuse, and the results are negative, then a healthcare provider may be obligated to not release any of that information to parents.
    • It is important to know your state's specific statutes.
    • Further information about adolescent consent and confidentiality issues can be found at www.cahl.org, the Web site for The Center for Adolescent Health and the Law.
  ▪ Confidentiality cannot be maintained when the adolescent poses risk of harm to himself or herself, or to others.

## Suggested Readings

Centers for Disease Control and Prevention. HPV vaccine questions and answers, June 2006. www.cdc.gov/std/hpv/STDFact-HPV-vaccine.htm

Centers for Disease Control and Prevention. STD treatment guidelines, 2006. MMWR 2006;55/NoRR-11.

Centers for Disease Control and Prevention. Update to CDC's STD treatment guidelines, 2006: fluoroquinolones no longer recommended for treatment of gonococcal infections. MMWR April 13, 2007.

Cheung A, et al. Guidelines for adolescent depression in primary care (GLAD-PC): II. Treatment and ongoing management. Pediatrics 2007;120(5):e1313–1326.

Diagnostic and Statistical Manual of Mental Disorders. 4th Ed. Text Revision.

English A, Ford CA. The HIPAA privacy policy rule and adolescents: legal questions and clinical challenges. Perspect Sex Reprod Health 2004;36(2):80–86.

Fisher M. Treatment of eating disorders in children, adolescents and young adults. Pediatr Rev 2006;27(1):5–16.

Greydanus DE, et al. Contraception in the adolescent: an update. Pediatrics 2001;107(3):562–573.

Hatcher RA, Zieman M, et al. A Pocketguide to Managing Contraception. Tiger, Georgia: Bridging the Gap Foundation, 2005.

Knight J, et al. Validity of the CRAFFT substance abuse screening test among adolescent clinic patients. Arch Pediatr Adolesc Med 2002;156:607–614.

Leslie L, et al. The Food and Drug Administration's deliberations on antidepressant use in pediatric patients. Pediatrics 2005;116(1):195–204.

Neinstein LS. Adolescent health care: a practical guide. 4th Ed. Philadelphia: Lippincott Williams & Wilkins, 2002.

Simon G, Savarino J, Operskalski B, et al. Suicide risk during antidepressant treatment. Am J Psychiatry. 2006;163(1):41–47.

The Center for Adolescent Health and the Law Web site: www.cahl.org

Vasa R, Carlino A, Pine D. Pharmacotherapy of depressed children and adolescents: current issues and potential directions. Bio Psychiatry 2006;11:1021–1028.

World Health Organization: Medical eligibility criteria for contraceptive use. 3rd Ed. 2004. http://www.who.int/reproductive-health/publications/mec/

# ALLERGIC DISEASES

Leonard B. Bacharier, Caroline C. Horner,
Elyra D. Figueroa, Karen DeMuth,
Avraham Beigelman, Anne E. Borgmeyer, Patti M. Gyr,
Eli Silver, Lila C. Kertz, and Sthorn Thatayatikom

## ALLERGIC RHINITIS

- Allergic rhinitis is a common disease that affects approximately 40% of children and may have a significant effect on quality of life.
- Children of parents with allergies and/or asthma are genetically predisposed to develop allergic rhinitis.

### Pathophysiology

- In the early phase, mediators (histamine, tryptase) are released from mast cells when allergen-specific immunoglobulin E (IgE) antibodies are cross-linked by allergens and cause acute mucosal edema, mucous secretion, vascular leakage, and stimulation of sensory neurons.
- In the late phase, recruitment of inflammatory cells (neutrophils, eosinophils, basophils) causes persistent inflammation, which may last for days.

### History

- Symptoms include rhinorrhea, nasal congestion, postnasal drainage, sneezing, and pruritus.
- Determine whether symptoms are present throughout the year (perennial rhinitis), only during a particular season (seasonal rhinitis), or perennially with seasonal worsening. Also, determine whether symptoms are worse in a specific environment, such as at home with a pet, at daycare, or at school.
- Identify measures that relieve symptoms, such as antihistamine usage and avoidance.
- Common accompanying complaints are snoring, sore throat, frequent clearing of throat, cough, and hoarseness.

### Physical Examination

- Close inspection of the skin, eyes, ears, nose, and throat is important.
- Many children often have dark discoloration below the lower eyelids (allergic shiners) and prominent creases in the lower eyelid skin (Dennie-Morgan lines). A child who frequently rubs his or her nose (allergic salute) may develop a resultant transverse nasal crease.
- Significant findings on nasal examination include pale, boggy turbinates as a result of edema and clear nasal discharge.
- Mouth breathing may be observed.
- Cobblestoning in the posterior pharynx is a sign of follicular hypertrophy of mucosal lymphoid tissue.

### Evaluation

- Skin testing for environmental aeroallergens is sensitive and provides immediate information.
- Serum allergen-specific IgE measurements are also available for common allergens. This testing is best used for children with dermatographism, with diffuse eczema, or who cannot discontinue the use of antihistamines or β-blockers.

- Other results suggestive of allergies are peripheral blood eosinophilia, elevated serum IgE, and eosinophils on nasal smear.
- Rhinoscopy to directly visualize the nasal mucosa and upper airway is seldom used in the pediatric population.
- Differential diagnosis
  - Other common causes of rhinitis are infectious, anatomic/mechanical, or nonallergic factors.
  - In younger children, it may be difficult to differentiate allergy symptoms from recurrent upper respiratory viral infections. In the presence of fevers, headache, myalgias, or purulent nasal discharge, an acute viral process or sinusitis should be considered.
  - Obstructive symptoms and unilateral purulent nasal discharge may suggest a foreign body.
  - History of mouth breathing and snoring may suggest adenoidal hypertrophy.
  - Presence of nasal polyps requires the exclusion of cystic fibrosis.

## Treatment

- Avoidance through environmental control
  - Effective, nonpharmacologic measures require a conscious effort from the parents to minimize allergen exposure.
  - For outdoor allergens, limit outdoor activity during peak pollen hours. Close windows and use air conditioning.
  - Homes cannot be made "allergen free," but exposure to major indoor allergens can be reduced.
  - House dust mite avoidance includes changing bedding weekly and washing in hot water (>130°F); placing dust mite impermeable covers on the pillows, mattresses, and box springs; using a high efficiency particulate air (HEPA) filter vacuum; and removing carpeting in the bedroom.
  - Removing the pet from the home is ideal. If patients reject this option, keeping the pet out of the bedroom and restricting the pet to certain areas may be helpful.
  - HEPA filters reduce the amount of some airborne allergens.
  - Limiting and repairing water damage inhibits mold growth.
- Pharmacotherapy (Table 11-1)
  - Intranasal corticosteroids are potent anti-inflammatory agents that relieve rhinorrhea, sneezing, pruritus, and congestion.
    - These agents are indicated for both perennial and seasonal allergic rhinitis.
    - To optimize benefits, administer daily.
    - Side effects include epistaxis, burning/stinging, and oropharyngeal irritation. Review of proper intranasal administration or temporary discontinuation usually resolves these problems.
  - Antihistamines reduce rhinorrhea, sneezing, and pruritus but have little effect on congestion.
    - First-generation antihistamines are sedating and are sold over-the-counter in many combination allergy medicines (chlorpheniramine and diphenhydramine). Most are well tolerated with the exception of sedation and potential anticholinergic effects.
    - Newer second-generation antihistamines (loratadine, desloratadine, cetirizine, fexofenadine) are less likely to cross the blood-brain barrier, minimizing sedation. Most require a prescription and provide once-a-day dosing.
    - Azelastine is the only topical (intranasal) antihistamine available.
  - The leukotriene receptor antagonist montelukast is approved as monotherapy for allergic rhinitis.
    - This drug is most effective in patients who suffer from nasal congestion.
    - It is well tolerated with minimal adverse effects and may be indicated in children as young as 6 months.
  - A short 3–5 day course of systemic corticosteroids may rarely be used for severe disease.
  - Topical and systemic decongestants (oxymetazoline hydrochloride, pseudoephedrine, and phenylephrine) are effective for short-term relief of symptoms, such

**TABLE 11-1    Medications Used in the Treatment of Allergic Rhinitis**

| First-Generation antihistamines | |
| --- | --- |
| Diphenhydramine (Benadryl, Benylin) | <12 yr: 5 mg/kg/day PO divided t.i.d./q.i.d.; not to exceed 300 mg/day (use in neonates and premature infants contraindicated)<br>>12 yr: 25–50 mg PO q4–6h; not to exceed 400 mg/day |
| Hydroxyzine (Atarax, Vistaril, Vistazine) | 2 mg/kg/day PO divided q6h |
| **Second-Generation antihistamines** | |
| Cetirizine (Zyrtec) | <6 mo: Not established<br>6–12 mo: 2.5 mg PO daily<br>12–24 mo: 2.5 mg PO daily or b.i.d.<br>2–5 yr: 2.5–5 mg PO daily<br>>6 yr: 5–10 mg PO daily |
| Fexofenadine (Allegra) | <6 mo: Not established<br>6–23 mo: 15 mg PO b.i.d.<br>2–11 yr: 30 mg PO b.i.d.<br>≥12 yr: 60 mg PO b.i.d.; 180 mg PO daily |
| Loratadine (Claritin)<br>Desloratadine (Clarinex) | Loratadine<br><2 yr: Not established<br>2–5 yr: 5 mg PO daily<br>>5 yr: 10 mg PO daily<br>Desloratadine<br><6 mo: Not established<br>6–11 mo: 1 mg PO daily<br>12 mo–5 yr: 1.25 mg PO daily<br>6–11 yr: 2.5 mg PO daily<br>≥12 yr: 5 mg PO daily |
| **Leukotriene receptor antagonists** | |
| Montelukast (Singulair) | <6 mo: Not established<br>6 mo–5 yr: 4 mg PO daily<br>6–15 yr: 5 mg PO daily<br>>15 yr: 10 mg PO daily |
| **Nasal corticosteroids** | |
| Budesonide (Rhinocort Aqua) | <6 yr: Not established<br>6–12 yr: 1–2 puffs/nostril daily or divided b.i.d.; titrate to lowest effective dose<br>≥12 yr: 1–4 puffs/nostril (32 μg/puff) daily or divided b.i.d. |
| Fluticasone furoate (Veramyst) | <2 yr: Not established<br>2–11 yr: 1 spray each nostril once daily<br>≥12 yr: 2 sprays each nostril once daily |
| Fluticasone propionate (Flonase) | <4 yr: Not established<br>≥4 yr: 1–2 puffs/nostril (50 μg/puff) daily or 1 puff/nostril b.i.d.; not to exceed 4 puffs/day (200 μg) |
| Mometasone furoate monohydrate (Nasonex) | <2 yr: Not established<br>2–11 yr: 1 spray daily<br>≥12 yr: 2 sprays daily |
| Triamcinolone (Nasacort AQ) | 6–12 yr: 1–2 sprays/nostril daily; start with 1 spray/day; max 2 sprays/nostril/day<br>≥12 yr: 1–2 sprays/nostril daily; start with 2 sprays/day; max 2 sprays/nostril/day |

as rhinorrhea and congestion. Restrict the use of topical decongestants to 3–5 days to avoid rhinitis medicamentosa.
- Intranasal mast cell stabilizers (Cromolyn) inhibit mast cell degranulation, are best used prophylactically, and are well tolerated with minimal adverse effects.
- Immunotherapy
  - The exact mechanism of immunotherapy remains unclear, but it reduces the levels of circulating specific IgE and increases allergen-specific IgG levels.
  - It is indicated in children who are not responsive to maximal pharmacotherapy and in some children with asthma.
  - Treatment is individualized and based on identified sensitizations to allergens. Immunotherapy requires commitment from the parents and child.
  - With the known risk of anaphylaxis, immunotherapy should be prescribed only by physicians trained in allergy and immunotherapy.

# ALLERGIC CONJUNCTIVITIS

- Allergic conjunctivitis is frequently seen concomitantly with allergic rhinitis.
- Pathophysiology is similar to that for allergic rhinitis and involves the same mediators and inflammatory cells.

## History and Physical Examination

- Diagnosis begins by history and physical examination.
- Allergic conjunctivitis is characterized by acute onset, bilateral involvement, clear watery discharge, and pruritus.
- On examination, there is bilateral hyperemia and edema of the conjunctivae.

## Evaluation

- Skin testing is the most sensitive diagnostic evaluation for identifying allergens.
- Ocular allergen challenge is sensitive but seldom used clinically.
- Differential diagnosis
  - Bacterial conjunctivitis is characterized by acute onset, thick purulent discharge, minimal pain, and history of exposure. It occurs with unilateral disease that may subsequently infect the contralateral side.
  - Viral conjunctivitis is characterized by acute/subacute onset, clear watery discharge, and history of recent upper respiratory infection.
  - Keratoconjunctivitis
    - Vernal keratoconjunctivitis is chronic bilateral inflammation of conjunctiva with the presence of giant papillae on the superior tarsal conjunctiva with ropy mucous discharge. Itching is the most common symptom, with photophobia, foreign body sensation, tearing, and blepharospasm as other reported symptoms.
    - Atopic keratoconjunctivitis is bilateral inflammation of conjunctiva and eyelids associated with atopic dermatitis. The most common symptom is bilateral itching of the eyelids, and symptoms are perennial.
    - Both vernal and atopic keratoconjunctivitis are sight-threatening disorders requiring immediate referral to an ophthalmologist.

## Treatment

- Identification and avoidance of the identified allergen is necessary.
- Artificial tear substitutes provide a barrier function, wash away allergens, and dilute inflammatory mediators.
- Topical antihistamines may provide relief of acute symptoms. They have a rapid onset of action.
- Mast cell stabilizers inhibit mast cell degranulation and the release of inflammatory mediators. Combination mast cell stabilizers/antihistamines are the most effective therapy (Table 11-2).

| TABLE 11-2 | Medications Used in the Treatment of Allergic Conjunctivitis |
|---|---|
| **Topical antihistamines/Mast cell stabilizers** | |
| Azelastine (Optivar)* | 1 gtts b.i.d. |
| Epinastine (Elestat)* | 1 gtts b.i.d. |
| Olopatadine (Patanol)* | 1 gtts b.i.d. |
| Ketotifen (Zaditor)* | 1 gtts q8–12h |
| *Use in children <3 yr of age is not established. | |

- Topical vasoconstrictors reduce injection but have little effect on pruritus or swelling. Continued use may cause conjunctivitis medicamentosa.
- Topical corticosteroids are usually not indicated for allergic conjunctivitis. Referral to an ophthalmologist is indicated for conditions requiring these agents.
- Topical medications are well tolerated. The difficulty of administrating eyedrops in a child and the frequency of dosing are the most common limiting factors.

## ATOPIC DERMATITIS (ECZEMA)

- Atopic dermatitis is a chronic relapsing and remitting inflammatory skin disease characterized by dermatitis with typical morphology and distribution.
- Eczema is a generic term for a constellation of clinical signs, whereas atopic dermatitis is a term that specifically connotes an allergic contribution to the etiology of the eczema.
- The overall prevalence of atopic dermatitis in the United States is 17% among school-aged children, leading to considerable disease-related morbidity, including irritability, secondary skin infections, sleep disturbance, school absenteeism, and poor self-image.

### History

- Age of onset is a consideration, with 45% of affected individuals manifesting atopic dermatitis in the first 6 months of life, 60% by the first year, and 85% by school age.
- Pruritus is a cardinal feature of eczema, often described as the "itch that rashes." Scratching leads to further compromise in the skin barrier and augments inflammation.
- Xerosis (dry skin) also involves nonlesional skin. (In other conditions, commonly mistaken for atopic dermatitis (seborrheic dermatitis, nummular eczema, and psoriasis), the uninvolved skin is generally healthy.)
- Patients may have a personal and family history of atopy (asthma, hay fever, food allergy).
- Exacerbating factors include food allergens (most frequently egg, milk, wheat, soy, peanut, tree nuts, shellfish) and inhalant allergens (e.g., pet dander, house dust mite).
- Systemic involvement, with failure to thrive, chronic diarrhea, and/or recurrent infections should prompt consideration of underlying systemic disease, such as immunodeficiency (e.g., Wiskott-Aldrich syndrome, Netherton syndrome, immune dysregulation polyendocrinopathy enteropathy X-linked (IPEX) syndrome, and hyper-IgE syndrome), or malabsorption (e.g., zinc deficiency or cystic fibrosis).

### Physical Examination

- Xerosis
- Morphology of lesions
  - Acute lesions: pruritic papules with excoriation and serous exudation
  - Chronic lesions: lichenified papules and plaques
  - Superficial linear abrasions from scratching
  - Indistinct lesional borders, unlike that of psoriasis

- Areas of involvement. Although atopic dermatitis may appear anywhere on the body, characteristic patterns include:
  - Infants: cheeks, forehead, and extensor surface of extremities
  - Children/adolescents: flexor surface of extremities popliteal and antecubital fossae, and ventral surface of wrists and ankles
  - Atypical areas: diaper region (as a result of a lack of access to scratch the area) and nasolabial folds (commonly involved in seborrheic dermatitis)

## Evaluation

- Diagnosis is based on clinical features. Skin biopsy is not essential for diagnosis. Identify factors that exacerbate atopic dermatitis.
- Food allergy
  - One third of children with moderate to severe atopic dermatitis experience worsening of eczema when exposed to food allergens.
  - Percutaneous skin tests, food-specific serum IgE, and oral food challenges may help identify specific foods.
- Aeroallergen sensitivity
- Infections
  - Bacteria. *Staphylococcus aureus* colonizes (cutaneous, nasal, or both) 80%–90% of individuals with atopic dermatitis, potentially leading to superinfection and/or production of superantigens and augmenting cutaneous inflammation.
  - Cutaneous viruses
    - Herpes simplex virus (eczema herpeticum). These vesicles and/or individual "punched out" lesions have an erythematous base. Confirm by herpes simplex virus polymerase chain reaction test or Tzanck smear from a newly unroofed vesicle.
    - Molluscum contagiosum
  - *Malassezia sympodialis* (formerly *Pityrosporum ovale*): Consider in individuals with recalcitrant eczema, especially with lesions concentrated on the head, neck, and upper torso. Sensitivity to *M. sympodialis* (by skin prick test or specific IgE determination) is diagnostic. Treatment is oral antifungal therapy (itraconazole).
- Differential diagnosis
  - Dermatologic disease: seborrheic dermatitis, psoriasis, nummular eczema, irritant or allergic contact dermatitis, keratosis pilaris, ichthyosis, lichen simplex chronicus, and Netherton syndrome
  - Infections: scabies, tinea corporis, tinea versicolor, and HIV-associated eczema
  - Metabolic disease: zinc or biotin deficiency and phenylketonuria
  - Immunodeficiency: see earlier discussion
  - Neoplastic disease: mycosis fungoides (cutaneous T-cell lymphoma) and Langerhans histocytosis

## Treatment

- Limiting exposure to triggers
  - Nonspecific irritants. Wear nonocclusive clothing, and avoid wool or synthetic material.
  - Allergens. Eliminate contact with established allergic triggers (food or aeroallergen) if identified.
- Topical therapy
  - Emollients. Rehydration of the skin is key to stopping the "itch-scratch" cycle by the "soak and seal" method. Daily baths with lukewarm water for 10–20 minutes followed by application of a thick emollient cream are necessary.
  - Topical steroids, which are the gold standard of therapy for treatment of acutely inflamed areas
    - Use mild to moderate potency steroids in children (e.g., hydrocortisone 1% ointment and triamcinolone 0.1% ointment, respectively).
    - Use only mild potency steroid on face, genital, and intertriginous areas.

- Topical calcineurin inhibitors, such as pimecrolimus and tacrolimus
  - Nonsteroidal topical agents are effective in treating atopic dermatitis and are approved for children 2 years of age and older.
  - A U.S. Food and Drug Administration "black box" warning exists for topical calcineurin inhibitors, recommending these drugs as second-line treatment options.
  - Wet-wrap therapy. This involves applying a damp wet layer of cotton dressing (or cotton pajamas) over the topical emollients and then placing a layer of dry clothing above.

- Antimicrobial therapy
  - Topical antiseptics (mupirocin, triclosan, or chlorhexidine) may be applied to open excoriated areas. Intranasal mupirocin may be used to eradicate nasal carriage of *S. aureus* if detected. Neomycin should be avoided because it can cause contact dermatitis.
  - Bleach baths, which may decrease colonization. Add 1–2 cups of household bleach per bathtub (adding a cup of table salt may diminish the stinging sensation).
  - Systemic antibiotics
    - If there is evidence of bacterial superinfection (e.g., honey-crusted lesions), systemic antistaphylococcal antibiotics are indicated; a 5- to 10-day course is usually sufficient.
    - Prophylactic therapy is not advised because of the emergence of bacterial resistance.

- Systemic corticosteroids. These agents are effective in short courses, but the systemic side-effect profile limits long-term applicability.
- Systemic antihistamines
  - The major therapeutic value of systemic antihistamines resides in the sedative effect of first-generation histamine blockers, which helps minimize scratching and discomfort at night. Nonsedating antihistamines provide a modest reduction in pruritus.
  - Topical antihistamines should be avoided because they may cause sensitization and worsen disease.
- Other therapies: ultraviolet light (PUVA), systemic cyclosporine, azathioprine, and immunotherapy

## Special Considerations

- Associated atopic disorders. Atopic dermatitis in early childhood may herald progression toward other allergic conditions. This is known as the atopic march (allergic rhinitis and asthma).
- Prevention
  - Exclusive breastfeeding for at least 4 months reduces the risk of atopic dermatitis, although the protective effect wanes by 3 years of age.
  - In infants with atopic dermatitis, consider delaying introduction of commonly allergenic food: cow's milk until 12 months; eggs until 24 months; and peanuts, tree nuts, and seafood until 36 months.

- Natural history. Among children with onset of atopic dermatitis before 2 years of age, 60% experience complete remission, 20% have intermittent symptoms, and 20% have persistent disease by 7 years of age.

# ASTHMA

## Definition

- Asthma is a reversible obstructive lung disease that is characterized by airway inflammation and hyperreactivity with airway mucosal edema, bronchoconstriction, and mucous plugging.
- Clinically, asthma presents with recurrent episodes of wheezing, coughing, and increased work of breathing.
- Diagnosis is based on previous history, presence of wheezing, coughing, and increased work of breathing that resolves in response to treatment with bronchodilators and

| TABLE 11-3 | Differential Diagnosis for Wheezing Not Responsive to Asthma Therapy |
|---|---|
| Infection | Mass |
| Foreign body | Bronchopulmonary dysplasia |
| Anatomic abnormalities | Congestive heart failure |
| Allergy | Cystic fibrosis |
| Sinusitis | Chronic aspiration |
| Vocal cord dysfunction | Gastroesophageal reflux disease |

corticosteroids. Many conditions may present with wheezing and must be considered, especially in patients who present with a first episode of wheezing and/or are not responsive to asthma therapy (Table 11-3).

## History

- History of current episode: precipitating factors, onset and progression of symptoms, treatment, and response to treatment
- Chronic history
  - Age of first episode, age at time of diagnosis, and course of the illness over time; typical signs and symptoms as well as precipitating factors (triggers)
  - Medication use: dosage, frequency, route, and schedule of all quick relief and control medications; effect of missed doses of medications; side effects; and adverse reactions
  - Assessment of chronic asthma severity (the intrinsic intensity of the disease process) to initiate therapy
    - Determine severity by quantifying frequency of daytime symptoms, nighttime symptoms, rescue β-agonist use, and interference with activity.
    - See Table 11-4, assessing both domains of impairment (frequency and intensity of symptoms and functional impairment the patient is currently experiencing or has recently experienced) and risk (the likelihood of either asthma exacerbations, progressive decline in lung function or growth, or risk of adverse effects of medications). This classification scheme is most appropriate for patients who are not receiving controller therapy.
  - Assessment of asthma control to adjust therapy
    - Determine number of school days missed because of asthma; number of previous emergency visits and admissions, including intensive care with or without intubation; prior use of oral steroids, including number of previous steroid bursts and date of last steroid course; and frequency of albuterol usage.
    - Use Table 11-5, assessing both domains of impairment and risk, to determine level of asthma control. This approach is most appropriate for patients already receiving controller therapy.
  - Environmental history: exposure to allergens (mold, pollen, animals, dust mites, cockroaches) and nonspecific airway irritants (smoke, odors)
  - Review of systems
    - Focus on allergy; eczema; infection, especially pneumonia; ear, nose, and throat, including otitis media, sinusitis, airway abnormalities, surgery and obstructive sleep apnea; and gastrointestinal, including gastroesophageal reflux, nutrition, and growth.
    - Previous testing (e.g., chest radiograph, pulmonary function testing, allergy testing, and sweat test) should be documented.
  - Family history: asthma, allergy, eczema, and cystic fibrosis
  - Social history to determine barriers to healthcare, particularly insurance coverage and transportation

TABLE 11-4

# Classifying Asthma Severity and Initiating Therapy in Children

## Classifying Asthma Severity and Initiating Therapy in Children

| Components of Severity | | Intermittent | | Persistent | | | | | |
|---|---|---|---|---|---|---|---|---|---|
| | | | | Mild | | Moderate | | Severe | |
| | | Ages 0–4 | Ages 5–11 | Ages 0–4 | Ages 5–11 | Ages 0–4 | Ages 5–11 | Ages 0–4 | Ages 5–11 |
| Impairment | Symptoms | ≤2 days/week | ≤2 days/week | >2 days/week but not daily | >2 days/week | Daily | Daily | Throughout the day | Throughout the day |
| | Nighttime awakenings | 0 | ≤2x/month | 1–2x/month | 3–4x/month | 3–4x/month | >1x/week but not nightly | >1x/week | Often 7x/week |
| | Short-acting beta₂-agonist use for symptom control | ≤2 days/week | ≤2 days/week | >2 days/week but not daily | >2 days/week but not daily | Daily | Daily | Several times per day | Often 7x/week |
| | Interference with normal activity | None | None | Minor limitation | Minor limitation | Some limitation | Some limitation | Extremely limited | Extremely limited |
| | Lung Function • FEV₁ (predicted) or peak flow (personal best) • FEV₁/FVC | N/A | Normal FEV₁ between exacerbations >80% >85% | N/A | >80% >80% | N/A | 60–80% 75–80% | N/A | <60% <75% |
| Risk | Exacerbations requiring oral systemic corticosteroids (consider severity and interval since last exacerbation) | 0–1/year (see notes) | 0–1/year (see notes) | ≥2 exacerbations in 6 months requiring oral systemic corticosteroids, or ≥4 wheezing episodes/1 year lasting >1 day AND risk factors for persistent asthma | ≥2x/year (see notes) Relative annual risk may be related to FEV₁ | | | | |

| Recommended Step for Initiating Therapy (See "Stepwise Approach for Managing Asthma" for treatment steps.) The stepwise approach is meant to assist, not replace, the clinical decisionmaking required to meet individual patient needs. | Step 1 (for both age groups) | | Step 2 (for both age groups) | | Step 3 and consider short course of oral systemic corticosteroids | Step 3: medium-dose ICS option and consider short course of oral systemic corticosteroids | Step 3 and consider short course of oral systemic corticosteroids | Step 3: medium-dose ICS option OR step 4 and consider short course of oral systemic corticosteroids |
|---|---|---|---|---|---|---|---|---|

In 2–6 weeks, depending on severity, evaluate level of asthma control that is achieved.
• Children 0–4 years old: If no clear benefit is observed at 4–6 weeks, stop treatment and consider alternative diagnoses or adjusting therapy.
• Children 5–11 years old: Adjust therapy accordingly.

Key: FEV₁, forced expiratory volume in 1 second; FVC, forced vital capacity; ICS, inhaled corticosteroids; ICU, intensive care unit; N/A, not applicable

**Notes:**
- Level of severity is determined by both impairment and risk. Assess impairment domain by caregiver's recall of previous 2–4 weeks. Assign severity to the most severe category in which any feature occurs.
- Frequency and severity of exacerbations may fluctuate over time for patients in any severity category. At present, there are inadequate data to correspond frequencies of exacerbations with different levels of asthma severity. In general, more frequent and severe exacerbations (e.g., requiring urgent, unscheduled care, hospitalization, or ICU admission) indicate greater underlying disease severity. For treatment purposes, patients with ≥2 exacerbations described above may be considered the same as patients who have persistent asthma, even in the absence of impairment levels consistent with persistent asthma.

*(continued)*

**TABLE 11-4** Classifying Asthma Severity and Initiating Therapy in Children *(Continued)*

## Classification of Asthma Severity ≥12 years of age

| Components of Severity | | Intermittent | Persistent | | |
|---|---|---|---|---|---|
| | | | Mild | Moderate | Severe |
| **Impairment** Normal FEV₁/FVC: 8–19 yr 85% 20–39 yr 80% 40–59 yr 75% 60–80 yr 70% | Symptoms | ≤2 days/week | >2 days/week but not daily | Daily | Throughout the day |
| | Nighttime awakenings | ≤2x/month | 3–4x/month | >1x/week but not nightly | Often 7x/week |
| | Short-acting beta₂-agonist use for symptom control (not prevention of EIB) | ≤2 days/week | >2 days/week but not daily, and not more than 1x on any day | Daily | Several times per day |
| | Interference with normal activity | None | Minor limitation | Some limitation | Extremely limited |
| | Lung function | • Normal FEV₁, between exacerbations • FEV₁ >80% predicted • FEV₁/FVC normal | • FEV₁ >80% predicted • FEV₁/FVC normal | • FEV₁ >60% but <80% predicted • FEV₁/FVC reduced 5% | • FEV₁ <60% predicted • FEV₁/FVC reduced >5% |
| **Risk** | Exacerbations requiring oral systemic corticosteroids | 0–1/year (see note) | ≥2/year (see note) → Consider severity and interval since last exacerbation. Frequency and severity may fluctuate over time for patients in any severity category. Relative annual risk of exacerbations may be related to FEV₁. | | |
| **Recommended Step for Initiating Treatment** (See "Stepwise Approach for Managing Asthma" for treatment steps.) | | Step 1 | Step 2 | Step 3 and consider short course of oral systemic corticosteroids | Step 4 or 5 and consider short course of oral systemic corticosteroids |
| | | In 2–6 weeks, evaluate level of asthma control that is achieved and adjust therapy accordingly. | | | |

Key: EIB, exercise-induced bronchospasm; FEV₁, forced expiratory volume in 1 second; FVC, forced vital capacity; ICU, intensive care unit

**Notes:**
- The stepwise approach is meant to assist, not replace, the clinical decisionmaking required to meet individual patient needs.
- Level of severity is determined by assessment of both impairment and risk. Assess impairment domain by patient's/caregiver's recall of previous 2–4 weeks and spirometry. Assign severity to the most severe category in which any feature occurs.
- At present, there are inadequate data to correspond frequencies of exacerbations with different levels of asthma severity. In general, more frequent and intense exacerbations (e.g., requiring urgent, unscheduled care, hospitalization, or ICU admission) indicate greater underlying disease severity. For treatment purposes, patients who had ≥2 exacerbations requiring oral systemic corticosteroids in the past year may be considered the same as patients who have persistent asthma, even in the absence of impairment levels consistent with persistent asthma.

From the National Heart, Lung, and Blood Institute, National Institutes of Health, Guidelines for the Diagnosis and Management of Asthma. NIH Publication No. 97-4051, July 1997.

## TABLE 11-5 Assessing Asthma Control and Adjusting Therapy in Children

### Assessing Asthma Control and Adjusting Therapy in Children

| Components of Control | | Well Controlled | | Not Well Controlled | | Very Poorly Controlled | |
|---|---|---|---|---|---|---|---|
| | | Ages 0-4 | Ages 5-11 | Ages 0-4 | Ages 5-11 | Ages 0-4 | Ages 5-11 |
| **Impairment** | Symptoms | ≤2 days/week but not more than once on each day | | >2 days/week or multiple times on ≤2 days/week | | Throughout the day | |
| | Nighttime awakenings | ≤1x/month | | >1x/week | ≥2x/month | >1x/week | ≥2x/week |
| | Interference with normal activity | None | | Some limitation | | Extremely limited | |
| | Short-acting beta₂-agonist use for symptom control (not prevention of EIB) | ≤2 days/week | | >2 days/week | | Several times per day | |
| | Lung function<br>• FEV₁ (predicted) or peak flow (personal best) | N/A | >80% | N/A | 60-80% | N/A | <60% |
| | • FEV₁/FVC | | >80% | | 75-80% | | <75% |
| **Risk** | Exacerbations requiring oral systemic corticosteroids | 0-1x/year | | 2-3x/year | ≥2x/year | >3x/year | ≥2x/year |
| | Reduction in lung growth | N/A | Requires long-term followup | N/A | | N/A | |
| | Treatment-related adverse effects | Medication side effects can vary in intensity from none to very troublesome and worrisome. The level of intensity does not correlate to specific levels of control but should be considered in the overall assessment of risk. | | | | | |
| **Recommended Action for Treatment**<br>(See "Stepwise Approach for Managing Asthma" for treatment steps.)<br><br>The stepwise approach is meant to assist, not replace, clinical decisionmaking required to meet individual patient needs. | | • Maintain current step.<br>• Regular followup every 1-6 months.<br>• Consider step down if well controlled for at least 3 months. | | Step up 1 step | Step up at least 1 step | • Consider short course of oral systemic corticosteroids;<br>• Step up 1-2 steps | |

• Before step up:
  — Review adherence to medication, inhaler technique, and environmental control.
  — If alternative treatment was used, discontinue it and use preferred treatment for that step.
• Reevaluate the level of asthma control in 2-6 weeks to achieve control;
  every 1-6 months to maintain control.
  Children 0-4 years old: If no clear benefit is observed in 4-6 weeks, consider alternative diagnoses or adjusting therapy.
  Children 5-11 years old: Adjust therapy accordingly.
• For side effects, consider alternative treatment options.

Key: EIB, exercise-induced bronchospasm; FEV₁, forced expiratory volume in 1 second; FVC, forced vital capacity; ICU, intensive care unit; N/A, not applicable

**Notes:**
- The level of control is based on the most severe impairment or risk category. Assess impairment domain by patient's or caregiver's recall of previous 2-4 weeks. Symptom assessment for longer periods should reflect a global assessment, such as whether the patient's asthma is better or worse since the last visit.
- At present, there are inadequate data to correspond frequencies of exacerbations with different levels of asthma control. In general, more frequent and intense exacerbations (e.g., requiring urgent, unscheduled care, hospitalization, or ICU admission) indicate poorer disease control.

*(continued)*

141

**TABLE 11-5** Assessing Asthma Control and Adjusting Therapy in Children *(Continued)*

| Components of Control | | | Classification of Asthma Control (≥12 years of age) | | | |
|---|---|---|---|---|---|---|
| | | | Well Controlled | Not Well Controlled | Very Poorly Controlled | |
| Impairment | Symptoms | | ≤2 days/week | >2 days/week | Throughout the day | |
| | Nighttime awakenings | | ≤2x/month | 1–3x/week | ≥4x/week | |
| | Interference with normal activity | | None | Some limitation | Extremely limited | |
| | Short-acting beta₂-agonist use for symptom control (not prevention of EIB) | | ≤2 days/week | >2 days/week | Several times per day | |
| | FEV₁ or peak flow | | >80% predicted/ personal best | 60–80% predicted/ personal best | <60% predicted/ personal best | |
| | Validated questionnaires | ATAQ | 0 | 1–2 | 3–4 | |
| | | ACQ | ≤0.75* | ≥1.5 | N/A | |
| | | ACT | ≥20 | 16–19 | ≤15 | |
| Risk | Exacerbations requiring oral systemic corticosteroids | | 0–1/year | ≥2/year (see note) | | |
| | | | | Consider severity and interval since last exacerbation | | |
| | Progressive loss of lung function | | Evaluation requires long-term followup care. | | | |
| | Treatment-related adverse effects | | Medication side effects can vary in intensity from none to very troublesome and worrisome. The level of intensity does not correlate to specific levels of control but should be considered in the overall assessment of risk. | | | |
| Recommended Action for Treatment (See "Stepwise Approach for Managing Asthma" for treatment steps.) | | | • Maintain current step.<br>• Regular followups at every 1–6 months to maintain control.<br>• Consider step down if well controlled for at least 3 months. | • Step up 1 step.<br>• Reevaluate in 2–6 weeks.<br>• For side effects, consider alternative treatment options. | • Consider short course of oral systemic corticosteroids.<br>• Step up 1–2 steps.<br>• Reevaluate in 2 weeks.<br>• For side effects, consider alternative treatment options. | |

*ACQ values of 0.76–1.4 are indeterminate regarding well-controlled asthma.

Key: EIB, exercise-induced bronchospasm; ICU, intensive care unit

**Notes:**

- The stepwise approach is meant to assist, not replace, the clinical decisionmaking required to meet individual patient needs.

- The level of control is based on the most severe impairment or risk category. Assess impairment domain by patient's recall of previous 2–4 weeks and by spirometry/or peak flow measures. Symptom assessment for longer periods should reflect a global assessment, such as inquiring whether the patient's asthma is better or worse since the last visit.

- At present, there are inadequate data to correspond frequencies of exacerbations with different levels of asthma control. In general, more frequent and intense exacerbations (e.g., requiring urgent, unscheduled care, hospitalization, or ICU admission) indicate poorer disease control. For treatment purposes, patients who had ≥2 exacerbations requiring oral systemic corticosteroids in the past year may be considered the same as patients who have not-well-controlled asthma, even in the absence of impairment levels consistent with not-well-controlled asthma.

ATAQ = Asthma Therapy Assessment Questionnaire©
ACQ = Asthma Control Questionnaire©
ACT = Asthma Control Test™
Minimal Important
Difference: 1.0 for the ATAQ; 0.5 for the ACQ; not determined for the ACT.

**Before step up in therapy:**

— Review adherence to medication, inhaler technique, environmental control, and comorbid conditions.

— If an alternative treatment option was used in a step, discontinue and use the preferred treatment for that step.

From the National Heart, Lung, and Blood Institute, National Institutes of Health, Guidelines for the Diagnosis and Management of Asthma. NIH Publication No. 97-4051, July 1997.

| TABLE 11-6 | Respiratory Rate for Children By Age |
|---|---|

| Age | Normal rate |
|---|---|
| <2 mo | 60 bpm* |
| 2–12 mo | 50 bpm |
| 1–5 yr | 40 bpm |
| 6–11 yr | 30 bpm |
| 12 and older | 20 bpm |

*Breaths per minute

## Physical Examination

- A rapid assessment should be initially performed to determine patients requiring immediate attention.
- Assessment should include color, vital signs, oxygen saturation, quality of air exchange, presence of wheezing or crackles, ratio of time spent in inspiration relative to expiration, accessory muscle use, ability to speak in sentences, and mental status.
- See Table 11-6 for a guide to normal respiratory rate by age.

## Laboratory Studies

- A chest radiograph is not routinely required but may be considered if this is the first episode of wheezing, the patient is febrile, there is marked asymmetry on chest examination, or there is poor response to treatment.
- Pulse oximetry can be used to estimate oxygen saturation.
- Arterial blood gas measurement should be considered in patients in severe distress or with increasing supplemental oxygen requirement. Capillary blood gas measurement is of limited value in evaluation of oxygenation.
- If the child is 7 years of age or older, peak flow monitoring can be helpful to assess the level of obstruction, severity of the exacerbation, and the response to treatment. If a personal best peak flow is not known, see Table 11-7 for predicted peak flow value by height.
- Spirometry is not usually performed in the inpatient or emergency department setting but should be considered if symptoms suggest vocal cord dysfunction or there is a discrepancy between physical assessment and clinical progress.
- Chest fluoroscopy or bronchoscopy should be considered if the history suggests possibility of foreign body aspiration.
- White blood cell (WBC) count, potassium, and glucose levels may be affected by β-agonists and oral steroids (elevated total WBC and blood glucose, low levels of potassium). Thus, these studies are likely be of little value during an acute exacerbation.
- A nasopharyngeal swab or aspirate may be helpful in identifying viral infection and to guide establishing cohorts of patients within the hospital.
- A sweat chloride test may be performed to evaluate for cystic fibrosis as the cause of chronic symptoms.

## Treatment During Acute Episode

- Oxygen should be administered to maintain oxygen saturation 90% and above.
  - If possible, obtain baseline oxygen saturation in room air before initiating oxygen. It is not unusual for oxygen saturation to drop transiently after albuterol treatments; this is likely due to ventilation-perfusion mismatch and usually resolves in 15 to 30 minutes.
  - Continuous oximetry is not typically necessary.
  - Check $SpO_2$ with any significant change in respiratory status. As symptoms improve, wean oxygen as tolerated.

| TABLE 11-7 | Predicted Peak Flow by Height |

| Predicted peak flow rate based on height | | | | |
|---|---|---|---|---|
| Height (cm) | Height (in) | Predicted Peak Flow | 80% Predicted | 50% Predicted |
| 120 | 47.0 | 210 | 170 | 100 |
| 126 | 49.5 | 240 | 190 | 120 |
| 128 | 50.0 | 250 | 200 | 130 |
| 130 | 51.0 | 260 | 210 | 130 |
| 132 | 52.0 | 270 | 220 | 130 |
| 134 | 53.0 | 280 | 220 | 140 |
| 136 | 53.5 | 290 | 230 | 140 |
| 138 | 54.5 | 300 | 240 | 150 |
| 140 | 55.0 | 310 | 250 | 150 |
| 142 | 56.0 | 320 | 250 | 160 |
| 144 | 56.5 | 330 | 260 | 160 |
| 146 | 57.5 | 330 | 260 | 160 |
| 148 | 58.0 | 340 | 270 | 170 |
| 150 | 59.0 | 350 | 280 | 180 |
| 152 | 60.0 | 360 | 290 | 180 |
| 154 | 60.5 | 370 | 300 | 180 |
| 156 | 61.5 | 380 | 300 | 190 |
| 158 | 62.0 | 390 | 310 | 200 |
| 160 | 63.0 | 400 | 320 | 200 |
| 162 | 64.0 | 410 | 330 | 200 |
| 164 | 64.5 | 410 | 330 | 200 |
| 166 | 65.5 | 430 | 340 | 210 |
| 168 | 66.0 | 440 | 350 | 220 |
| 170 | 67.0 | 450 | 360 | 220 |
| 172 | 68.0 | 460 | 370 | 230 |
| 174 | 68.5 | 460 | 370 | 230 |
| 176 | 69.0 | 470 | 380 | 240 |
| 178 | 70.0 | 480 | 390 | 240 |
| 180 | 71.0 | 490 | 390 | 250 |

Adapted from Murray AB, Cook CD. Measurement of peak expiratory flow rate in 220 normal children ages 4.5–18.5 yr old. J Pediatr 1963;62:186–189.

- Inhaled $\beta_2$-agonists reverse airflow obstruction quickly.
  - If exacerbation is mild, two to four puffs of albuterol by metered dose inhaler (MDI) may be given with spacer every 20 minutes for 1 hour as initial therapy. Albuterol may also be given via nebulizer.
  - See Table 11-8 for emergency dosing of albuterol and protocol guiding emergency department care.
  - During hospitalization, albuterol nebulization treatments (2.5–5 mg) are provided every 1–2 hours and gradually weaned to every 4 hours as the patient's symptoms and status improve.
    - In mild to moderate exacerbations, MDI plus valved holding chamber is as effective as nebulized therapy with appropriate administration technique and coaching by trained personnel.
    - Patients whose clinical status tolerates albuterol treatments every 4 hours are usually discharged home.

**TABLE 11-8   Emergency Dosing of Albuterol**

| kg | Albuterol (mg) | Albuterol (mL) | Atrovent (μg)* | Total volume |
|---|---|---|---|---|
| **Short albuterol treatments**<br>(O₂: 7 L/min; may increase to keep saturation >95%) | | | | |
| 10–30 | 2.5 | 0.5 | 1 vial | 3.0 mL |
| 30–50 | 5.0 | 1.0 | 1 vial | 3.5 mL |
| >50 | 10.0 | 2.0 | 1 vial | 4.5 mL |

| kg | Albuterol (mg) | Albuterol (mL) | Normal saline (mL)* | Total volume |
|---|---|---|---|---|
| **Continuous albuterol treatments**<br>(O₂: 5 L/min; may increase to keep saturation >95%) | | | | |
| 10–30 | 2.5 | 0.5 | 1 vial | 8.0 mL |
| 30–50 | 5.0 | 1.0 | 1 vial | 8.0 mL |
| >50 | 10.0 | 2.0 | 1 vial | 8.0 mL |

*Only give Atrovent in first two treatments.

- Systemic corticosteroids 2 mg/kg/day (60 mg maximum dose) are given promptly on presentation and typically continued daily for 5 days, typically administered in the morning.
  - Oral dosing is preferred, but intravenous (IV) therapy may be appropriate if the patient is vomiting or intensive care therapy seems likely. If IV Solu-Medrol is necessary, it is recommended to divide dose for every 6 hour administration.
  - Tapering corticosteroids over a longer period of time is recommended for severe exacerbations or if recent (<1 month) course of oral corticosteroids.
- Ipratropium bromide (Atrovent) 0.5 mg may provide additional bronchodilator effect when added to nebulized albuterol treatments during the first 24 hours of the exacerbation. There is no evidence that use after the first 24 hours provides additional benefit.
- Adjunctive treatments, such as IV magnesium sulfate or helium-oxygen mixtures (Heliox), may be considered in severe exacerbations if patients are unresponsive to the initial treatments listed above.
- Antibiotics have not been shown to be effective when administered routinely for acute asthma exacerbation but may be prescribed for coexisting conditions, such as pneumonia or bacterial sinusitis.
- Medications previously prescribed for control of chronic asthma should be continued during the acute episode to reinforce schedule and technique. If asthma history indicates lack of control with current regimen, see later discussion of Daily Management of Pediatric Asthma for options to optimize home plan to achieve better control.
- Treatments not recommended in the hospital setting include methylxanthine infusions, aggressive hydration, chest physical therapy, mucolytics, and sedation.
- Discharge plan after acute episode
  - Patients discharged home from the emergency department may be given a short term Asthma Action Plan (Figure 11-1) with directions to return to the primary care provider in 3–5 days.
  - Patients discharged home from the inpatient area should be given an Asthma Action Plan and an appointment with their primary care physician 5–7 days after discharge (see Figure 11-1).
  - Patients and families should be educated in the use of the Asthma Action Plan and medication administration. Patients should have prescriptions and all needed equipment (e.g., spacers, nebulizer) before discharge. Patients may use albuterol MDI using appropriate spacer on the day of discharge.

# Asthma Action Plan

**Green Zone:** Well
- no signs of asthma
- able to do normal activities
- no problems while sleeping

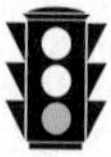

- Peak flow above: _____
  (above 80% of best)

*rinse mouth after this medicine

☐ Give your child these medicines every day:

| Medicine: | How much: | When: |
|---|---|---|
| _____ | _____ | _____ |
| _____ | _____ | _____ |
| _____ | _____ | _____ |
| _____ | _____ | _____ |
| _____ | _____ | _____ |

**Yellow Zone:** Caution!

- **Early signs of Asthma:**
- coughing
- wheezing
- tightness of chest
- unable to sleep at night
- cold symptoms

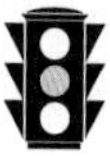

- Peak flow: _____
  (50-80% of best)

☐ **First** — give your child:
  ☐ **Albuterol**   2–4 puffs or 1 nebulizer   1–3 times in first hour
  _____

☐ **Next**— If signs of asthma return, you may give:
  ☐ **Albuterol**   2–4 puffs or 1 nebulizer   every 4 hours as needed
  ☐ Continue other Green Zone medicines.

☐ **Call** your Doctor or Nurse if:
  ☐ Not in the Green Zone after the first hour.
  ☐ Albuterol needed more than every 4 hours.
  ☐ Albuterol needed every 4 hours for more than 1 day.

**Red Zone:** EMERGENCY!

- **Late signs of Asthma:**
- very hard time breathing
- trouble talking or walking
- constant coughing
- use of neck or stomach muscles to breathe
- lips or nails blue

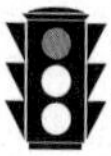

- Peak flow below: _____
  (below 50% of best)

☐ **First** — give your child:
  ☐ **Albuterol**   4–6 puffs or 1 nebulizer   **Immediately**

☐ **Call** your Doctor or Nurse.

☐ If you cannot reach your doctor or nurse, give:
  ☐ **Albuterol**   4–6 puffs or 1 nebulizer   **Immediately**
  _____ (oral steriod)   **Immediately**

☐ **Then go to the nearest emergency room or call 911.**

_Patient/Parent/Guardian Signature_        _Date_

_RN/MD Signature_        _Date_

| Phone number of Doctor or Nurse: |
|---|
| Day: _____ |
| Night: _____ |

Rev. 4/06
Copyright © 1995 St. Louis Children's Hospital

**Figure 11-1.** St. Louis Children's Hospital Asthma Action Plan.

■ It is usually recommended that the patient receive albuterol every 4–6 hours for 1 week or until follow-up appointment.

## Daily Management of Pediatric Asthma

### Control of Asthma

■ The following goals of therapy have been established by the National Heart, Lung, and Blood Institute (NHLBI).

- Reduce impairment: frequency and intensity of symptoms as well as the functional impairment the patient is currently experiencing (or has recently experienced)
  - Prevent asthma symptoms.
  - Reduce need for inhaled short-acting β-agonist (≤2 days per week).
  - Maintain normal lung function.
  - Exercise and go to school regularly.
  - Meet patients' and families' expectations of and satisfaction with asthma care.
- Reduce risk: likelihood of asthma exacerbations, progressive decline in lung function or growth, or risk of side effects of medications
  - Prevent recurrent exacerbations and minimize emergency visits or hospital admissions.
  - Prevent loss of lung function and reduced lung growth.
  - Provide optimal pharmacotherapy with no side effects from asthma medication.

- The NHLBI's Stepwise Approach for Managing Asthma should serve as a guideline for decision making to meet the individual needs of the patient (Figure 11-2).
- Provide a written Asthma Action Plan that includes medications used daily for control as well as quick relief medications for acute episodes. This plan serves as a guide for self-monitoring and self-management (see Figure 11-1).
- Severe exacerbations can occur in patients at any level of asthma severity or control. Patients at high risk for asthma-related death require special attention, including intensive education, monitoring, and care. Such patients should be encouraged to seek care early during an exacerbation. Risk factors for asthma-related death include:
  - Previous severe exacerbation
  - Two or more hospitalizations or 3 emergency department visits in the past year
  - Use of >2 canisters of short-acting β-agonist (SABA) per month
  - Poor perception of airway obstruction or worsening asthma
  - Low socioeconomic status or inner city residence
  - Illicit drug use
  - Major psychosocial problems or psychiatric disease
  - Comorbidities, such as cardiovascular disease or other chronic lung disease

### Controlling Precipitating Factors (Triggers)
- Take history to identify factors that precipitate asthma and recommend controls.
- Prioritize based on family's individual situation.
- Give written recommendations to patient and family.
- Allergens
  - Molds. Avoid opening doors and windows. Use air conditioning and dehumidifiers.
  - Dust mites. Use allergen-impermeable mattresses and pillow covers and wash linens in hot water. Minimize carpeting. Vacuum once weekly.
  - Animals. Do not have feathered or furry animals in the home. Avoid feathers.
  - Cockroaches. Rid home of roaches. Store food in closed containers.
- Weather. Stay indoors if there is changing weather or poor air quality.
- Colds and viruses. Influenza vaccination annually.
- Irritants. Do not smoke in the house or car. Avoid perfumes and strong odors.
- Exercise. Work out a medical plan to allow exercise. Have quick-relief medicine available during exercise.

## Patient Education
- Individualized education of the patient and family is crucial to successful self-management of asthma.
- Assessment of understanding of the Asthma Action Plan (see Figure 11-1), correct medication administration technique, and correct use of the peak flow meter (when applicable) should be reinforced at each visit. Reeducate family as needed, especially when changes are made to the management plan.
- Psychosocial issues should be addressed, and patients and families should be referred to support agencies when needed.

**Step up if needed** (first check inhaler technique, adherence, environmental control, and comorbid conditions)

**Assess control**

**Step down if possible** (and asthma is well controlled at least 3 months)

## Children 0–4 Years of Age

| | Step 1 | Step 2 | Step 3 | Step 4 | Step 5 | Step 6 |
|---|---|---|---|---|---|---|
| | Intermittent Asthma | Persistent Asthma: Daily Medication | | | | |
| | | Consult with asthma specialist if step 3 care or higher is required. Consider consultation at step 2. | | | | |
| **Preferred** | SABA PRN | Low-dose ICS | Medium-dose ICS | Medium-dose ICS + LABA or Montelukast | High-dose ICS + LABA or Montelukast | High-dose ICS + Oral corticosteroids ICS + LABA or Montelukast |
| **Alternative** | | Cromolyn or Montelukast | | | | |

**Quick-Relief Medication**

**Each Step: Patient Education and Environmental Control**

- SABA as needed for symptoms. Intensity of treatment depends on severity of symptoms.
- With viral respiratory symptoms: SABA q 4–6 hours up to 24 hours (longer with physician consult). Consider short course of oral systemic corticosteroids if exacerbation is severe or patient has history of previous severe exacerbations

Caution: Frequent use of SABA may indicate the need to step up treatment. See text for recommendations on initiating daily long-term control therapy.

## Children 5–11 Years of Age

| | Step 1 | Step 2 | Step 3 | Step 4 | Step 5 | Step 6 |
|---|---|---|---|---|---|---|
| | Intermittent Asthma | Persistent Asthma: Daily Medication | | | | |
| | | Consult with asthma specialist if step 4 care or higher is required. Consider consultation at step 3. | | | | |
| **Preferred** | SABA PRN | Low-dose ICS | Low-dose ICS + LABA, LTRA, or Theophylline OR Medium-dose ICS | Medium-dose ICS + LABA | High-dose ICS + LABA | High-dose ICS + LABA + Oral corticosteroids |
| **Alternative** | | Cromolyn, LTRA, Nedocromil, or Theophylline | | Medium-dose ICS + LTRA or Theophylline | High-dose ICS + LTRA or Theophylline | High-dose ICS + LTRA or Theophylline + oral corticosteroids |

**Quick-Relief Medication**

**Each Step: Patient Education, Environmental Control, and Management of Comorbidities**

**Steps 2–4:** Consider subcutaneous allergen immunotherapy for patients who have persistent, allergic asthma.

- SABA as needed for symptoms. Intensity of treatment depends on severity of symptoms: up to 3 treatments at 20-minute intervals as needed. Short course of oral systemic corticosteroids may be needed.

Caution: Increasing use of SABA or use >2 days a week for symptom relief (not prevention of E(I)B) generally indicates inadequate control and the need to step up treatment

## Notes

- The stepwise approach is meant to assist, not replace, the clinical decisionmaking required to meet individual patient needs.
- If an alternative treatment is used and response is inadequate, discontinue it and use the preferred treatment before stepping up.
- If clear benefit is not observed within 4–6 weeks, and patient's/family's medication technique and adherence are satisfactory, consider adjusting therapy or an alternative diagnosis.
- Studies on children 0–4 years of age are limited. Step 2 preferred therapy is based on Evidence A. All other recommendations are based on expert opinion and extrapolation from studies in older children.
- Clinicians who administer immunotherapy should be prepared and equipped to identify and treat anaphylaxis that may occur.

**Key: Alphabetical listing is used when more than one treatment option is listed within either preferred or alternative therapy.** ICS, inhaled corticosteroid; LABA, inhaled long-acting beta2-agonist; LTRA, leukotriene receptor antagonist; oral systemic corticosteroids; SABA, inhaled short-acting beta2-agonist

- The stepwise approach is meant to assist, not replace, the clinical decisionmaking required to meet individual patient needs.
- If an alternative treatment is used and response is inadequate, discontinue it and use the preferred treatment before stepping up.
- Theophylline is a less desirable alternative due to the need to monitor serum concentration levels.
- Steps 1 and 2 medications are based on Evidence A. Step 3 ICS and ICS plus adjunctive therapy are based on Evidence B for efficacy of each treatment and extrapolation from comparator trials in older children and adults—comparator trials are not available for this age group; steps 4–6 are based on expert opinion and extrapolation from studies in older children and adults.
- Immunotherapy for steps 2–4 is based on Evidence B for house-dust mites, animal danders, and pollens; evidence is weak or lacking for molds and cockroaches. Evidence is strongest for immunotherapy with single allergens. The role of allergy in asthma is greater in children than adults.
- Clinicians who administer immunotherapy should be prepared and equipped to identify and treat anaphylaxis that may occur.

**Key: Alphabetical listing is used when more than one treatment option is listed within either preferred or alternative therapy.** ICS, inhaled corticosteroid; LABA, inhaled long-acting beta2-agonist; LTRA, leukotriene receptor antagonist; SABA, inhaled short-acting beta2-agonist

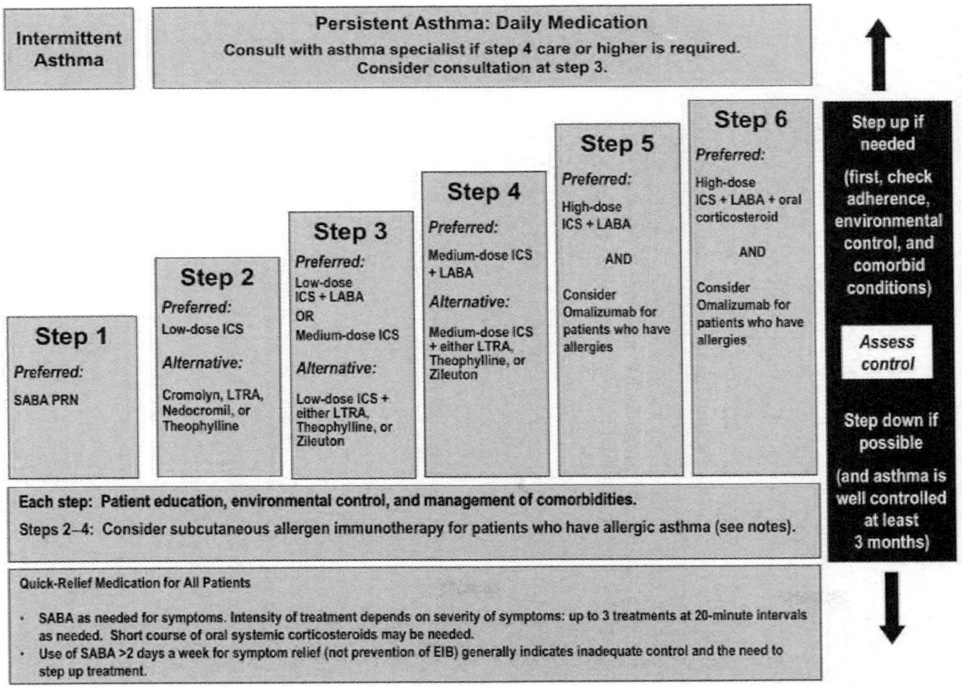

**Figure 11-2.** Stepwise approach to management of asthma in children. From the National Heart, Lung, and Blood Institute, National Institutes of Health, Guidelines for the diagnosis and management of asthma. NIH Publication No. 97-4051, July 1997.

# URTICARIA AND ANGIOEDEMA

- Urticaria (hives) are raised, well confined, pruritic skin lesions with central clearing that blanch with pressure and are surrounded with erythema.
  - Individual lesions last <24 hours and resolve without leaving any sequelae.
  - Urticaria is said to affect approximately 15%–25% of people during their lifetime.
- Angioedema is deeper localized swelling without overlying erythema and although it can occur anywhere it typically affects the tongue, lips, or eyelids.
- Urticaria and angioedema are both caused by release of mediators from mast cells in the skin and sub-subcutaneous tissue.

## Acute Urticaria (With or Without Angioedema)

- Episodes of urticaria lasting <6 weeks

### Etiology

- Responses to underlying infections: Epstein-Barr virus (EBV), viral hepatitis, respiratory viruses, enteroviruses, and parasitic infections. In children, acute urticaria is most commonly caused by an infectious etiology.
- Food: milk, egg, soy, wheat, peanuts, tree nuts, fish, and shellfish
- Insect stings or bites (bee, wasps, hornets, yellow jackets, and fire ants)
- Medications: most commonly antibiotics. Other medications that can cause non-IgE mediated mast cell degranulation include opiates, nonsteroidal anti-inflammatory drugs (NSAIDs), IV contrast media, and alcohol.
- Allergen exposure (contact or inhalation): animal dander, grasses, weeds, and latex.

### Evaluation

- The most valuable step is a detailed history and physical examination to identify one of the causes described above.
- Specific tests for infectious etiologies as suggested by history are necessary.
- Skin prick testing or specific IgE (ImmunoCAP) for food, inhalant allergens, or drugs as guided by clinical history and availability of testing are also necessary.

### Treatment

- In the presence of systemic symptoms consistent with anaphylaxis (hypotension, respiratory symptoms, or central nervous system symptoms), treatment should include epinephrine (0.01 mg/kg of a 1:1,000 solution intramuscular maximal dose 0.5 mg). See the "Anaphylaxis" section for further details.
- The mainstays of treatment are $H_1$ antihistamines. The first line should include the nonsedating $H_1$-antihistamines, such as cetirizine (minimally sedating), fexofenadine, loratadine, and desloratadine.
- If an avoidable cause of acute urticaria (e.g., food allergy) is identified, it should be avoided.
- Glucocorticoids are not typically part of the routine treatment of children with acute urticaria; however, a short course of oral glucocorticoids can be considered in episodes that have not responded quickly or completely to antihistamines.

## Chronic Urticaria (With or Without Angioedema)

- Episodes of urticaria occurring on a daily (or near daily) basis for >6 weeks

### Etiology

- A precise etiology cannot be determined in 60%–80% of the children with chronic urticaria. Types of chronic urticaria include:
  - Chronic autoimmune urticaria. In individuals with positive autologous skin tests, this is because of autoantibodies against the high-affinity IgE receptor on mast cells.
  - Papular urticaria. This is because of immunologic hypersensitivity to the saliva of the biting insects.

- Physical urticaria. Physical triggers may include mechanical (dermatographism and delayed pressure urticaria), thermal (cold- and heat-induced urticaria), exercise/sweating (cholinergic urticaria), vibration, UV radiation (solar urticaria), and water (aquagenic).
- Urticarial vasculitis. This is typified by lesions that last >24 hours and leave bruising or hyperpigmented lesions.
- Urticaria pigmentosa. Mastocytosis is typified by red-brown macules that urticate when scratched.
- Others. These types of urticaria include Muckle-Wells syndrome and familial cold-induced urticaria.

### Evaluation
- A detailed history and physical examination is critical to identify one of the above described forms of disease. Special consideration should be given to the duration of each specific wheal. Wheals that last >24 hours could be either urticarial vasculitis or delayed-pressure urticaria.
- Challenge tests for physical urticaria include dermatographism (an immediate wheal-and-flare response on stroking the skin), ice cube test (cold urticaria), or pressure.
- A skin biopsy should be performed if the diagnosis is suspicious of vasculitis or mastocytosis.
- An autologous serum skin prick test screens for the presence of autoantibodies against the high-affinity IgE receptor.
- In the absence of an identified trigger, laboratory screening may be sent to identify an underlying disease, such as systemic lupus erythematosus (complete blood count with differential, erythrocyte sedimentation rate, antineutrophil antibody test, C3, C4, and urinalysis), hepatitis (liver enzymes), thyroid disease (thyroid-stimulating hormone, thyroid autoantibodies), and mastocytosis (serum tryptase levels).

### Treatment
- Treat any identified underlying causes of disease.
- $H_1$ antihistamines (see Acute Urticaria, Treatment)
  - The dose should be titrated to the lowest dose needed for symptom control.
  - First-generation $H_1$ antihistamines (e.g., hydroxyzine, diphenhydramine (Benadryl), cyproheptadine) may be added for breakthrough lesions. Of note, cyproheptadine is the preferred antihistamine in cold-induced urticaria.
- $H_2$ blocking agents (e.g., ranitidine, cimetidine) in combination with $H_1$ antihistamines may provide additional benefits.
- Doxepin is a tricyclic antidepressant with a potent blocking effect on both the $H_1$ and $H_2$ receptors. Sedation may limit its usefulness.
- Leukotriene antagonists (e.g., zafirlukast and montelukast) may have additional benefits when used in combination with antihistamines.
- Oral glucocorticoids, although effective, should be reserved for individuals who cannot be controlled with combinations of the above medications and only used in short courses to limit side effects.
- Other experimental therapeutic approaches (evaluated mainly on adults) include cyclosporine, sulfasalazine, hydroxychloroquine, and levothyroxine in individuals with antithyroid antibodies (even if the patient is euthyroid).

## Angioedema (Without Urticaria)

- Angioedema unaccompanied by urticaria should prompt evaluation for specific underlying causes.
- Hereditary angioedema (HAE), or C1 esterase inhibitor deficiency, is an autosomal dominant condition. In 85% of cases, the cause is deficiency of the C1 esterase inhibitor, and in 15% of cases, the cause is a nonfunctional C1 esterase inhibitor protein.
- Acquired C1 esterase inhibitor deficiency is very rare in children and usually associated with B-cell proliferation disorders. The C1q level is reduced in individuals with acquired C1 esterase inhibitor deficiency, but not HAE.
- Symptoms are recurrent episodes of nonpruritic angioedema and abdominal pain.

- Screening test is a complement C4 level. If the C4 level is reduced, evaluation of C1 esterase inhibitor levels and functional assays should be performed.

### Treatment

- Acute management involves supportive measures, especially airway management; fresh frozen plasma; and replacement C1-esterase inhibitor and bradykinin pathway inhibitors. Although these inhibitors are not currently licensed in the United States, they are useful in aborting acute attacks.
- Preventive measures involve attenuated anabolic steroids, which are effective in preventing episodes of HAE; however, their side effects may limit their usefulness in women and children. They are not effective in the acute management of HAE.
- If angiotensin-converting enzyme inhibitors are identified as the cause of angioedema, a different class of therapeutic drug should be chosen.

## FOOD ALLERGY

### Definition

- Food allergy describes a hypersensitivity reaction to a food protein as a result of an immunologic mechanism. The term adverse food reaction refers to any untoward reaction to a food or food component, regardless of the pathophysiologic mechanism involved.
- Adverse immunologic food reactions are classified as IgE-mediated or non–IgE-mediated, with the majority being IgE-mediated.

### Epidemiology

- Allergy to one or more foods occurs in 6%–8% of children and 1%–2% of adults. The majority of food allergic reactions present before 12 months of age.
- Eight foods are responsible for the majority of documented food reactivity (Table 11-9), although numerous other foods have been shown to trigger allergic reactions.

### Clinical Presentation

- As Table 11-10 shows, the clinical manifestations of food allergy can vary, depending on the underlying pathophysiologic process.

### IgE-Mediated Food Allergy

- Cutaneous reactions in the form of acute onset urticaria and/or angioedema are the most common manifestations in IgE-mediated food hypersensitivity reactions.
- Gastrointestinal symptoms may include nausea, abdominal pain, abdominal cramping, vomiting, and/or diarrhea.
- Respiratory symptoms such as cough and wheeze are common. Inhalation of food allergens via cooking (e.g., fish) or exposure to airborne particles (e.g., peanut dust) may also trigger acute bronchospasm.
- Isolated rhinoconjunctival symptoms are uncommon.
- Anaphylaxis resulting from exposure (typically ingestion) to food allergens has been estimated to account for up to 50% of all anaphylaxis cases seen in the emergency department. There is an increased incidence of food-induced anaphylaxis when asthma exists as a comorbid condition.

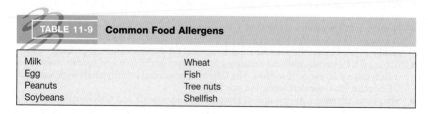

| TABLE 11-9 | Common Food Allergens |
| --- | --- |
| Milk | Wheat |
| Egg | Fish |
| Peanuts | Tree nuts |
| Soybeans | Shellfish |

| TABLE 11-10 | Characteristics of Adverse Food Reactions Based on Mechanism | |
|---|---|---|
| | **IgE-Mediated** | **Non–IgE-Mediated** |
| Onset | Rapid in onset, occurring within several minutes to 2 hr after ingestion | Subacute and/or chronic symptoms, delayed in onset by 4–48 hr |
| Mechanism | Results from mediator release from tissue mast cells and circulating basophils | Multiple mechanisms, including immunologic (e.g., celiac disease, eosinophilic gastrointestinal disorders), pharmacologic (e.g., caffeine, histamine), metabolic (e.g., phenylketonuria, lactose intolerance), additives (e.g., MSG, tartrazine) and toxic (e.g., staphylococcal food poisoning) |
| System(s) involved | Cutaneous, gastrointestinal, respiratory, ocular, cardio-vascular, and/or multisystem (anaphylaxis) | Usually isolated to the gastrointestinal tract |

- Atopic dermatitis may be exacerbated by consumption of food allergens.
  - Approximately 40% of children with atopic dermatitis have food allergy (see the "Atopic Dermatitis" section).
  - Elimination of the suspected food (following appropriate evaluation, see later discussion) often improves symptoms.
- Oral allergy syndrome presents as immediate onset of oropharyngeal pruritus and mild edema of the lips and/or tongue in patients with pollen allergy. Symptoms occur after consuming cross-reactive (and often heat-labile) proteins in fresh, uncooked fruits or, less often, vegetables.
  - Apple, pear, cherry, carrot, celery, and potato are cross-reactive with birch pollen.
  - Melons and banana have cross-reactivity with ragweed.

### Non–IgE-Mediated Food Hypersensitivity
- Food protein–induced enterocolitis presents in early infancy, usually before 3 months of age, with poor weight gain along with vomiting and diarrhea after consuming cow-and/or soy-based formula. Stool contains occult blood, neutrophils, eosinophils, and reducing substances. Tolerance to the food(s) usually occurs by 12–24 months.
- Food-induced colitis presents with painless rectal bleeding as in food-induced enterocolitis, but patients are not generally as ill and tend to have appropriate weight gain. Tolerance to the food generally develops by 12–24 months of age.
- Allergic eosinophilic gastroenteropathy is a result of infiltration of eosinophils in the gastric and/or intestinal walls. Symptoms include postprandial nausea and vomiting, abdominal pain, malabsorption, and weight loss.
- Celiac disease results from intestinal damage and villous atrophy because of a cell-mediated immune response to gliadin found in wheat, rye, barley, and oats.
  - Clinical symptoms include diarrhea (usually steatorrhea), abdominal distension, weight loss, and occasional nausea and vomiting.
  - Diagnosis is made via intestinal biopsy. Presence of IgA tissue transglutaminase antibodies is highly specific for celiac disease.
  - Elimination of gluten-containing food produces normalization of mucosal histology.

## History
- The diagnosis of a food allergy requires a thorough clinical history of the event.

- The history must include the following:
  - The specific food or ingredient thought to provoke the reaction
  - All other food and medication consumed at the same time
  - Quantity of food consumed
  - Method of food preparation, including possibility of cross-contamination with other food
  - Amount of time between consumption and reaction
  - Symptoms that occurred on other occasions when the food was consumed, both previously and since the event
  - Intervention administered to resolve symptoms
  - Amount of time until resolution of symptoms

## Laboratory Studies

- Once a history of IgE-mediated reactivity has been established, diagnostic testing should be used.
- Epicutaneous skin testing is an excellent way of excluding IgE-mediated food allergies because this approach has a >95% negative predictive value. However, positive skin tests to food have approximately a 50% positive predictive value, reflecting a high prevalence of asymptomatic allergic sensitization.
- An alternative approach for the detection of food allergen-specific IgE uses in vitro testing (e.g., ImmunoCAP system). These assays provide a quantitative measure of allergen-specific IgE and may provide guidance as to the timing of an oral food challenge (see later discussion).

## Oral Food Challenges

- Confirmation of a food allergy may require an oral food challenge, during which the patient consumes the food in question under direct medical supervision, starting with very small quantities and increasing toward a standard portion of the food.
- Timing of oral challenges may be guided by allergen-specific IgE levels. Table 11-11 provides values for food-specific IgE levels and their positive and negative predictive values for outcomes of oral food challenges. Oral challenges are often recommended when milk-, egg-, or peanut-specific IgE levels fall below 2 kU/L because approximately 50% of children exhibit tolerance to the food at that level.
- If a food challenge is indicated, the double-blind placebo-controlled method is considered to be the gold standard for the diagnosis of food allergy.
  - This should be performed by an allergist in a setting with the personnel and equipment necessary for treatment of a potential anaphylactic reaction.
  - A single-blind graded challenge may be appropriate in confirming or refuting histories suggestive of food allergy. Single-blind challenges are particularly useful in young children whose response is not influenced by knowledge of consumption of the suspected food allergen.

| TABLE 11-11 | Positive and Negative Predictive Values for Food-Specific IgE Levels | |
|---|---|---|
| Food | >95% Positive predictive value | >95% Negative predictive value |
| Egg | 6 kU/L | — |
| Milk | 32 kU/L | 0.8 kU/L |
| Peanut | 15 kU/L | Best value = 85% at 0.35 kU/L |
| Fish | 20 kU/L | 0.9 kU/L |
| Soy | Best value = 50% at 65 kU/L | 2 kU/L |
| Wheat | Best value = 75% at 100 kU/L | 5 kU/L |

Adapted from Sampson H, Ho D. J Allergy Clin Immunol 1997;100:444–451.

## Treatment

■ Management of food allergy is based on avoidance of food allergens and preparation for adverse reactions.

■ Total and strict avoidance of all forms of the food, both as major and minor ingredients, is necessary. Many patients report tolerating consumption of products with the allergen as an ingredient (e.g., egg-containing baked goods), but this is highly variable. Such practices expose individuals to potential adverse reactions.

■ A form of immediately available self-injectable epinephrine, such as EpiPen or Twinject, is appropriate for patients with an IgE-mediated food allergy. Extensive education regarding use of epinephrine should be provided at each office visit and offered to all caregivers, including day care providers and teachers.

■ Educational resources, including instructions for reading ingredient labels and support groups for people with food allergies, should be made available. The Food Allergy and Anaphylaxis Network (www.foodallergy.org) is an excellent resource.

■ Symptomatic food sensitivity is often lost over time with milk (85% by 5 years) and egg allergy (60% by 5 years). In contrast, sensitivity to peanuts, tree nuts, and seafood is often lifelong.


# ANAPHYLAXIS

■ Anaphylaxis is an acute, life-threatening allergic reaction caused by an IgE-dependent mechanism.

■ An anaphylactoid reaction presents with the same clinical manifestations but is not IgE-mediated.

## Etiology

■ The most common causes of anaphylactic reactions in children are food and drugs.

■ Most likely food: peanuts, tree nuts, milk, eggs, fish, and shellfish
■ Most likely drugs: penicillin, cephalosporins, sulfonamides, and NSAIDs

■ One risk factor for fatal anaphylaxis is a history of asthma. The most important risk factor for fatal anaphylaxis is failure to inject epinephrine appropriately or promptly in the early part of a reaction.

■ Usual causes of anaphylactoid reactions in children include opioids, muscle relaxants, vancomycin, and radiocontrast media.

## Pathophysiology

■ Onset of anaphylaxis occurs in minutes to several hours. Degranulation of mast cells and basophils precipitated by the cross-linking between allergen-specific IgE and the allergen releases biochemical mediators such as histamine, leukotrienes, tryptase, prostaglandins, and histamine-releasing factor.

■ Histamine activation of $H_1$ and $H_2$ receptors causes flushing, headache, and hypotension. Activation of $H_1$ receptors alone contributes to rhinorrhea, tachycardia, pruritus, and bronchospasm.

## Diagnosis

■ Anaphylaxis usually is diagnosed when two or more organ systems are involved. Systems frequently affected include skin, respiratory, gastrointestinal, and cardiovascular.

■ Frequent manifestations are urticaria, angioedema, wheezing, shortness of breath, vomiting, and hypotension, among others.

■ A laboratory test can help with the diagnosis of anaphylaxis, especially if the patient presents with hypotension alone. This test is a serum beta-tryptase level.

■ If anaphylaxis is present, the serum beta tryptase will be elevated and will peak 1–2 hours after the onset of anaphylaxis. The serum beta tryptase will then remain elevated for 4–6 hours.

- Serum beta tryptase levels can be normal in mild reactions or in food-induced anaphylaxis.

## Treatment

### Acute Therapy
- Assess and maintain airway, breathing, and circulation.
- Give intramuscular epinephrine (1:1000 dilution) 0.01 mg/kg in children (maximum dose 0.3 mg) into the anterolateral thigh (preferred) or the deltoid. An epinephrine autoinjector (e.g., EpiPen 0.3 mg for children >25 kg or EpiPen Jr 0.15 mg for children between 10 and 25 kg) may be injected through clothing into the anterolateral thigh alternatively. Repeat every 5 minutes as necessary.
- Place the patient in the supine position with elevated lower extremities (or in the left lateral position for vomiting patients).
- Administer supplemental oxygen as needed.
- Administer IV saline 20 mL/kg in the first 5–10 minutes if there is hypotension despite epinephrine.
  - If persistent or severe hypotension continues, multiple fluid boluses of 10–20 mL/kg up to 50 mL/kg may be administered over the first 30 minutes.
  - For refractory hypotension after fluid resuscitation and epinephrine administration, dopamine, noradrenaline, or vasopressin may be required to maintain a systolic blood pressure of >90 mm Hg.
- Diphenhydramine may be administered at 1–2 mg/kg/dose (up to 50 mg) orally or intravenously. Antihistamine should not be used without epinephrine in anaphylaxis management.
- Ranitidine 1 mg/kg in children (up to 50 mg) orally or intravenously may be added.
- Administer an inhaled $\beta_2$-agonist (albuterol or levalbuterol) for resistant bronchospasm.
- In a patient receiving β-blockers, consider glucagon 20–30 μg/kg (up to 1 mg in children) injected over 5 minutes intravenously every 20 minutes if initial administration of epinephrine is ineffective. Follow with an infusion of 5–15 μg/min.
- Corticosteroids are not useful acutely but may inhibit a biphasic or protracted response.
  - Methylprednisolone 1–2 mg/kg may be given intravenously.
  - Oral prednisone 1–2 mg/kg (up to 60 mg) may also be considered.

### Observation
- Even though the majority of patients who have anaphylactic events respond rapidly to treatment and do not relapse, observation for 4–6 hours postanaphylaxis is suggested because biphasic reactions can occur or the effect of epinephrine may wane.
- Hospitalization in patients with moderate to severe symptoms is appropriate.

### Discharge and Follow-up
- Epinephrine autoinjectors (dosage described in "Treatment" section) with instruction in administration should be prescribed for all patients experiencing an anaphylactic reaction to an allergen present in a community setting. Discharge medications such as diphenhydramine and oral prednisone can be continued for 24–72 hours.
- Education materials should be provided to all patients before discharge home. Patients should be educated about how to avoid the anaphylactic allergen if identified, particularly in food anaphylaxis (resources available from the Food Allergy and Anaphylaxis Network, www.foodallergy.org).
- An anaphylaxis action plan should be formulated. This plan should include the child's name, allergens, parental contact information, when and how to use an epinephrine autoinjector, antihistamine dose, and when to seek emergency help.
- Referral to an allergy specialist should be arranged for a complete evaluation.

## Suggested Readings
Leung DYM, Sampson HA, Geha RS, et al, eds. Pediatric Allergy: Principles and Practice. St. Louis: Mosby, 2003.
National Heart, Lung, and Blood Institute, National Institutes of Health, Guidelines for the Diagnosis and Management of Asthma. NIH Publication No. 97-4051, July 1997.

# ELECTROCARDIOGRAM INTERPRETATION

- Electrocardiography is critical in the diagnosis of electrical disorders of the heart. It may serve as a useful screening tool in the evaluation of patients of suspected structural defects or abnormalities of the myocardium.
- Newborns have a large variability in electrocardiogram (ECG) voltages and intervals due in large part to hemodynamic and myocardial adaptations that are needed once the placenta is no longer part of the circulatory system.
- Changes continue, albeit at a slower pace, from infancy through adolescence.
- Algorithms used to interpret ECGs in adults cannot be used in children. This section is a basic, although incomplete, guide to the pediatric ECG.

## Rate

- The usual recording speed is 25 mm/sec; each little box (1 mm) is 0.04 seconds and each big box (5 mm) is 0.2 seconds.
- With a fast heart rate, count the R-R cycles in 6 large boxes (1.2 seconds) and multiply by 50.
- With a slow heart rate, count the number of large boxes between R waves and divide into 300 (1 box = 300, 2 boxes = 150, 3 boxes = 100, 4 boxes = 75).
- Table 12-1 lists normal heart rates.

## Rhythm

- Are the QRS deflections regular? Variation in the rate up and down in concert with respirations is normal (sinus arrhythmia) and can be pronounced in young healthy hearts.
- Irregular QRS pattern suggests the possibility of an atrial arrhythmia. With pauses and narrow QRS, look for evidence of atrial premature contractions with P waves of different appearance and/or axis as compared with sinus beats. The early P wave may not conduct, leading to longer pauses (blocked atrial premature contractions).
- The QRS may be prolonged if conduction down the atrioventricular (AV) node is delayed (aberrant conduction). Wide QRS complexes with pauses may represent premature contractions from a ventricular focus, especially if the T-wave morphology is also altered with the opposite axis.
- Look for a P wave before each QRS at an expected interval, usually between 100 and 150 milliseconds. The P wave should be upright in I and aVF for the typical location of sinus node. The sinus P wave is up in leads I, II, aVF, pure negative in aVR, and usually biphasic in lead $V_1$—first positive, then negative.
  - Inverted P waves associated with slower heart rates, along with a low atrial rhythm, are a normal finding.
  - Inverted P waves associated with tachycardias are abnormal and may be ectopic atrial tachycardia or other forms of supraventricular tachycardia (SVT).

## PR Interval

- The PR interval represents atrial depolarization.
- Table 12-2 lists the mean and upper limits of normal PR intervals by age and heart rate.

| TABLE 12-1 | Normal Heart Rates in Children* |
|---|---|
| **Age** | **Heart rate (beats/ min)** |
| 0–1 mo | 145 (90–180) |
| 6 mo | 145 (105–185) |
| 1 yr | 132 (105–170) |
| 2 yr | 120 (90–150) |
| 4 yr | 108 (72–135) |
| 6 yr | 100 (65–135) |
| 10 yr | 90 (65–130) |
| 14 yr | 85 (60–120) |

*Recorded on ECG, with mean and ranges.
*Source*: Park MK, et al. How to read pediatric ECGs. 4th Ed. Philadelphia: Mosby, 2006:46.

## QRS Axis and Duration

- The QRS axis shows the direction of ventricular depolarization.
  - Left axis deviation can suggest left ventricular hypertrophy or left bundle branch block (LBBB).
  - Right axis deviation can suggest right ventricular hypertrophy or right bundle branch block (RBBB).
- Table 12-3 gives the mean QRS axis values by age.
- The QRS duration represents ventricular depolarization. Normal times for depolarization depend on age. A prolonged QRS may indicate bundle branch block, hypertrophy, or arrhythmia.
- Table 12-4 lists the normal QRS durations by age.

## ECG Abnormalities

### Ventricular Hypertrophy
- The ECG is only a screening tool for hypertrophy, with high false-negative and false-positive rates, especially in infants. The QRS axis shifts toward the hypertrophied ventricle.
- In children >3 years of age, the usual QRS is between 20° and 120°. The QRS voltage changes increase in leads toward which the electrical depolarization is directed and decrease in leads in the opposite direction.
- In right ventricular hypertrophy, increased R waves may be present in $V_1$ with an increased R/S ratio in $V_1$ and decreased R/S ratio in $V_6$. An upright T wave in $V_1$ between 7 days and 7 years of age is also suggestive of right ventricular hypertrophy.
- In left ventricular hypertrophy, increased R waves may be present in $V_5$, $V_6$, I, II, III, or aVF. The R/S ratio may be decreased in $V_1$ or $V_2$. Inverted T waves in I, aVF, $V_5$, or $V_6$ suggest a "strain" pattern, indicating abnormal repolarization.

### Bundle Branch Blocks
- In RBBB, late depolarization in the right ventricle leads to rightward QRS axis as well as a widened QRS with wide and slurred S in I, $V_5$, and $V_6$. R' is slurred in aVR, $V_1$, and $V_2$. (Last activated chamber is anterior and rightward.)
- In LBBB, late depolarization in the left ventricle leads to leftward QRS axis, widened QRS with slurred and wide R waves in I, aVL, $V_5$, and $V_6$. Wide S waves are seen in $V_1$ and $V_2$. Q waves may be absent in I, $V_5$, and $V_6$. (Last activated chamber is posterior and leftward.)
- In the setting of bundle branch blocks, the usual criteria for ventricular hypertrophy do not apply.

**TABLE 12-2** Normal PR Intervals

| Heart rate (beats/min) | Age | | | | | | | |
|---|---|---|---|---|---|---|---|---|
| | 0–1 mo | 1–6 mo | 6–12 mo | 1–3 yr | 3–8 yr | 8–12 yr | 12–16 yr | Adult |
| <60 | — | — | — | — | — | 0.16(0.18) | 0.16(0.19) | 0.17(0.21) |
| 60–80 | 0.10(0.12) | — | — | — | 0.15(0.17) | 0.15(0.17) | 0.15(0.18) | 0.16(0.21) |
| 80–100 | 0.10(0.12) | — | — | — | 0.14(0.16) | 0.15(0.16) | 0.15(0.17) | 0.15(0.20) |
| 100–120 | 0.10(0.11) | — | — | (0.15) | 0.13(0.16) | 0.14(0.15) | 0.15(0.16) | 0.15(0.19) |
| 120–140 | 0.10(0.11) | 0.11(0.14) | 0.11(0.14) | 0.12(0.14) | 0.13(0.15) | 0.14(0.15) | — | 0.15(0.18) |
| 140–160 | 0.09(0.11) | 0.10(0.13) | 0.11(0.13) | 0.11(0.14) | 0.12(0.14) | — | — | (0.17) |
| 160–180 | 0.10(0.11) | 0.10(0.12) | 0.10(0.12) | 0.10(0.12) | — | — | — | — |
| >180 | 0.09 | 0.09(0.11) | 0.10(0.11) | — | — | — | — | — |

*Source:* Park MK, et al. How to read pediatric ECGs. 4th Ed. Philadelphia: Mosby, 2006:49.

| TABLE 12-3 | Normal QRS Axis Ranges by Age |
| --- | --- |
| **Age** | **Mean value (Range)** |
| 0–1 month | +110 degrees (+30 to +180) |
| 1–3 months | +70 degrees (+10 to +125) |
| 3 months–3 yr | +60 degrees (+5 to +110) |
| >3 yr– | +60 degrees (+20 to +120) |
| Adult | +50 degrees (−30 to +105) |

*Source*: Park MK, et al. How to read pediatric ECGs. 4th Ed. Philadelphia: Mosby, 2006:50.

### QT Prolongation

■ Long QT syndrome is an important cause of sudden death. Determination of the QT interval is important, especially in patients with syncope or seizures.
■ The QT interval is measured in milliseconds (usually in lead II) from the start of the QRS complex to the end of the T wave.
■ The U wave, which may occur after the T wave, should be included only if it is at least one half the amplitude of the T wave.
■ The QT interval is adjusted for heart rate (QTc) by dividing by the square root of the preceding RR interval:

$$\text{Bazett formula: } QTc = QT \text{ interval}/\sqrt{(RR \text{ interval})}$$

■ The QTc is usually <0.44 seconds (95th percentile).
■ Patients with long QT syndrome may also have notched, bifid, or biphasic T wave.
■ Figure 12-1 shows an ECG of a teenage patient with a presenting complaint of seizures.
■ The Schwartz criteria use ECG and clinical criteria to determine a probability of a patient having prolonged QT syndrome (Table 12-5) (Schwartz, et al.).

## ARRHYTHMIA

### General Principles

■ Arrhythmias other than sinus abnormalities are uncommon in children.
■ Children with congenital heart disease or heart surgery are more likely to have arrhythmias.
■ This section presents the basic presentation and therapy of arrhythmias in children, but it is not a complete description.

| TABLE 12-4 | Normal QRS Duration | | | | | | | |
| --- | --- | --- | --- | --- | --- | --- | --- | --- |
| Age | 0–1 mo | 1–6 mo | 6–12 mo | 1–3 yr | 3–8 yr | 8–12 yr | 12–16 yr | Adult |
| Normal (mean in seconds) | 0.05 | 0.055 | 0.055 | 0.055 | 0.06 | 0.06 | 0.07 | 0.08 |
| Upper limit of normal | 0.07 | 0.075 | 0.075 | 0.075 | 0.075 | 0.085 | 0.085 | 0.10 |

*Source*: Park MK, et al. How to read pediatric ECGs. 4th Ed. Philadelphia: Mosby, 2006:52.

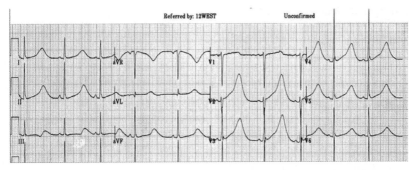

**Figure 12-1.** Electrocardiogram showing a sinus rhythm and corrected QTc of 700 milliseconds.

## Diagnosis

### Clinical Presentation and History
- Palpitations, syncope, and shock
- Complaints of heart racing or fluttering
- Syncope occurring in the midst of exercise
- Abrupt syncope with no premonitory symptoms
- Prior history of congenital heart disease or heart surgery
- Brought on by sudden startle such as alarm clock without preceding symptoms; think long QT syndrome

### Physical Examination
- Possible murmur, irregular rhythm, tachycardia, hypotension, or poor oxygen saturation
- Edema and poor perfusion in the extremities if in heart failure or shock
- Possible loss of consciousness

**TABLE 12-5** **Schwartz Criteria Including ECG Findings, Clinical Findings, and Family History**

| ECG Findings | Points |
|---|---|
| QTc >480 msec | 3 |
| QTc 460–470 | 2 |
| QTc >450 msec (men) | 1 |
| Torsades de pointes (ventricular tachycardia) | 2 |
| T wave alternans | 1 |
| Notched T wave >3 leads | 1 |
| Bradycardia for age | 0.5 |
| **Clinical Findings** | **Points** |
| Syncope with stress | 2 |
| Syncope without stress | 1 |
| Congenital deafness | 0.5 |
| **Family History** | **Points** |
| Definite long QT syndrome | 1 |
| Sudden cardiac death before age 30 yr in immediate family | 0.5 |
| **Total Points:** | |

| | |
|---|---|
| <1 | low probability |
| 2–3 | intermediate |
| >4 | high |

### Differential Diagnosis: ECG Findings

- The differential diagnosis of tachycardia starts with determining whether the tachycardia is regular or irregular and the width of the QRS.
- Narrow complex regular tachycardia
  - P before QRS
    - Sinus tachycardia
    - Ectopic atrial tachycardia (regular)
    - Persistent junctional reciprocating tachycardia (very slow SVT)
  - P within QRS
    - AV node reentry tachycardia: uncommon in children <2 years of age but typical in teenagers
    - Junctional ectopic tachycardia: typically occurs postoperatively, after congenital heart surgery
  - P behind QRS: reentry pathway (Figure 12-2)
    - Occurs especially with preexcitation when the patient is in sinus rhythm (Wolff-Parkinson-White [WPW] syndrome) (Figure 12-3)
    - Can present at any age
  - More Ps than QRSs
    - Atrial flutter
    - Ectopic atrial tachycardia (regular)
    - Coarse atrial fibrillation ("fib-flutter")
- Narrow complex irregular tachycardia
  - Atrial fibrillation
  - Ectopic atrial tachycardia (irregular)
  - Atrial flutter with variable AV conduction
- Wide complex regular tachycardia
  - Usually ventricular tachycardia
  - **V**entricular >**A**trial depolarizations, which are diagnostic
  - 1:1 **V**entricular:**A**trial depolarizations unusual

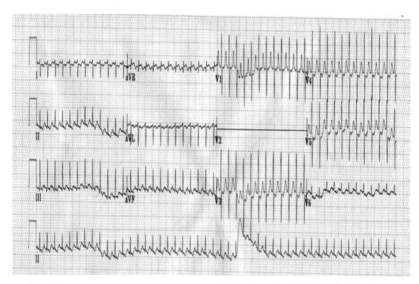

**Figure 12-2.** Electrocardiogram showing a narrow complex regular tachycardia from a supraventricular tachycardia pathway. The tracing shows a retrograde (inverted/nonsinus) P wave after each QRS. This tachycardia stops and starts suddenly. It is common in infants and young children and in patients with Wolff-Parkinson-White syndrome during sinus rhythm.

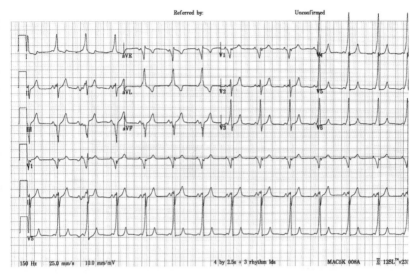

**Figure 12-3.** Electrocardiogram showing a sinus rhythm with preexcitation from a pathway that causes depolarization of some of the ventricular mass before depolarization through the usual delay via the atrioventricular node (Wolff-Parkinson-White syndrome). The delta waves are seen at the start of the QRS complex leading to a short PR interval. This tracing could be from the patient in Figure 12-2.

- SVT (any type) with aberrancy or preexisting bundle branch block
- Antidromic reentry pathway (atrium-to-ventricle down WPW pathway and ventricle-to-atrium via AV node)
- Wide complex irregular tachycardia (Figure 12-4)
    - Ventricular fibrillation/fast polymorphic ventricular tachycardia
    - Torsades de pointes
    - Atrial fibrillation with WPW
    - Ectopic atrial tachycardia, irregular, with aberrancy

## Treatment (Acute)

### Initial Therapy
- Do not forget ABCs.
- Assess the hemodynamic status of the patient.
- Attach monitor/defibrillator leads.
- Give oxygen.

### Therapy to Terminate the Arrhythmia
- Probable narrow complex regular SVT (heart rate usually >220 beats/min in infants and >180 beats/min in children)
    - Consider vagal maneuvers but do not delay further treatment.
    - Give adenosine rapid IV push dose of 0.1 mg/kg up to 6 mg.
        - Record hard-copy ECG during treatment.
    - If the first dose is not effective, repeat using dose of 0.2 mg/kg up to 12 mg (maximum adult [teenager] dose).
- Wide complex tachycardia: unconscious patient who is in shock
    - Use synchronized cardioversion at 0.5–1 J/kg.
    - If not effective, repeat cardioversion with 2–4 J/kg.

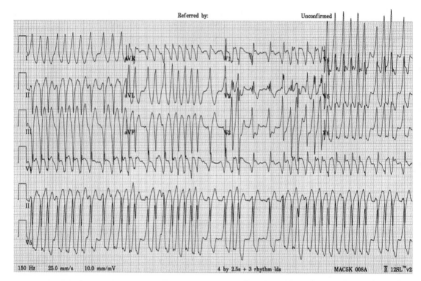

**Figure 12-4.** Electrocardiogram showing an irregular wide complex tachycardia from atrial fibrillation that is conducted rapidly down the aberrant pathway. Adenosine should not be used because it may lead quickly to ventricular fibrillation by enhancing conduction down the pathway.

- Wide complex, regular tachycardia: awake but unstable patient
  - A trial of adenosine may be considered.
  - If hemodynamically unstable but awake, consider sedation for synchronized cardioversion, but do not delay if the patient is deteriorating.

## NEWBORN WITH HEART DISEASE

### General Principles

- Congestive heart failure is the inability of the heart to meet the metabolic demands of the body and may progress to shock.
- The incidence of congenital heart disease in newborns is 5–9 per 1,000 live births.
- The development of symptoms at 6–48 hours of age raises the possibility of ductal-dependent cardiac disease.

### Diagnosis

*Clinical Presentation and History*

- The presentations of congenital heart disease in newborns are presented in Table 12-6.
- Many infants with congenital heart disease are diagnosed prenatally with ultrasound and fetal echocardiograms.
  - However, newborns who do not have a prenatal diagnosis may have a history of central cyanosis, apnea, tachycardia, tachypnea, hepatomegaly, peripheral edema, or poor feeding. Symptoms from left-to-right intracardiac shunts often develop in the first month of life.
  - Peripheral edema or hydrops is less common and suggests long-standing fetal heart failure.

| TABLE 12-6 | Clinical Presentations of Congenital Heart Disease in Newborns |
|---|---|
| Cyanosis | Because of right-to-left shunts or inadequate mixing of systemic and pulmonary circulations |
| Shock | Usually because of loss of ductal dependent systemic blood flow in obstructive left heart lesions |
| Congestive Heart Failure | Presents at different times, usually caused by large left-to-right shunts or poor pump function |
| Murmur | Interpreted in the clinical context |
| Arrhythmia | Usually insignificant unless incessant (prolonged supraventricular tachycardia or congenital complete heart block) |

### Physical Examination

- A basic physical examination and readily available testing should identify most newborns with major congenital heart defects. This screening process allows the timely institution of therapy before a definitive diagnosis is made by consultation with cardiology and echocardiography.
- Special attention should be paid to the presence or absence of murmurs, the nature of $S_2$ sounds (single and loud, fixed split, physiologically split), the character and amplitude of four external pulses and perfusion, and the presence of hepatosplenomegaly.
- Examination findings
  - Bounding right brachial and no femoral pulses: coarctation of aorta
  - Gallop and big liver with murmur: big shunt/congestive heart failure
  - No murmur, symmetric diminished pulses, and shock: ductal dependent systemic blood flow (e.g., hypoplastic left heart)
- Oxygen saturation in right arm compared with leg
  - Normal: no difference
  - Leg lower than right arm: differential cyanosis
    - Ductal-dependent systemic blood flow (coarctation of aorta, interrupted aortic arch, critical aortic stenosis)
    - Pulmonary hypertension with right-to-left shunt at patent ductus arteriosus (PDA)
  - Right arm lower than leg: reverse differential cyanosis
    - Transposition of great vessels with arch obstruction or pulmonary hypertension
  - The presence of differential or reverse differential cyanosis by oximetry is diagnostic of right-to-left shunting. However, because of the high affinity of fetal hemoglobin for oxygen, the **lack** of differential cyanosis by oximetry does not rule out right-to-left shunting (i.e., it is possible to flunk a hyperoxia test with $PO_2 = 90$ mm Hg on 100% $FiO_2$ and still have an oxygen saturation >95%).

### Diagnostic Studies

- ECG
  - Primary arrhythmias (fast or slow): SVT or complete heart block
  - Superior axis (negative in aVF): AV canal or tricuspid atresia
- Hyperoxia test: baseline postductal arterial blood gas (ABG) for $PaO_2$. Give 100% $FiO_2$ for 10 minutes. Draw repeat ABG for $PaO_2$ (Table 12-7).
  - $PaO_2$ <200 mm Hg: abnormal
  - $PaO_2$ <70 mm Hg: almost always heart disease
  - $PaO_2$ <30 mm Hg: most often transposition of the great vessels

### Imaging

- Chest radiograph (exclude major lung disease)
  - Reduced pulmonary blood flow: tetralogy of Fallot, pulmonary atresia
  - Increased pulmonary blood flow: transposition of great vessels, ventral septal defect

| TABLE 12-7 | Hyperoxia Test | | | |
|---|---|---|---|---|
| | $FiO_2 = 0.21$ $PaO_2$ (mm Hg; % saturation) | | $FiO_2 = 1.00$ $PaO_2$ (mm Hg; % saturation) | $PaCO_2$ (mm Hg) |
| Normal | 70 (95) | | >200 (100) | 40 |
| Pulmonary disease | 50 (85) | | >150 (100) | 50 |
| Neurologic disease | 50 (85) | | >150 (100) | 50 |
| Methemoglobinemia | 70 (95) | | >200 (100) | 35 |
| Cardiac disease | | | | |
|   Parallel circulation | <40 (<75) | | <50 (<85) | 35 |
|   Restricted PBF | <40 (<75) | | <50 (<85) | 35 |
|   Complete mixing without PBF | 50–60 (85–93) | | <150 (<100) | 35 |
| PPHN | Preductal | Postductal | | |
|   PFO (no right-to-left shunt) | 70 (95) | <40 (<75) | Variable | 35–50 |
|   PFO (right-to-left shunt) | <40 (<75) | <40 (<75) | Variable | 35–50 |

*PPHN,* persistent pulmonary hypertension of the newborn
*PFO,* patent foramen ovale
*PBF,* pulmonary blood flow
From Chang AC et al, ed. Pediatric Cardiac Intensive Care. Williams & Wilkins, 1998:155.

- Hyaline membrane disease appearance in term infant: obstructed total anomalous pulmonary venous connection
- Recognizable shapes (boot: tetralogy of Fallot; snowman: obstructed total anomalous pulmonary venous connection; egg-on-a-string: transposition of great vessels)
- Echocardiography
  - Often makes a definitive diagnosis
  - Requires significant skill and experience in children; may not be helpful if obtained in a laboratory that scans mostly adults

## Treatment (see "Management of Children With Single Ventricles" section in Chapter 8, Critical Care)

- The newborn with cyanosis or shock with suspected heart disease can be stabilized and transported before a definitive anatomic diagnosis is made. It is not necessary to make an exact anatomic diagnosis before deciding to initiate prostaglandin $E_1$ therapy but only to determine that there is a high probability of ductal-dependent congenital heart disease.
- Urgent cardiology consultation is indicated.

### Medications

- Institution of a continuous infusion of prostaglandin at 0.1 μg/kg/min is usually beneficial. Usual doses are 0.02–0.10 μg/kg/min; the only approved dose is 0.10 μg/kg/min.
- Supplemental oxygen should be avoided if oxygen saturations are >80%–85%.
- Prostaglandin therapy should be avoided in the presence of pulmonary venous obstruction that may occur in total anomalous pulmonary venous connection. This should be suspected if the chest radiograph has a diffuse reticular pattern fanning out from the hilum and obscuring the heart border. Increased pulmonary blood flow from prostaglandin treatment may aggravate pulmonary edema in this setting.

*Nonoperative: Mechanical Ventilation*
■ See Management of Children With Single Ventricles in Chapter 8, Critical Care).
■ Intubation with mechanical ventilation should be considered for transportation of neonates on prostaglandin, especially if apnea is noted.
■ Mechanical ventilation may also be of benefit for infants in shock by decreasing the work of breathing and thereby decreasing metabolic demands.
■ Hyperventilation should be avoided.

## CHEST PAIN

■ Chest pain is a common complaint in the pediatric population, but cardiac disease is an uncommon cause of pediatric chest pain. In a prospective emergency department study, only 4% of children with chest pain had cardiac disease (Selbst, et al).
   ■ Musculoskeletal disorders are the most common identifiable cause of chest pain in children.
   ■ Gastrointestinal causes are suggested by an association with eating or vomiting.
   ■ Pain that awakens a child is more likely to be organic.
   ■ Cardiac causes are especially unlikely in an adolescent with a longstanding history of chest pain.
   ■ Exercise-induced bronchospasm or vocal cord dysfunction should be considered with exertional pain accompanied by difficulty breathing, noisy breathing, wheezing, or cough.

### Diagnosis

*Clinical Presentation and History*
■ Chest pain that is seen in patients with known or suspected congenital heart disease, primarily exertional pain, or severe pain of acute onset requires more extensive evaluation.
■ History. The following historical information should be sought:
   ■ History of structural heart disease, especially aortic stenosis
   ■ Cardiomyopathy/myocarditis: exercise intolerance, family history of sudden unexpected death, murmur, gallop rhythm, hepatomegaly, tachycardia, or tachypnea
   ■ Tachyarrhythmia: tachycardia preceding the pain, rapid onset, and rapid resolution
   ■ Pericarditis: fever, recent viral illness, and pain worse in the supine position, which is decreased by leaning forward

*Physical Examination*
■ Tenderness on palpation or pain accentuated by inspiration, which suggests a musculoskeletal cause
■ Surgical scar, murmur, gallop rhythm, muffled heart sounds, tachycardia, tachypnea, or hepatomegaly that suggests cardiac disease
■ Rales, wheezes, or differential breath sounds with pulmonary disease

*Diagnostic Studies*
■ Troponin is rarely indicated.
   ■ Coronary artery disease is rare in children.
   ■ Troponin levels may be elevated in myocarditis.
■ ECG
   ■ Hypertrophy or T-wave changes may be seen with hypertrophic cardiomyopathy or aortic stenosis.
   ■ Preexcitation (WPW syndrome) raises the possibility of SVT.
   ■ Low voltages or ST elevation occurs with pericarditis.
■ Chest radiograph: should be considered with more acute presentation or ill-appearing child
   ■ Cardiomegaly may be present in cardiomyopathy, pericardial effusion, or structural heart disease.
   ■ Infiltrates, pleural effusion, or pneumothorax suggest respiratory disease.

## Treatment

*Medications*
- Short courses of nonsteroidal anti-inflammatory drugs can be used for musculoskeletal pain.
- β-agonists and steroids can be used for wheezing or asthma.

*Referrals*
- If cardiac disease is suspected based on the initial evaluation, cardiology consultation should be sought before ordering additional tests.

# SYNCOPE

## Definition and Epidemiology

- Syncope, defined as the sudden loss of consciousness and postural tone, occurs at least once in 15%–25% of children and adolescents.
- Despite its frequent occurrence, syncope creates significant anxiety for families and caregivers.
- In a study of children presenting to a tertiary care center for syncope, an average of four diagnostic tests were obtained, with an average cost for testing of $1055 per patient. Only 3.9% of the tests were diagnostic (Steinberg, et al).
- Anxiety and depression may be associated with recurrent syncope (Kouakam, et al).

*Etiology*
- Neurally mediated (vasovagal) mechanisms cause the vast majority of syncope in children.
- Cardiac causes are uncommon.
- Breath-holding spells are frequently seen in early childhood and are usually classified as pallid or cyanotic (Table 12-8).

## Diagnosis

*Clinical Presentation and History*
- The history before the event is most important, although parents focus on the history after the syncope. Seek history from other observers, such as friends, teachers, and coaches.
- If the event occurred at a sporting event, determine whether the episode/symptoms occurred after participating in an activity (e.g., standing on sidelines) or while engaging in a vigorous activity (suggestive of a cardiac cause).
- Neurally mediated syncope is often characterized by presyncopal symptoms such as dizziness, "head rush," diaphoresis, visual blurring, facial pallor, abdominal pain/nausea, warm or cold sensation, and tachycardia, which last for seconds to minutes.
  - There is often a history of positional presyncopal symptoms.

| TABLE 12-8 | Pallid vs Cyanotic Breath-Holding Spell |
|---|---|
| **Pallid** | **Cyanotic** |
| Precipitated by sudden, unexpected, unpleasant stimulus, frequently a mild head injury | Violent crying (temper tantrum) |
| Crying not prominent | Breath holding (apnea) in expiration |
| Pallor and diaphoresis are common | |
| Bradycardia with excessive vagal tone | |

| TABLE 12-9 | Common Situations for Neurally Mediated Syncope |
| --- | --- |

- Noxious stimuli such as blood drawing
- Hair combing by someone else
- Shower, hot bath, especially in morning, before breakfast
- Micturition, defecation with Valsalva maneuver
- Hyperventilation
- Standing in line, kneeling in church

■ Loss of consciousness usually lasts for 5–20 seconds, but there may be 5 minutes to several hours of fatigue, weakness, dizziness, headache, or nausea.
■ Table 12-9 lists common situations for neurally mediated syncope.
- Always seek historical red flags that would suggest a seizure when a child presents with syncope (Table 12-10).
- Always seek historical red flags and family history that would suggest a cardiac cause (Tables 12-11 and 12-12).

### Physical Examination
- Orthostatic changes in heart rate and blood pressure: neurally mediated syncope
- Right ventricular heave or loud second heart sound in pulmonary hypertension
- Systolic murmur in left ventricular outflow tract obstruction. Auscultate for murmur in supine and standing positions to look for dynamic obstruction, suggesting hypertrophic cardiomyopathy.

### Diagnostic Testing
- Laboratory testing. None is required for cardiac or neurally mediated causes of syncope. If there is concern that a syncopal episode was a seizure, check bedside glucose, electrolyte profile, including magnesium and phosphorus.
- ECG. Perform in all patients. It is inexpensive and a reasonable screen given the low incidence of cardiac disease in children with syncope.
  ■ Determine corrected QT interval: long QT syndrome
  ■ Left ventricular hypertrophy, T-wave abnormalities: abnormal in 80% of patients with hypertrophic cardiomyopathy
  ■ Right ventricular hypertrophy: pulmonary hypertension
  ■ Preexcitation: WPW syndrome
  ■ Right bundle branch block with ST elevation in leads $V_1$-$V_3$: Brugada syndrome, a rare cause of ventricular arrhythmias
  ■ Complete heart block: rare without a history of congenital heart defect
- Echocardiography. This is usually indicated after consultation with cardiology with atypical history, abnormal cardiac examination, or abnormal ECG.
- Tilt table testing. This is unlikely to be useful because it has 90% specificity but only 60% sensitivity for neurally mediated syncope. Therefore, it is not a good screening test.

| TABLE 12-10 | Historical Red Flags in Syncope That Suggest a Seizure |
| --- | --- |

- History of seizure disorder
- Shaking of extremities during a syncopal episode
- Drooling, loss of bowel or bladder control during a syncopal episode
- Eyes open during the unresponsive episode.
- Prolonged postictal confusion (mental status recovers promptly in syncope but may be abnormal for awhile in seizure)

**TABLE 12-11** **Historical Red Flags That Suggest a Cardiac Cause of Syncope**

- Occurring in the midst of exercise
- Abrupt syncope with no premonitory symptoms
- Prior history of congenital heart disease or heart surgery, especially aortic stenosis or single ventricle
- Brought on by sudden startle, such as by an alarm clock, without preceding symptoms—long QT syndrome
- Acute or subacute history of exercise intolerance between spells—cardiomyopathy, myocarditis

## Treatment

### Behavioral

- Education and reassurance is usually the only treatment needed for patients with vaso-vagal (neurally mediated) syncope. Talk with patient and parents about situations when syncope is common and advise the patient to sit or lie down when they experience pre-syncopal symptoms.
- A randomized study in adults showed that water before tilt testing enhanced tolerance of upright positioning (Lu, et al).
- Increased intake of fluid and salt especially before and during physical activity to enhance preload is the primary treatment. Advise the patient to drink enough flu-ids to make the urine appear clear and to avoid fluids with caffeine. It may be help-ful to write a note to allow a water bottle at school and more frequent restroom breaks.
- Isometric maneuvers such as tensing muscles in the arms or legs with prodromal symp-toms may decrease the incidence of syncope (Brignole, et al).

### Medications

- A number of drugs have been used in patients with recurrent syncope, but data regard-ing efficacy are limited (Calkins).
    - Fludrocortisone has been used commonly in children, but a recent double-blind placebo-controlled trial in children found that patients on a placebo had fewer re-currences as compared with the active treatment group (Salim, et al).
    - Beta blockers have proven ineffective in placebo-controlled randomized trials. Smaller studies support the use of selective serotonin reuptake inhibitors. Midodrine (direct vasoconstrictor) may be effective; however, it may cause hypertension (i.e., treatment is worse than the disease).

### Referrals

- If cardiac disease is suspected based on the initial evaluation, cardiology consultation should be sought before ordering additional tests.

**TABLE 12-12** **Family History That Suggests a Cardiac Cause of Syncope**

- Premature and unexplained sudden death
- Cardiomyopathy
- Arrhythmias, especially long QT syndrome
- Implanted defibrillator
- Congenital deafness (long QT syndrome), seizures

# HEART MURMURS

## General Principles

- Heart murmurs are common in children. At least 50% of children will have a murmur noted at some time.
- The vast majority of heart murmurs in childhood are innocent or functional in nature.
  - These murmurs occur in the absence of anatomic or physiologic abnormalities of the heart and therefore have no clinical significance.
  - The age at onset is most frequently 3–8 years.

## Diagnosis

### Clinical Presentation and History

- Pathologic murmurs should be suspected when other features of heart disease are present, including poor growth/failure to thrive, tachypnea/tachycardia, and central cyanosis.
- Murmurs may occur with a history of poor feeding in infants, with activity intolerance, or with a family history of congenital heart defects or cardiomyopathy.

### Physical Examination

- With training and experience, the physical examination can be sensitive and specific.
- Innocent murmurs usually occur during early to midsystole (they are never diastolic), are short in duration, have a crescendo-decrescendo contour, and are usually <3/6 in intensity.
- Innocent murmurs are often louder in the supine position, or with fever, anemia, or other conditions that lead to increased cardiac output.
- The venous hum is an innocent continuous murmur best heard in the infraclavicular area. This hum should disappear when the patient is supine and with compression of the neck veins.
- Examination findings. The intensity (loudness) of a murmur does not necessarily correlate with the severity of the condition. The examination of a child with a murmur should go beyond listening to the murmur.
  - Identify $S_1$: produced by closure of the mitral and the tricuspid valve in that order. This signals the beginning of systole.
  - Identify $S_2$: produced by closure of the aortic ($A_2$) and the pulmonic ($P_2$) valves. The $A_2$–$P_2$ interval widens with inspiration and narrows with expiration (physiologic splitting of $S_2$).
  - Assess skin color, respiratory effort, and respiratory and heart rate.
  - Perform a precordial examination by inspection and palpation.
    - Right ventricular heave (lift) from volume overload (atrial septal defect), or a pressure overload (large ventral septal defect, pulmonary hypertension, pulmonary stenosis)
    - Left ventricular heave (lift): aortic stenosis
    - A thrill with grade 4 or 5 murmur, which is usually pathologic
  - Auscultate lung fields.
  - Palpate abdomen. Hepatomegaly may suggest congestive heart failure.
  - Palpate peripheral pulses. Differential pulses occur in coarctation of the aorta.
  - Measure blood pressure. Differential blood pressure occurs in coarctation of the aorta.
  - Table 12-13 includes features of murmurs that may be pathologic.
  - The timing and location of pathologic murmurs can help narrow the differential diagnosis (Tables 12-14 through 12-19).

## Treatment

- Treatments vary depending on the condition.
- Initiate ABCs if necessary to stabilize the patient.
- If cardiac disease is suspected based on the initial evaluation, seek cardiology consultation before ordering additional tests.

**TABLE 12-13** Features That May Suggest a Pathologic Murmur

- All diastolic murmurs
- All holosystolic murmurs
- Late systolic murmurs
- Presence of a thrill

**TABLE 12-14** Characteristics of Systolic Murmurs Along Right Upper Sternal Border

| Lesion | Timing, quality | Heard best | Transmits to | Comments |
|---|---|---|---|---|
| Aortic valve stenosis | Ejection | 2nd left intercostal space | Neck, left upper sternal border, apex | +/− thrill, ejection click, left ventricular lift, possible single $S_2$ |
| Subaortic stenosis | Ejection | — | — | No click |
| Supravalvular aortic stenosis | Ejection | — | Back | No click, +/− thrill, associated with Williams syndrome |

**TABLE 12-15** Characteristics of Systolic Murmurs Along Left Upper Sternal Border

| Lesion | Timing, quality | Heard best | Transmits to | Comments |
|---|---|---|---|---|
| Pulmonic valve stenosis | Ejection | — | Back | +/− thrill, $S_2$ may be widely split if mild, +/− variable ejection click at 2nd left intercostal space |
| ASD | Ejection, soft | 2nd left intercostal space | — | Widely split, fixed $S_2$, +/− diastolic murmur |
| Pulmonary artery stenosis | Ejection | — | Back and both lung fields | $P_2$ may be loud |
| Tetralogy of Fallot | Long ejection murmur | Mid-left sternal border or left upper sternal border | — | +/− thrill, single $S_2$ |
| Coarctation of the aorta | Ejection | Left interscapular area | — | Pulse and blood pressure disparity |
| Patent ductus arteriosus in neonates | High frequency, rocky | Left infraclavicular area | — | Bounding pulses |

| TABLE 12-16 | Characteristics of Systolic Murmurs Along Left Lower Sternal Border |

| Lesion | Timing, quality | Heard best | Transmits to | Comments |
|---|---|---|---|---|
| Ventral septal defect (VSD) | Regurgitant, harsh, systolic, may be holosystolic | Localized and short if small, muscular | Lower right of sternum, left upper if outflow | May be soft with loud $P_2$ and right ventricular lift if large |
| Complete atrioventricular (AV) canal | As with VSD | — | Apical murmur with AV regurgitation, diastolic rumble, may have gallop | |
| Subaortic stenosis with hypertrophic cardiomyopathy | Ejection | Left lower sternal border or apex, medium pitch | — | +/− thrill, Valsalva increases murmur, squatting decreases murmur |
| Tricuspid regurgitation | Regurgitant systolic | — | — | Multiple sounds: split $S_1$, $S_3/S_4$ in Ebstein anomaly |

| TABLE 12-17 | Characteristics of Systolic Murmurs at Apex |

| Lesion | Timing, quality | Heard best | Transmits to | Comments |
|---|---|---|---|---|
| Mitral regurgitation | Plateau-type blowing | Apex to mid-precordium | Left axilla, back | Diastolic rumble if severe |
| Mitral valve prolapse | Midsystolic click with late systolic murmur if mitral regurgitation present | — | Click moves toward $S_2$ (squatting) and toward $S_1$ (standing) | |

| TABLE 12-18 | Characteristics of Diastolic Murmurs |

| Lesion | Timing, quality | Heard best | Transmits to | Comments |
|---|---|---|---|---|
| Aortic regurgitation | Early, decrescendo, high pitched | 3rd left intercostal space | Apex | Short and loud if severe |
| Pulmonary regurgitation | Early, medium pitched | 2nd left intercostal space | Along left sternal border | Short and loud if severe |
| Mitral stenosis | Mid to late, crescendo low pitched rumble | Apex | | Soft or loud $S_2$ |

| TABLE 12-19 | Characteristics of Continuous Murmurs | | |
|---|---|---|---|
| Lesion | Timing, quality | Heard best | Comments |
| Patent ductus arteriosus | Louder in systole, machinery | Left mid to upper sternal border | Bounding pulse if large |
| Coronary to right heart fistula | | Left sternal border | Rare cause of murmur |
| Cerebral arteriovenous fistula | Louder in diastole | Infraclavicular | Bruit in head |

# CONGESTIVE HEART FAILURE

## General Principles

- Congestive heart failure in pediatrics is defined as inadequate delivery of oxygen and nutrients to the tissues to meet the metabolic demands of a growing infant or child.
- The most common causes of congestive heart failure vary depending on the age of the patient (Table 12-20).

## Diagnosis

### Clinical Presentation and History
- Tachypnea and tachycardia are cardinal symptoms of congestive heart failure.
- With chronic heart failure, infants often have poor feeding, inadequate weight gain, and irritability. Older children often have decreased exercise tolerance, anorexia, and vomiting.

| TABLE 12-20 | Common Causes of Congestive Heart Failure By Age | | |
|---|---|---|---|
| Fetus | Newborn | Young infant | Older child |
| Tachyarrhythmias | Structural heart disease, especially hypoplastic left heart, critical aortic stenosis and coarctation, and obstructed pulmonary venous return (see "Newborn With Heart Disease" section) | Left-to-right shunts: ventricular septal defects | Cardiomyopathy |
| Anemia—parvovirus | Patent ductus arteriosus in the preterm infant | Coarctation of the aorta | Myocarditis/pericarditis with pericardial effusion |

*Physical Examination*
- Surgical scar, murmur, gallop rhythm, muffled heart sounds, tachycardia, tachypnea, or hepatomegaly, which may suggest cardiac disease
- Edema and poor perfusion in extremities

*Diagnostic Studies*
- Laboratory studies
  - A brain natriuretic peptide (BNP) level has been established in adults as an adjunct in the diagnosis of congestive heart failure.
    - In adults with dyspnea, a BNP cutoff value of 100 pg/mL had a sensitivity of 90% and specificity of 76% for identifying those with heart failure (Maisel, et al).
- ECG
  - This is used primarily to rule out a tachyarrhythmia.
  - Low QRS voltages and ST-T wave changes may suggest myocardial or pericardial disease.
- Imaging
  - Chest radiography: important initial test in differential diagnosis that includes cardiac and respiratory disease
    - Cardiomegaly or increased pulmonary vascular markings suggests cardiac disease.
  - Echocardiography
    - Often makes a definitive diagnosis
    - Requires significant skill and experience in children; may not be helpful if obtained in a laboratory that tests mostly adults

## Treatment (see "Management of Children With Single Ventricles" section in Chapter 8, Critical Care)

- Management is guided by consultation with a pediatric cardiologist and depends on the etiology of heart failure, hemodynamic status, and clinical symptoms. Specific guidelines are beyond the scope of this text.
- Surgical or catheter based intervention is usually undertaken for structural heart defects.
- Pharmacologic treatment may include diuretics, systemic vasodilators, β-blockers, and inotropic agents.
- In the emergency department, for patients with probable new congestive heart failure and marked dyspnea, an IV dose of furosemide (Lasix) of 1 mg/kg up to 40 mg can be given while arrangements are made for pediatric cardiology consultation.

### Suggested Readings

Brignole M, et al. Isometric arm counter-pressure maneuvers to abort impending vasovagal syncope. J Am Coll Cardiol 2002;40:2053–2059.

Calkins H. Pharmacologic approaches to therapy for vasovagal syncope. Am J Cardiol 1999;84:20Q–25Q.

Kouakam C, et al. Prevalence and prognostic significance of psychiatric disorders in patients evaluated for recurrent syncope. Am J Cardiol 2002;89:530–535.

Lu CC, et al. Water ingestion as prophylaxis against syncope. Circulation. 2003;108: 2660–2665.

Maisel AS, et al. Rapid measurement of B-type natriuretic peptide in the emergency diagnosis of heart failure. N Engl J Med 2002;347:161–167.

Newburger JW, et al. Noninvasive tests in the initial evaluation of heart murmurs in children. N Engl J Med 1983;308:61.

Salim MA, et al. Effectiveness of fludrocortisone and salt in preventing syncope recurrence in children. J Am Coll Cardiol 2005;45:484–488.

Schwartz PJ, et al. Diagnostic criteria for the long QT syndrome. Circulation 1993;88:782–784.

Selbst SM, et al. Pediatric chest pain: a prospective study. Pediatrics 1988;82:319–323.

Steinberg LA, et al. Syncope in children: diagnostic tests have a high cost and low yield. J Pediatr 2005;146:355–358.

# DERMATOLOGIC DISEASES
### Kara Sternhell Nunley and Susan J. Bayliss

**13**

- Skin disorders are one of the most common problems in pediatrics.
- Never underestimate parental concerns about their child's skin. Unlike many disease processes, the skin is visible and noticeable to parents and others.
- Examination of the skin requires observation and palpation of the entire skin surface under good light. Do not forget to look at the eyes and mouth for mucous membrane involvement.
- Examination should include onset, duration, and inspection of a primary lesion. It is also important to note secondary changes, morphology, and distribution of the lesions.

## NEONATAL DERMATOSES

### Cutis Marmorata

- Transient, blanchable, reticulated mottling occurs on the skin exposed to a cool environment.
- No treatment is necessary; the condition generally resolves by 1 year of age.
- If it persists, consider hypothyroidism, heart disease, or other associated abnormalities.

### Erythema Toxicum Neonatorum

- Scattered erythematous papules and pustules may occur anywhere on the body (Figure 13-1).
- This self-limited condition generally appears in the first week of life and resolves within 1 month.

### Transient Neonatal Pustular Melanosis

- Pustular lesions rupture easily and leave hyperpigmented macules on the neck, chin, forehead, lower back, and shins (Figure 13-2).
- Almost always present at birth, this condition is more common in dark-skinned infants.
- It is self-limited. Pustules resolve within days, but hyperpigmentation may take months to resolve.

### Acne Neonatorum

- Comedones, pustules, and papules on the face resemble acne vulgaris (Figure 13-3).
- Generally develops at 2–3 weeks of age and resolves within 6 months.
- No treatment is usually necessary; wash face with baby soap. In severe cases, referral to a pediatric dermatologist may be warranted.

### Milia

- These 1–2 mm pearly white papules are found most commonly on the face (Figure 13-4) but may occur anywhere. On the palate, they are known as "Epstein pearls."
- They may be present at birth.
- They usually resolve without treatment by 2–6 months of age.

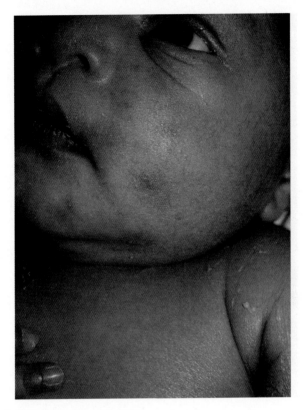

**Figure 13-1.** Erythema toxicum neonatorum.

## Miliaria

- This sweat retention as a result of plugging of sweat glands is worsened by heat and humidity.
  - Miliaria crystallina are 1–2 mm vesicles without erythema in intertriginous areas, neck, and chest.
  - Miliaria rubra are erythematous papules in the same distribution that result from obstruction deeper in the epidermis.
- This condition resolves without treatment in a dry environment.

## Harlequin Color Change

- This transient erythematous flush occurs on the dependent half of the body when the infant is placed on his or her side.
- This self-limited condition generally resolves within minutes but may recur.

## Subcutaneous Fat Necrosis

- Erythematous subcutaneous nodules and plaques may be fluctuant.
- They appear at 1–6 weeks of life and generally resolve without treatment in 2–6 months. Fluctuant nodules require drainage.

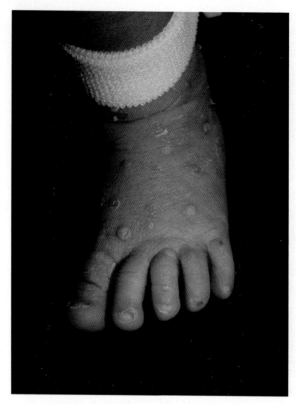

**Figure 13-2.** Transient neonatal pustular melanosis.

- They may be associated with significant hypercalcemia as well as localized calcification, so infants should be monitored for hypercalcemia for at least 6 months after appearance of extensive lesions.

## BIRTH MARKS

### Mongolian Spots (Dermal Melanosis)

- These blue-gray poorly circumscribed macules often occur in lumbosacral area or lower extremities (Figure 13-5).
- More common in pigmented skin, they are present from birth.
- Lumbosacral lesions tend to fade during childhood; however, lesions in other locations usually do not fade.

### Café-au-Lait Macules

- These light brown macules (Figure 13-6) can occur anywhere on the body.
- They may occur in isolation or in association with a syndrome.
  - The presence of six or more macules >0.5 cm in diameter in prepubertal children or >1.5 cm in postpubertal, as well as inguinal or axillary freckling, is suggestive of neurofibromatosis 1.
  - Large truncal macules may be associated with McCune-Albright syndrome.

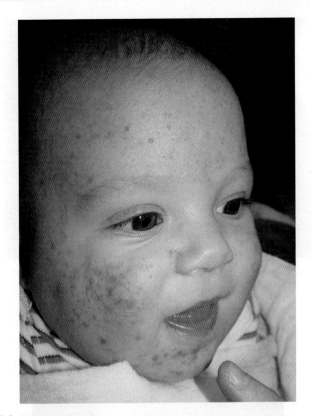

**Figure 13-3.** Acne neonatorum.

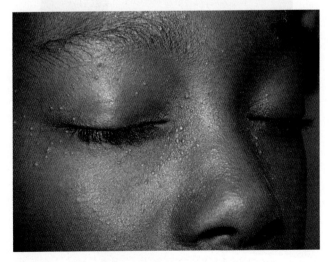

**Figure 13-4.** Milia.

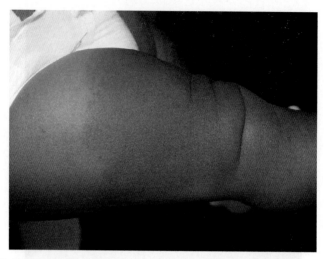

**Figure 13-5.** Mongolian spots (Dermal Melanosis).

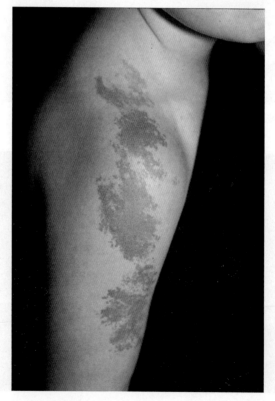

**Figure 13-6.** Café-au-Lait macules.

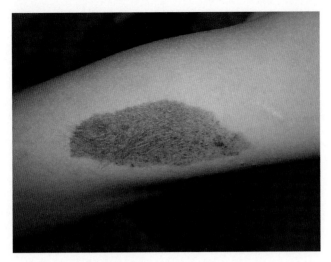

**Figure 13-7.** Congenital melanocytic nevi.

## Congenital Melanocytic Nevi

■ These brown pigmented macules or plaques may have dark brown or black papules or other irregular pigmentation within the lesions (Figure 13-7). They may cover large areas of skin.
■ Lesions are present at birth; small congenital melanocytic nevi may become more noticeable within the first year of life.
■ The small increased risk of melanoma development within lesions makes close follow-up important.
■ Decisions about excision versus observation vary with the size and site of the lesion.

## Nevus Sebaceous

■ This hairless, yellow-colored plaque tends to have an irregular surface.
■ Located on the scalp (Figure 13-8), it becomes less prominent after the newborn period but later grows and becomes more papular or verrucous around puberty, when hormone levels increase.
■ Treatment is surgical excision or observation.
   ■ Surgery is often deferred until puberty when the lesion begins to grow.
   ■ The plaque should be followed by clinical observation until excision because there is a low, but increased, risk of benign tumors within the lesion.

## Aplasia Cutis Congenita

■ This is an absence of skin with scar formation in a localized area, most commonly on the scalp (Figure 13-9).
■ Defects are present from birth.
■ Larger or multiple lesions may be associated with other congenital anomalies or a genetic syndrome.
■ Small defects often heal on their own, leaving scar tissue. Larger defects may require skin grafting or other surgical intervention.

## Port Wine Stain

■ This pink, red, or purple blanchable macule is caused by capillary malformations (Figure 13-10).

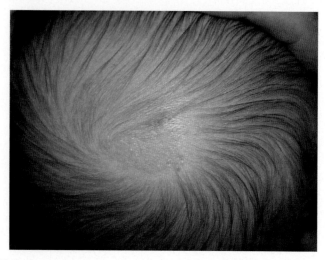

**Figure 13-8.** Nevus sebaceous.

■ Lesions in cranial nerve V1 or V2 distribution on the face should be evaluated for associated glaucoma and/or Sturge-Weber syndrome. These lesions persist and generally become darker and more populus with age.
■ Therapy is pulsed-dye laser treatment.

## Salmon Patch/Nevus Simplex ("stork bite")

■ These are pink macular patches (Figure 13-11), generally on the scalp or neck.
    ■ Lesions on the eyelids usually improve at 1 year and fade by 3 years.
    ■ Those on the nape of the neck tend to persist.

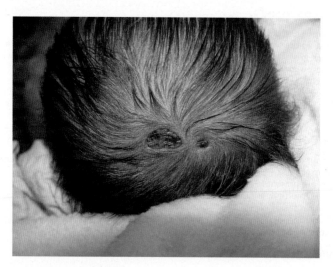

**Figure 13-9.** Aplasia cutis congenita.

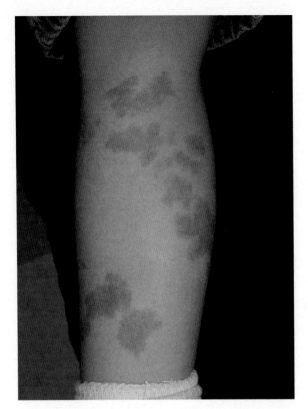

**Figure 13-10.** Port wine stain.

## Hemangiomas

*Appearance*
- Superficial: bright red vascular plaques or nodules
- Deep: bluish purple nodules, sometimes with overlying telangiectatic markings (Figure 13-12)

*Course*
- Lesions may or may not be noticeable at birth.
    - They generally appear as faint vascular markings at first and then enlarge and develop characteristic appearance over 2–4 months.
    - They then stabilize in size and appearance at 6–12 months. Most involute by 5–10 years of age, but many leave behind residual markings or fibrous tissue.

*Complications and Associations*
- Kasabach-Merritt syndrome: sudden growth of a lesion accompanied by platelet sequestration, leading to thrombocytopenia
- Disseminated neonatal hemangiomatosis: multiple scattered small hemangiomas on the skin. This condition is often accompanied by internal involvement with hemangiomas in liver, brain, or gastrointestinal tract.

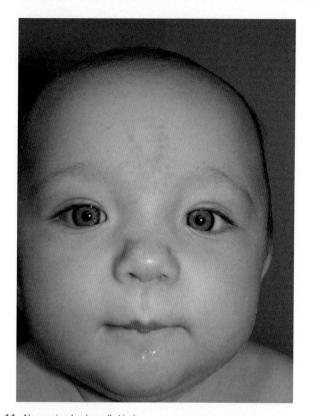

**Figure 13-11.** Nevus simplex (angel's kiss).

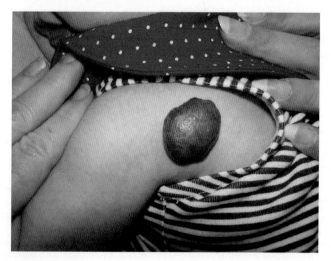

**Figure 13-12.** Hemangioma.

- PHACES syndrome: **p**osterior fossa malformations, **h**emangiomas, **a**rterial anomalies, **c**oarctation of the aorta, **e**ye anomalies, and **s**ternal cleft
- Chin and neck hemangiomas: may be associated with tracheal involvement
- Sacral hemangiomas: may be associated with tethered cord or spinal dysraphism
- Ulceration: may occur in any hemangioma, but is more common around the mouth and diaper area. Treatment is oral steroids, laser, or topical/oral antibiotics and occlusive dressing.

## ACNE VULGARIS

- The etiology of acne is multifactorial. Causes include follicular plugging, increased sebum production, *Propionibacterium acnes* overgrowth, and inflammation.

### Classification

- Comedonal: open comedones (blackheads) and closed comedones (whiteheads) (Figure 13-13A)
- Inflammatory: erythematous, inflammatory papules and pustules in addition to comedones
- Cystic: nodules and cysts on face, chest, and back (Figure 13-13B)

### Treatment

- General skin care: washing of face with soap or acne wash 2–3 times per day. Avoid scrubbing and excessive washing.
- Comedonal acne: topical benzoyl peroxide, topical retinoid, or topical antibiotic
  - Mild: sample regimen for mild comedonal acne is benzoyl peroxide 5% OR adapalene cream at night and clindamycin 1% solution each day.
    - Benzoyl peroxide and retinoids can be irritating. Advise patients to use only a pea-sized amount on the face. Use every other day initially if redness/drying occurs, and then increase to daily as tolerance develops.
    - Benzoyl peroxide 2.5% and 5% products are as effective as 10% preparations. Benzoyl peroxide products should not be used at the same time as a topical retinoid.
    - Topical retinoids come in a variety of strengths: adapalene 0.1% (least potent and least irritating); tretinoin 0.025%, 0.05%, and 0.1%; and tazarotene 0.05% and 0.1% (most potent but most irritating). Start with the least potent for patients with dry or sensitive skin and work up as tolerated.
    - Products combining a topical antibiotic and benzoyl peroxide are available to simplify regimens.
  - Inflammatory acne
    - Add oral antibiotic (doxycycline, minocycline, tetracycline) to topical regimen for comedonal acne. Oral antibiotics should be continued for 2–3 months minimum.
    - Advise patients to use sunscreen and take antibiotics with a large glass of water to minimize risks of photosensitivity and esophagitis.
  - Cystic/nodular or scarring acne
    - Refer to dermatologist for possible systemic retinoid therapy (isotretinoin).
    - This requires monitoring of lipid profile, aspartate aminotransferase, alanine aminotransferase, and strict contraception in females because the agent is teratogenic.
  - For females, consider an endocrine workup if early presentation is accompanied by other virilizing signs to look for androgen excess disorder or if acne is accompanied by hirsutism and irregular periods to look for polycystic ovary syndrome.

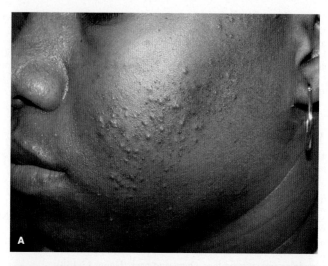

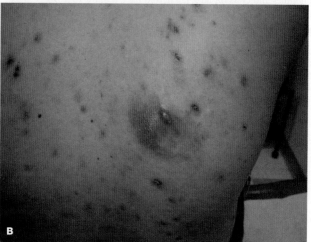

**Figure 13-13.** Acne vulgaris. **A.** Comedonal Acne. **B.** Cystic acne.

## ATOPIC DERMATITIS

### Definition

- This condition is characterized by pruritic, erythematous papules and plaques.
- Secondary changes include lichenification and postinflammatory hyperpigmentation or hypopigmentation.

### Epidemiology

- There is a strong association with personal or family history of asthma and allergic rhinitis.
- Most eczema improves by 10 years of age.

- Severe, recalcitrant eczematous dermatitis may be associated with immunodeficiencies, including hyper-IgE syndrome, Wiskott-Aldrich syndrome, and severe combined immunodeficiency syndrome.
- Children with eczema are prone to viral superinfection (e.g., herpes simplex virus [HSV], molluscum contagiosum) and colonization with *Staphylococcus aureus*.

## Subtypes

- Infantile
  - From 2 months to 2 years
  - Commonly involves cheeks (Figure 13-14A), scalp, trunk, and extensor surfaces of the extremities
- Childhood
  - From 2 years to adolescence
  - Commonly involves flexural surfaces, including antecubital, popliteal fossae, neck, wrists, and feet (Figures 14B, C)
- Adolescent/Adult
  - Flexural surfaces; may be limited to hands and/or face
- Nummular
  - Coin-shaped erythematous, oozing plaques that may have papules or vesicles at the periphery
  - Often occur on hands, arms, or legs (Figure 13-14D)
- Dyshidrotic
  - Bilateral hand and/or foot dermatitis
  - Intensely pruritic with small vesicles along sides of fingers and toes

## Treatment

- General skin care. Tell patients to:
  - Limit bathing to once daily in lukewarm water. Use mild soaps (e.g., Dove, Aveeno) only in small amounts and in the area necessary.
  - Apply moisturizers immediately after bathing. Ointments (e.g., petroleum jelly [Vaseline] or Aquaphor) or thick creams (e.g., Eucerin) are more effective than lotions.

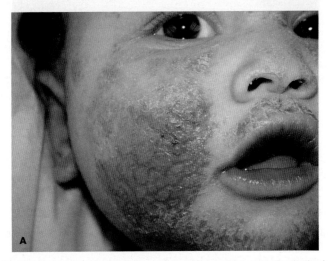

**Figure 13-14.** Atopic dermatitis. **A.** Infantile eczema with oozing plaques on the cheeks. *(continued)*

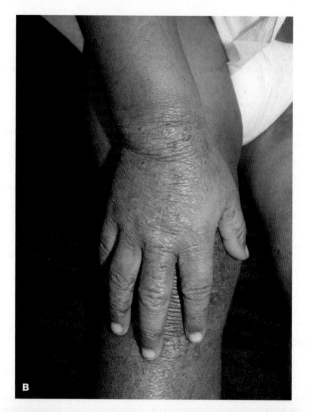

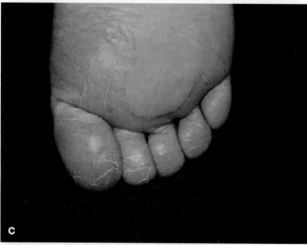

**Figure 13-14.** *(continued)* **B.** Childhood eczema-lichenified plaques with excoriations. **C.** Juvenile plantar dermatosis (foot eczema).

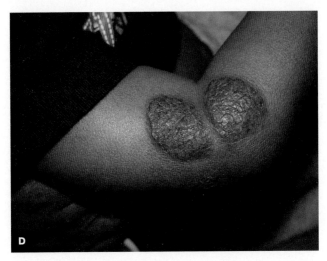

**Figure 13-14.** *(continued)* **D.** Nummular eczema.

- Education of patients, including emphasizing the chronicity of disease and the need for consistent application of prescribed treatment, which can improve compliance and outcomes.
- Topical steroids
  - Classification
    - Low-strength (e.g., hydrocortisone 1% or 2.5% ointment): can be used for mild to moderate disease
    - Midstrength (e.g., triamcinolone 0.1% ointment): can be used for limited amounts of time on more severe, localized areas of disease. These agents can cause atrophy if used inappropriately.
    - High-strength (e.g., fluocinonide or clobetasol ointment) may be needed for palmar and plantar dermatitis. Referral to a pediatric dermatologist may be appropriate if high-strength steroids are required.
  - Avoid using topical steroids on the face and intertriginous areas. Risks of topical steroids, including skin atrophy, striae, and hypopigmentation, should be discussed with patients.
- Immunomodulators
  - Topical tacrolimus (0.03% or 0.1%) or topical pimecrolimus (1%) may be useful in limited areas such as the face, where topical steroids may cause undesirable side effects with prolonged use.
  - These agents should only be used in children over age 2 years.
- Antihistamines. Oral diphenhydramine, hydroxyzine, or cetirizine are often useful to control pruritus. These agents may cause sedation, restricting their use to nighttime.
- Systemic steroids
  - These may be used in short bursts for severe exacerbations.
  - Regular or long-term use is not recommended.
- Antibiotics
  - *S. aureus* is the most common cause of bacterial superinfection. Topical antibiotics or oral antibiotics may be necessary depending on the severity of infection. Methicillin-resistant *S. aureus* is becoming more prevalent. Cultures to determine antibiotic susceptibility should be performed.
  - Avoid neomycin/polymyxin/bacitracin (Neosporin) because neomycin and bacitracin are a common cause of contact dermatitis.

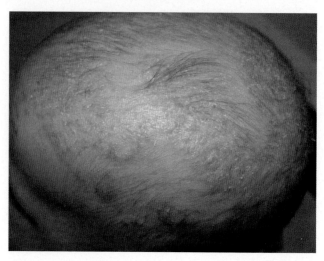

**Figure 13-15.** Seborrheic dermatitis.

## SEBORRHEIC DERMATITIS

- This is characterized by erythematous patches covered by thick, yellow scale.
- "Cradle cap" occurs on the scalp of infants (Figure 13-15).
  - It is most common at 2–10 weeks and may last for 8–12 months.
  - Treatment involves hydrocortisone 0.5% –1% ointment.
- The adolescent/adult form is characterized by dryness and flaking in scalp, eyebrows, nasolabial folds, and chest. Treatment involves:
  - Shampoos: sulfur or salicylic acid (T-gel), selenium sulfide 2.5% (Selsun), or keto-conazole 2% (Nizoral) on affected areas, including face and body
  - Low-strength topical steroid (hydrocortisone 1% cream) for 5–7 days if needed
- Blepharitis is characterized by flaking along eyelids. Treatment involves warm water compresses and baby shampoo eyelid scrubs.

## CONTACT DERMATITIS

- The lesions of contact dermatitis are erythematous papules and vesicles with oozing and crusting. Pruritus may be intense. This is a type IV (delayed/cell mediated) hypersensitivity reaction.
- Common causes include poison ivy/oak, nickel, cosmetics and fragrances, topical medications, and tape or other adhesives (Figures 13-16A, B). The distribution often gives clues to the causative agent (e.g., exposed areas for poison ivy, umbilicus for nickel, eyelids and face for nail polish or other cosmetics).
- This may be accompanied by eczematous dermatitis at sites far from initial exposure.
- Treatment
- Calamine lotion t.i.d. for oozing plaques
  - High-strength topical steroids b.i.d. for 5–7 days (avoid face, intertriginous areas)
  - Oral antihistamines for pruritus
  - Systemic steroids: short burst (2–3 week taper) for severe eruptions
  - Referral to a dermatologist for skin patch testing if the condition is recurrent and no causative agent can be identified

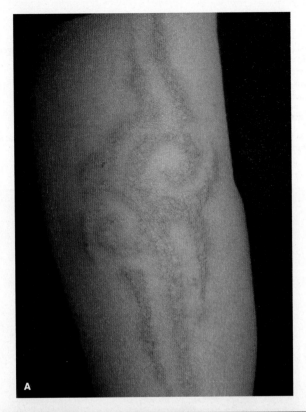

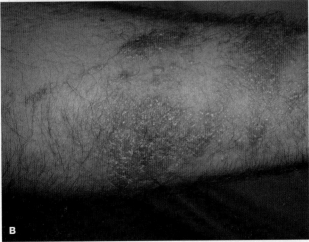

Figure 13-16.  Contact dermatitis. **A.** Henna tattoo allergy. **B.** Poison Ivy.

# TINEA

- Fungal infections can occur on the scalp (tinea capitis) (Figures 13-17A, B), body (tinea corporis) (Figure 13-18), feet (tinea pedis), groin (tinea cruris), and nails (onychomycosis).
- They are most often caused by *Microsporum* and *Trichophyton* species.
- They are transmitted by contact with affected individuals, cats, or dogs.
- Diagnosis may be made by clinical appearance, potassium hydroxide slide "prep" showing branching hyphae, or fungal culture.

## Clinical Presentation

- Skin infections are characterized by annular, scaly plaques with central clearing and erythematous papular border.

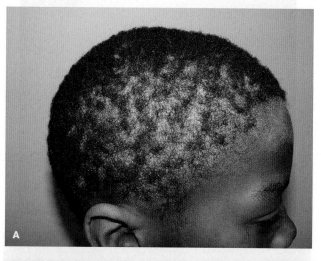

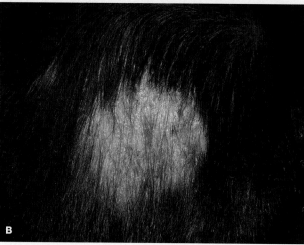

**Figure 13-17. A, B.** Tinea capitis.

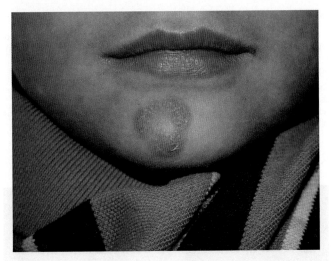

**Figure 13-18.** Tinea corporis.

- Scalp infections are characterized by scaling and patchy hair loss. They may be confused with seborrheic dermatitis if there is minimal hair loss and inflammation. A kerion is a sharply demarcated, painful, inflammatory mass.
- Nail infections are characterized by yellow-white discoloration of the distal nail, nail thickening, and subungual debris. They are often associated with tinea pedis when occurring on the feet.

## Treatment

- Skin infections: topical antifungals (e.g., miconazole, clotrimazole) b.i.d. for 3–4 weeks or until scaling clears
- Scalp infections: topical antifungals ineffective when used alone; requires systemic antifungal treatment with griseofulvin for 6 weeks minimum (see formulary for dosing) and selenium sulfide 2.5% or ketoconazole 1%–2% shampoo 2–3 times per week
- Nail infections: generally require prolonged systemic antifungal therapy (6 months for fingernails and 12–18 months for toenails)

# WARTS

- Caused by human papillomavirus infection of keratinocytes

## Classification

- Verruca vulgaris
  - These round papules have an irregular, papillomatous surface that disrupts skin lines (Figure 13-19A).
  - They are common on the hands but may occur anywhere.
- Flat warts
  - These are skin-colored slightly raised, flat-topped papules (Figure 13-19B).
  - They often occur in groups on the legs and face.
- Plantar warts
  - These are flat hyperkeratotic papules on plantar feet. Thrombosed capillaries may appear as black dots.
  - They may be painful.

## Treatment

- Most warts resolve spontaneously within 2 years. Therapeutic methods include:
  - Topical keratolytics (e.g., salicylic acid). These are available over-the-counter; however, they may be slow to work
  - Liquid nitrogen cryotherapy
- For flat warts on legs, patients should avoid shaving because microtrauma can lead to new lesions.
- For refractory lesions, more intensive intervention, including laser therapy or surgical removal, may be considered.

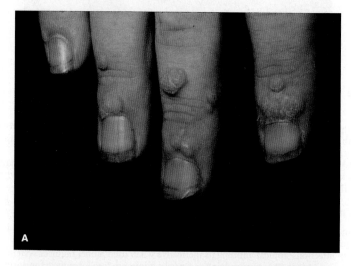

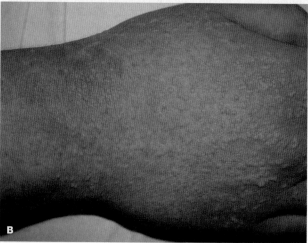

**Figure 13-19.** Warts. **A.** Verrucae vulgaris. **B.** Flat warts. *(continued)*

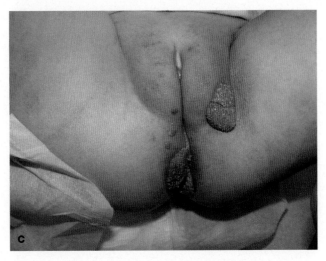

**Figure 13-19.** *(continued)* **C.** Genital warts (Condyloma acuminata).

■ Anogenital warts (Figure 13-19C) require different treatment methods. These may be caused by autoinoculation or vertical transmission during childbirth, but should prompt consideration of screening for sexual abuse in a child who is not sexually active.

## MOLLUSCUM CONTAGIOSUM
■ These are skin-colored pearly papules with central umbilication. If they become in-flamed, they may become red and increase in size (Figure 13-20).
■ This condition is caused by a poxvirus. It is thought to be transmitted by swimming, bathing, or other close contact with an infected person.
■ Treatment
   ■ Lesions are generally self-limited, and the condition often resolves in 6–9 months.
   ■ For extensive or persistent lesions, curettage, topical canthadrin (blistering agent), or liquid nitrogen may be effective.

## ERYTHEMA MULTIFORME

### Erythema Multiforme Minor
■ This condition is characterized by erythematous papules that evolve into target lesions with dusky centers. Some oral lesions may be present (Figure 13-21).
■ The most common precipitant is HSV infection. It may also be drug-induced.

*Treatment*
■ Antihistamines provide symptomatic relief.
■ Systemic steroids may be helpful if given early.
■ Prophylactic acyclovir may be useful to prevent recurrent HSV-related disease.

### Erythema Multiforme Major (Stevens-Johnson Syndrome and Toxic Epidermal Necrolysis)
■ In Stevens-Johnson syndrome (SJS) and toxic epidermal necrolysis (TEN), marked ery-thema or target lesions rapidly progress to blistering and epidermal sloughing.

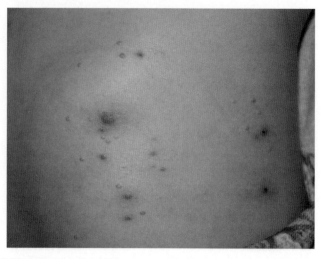

**Figure 13-20.** Molluscum contagiosum.

- Mucosal involvement with erosions and crusting of the oral, ocular, and genital mucosa is prominent.
  - Patients may also have fever and lymphadenopathy.
- Percent body surface area denuded:
  - <10%: SJS
  - 10%–30%: SJS/TEN overlap
  - >30%: TEN
- Common precipitants:
  - Drugs: antibiotics (penicillin, sulfa, doxycycline, sulfonamides, tetracycline), anticonvulsants, nonsteroidal anti-inflammatory drugs
  - *Mycoplasma pneumoniae* infection

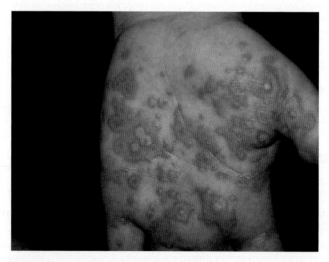

**Figure 13-21.** Erythema multiforme with typical target lesions.

*Treatment*
- Discontinue all possible precipitating medications.
- Replace fluid losses and provide adequate nutrition.
- Administer local wound care. Débridement is not recommended.
- Give antibiotics as needed for superinfection. Avoid prophylactic antibiotics.
- Consider systemic steroids, which may be beneficial early in the course of the disease.
- Intravenous immune globulin has been shown to be beneficial in some cases of TEN.

## Suggested Readings

Conlon JD, Drolet BA. Skin lesions in the neonate. Pediatr Clin North Am 2004 Aug;51(4):863–88, vii–viii.

Eichenfield LF, Hanifin JM, Luger TA, et al. Consensus conference on pediatric atopic dermatitis. J Am Acad Dermatol 2003 Dec;49(6):1088–1095.

Mallory S, et al. Illustrated Manual of Pediatric Dermatology. New York: Taylor & Francis, 2005.

Metry DW, Jung P, Levy ML. Use of intravenous immunoglobulin in children with Stevens-Johnson syndrome and toxic epidermal necrolysis: seven cases and review of the literature. Pediatrics 2003 Dec;112(6 Pt 1):1430–1436.

Paul C, Cork M, Rossi AB, et al. Safety and tolerability of 1% pimecrolimus cream among infants: experience with 1133 patients treated for up to 2 years. Pediatrics 2006 Jan;117(1):e118–128. Epub 2005 Dec 15.

## 14 ENDOCRINE DISEASES
### Ana Maria Arbelaez, Arpita Kalla Vyas, and Stacie P. Shepherd

## DIABETES MELLITUS

### Definition

- Diagnostic criteria are symptoms of diabetes mellitus (DM) and random plasma glucose of ≥200 mg/dL, fasting plasma glucose of ≥126 mg/dL, or a 2-hour plasma glucose of ≥200 mg/dL on an oral glucose tolerance test in the absence of acute illness.
- Asymptomatic children should receive a provisional diagnosis of diabetes and have confirmatory testing with repeat testing on a different day.
- Patients with fasting blood glucose of 100–125 mg/dL with symptoms of diabetes should have an oral glucose tolerance test (1.75 gr/kg glucose, up to maximum of 75 gr).

#### Type 1 Diabetes Mellitus
- Autoimmune disease resulting from destruction of pancreatic beta cells
- Characterized by absolute insulin deficiency
- Classic clinical symptoms include polyuria, polydipsia, and weight loss
- Urgent referral of all patients with new-onset type 1 diabetes for initiation of insulin therapy and intensive education
- Wearing medic alert bracelets by patients with this diagnosis is important.

#### Type 2 Diabetes Mellitus
- Characterized by peripheral insulin resistance, impaired regulation of hepatic glucose production, and declining β-cell function, eventually leading to β-cell failure.
- Risk factors are obesity and family history
- Increased incidence in American Indian, African American, Latino, and Asian children of lower body weight
- Screening of children at high risk for type 2 diabetes with a fasting plasma glucose every 1–2 years

### Treatment

- Starting daily dosages for subcutaneous (SC) insulin, which are adjusted based on patient requirements, at onset of DM
  - < 3yr = 0.3–0.4 U/kg/day
  - 3–6 yr = 0.5 U/kg/day
  - 7–10 yr = 0.6–0.8 U/kg/day
  - 11–14 yr = 0.8–1 U/kg/day
  - >14 yr = 1–1.5 U/kg/day
- Blood glucose monitoring. It should be done before meals, bedtime, or if symptoms of low blood glucose occur. Middle-of-the-night (2 AM) glucose levels should be obtained at the onset of therapy with changes of PM or basal insulin doses.
- Insulin administration (for time course of insulin preparations, see Table 14-1)
  - Twice-daily injections:
    - ⅔ total dose in AM: ⅓ Lispro or Aspart, ⅓ NPH
    - ⅓ total dose in PM: ½ Humalog or NovoLog, ½ NPH
  - Basal bolus regimen—preferred insulin regimen in children:
    - Allows for greater glycemic control and greater flexibility
    - Once-daily basal insulin as insulin glargine (Lantus): ½ total daily dose

| TABLE 14-1 | Time Course of Action of Human Insulin Preparations | | |
|---|---|---|---|
| **Insulin** | **Onset** | **Peak** | **Maximum** |
| Lispro (Humalog)/Aspart (Novolog) | <15 min | 30–90 min | 4–6 hr |
| Regular | 30 min | 2–3 hr | 6–8 hr |
| NPH | 2–4 hr | 6–10 hr | 14–18 hr |
| 70/30 70NPH/30 Regular | 30–60 min | dual | 14–18 hr |
| Glargine (Lantus) | 2 hr | none | 24 hr |

- Remaining total daily dose: short-acting insulin (Lispro or Aspart) with meals—based on carbohydrate intake
- Basal insulin is provided by short-acting insulin via subcutaneous infusion (80% of basal insulin/24 hours). Before initiating pump therapy, patients should have adequate pump training, often including a trial with a saline pump. Mealtime boluses of short-acting insulin are given via the pump based on carbohydrate intake. With only short-acting insulin present, disruption of insulin delivery can be associated with ketosis and even diabetic ketoacidosis in a period of several hours; equivalent glycemic control can be obtained with basal bolus insulin and insulin pump with good compliance.

- Dietary recommendations
  - Caloric requirements:
    - Up to age 10: 1,000 kcal + 100 kcal/yr
    - After age 10: for females: 45 kcal/kg/day; for males: 55 kcal/kg/day
  - Tight dietary control is best achieved when patients count carbohydrates. 1 carbohydrate unit = 15 gm of carbohydrate

- Hemoglobin (Hgb) $A_{1c}$ levels. These give an average of blood glucose levels over the 3 months preceding measurement (Table 14-2) and should be monitored every 3–4 months. Target Hgb $A_{1c}$ depends on developmental stage/age.

## Complications: Hypoglycemia

- Hypoglycemia is the most common complication of diabetes management and is the limiting factor of adequate glycemic control.
- Symptoms are shakiness, sweatiness, nervousness, headache, irritability, confusion, and seizures.
- Treat mild-to-moderate hypoglycemia with 15 grams of fast-acting sugar, such as juice or glucose tablets. Recheck blood glucose 15 minutes later.
- Treat severe hypoglycemia (loss of consciousness or seizures) with glucagon 1 mg intramuscularly (if <20 kg, give 0.5 mg intramuscularly).

| TABLE 14-2 | Hemoglobin $A_{1c}$ Values and Corresponding Blood Glucose Levels |
|---|---|
| **Hemoglobin $A_{1c}$ (%)** | **Average blood glucose (mg/dL)** |
| 4–6 | Nondiabetic |
| 6 | 120 (excellent) |
| 7 | 150 (very good) |
| 8 | 180 (good) |
| 9 | 210 (fair) |
| 10 | 240 (poor) |

■ Hypoglycemia unawareness is the lack of hypoglycemic symptoms and adequate responses to hypoglycemia. This may develop in patients with tight diabetes control and recurrent hypoglycemia or after exercise.

# DIABETIC KETOACIDOSIS

■ Diabetic ketoacidosis (DKA) is characterized by serum glucose >200 mg/dL, ketonemia (>3 mmol/L) or ketonuria, and serum pH <7.3 or serum bicarbonate <15 mEq/L.

## Etiology

■ Type 1 DM: new onset, insulin omission, illness
■ Type 2 DM: severe illness, traumatic stress, or use of some antipsychotic agents

## Clinical Presentation

■ Patients with a range of symptoms that may be present with mild to severe DKA: vomiting, deep-sighing respirations (Kussmaul) with acetone odor, abdominal pain, and somnolence or loss of consciousness
■ Those with new-onset DM or ongoing poor glycemic control: also a history of polyuria, polydipsia, polyphagia, nocturia, and weight loss

## Laboratory Studies

■ Rapid assessment: blood glucose and urine ketones
■ Initial studies: basic metabolic profile (BMP), venous blood gas, complete blood count (CBC), Hgb $A_{1c}$, urinalysis, electrocardiogram (ECG) if potassium is abnormal, blood and urine culture if temperature >38.5°C or signs of infection
  ■ Anion gap (mEq): $(Na - (Cl + HCO_3)$, normal: 8–12
  ■ Corrected Na: $Na + [(glucose - 100)/100] \times 1.6$
  ■ Plasma osmolarity: $2(Na) + Glucose/18 + $ blood urea nitrogen/2.8
    • Patients with DKA have plasma osmolarity >300 mOsm/L

## Treatment (Figure 14-1)

### Mild Diabetic Ketoacidosis or Ketosis

■ Characteristics include no vomiting, pH >7.3, $HCO_3$ >15 mmol/L, and moderate to large ketones.
■ Often outpatient treatment is appropriate.
■ Blood sugar and ketones should be monitored before each injection.
■ Give additional short-acting insulin (Lispro and Aspart) every 2–3 hours.
  ■ Moderate urine ketones: usually 5%–10% of total daily dose
  ■ Large urine ketones: usually 10%–20% of total daily dose

■ If blood sugar is <150 mg/dL, it may be necessary to give additional sugary drinks to bring the blood sugar up before additional insulin.
■ Increase oral fluid intake to compensate for increased urinary losses and to help clear ketones.
■ If patient is on an insulin pump and unable to clear ketones, always give the additional bolus of short-acting insulin by injection and change the pump site.
■ If concomitant hypoglycemia results from gastrointestinal (GI) disease, consider subcutaneous glucagon rescue therapy with 1 unit (10 μg)/yr of age, starting at 2 units and up to 15 units (150 μg).
■ If patients are unable to clear ketones, or they have labored breathing, confusion, or lethargy, refer them to the emergency department for further care.

### Moderate Diabetic Ketoacidosis

■ Characteristics include persistent emesis, high levels of ketones, pH 7.2–7.3, and $HCO_3$ 10–15 mmol/L.

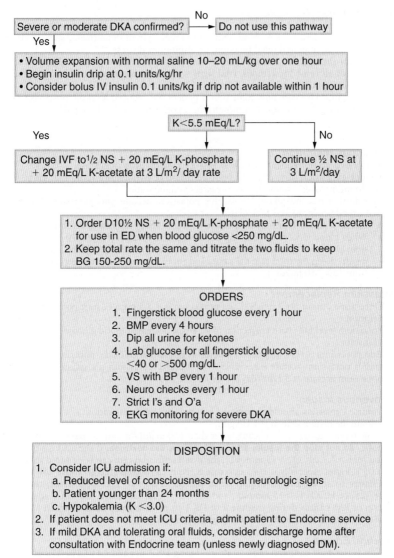

No

Severe or moderate DKA confirmed? ⟶ Do not use this pathway

Yes ↓

• Volume expansion with normal saline 10–20 mL/kg over one hour
• Begin insulin drip at 0.1 units/kg/hr
• Consider bolus IV insulin 0.1 units/kg if drip not available within 1 hour

K<5.5 mEq/L?

Yes

Change IVF to ½ NS + 20 mEq/L K-phosphate + 20 mEq/L K-acetate at 3 L/m²/ day rate

No

Continue ½ NS at 3 L/m²/day

1. Order D10½ NS + 20 mEq/L K-phosphate + 20 mEq/L K-acetate for use in ED when blood glucose <250 mg/dL.
2. Keep total rate the same and titrate the two fluids to keep BG 150-250 mg/dL.

ORDERS
1. Fingerstick blood glucose every 1 hour
2. BMP every 4 hours
3. Dip all urine for ketones
4. Lab glucose for all fingerstick glucose <40 or >500 mg/dL.
5. VS with BP every 1 hour
6. Neuro checks every 1 hour
7. Strict I's and O'a
8. EKG monitoring for severe DKA

DISPOSITION
1. Consider ICU admission if:
   a. Reduced level of consciousness or focal neurologic signs
   b. Patient younger than 24 months
   c. Hypokalemia (K <3.0)
2. If patient does not meet ICU criteria, admit patient to Endocrine service
3. If mild DKA and tolerating oral fluids, consider discharge home after consultation with Endocrine team (unless newly diagnosed DM).

**Figure 14-1.** Algorithm showing the management of diabetic ketoacidosis (DKA).

■ Often, patients are managed in the emergency department or short-stay unit.
■ Intravenous (IV) hydration is often necessary.
■ Give short-acting insulin every 2–3 hours, 10%–20% of total daily dose, or regular insulin q 2–4 hours.
■ Admit if not resolving after 3–4 hours (i.e., $HCO_3$ not rising and/or unable to take oral fluids), newly diagnosed, or if the ability of caregivers is questionable.

*Severe Diabetic Ketoacidosis*
- Characteristics include high levels of ketones, pH <7.1, $HCO_3$ <10 mmol/L, pH <7.2, or mild to moderate DKA along with other organ system impairment, such as altered mental status, impaired renal function, or respiratory distress.
- Admit for therapy and intensive monitoring (fingerstick blood glucose q1h, BMP q4h, dipstick of all urine for ketones, vital signs with blood pressure q1h, neurology checks q1h, strict input/output).
- Consider intensive care unit admission if patient has reduced level of consciousness or focal neurologic signs, age <24 months, or a potassium level <3.0 mg/dL.

## Complications

*Intravenous Hydration*
- Simple hydration frequently causes a 180–240 mg/dL drop in glucose.
- Volume expansion (first phase [if poor perfusion or hypotension]): normal saline (NS) 10–20 mL/kg over 1 hour and then reassess volume status.
- Rehydration (second phase): ½NS plus potassium acetate plus potassium phosphate (see later discussion) at 3 L/m²/day.
  - Decrease to 2.5 L/m²/day if there are concerns about the risk of cerebral edema.
  - When blood glucose is <250 mg/dL, change to D5 ½NS. (Have D10 ½NS + potassium acetate + potassium phosphate available for use when blood glucose <250 mg/dL. Keep the total rate the same, and titrate the two fluids to keep blood glucose from 150–250 mg/dL.)

*Potassium Replacement*
- Once urine output is established and potassium is <5.5 mEq/L, start potassium administration.
- Potassium level falls with correction of acidosis, decreased blood glucose, and initiation of insulin.
- Add potassium 30–40 mEq/L to IV fluids as potassium chloride, potassium phosphate, and/or potassium acetate (i.e., ½NS + 20 mEq/L, potassium phosphate + 20 mEq/L potassium acetate at 3 L/m²/day).

*Intravenous Insulin*
- Volume expansion should be initiated before insulin administration.
- Initiate the insulin drip at 0.1 U/kg/hr.
- If the blood glucose is decreasing faster than 150 mg/dL/hr and the patient remains acidotic, **do not stop the insulin drip, but increase the dextrose.** If the acidosis is resolving (pH >7.3, $HCO_3$ >15 mmol/L), the insulin infusion rate can be reduced to 0.08 or 0.05 U/kg/hr, especially if 10% dextrose is required to keep glucose above 150 mg/dL.
- Change to subcutaneous insulin when patient is able to take oral fluids, the pH is >7.25, or $HCO_3$ is >15 mmol/L, and the anion gap has closed. Consider administration of PM Lantus during treatment of DKA to provide basal insulin, which facilitates discontinuation of insulin drip at the appropriate time.

*Cerebral Edema*
- This is the most common cause of death during DKA in children (0.4%–1% of cases).
- Anticipate cerebral edema in the first 24 hours after initiation of treatment. Always have mannitol available during the first 24 hours in patients with severe DKA.
- Symptoms are change in affect, altered level of consciousness, irritability, headache, equally dilated pupils, delirium, incontinence, emesis, bradycardia, and papilledema.
- Treatment
  - Cerebral edema is a medical emergency, and immediate intervention is necessary.
  - Cerebral edema is a clinical diagnosis. Brain computed tomography (CT) is not indicated before treatment or to establish diagnosis, but consider CT to evaluate for thrombosis or infarction in addition to cerebral edema.
  - Mannitol 0.5–1 gm/kg IV push.
  - Decrease IV infusion rate.
  - Consider hyperventilation and dexamethasone.

# HYPOGLYCEMIA

■ There is a normal process of adaptation during fasting to maintain englycemia fuel supply to the brain.
■ Normal fasting adaptation includes (1) hepatic glycogenolysis (when glycogen stores are depleted: >4 hour fast in infants and >8 hour fast in children), (2) hepatic gluconeogenesis, and (3) hepatic ketogenesis.
   ■ These are mediated by a series of counterregulatory hormones: insulin, which suppresses all three metabolic systems, epinephrine, which activates all three metabolic systems and suppresses insulin; cortisol, which activates gluconeogenesis; glucagon, which activates glycogenolysis; and growth hormone, which activates ketogenesis.
■ Hypoglycemia does not represent a single entity but a defect in these major adaptive pathways.

## Definition

■ There is controversy in the precise definition for newborns. An arbitrary level of 40 mg/dL or less has been used as the classic standard for hypoglycemia based on the fact that healthy newborns are able to maintain blood glucose concentrations above 40 mg/dL after 12 hours of life.
■ Because of concerns of hypoglycemic brain injury, many authors prefer to use a blood glucose level below 50 mg/dL as a reasonable definition for hypoglycemia.

## Clinical Presentation

■ Infants: cyanotic spells, apnea, respiratory distress, refusal to feed, subnormal temperature, floppy spells, myoclonic jerks, somnolence, seizures
■ Children: tachycardia, anxiety, irritability, hunger, sweating, shakiness, stubbornness, sleepiness, seizures

## History

■ A good history is crucial when evaluating hypoglycemia.
■ Information to know is the age of patient, gestational age and birth weight (for infants), length of the fasting period, triggering event (e.g., fructose ingestion), glucose infusion rate (GIR), perinatal history, and comorbidities (e.g., liver disease, midline defects).

## Laboratory Studies

■ An actual laboratory blood glucose measurement, not a glucometer result, to confirm true hypoglycemia is very important.
■ The critical sample to diagnose the underlying cause generally must be obtained during a hypoglycemic episode or during a formal fast. This sample is obtained when blood glucose levels fall below 50 mg/dL.
   ■ Samples for blood glucose, serum $HCO_3$, insulin, C peptide, β-hydroxybutyrate, lactate, free fatty acids, cortisol, growth hormone, and plasma $NH_3$ are obtained.
   ■ Urine for ketones is also obtained immediately following the hypoglycemia.
   ■ In patients who are being worked up for hypoglycemia, depending on the suspected diagnosis, also obtain the blood samples for plasma total and free carnitine, urinary organic acid profile, and plasma acylcarnitine profile (always do so before a formal fast).
   ■ During a normal response to a blood glucose level below 50 mg/dL, the insulin level should be undetectable (<2 uU/mL), β-hydroxybutyrate increased (2–5 mM), lactate reduced (<1.5 mM), free fatty acids increased (1.5–2 mM), and all the counterregulatory hormones increased.

## Evaluation (Figure 14-2)

### *Transient Hypoglycemia of Infancy: Transient Neonatal Hyperinsulinism*
- Infants of diabetic mothers
  - This manifests as transient hypoglycemia as a result of hyperinsulinemia following chronic exposure to elevated blood glucose in utero. Infants are usually macrosomic, and the hypoglycemia can last 3–7 days.
  - Treatment consists of frequent feeds or if needed, supplemental IV glucose at a rate not to exceed 5–10 mg/kg/min.
- Intrauterine growth retardation and perinatal stress
  - This can manifest as hypoglycemia. It usually persists for >5 days of life, and insulin levels can be inappropriately elevated.
  - Treatment involves frequent feedings, or most infants are responsive to diazoxide (5–15 mg/kg/day).
- Infants taking β-blockers, which causes hypoketotic hypoglycemia because of suppression of lipolysis

### *Persistent Hypoglycemia of Infancy or Childhood*
- Hypoglycemia with lactic acidosis: inborn errors of metabolism
  - Glycogen storage disease type 1 (glucose-6-phosphatase deficiency)
    - Infants can develop hypoglycemia on day of life 1, although because of frequent feeds, this can go undiagnosed for months. Fasting tolerance is usually very short (2–4 hours).
    - Associated conditions include lactic acidemia, tachypnea, hepatomegaly, hyperuricemia, growth failure, hypertriglyceridemia, and neutropenia.
    - Treatment consists of frequent carbohydrate feeds, uncooked cornstarch (>1 year of age), limited fructose and galactose intake, and granulocyte-macrophage colony-stimulating factor.
  - Defects in hepatic gluconeogenesis (fructose-1,6-diphosphatase deficiency)
    - Patients usually develop hypoglycemia after fasting for 8–10 hours or after fructose ingestion.
    - Associated conditions include lactic acidemia and hepatomegaly.
  - Galactosemia (galactose-1-phosphate uridyl transferase deficiency)
    - This usually presents with jaundice without hepatomegaly and neonatal *Escherichia coli*-related sepsis.
    - Later on in life, patients can develop hepatomegaly, cataracts, developmental delay, ovarian failure, and Fanconi syndrome.
    - Treatment consists of galactose-restricted diet.
  - Hypoglycemia with lactic acidosis: alcohol intake
  - Normal newborns. Infants have poor ability to make ketones and gluconeogenesis in first 24 hours of life
- Hypoglycemia with ketosis
  - Inborn errors of metabolism: glycogen storage disease types 3, 6, and 9 (debrancher, liver phosphorylase, or phosphorylase kinase deficiencies)
    - Fasting tolerance is usually 4–6 hours.
    - Patients can present with failure to thrive, hepatomegaly, cardiomyopathy, and myopathy.
    - Treatment consists of frequent feedings, low free sugar diet, uncooked cornstarch.
  - Cortisol and growth hormone deficiency (hypopituitarism)
    - It has an incidence of hypoglycemia of approximately 20%, which beyond the neonatal period is usually associated with ketosis.
    - Fasting tolerance is usually 8–14 hours.
    - Treatment is adequate replacement therapy (9–13 mg/m$^2$/day for hydrocortisone and 0.3 mg/kg/week for growth hormone).
  - Ketotic hypoglycemia

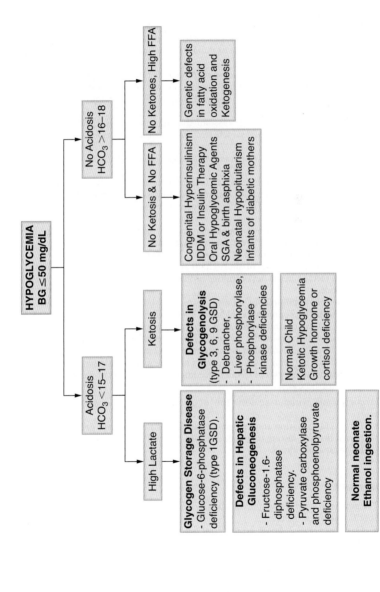

**Figure 14-2.** Algorithm showing the management of hypoglycemia.

- This occurs more commonly during the toddler and preschool age during periods of intercurrent illness, with poor oral intake or fasting periods of 10–12 hours. It is a diagnosis of exclusion.
- Treatment involves frequent carbohydrate intake during periods of illness and avoidance of a prolonged overnight fast.

- Hypoglycemia without acidosis (no ketosis; no elevated free fatty acids)
  - Congenital hyperinsulinism
  - It is the most common cause of persistent hypoglycemia of the newborn.
  - Time of onset, clinical features, fasting tolerance (0–6 hours) and therapy depend on the severity and type of disease or mutation. Patients usually do not present with failure to thrive.
  - Patients usually have high glucose requirements (10–30 mg/kg/min).
  - Patients respond to a glucagon stimulation (0.03 mg/kg to a maximum of 1 mg IV) with an increase in glucose >30 mg/dL within 15–30 minutes.
  - The different types are:
    - Recessive mutations of potassium channel genes (SUR 1, Kir6.2). Treatment is octreotide and subtotal pancreatectomy (98%); patients are unresponsive to diazoxide.
    - Dominant mutation of potassium channel genes. Treatment is subtotal pancreatectomy (98%).
    - Focal hyperinsulinism: focal loss of heterozygosity for maternal 11p and expression of paternally transmitted potassium channel mutations of either SUR 1 or Kir6.2. Treatment is focal resection; patients are unresponsive to diazoxide.
    - Dominant mutations of glutamate dehydrogenase: hyperinsulinism hyperammonemia syndrome. Treatment is diazoxide.
    - Dominant mutations of glucokinase. Treatment is diazoxide.
    - Recessive mutations of short-chain acyl CoA dehydrogenase (SCHAD): abnormal metabolites in acyl-carnitine profile and urine organic acids. Treatment is diazoxide.
  - Neonatal hypopituitarism. Clinical features associated with this condition are midline defects, microphallus, cholestatic liver dysfunction, and jaundice.
  - Furtive insulin or oral insulin secretagogue administration is characterized by hypoglycemia with high insulin levels but low C-peptide. When this is suspected, social work should be involved in evaluation of the case.
  - Post-Nissen dumping syndrome occurs in some infants following surgery for reflux.
    - Treatment consists of frequent feedings, and inhibitors of gastric motility as well as acarbose may be useful.

- Hypoglycemia without acidosis (no or abnormally low ketosis but high free fatty acids)
  - Fatty acid oxidation and ketogenesis defects. Patients do not present in the neonatal period because fasting tolerance is 12–16 hours. The first episode is usually triggered by nonspecific illness.

## Treatment

- The goal is to keep blood glucose above 70 mg/dL after a 10-hour fast.
- Specific therapies include:
  - Dextrose: IV 0.2 gm/kg bolus (2 mL/kg of 10% dextrose), followed by 10% dextrose continuous infusion (5 mL/kg/hr of 10% dextrose is approximately a GIR of 8 mg/kg/min in a newborn).
  - Glucagon (only if insulin induced): 0.5 mg SQ or IV if <20 kg, 1 mg SQ or IV if >20 kg.
  - Diazoxide: 5–15 mg/kg/day divided into 2–3 doses. Start with maximum dose. Side effects: fluid retention and congestive heart failure.

- Octreotide: start at 2–10 µg/kg/day may increase up to 50 µg/kg/day SQ divided q6–8h or continuous IV. Tachyphylaxis is a common problem, and this can cause suppression of other hormones such as glucagon, cortisol, growth hormone, and thyroid-stimulating hormone.
- Uncooked cornstarch (glycogen storage disease type 1): 1–2 g/kg/dose in older infants.
- Carnitine (for CPT1 defect): 100 mg/kg/day divided 3–4 doses

# ADRENAL INSUFFICIENCY

- Adrenal insufficiency may be primary (as a result of disorder of the adrenal gland) or secondary (as a result of congenital anomalies or acquired insults to the hypothalamus or pituitary).
- Onset may be rapid or slow.
- A high index of suspicion is crucial because presenting symptoms may be subtle and may range from vague symptoms of weight loss, fatigue, and weakness to acute vascular collapse. Early diagnosis may be life saving.
- Laboratory abnormalities include hyponatremia (90%), hyperkalemia (60%) if primary adrenal insufficiency, hypercalcemia, metabolic acidosis, anemia, lymphocytosis, eosinophilia, and azotemia.

## Etiology

- Primary acute adrenal insufficiency: Waterhouse-Friderichsen syndrome (septicemia with subsequent bilateral adrenal infarcts), infection (tuberculosis, histoplasmosis, cytomegalovirus, HIV), medications (ketoconazole)
- Primary chronic adrenal insufficiency: autoimmune (polyglandular autoimmune syndrome), congenital adrenal hyperplasia, congenital adrenal hypoplasia, Wolman disease (lysosomal storage disease that includes calcification of the adrenals), adrenoleukodystrophy, congenital unresponsiveness to ACTH
- Secondary adrenal insufficiency: isolated ACTH deficiency, radiation, craniopharyngioma, septo-optic dysplasia, iatrogenic (chronic steroid therapy). Traumatic, hemorrhagic, or autoimmune insults to the pituitary are associated with deficiencies of growth hormone and gonadotropin as well as ACTH and thyrotropin.

## Clinical Presentation

- Signs
    - General: weight loss, hypotension/shock, vitiligo
    - Primary adrenal insufficiency only: hyperpigmentation of extensor surfaces, hand creases, gingival, lips, areola, scars
- Symptoms: weakness, fatigue, anorexia, nausea, vomiting, salt craving, postural dizziness

## History

- There should be a high suspicion for adrenal insufficiency if there is/are:
    - History of steroid use
    - Other autoimmune endocrine disorders (especially hypoparathyroidism, mucocutaneous candidiasis, type 1 DM)
    - Family history of autoimmune endocrinopathies

## Laboratory Studies

- Random plasma cortisol levels are not very useful except in infants, in patients in shock, or during a crisis if treatment is emergent.

- Initial diagnostic procedures could include 8 AM serum cortisol, ACTH, and electrolytes.
  - An early morning serum cortisol value >11 μg/dL (300 nmol/L) makes it unlikely that the patient has clinically important hypothalamic-pituitary-adrenal insufficiency.
  - A value <3 μg/dL (80 nmol/L) makes adrenal insufficiency very likely if the patient has presumed normal circadian rhythmicity.
  - If the patient's condition permits waiting to initiate therapy, perform an **ACTH stimulation test** with cosyntropin, 250 μg IV, and monitor plasma cortisol levels at time = 0, 30 min, and 60 min. Some studies have shown that a low dose 1 μg/1.73 m² cosyntropin test provides a better test to assess hypothalamopituitary disease in preterm infants or patients that had been on dexamethasone treatment. A serum cortisol value of ≥20 μg/dL (550 nmol/L) at 30 or 60 minutes indicates a normal response.
  - Dexamethasone can be given if emergent therapy is necessary, and ACTH stimulation testing can be performed shortly after.
- Secondary adrenal insufficiency can be diagnosed using the insulin tolerance test or metyrapone test with the help of an endocrinologist.

## Treatment

### Acute Adrenal Insufficiency
- Rapid volume expansion with NS or D₅NS if there is concomitant hypoglycemia
- Close monitoring of electrolytes and blood glucose
- Hydrocortisone at 50 mg/m² IV bolus; then 50 mg/m²/day divided q4–6h

### Chronic Adrenal Insufficiency
- Physiological replacement (hydrocortisone 10–20 mg/m²/day PO divided q8h; the best dose is the lowest the patient can support without symptoms)
- Fludrocortisone 0.1 mg/day PO in primary adrenal insufficiency. Increase dose if needed
- Minor illness (nausea, emesis, fever). Triple total daily corticosteroid dose and divide three times daily or give hydrocortisone 30–50 mg/m²/day IV for 48 hours or until symptoms resolve. Patients should have injectable corticosteroid available and be instructed in intramuscular use for emesis or emergencies (dexamethasone 1 mg/m²/day).
- Major stress (severe illness, general anesthesia, bone fracture). Give hydrocortisone 50–100 mg/m²/day IV divided q6–8h
- Chronic supraphysiologic doses of corticosteroids
  - Decreasing to physiologic doses can be done at any rate followed by careful slow decreases in steroids below physiologic doses because of concern of adrenal insufficiency.
  - The patient should receive stress dosing during times of illness if below stress dosing or off of steroids until an ACTH/cosyntropin (Cortrosyn) test verifies adrenal sufficiency.
  - A MedicAlert bracelet must be worn by a patient with this diagnosis.
- Postoperatively (for pituitary lesions). A cortisol value >8 μg/dL 24 hours after stopping dexamethasone or hydrocortisone is reassuring. The patient will still need a ACTH/cosyntropin stimulation test approximately 1 month after surgery.

### Corticosteroid Potencies
- The relative potencies of corticosteroids vary, and this must be considered (Table 14-3).

## CONGENITAL ADRENAL HYPERPLASIA

- Congenital adrenal hyperplasia (CAH) is the most common cause of genital ambiguity in the newborn.
- It has an autosomal recessive inheritance.
- It is caused by deficiency in one of the enzymes of the corticosteroid biosynthetic pathway (Table 14-4).

**TABLE 14-3** **Relative Potencies of Systemic Corticosteroids**

| Drug | Glucocorticoid effect | Mineralocorticoid effect | Biological half-life (hr) |
|---|---|---|---|
| Hydrocortisone | 1 | 1 | 8–12 |
| Prednisone/Prednisolone | 4 | 0.3 | 18–36 |
| Methylprednisolone | 5 | 0 | 18–36 |
| Dexamethasone | 25–40 | 0 | 36–54 |
| Fludrocortisone | 10–15 | 125 | 18–36 |

- The primary defect is the inability to synthesize adequate cortisol, resulting in excessive corticotropin-releasing hormone and ACTH, causing the adrenal glands to become hyperplastic.
- Increased trophic hormone stimulation leads to excessive adrenal androgen production (androstenedione), which is peripherally converted to testosterone, leading to virilization.

**TABLE 14-4** **Enzyme Defects and Phenotype of Congenital Adrenal Hyperplasia**

| Enzyme deficiency | Female phenotype | Male phenotype | Treatment | 17-OHP | K | Na | Others |
|---|---|---|---|---|---|---|---|
| **21-OH Deficiency (90%)** | | | | | | | |
| Classic salt-wasting | Virilized/ ambiguous genitalia | Normal genitalia/ salt-losing crisis at 1–2 wk old | GC, MC; NaCl in infants | ↑ (usually >2,000 ng/dL) | ↑ | ↓ | Acidosis, decreased glucose |
| Classic simple virilization | Virilized/ ambiguous genitalia | Phenotyp-ically normal | GC, ± MC | ↑ (usually >2,000 ng/dL) | N | N | |
| Nonclassic | Premature adrenarche, irregular menses, advanced bone age | Premature adrenarche, advanced bone age | GC | Modest ↑ high on ACTH stimulation | N | N | |
| 11β-OH deficiency (5%) | Hypertension, hypokalemia, virilization | Hypertension, hypokalemia (not as neonate) | GC, treat hyperten-sion | | ↓ | N | ↑DOC |
| 17α-OH deficiency (1%) | Hypertension, absence of adrenarche/ puberty | Hypertension, ambiguous genitalia | GC, sex steroids, treat hyper-tension | | ↓ | N | ↓sex steroids, cortisol, ↑DOC |

*21-OH,* 21-hydroxylase; *11β-OH,* 11β-hydroxylase; *17α-OH,* 17α-hydroxylase; *17-OHP,* 17-hydrox-yprogesterone; *DOC,* deoxycorticosterone; *N,* normal; *GC,* glucocorticoids (hydrocortisone 10–20 mg/m²/day divided t.i.d.); *MC,* mineralocorticoids (fludrocortisone typically 0.1 mg daily); *NaCl,* sodium chloride supplements typically 1–2 gm or 17–34 mEq of sodium daily.

- Steroidogenic defects that interrupt aldosterone synthesis result in an inability to maintain sodium balance, and if not diagnosed promptly, this can lead to hyponatremic dehydration, shock, and death.
- Newborn screening
  - Most states perform routing screening by assay of 17-hydroxyprogesterone (17-OHP) obtained by heel puncture at 2–4 days of life. Screening before 36 hours of life leads to a high false-positive rate.
  - Assays vary widely, and 17-OHP levels can be affected by gestational age, severe illness, and stress.
  - If ambiguous genitalia, decreased alertness, poor weight gain, or highly elevated 17-OHP is evident on screening, the infant should be immediately referred to a pediatric endocrinologist and admitted. An elevated 17-OHP on screening should be confirmed with a laboratory serum 17-OHP and electrolytes should be followed until diagnosis of CAH is excluded.

# GLUCOCORTICOID EXCESS (CUSHING SYNDROME)

- Causes are iatrogenic, ACTH-secreting adenoma, ectopic ACTH-secreting tumor, adrenocortical adenoma, adrenocortical carcinoma, McCune-Albright syndrome, and multiple endocrine neoplasia 1.
- Most sensitive indicators of glucocorticoid excess are excessive weight and impaired linear growth.
- Other clinical manifestations include moon face, buffalo hump, obesity, hypertension, thinning of the skin, violaceous striae, bruising, and hirsutism.
- Initial evaluation is 24-hour urinary free cortisol (in excess of 70–80 $\mu g/m^2$ in children is consistent with glucocorticoid excess) or salivary cortisol at 2300 hours (normal concentration is <0.28 $\mu g/dL$).
- An overnight low-dose dexamethasone suppression test can also be performed as an outpatient study: dexamethasone, 1 mg or 0.3 mg/m$^2$, give orally at 2300 hours and measure 0800 serum cortisol.

# DIABETES INSIPIDUS

## Definition

- Insufficient antidiuretic hormone (ADH) or renal unresponsive to ADH due to ADH receptor defect.
  - This causes a syndrome of polyuria and polydipsia, which are characteristic of diabetes insipidus (DI).
  - With an intact thirst mechanism, copious water drinking (>2 L/m$^2$/day) maintains normal osmolalities. However, problems with thirst mechanism or insufficient water intake lead to hypernatremic dehydration.

## Etiology (Table 14-5)

### Clinical Presentation and Laboratory Studies
- Clinical characteristics: polyuria, polydipsia (water intake >2 L/m$^2$/day)
- Urine osmolality <300 mOsm/kg and serum osmolality >300 mOsm/kg
  - Serum sodium and serum osmolality are usually normal or slightly elevated in children with uncomplicated DI and free water access.
  - Urine specific gravity: <1.005
- Water deprivation test: used to confirm the diagnosis of diabetes insipidus (Table 14-6)
  - Begin the test in the morning after 24 hours of adequate hydration and after patient empties his or her bladder.
  - Weigh the patient and give no fluid until completion of test.
    - Measure weight and urine volume and specific gravity hourly.
    - Check urine and serum osmolality and serum sodium every 2 hours.
  - Terminate the test if weight loss approaches 3% to 5% of initial body weight.

**TABLE 14-5** **Etiology of Diabetes Insipidus**

**Central Causes**
Congenital: autosomal dominant, DIDMOAD
Trauma/injury: injury to the sella turcica, intraventricular hemorrhage
Surgery: pituitary–hypothalamic surgery/ neurosurgical
Tumors: craniopharyngioma, germinoma
Infection: tuberculosis, meningitis, listeria
Infiltrations: sarcoidosis, Langerhans histiocytosis

**Nephrogenic Causes**
Electrolyte disturbances; hypokalemia, hypercalcemia
Nephrocalcinosis
Congenital: X-linked recessive
Chronic renal failure, polycystic kidney disease
Drugs: demeclocycline, lithium

*DIDMOAD,* diabetes insipidus, diabetes mellitus, optic atrophy, deafness.

- Vasopressin test: used to differentiate between a nephrogenic and central etiology (Table 14-7)
    - Give vasopressin 0.05–0.1 U/kg subcutaneously at the end of water deprivation test after measuring vasopressin level.
    - Monitor urine output, concentration, and water intake (water intake is limited to documented output during deprivation test).

## Treatment

### *Central Diabetes Insipidus*
- Provide fluid replacement.
- Aim for limited salt delivery to reduce driving up urine output (¼NS with dextrose and as required additives are usually good maintenance fluid for patient with DI). Use urine replacement with enteral water or 5% dextrose plus water via IV route.
- Patients with intact thirst mechanisms maintain serum osmolality and sodium normal provided free access to water.
- Those with nonintact thirst mechanisms should be restricted to about 1 L/m$^2$/day of fluid if they are taking desmopressin (DDAVP).

**TABLE 14-6** **Water Deprivation Test**

| Condition | Urine osmolality (mOsm/kg) | Plasma osmolality (mOsm/kg) | Specific gravity | Urine: plasma osmolality ratio | Urine volume | Weight loss |
|---|---|---|---|---|---|---|
| Normal/ psychogenic polydipsia | 500–1,400 | 288–291 | 1.010 | >2 | Decreased | No change |
| Central/ nephrogenic diabetes insipidus | <300 | >300 | <1.005 | — | Increased | ≥5% |

| TABLE 14-7 | Vasopressin Test | | |
|---|---|---|---|
| Condition | Urine specific gravity | Urine volume | Fluid intake |
| Central diabetes insipidus | >1.010 | Decreased | Decreased |
| Nephrogenic diabetes insipidus | <1.005 | No change | No change |

- Monitor status.
  - Urine output and specific gravity. This helps determine dosing of DDAVP (breakthrough is urine specific gravity <1.005 and urine output > input).
  - Sodium level. This also helps determine status of DI; aim to maintain sodium level 140–150 mEq if thirst is not intact and 135–145 mEq for intact thirst.
  - Formula to correct free water deficit: if Na 145–170 mEq: 4 mL × (current sodium − desired sodium) × weight (kg) × 0.6/24 hours or 48 hours if Na ≥170 mEq: 3 mL × (current sodium − desired sodium) × weight (kg) × 0.6/24 hours or 48 hours
  - DDAVP. Titrate to allow 1–2 hours of breakthrough urine output per day. It is available in the following forms:
    - Subcutaneous: most potent (4 μg/mL)
    - Inhaled: 10-fold less potent than subcutaneous (10 μg/mL)
    - Oral: 100–200 fold less potent than subcutaneous (0.1 mg, 0.2 mg tablets)
- Administer vasopressin drip.
- Start at 0.5 mU/kg/hr and titrate up.
  - 1.5 mU/kg/hr usually achieves twice normal vasopressin needed for maximal antidiuretic effect
  - Very short half-life (5–10 minutes)
  - It is important to restrict the patient to 1 L/m$^2$/day of IV fluids when continuous vasopressin is administered to prevent hyponatremia.

### Nephrogenic Diabetes Insipidus
- Thiazide diuretics
- Nonsteroidal anti-inflammatory drugs
- Amiloride

### Triphasic Response (After Pituitary Stalk Transection)
- Usually post–central nervous system (CNS) surgery or head injury
  - Initial DI (occurring within the first few hours ) followed by syndrome of inappropriate secretion of ADH (SIADH) phase (lasting up to 5–10 days), followed finally by central DI disorder
  - Occurs after an acute injury to neurohypophysis without transection of the septum (basal skull fracture or status posttransection of the stalk during CNS surgery)
- Treatment
  - Restrict fluids to 1 L/m$^2$/day of ½NS plus 5% dextrose.
  - Replace output in excess of 1 L/m$^2$/day with mL/mL of 5% dextrose plus water or enteral water.
  - Monitor strict input/output charts and electrolytes regularly.

## HYPOTHYROIDISM
- Primary (thyroid gland dysfunction: elevated thyroid-stimulating hormone (TSH), low free thyroxine)
  - Congenital
  - Familial: Pendred syndrome, which consists of goiter and eight nerve deafness, is inherited as an autosomal recessive trait. The disorder is mapped to chromosome 7.

- Atrophic autoimmune thyroiditis: serum positivity for thyroid peroxidase antibodies
- Hashimoto thyroiditis: goiter, positive serum thyroid peroxidase antibodies and thyroid-stimulating hormone-binding inhibitory immunoglobulin (TBII), more common in Turner syndrome
- Iodine deficiency: presents with a goiter
- Treatment for hyperthyroidism or radiotherapy of neck for lymphoma, leukemia
- Drugs: amiodarone, iodine-containing medication
- Secondary (low TSH and normal or low free thyroxine)
  - Pituitary or hypothalamic disease

# CONGENITAL HYPOTHYROIDISM

## Epidemiology and Etiology

- This condition occurs in 1 in 4,000 births.
- Thyroid dysgenesis/agenesis, hypoplasia, ectopic presence (75%)
- Dyshormogenesis (10%): may resolve; usually organification defect
- Transient hypothyroidism (10%): maternal thyroid antibodies, iodine deficiency/excess
- Hypothalamic: pituitary TSH deficiency (5%)

## Clinical Presentation

- No symptoms (most infants)
- Possible symptoms
  - Wide cranial suture, delayed skeletal maturation
  - Umbilical hernia
  - Prolonged jaundice
  - Hypotonia, puffy hands and feet, macroglossia
  - Hoarse cry
  - Goiter (dyshormogenesis; transient only)

## Laboratory Studies

- >15 million neonates worldwide are screened for hypothyroidism using newborn screening protocols.
  - If the screen is abnormal, obtain serum TSH and free thyroxine ($T_4$).
  - If the newborn screen is normal, consider recheck at 2–6 weeks in infants with Downs syndrome, family history of dyshormogenesis, or maternal thyroid disorder.
- Presume disease if after 2 days of life, the serum TSH is >20–25 mU/L in a well term infant. TSH peaks at delivery and remains elevated for 2–5 days, which stimulates the rise of $T_4$ 2–6 fold. $T_4$ remains elevated for several weeks.
- Sick or very premature infants must be evaluated with free $T_4$ and TSH when clinically stable.
- For low $T_4$ and normal TSH, consider thyroid-binding globulin deficiency versus hypothalamic/pituitary disturbance (TSH/TRH deficiency).

## Treatment

- Institute treatment as soon as the diagnosis is confirmed to optimize neurologic development.
- Monitor TSH and free $T_4$ 1–3 times monthly during the first year of treatment. Aim for free $T_4$ at the upper end of normal.
- Give thyroxine treatment orally 10–15 microgram/kg/day (starting dose usually 37.5 μg once daily). For infants with Down syndrome, start at a low dose 25 μg once daily.
- There is decreased absorption of thyroxine with soy formula as well as with iron and calcium supplements.

# ACQUIRED HYPOTHYROIDISM

## Clinical Presentation

- Growth deceleration (one of earlier markers)
- Delayed ossification
- Dry skin; dry, brittle, thin hair
- Cold intolerance
- Low energy
- Constipation
- Proximal myopathy, ataxia, slow reflexes
- Headache, precocious puberty, and galactorrhea (seen in pituitary disease)
- Possible hypercalcemia, hypercholesterolemia, and hyperprolactinemia

## Laboratory Studies

- Obtain a thyroid function test.
- If TSH is low or normal in light of a low free $T_4$, then investigate for pituitary disease.

## Treatment

- For infants, use 10–15 microgram/kg/day of thyroxine orally (starting dose usually 37.5 μg once daily).
- In older children, consider starting dose of 1.75 μg/kg/day of thyroxine orally. (Tablets are available in various sizes ranging from 25–200 μg/pill.)
- For infants and children with Down syndrome, consider starting thyroxine dose of 25 μg once daily
- It is necessary to assess compliance when reviewing abnormal thyroid function tests while on therapy.

# HYPERTHYROIDISM

## Etiology

- Graves disease (most common cause in childhood)
  - Diffuse toxic goiter, proptosis, and pretibial myxoedema
  - Female > male
  - HLA $B_8$, $DW_3$ association
  - Thyroid-stimulating antibody present
  - May have other autoimmune association: vitiligo, DM type 2, idiopathic thrombocytopenic purpura, rheumatic fever, Addison disease
- Solitary nodule/adenoma (fine needle aspiration or biopsy warranted to rule out cancer): Plummer disease, toxic uninodular goiter
- De Quervain thyroiditis: acute disease with tender goiter and elevated total triiodothyronine ($T_3$)
- Subacute thyroiditis: viral origin (mumps, coxsackie, adenovirus)
- Reidel thyroiditis: dense thyroid fibrosis, including neck vessels and trachea
- Tumors: ovarian tumors, choriocarcinoma, hydatidiform mole
- Transient neonatal: secondary to transmission of stimulating antibodies in maternal Graves disease, lasts 6–12 weeks

## Clinical Presentation

- General symptoms and signs
  - Increased appetite, short attention span
  - Hyperactivity
  - Tachycardia, palpitation, dyspnea
  - Goiter

- Smooth skin, increased sweating, tremor
- Hypertension, cardiomegaly, atrial fibrillation
- Eye signs: exophthalmos, lid retraction, lid lag, impaired convergence
- Thyroid storm
    - Acute onset
    - Presenting symptoms: tachycardia, high-grade fever, hypertension, restlessness
    - Progression to delirium, coma and death if not treated rapidly
- Neonatal hyperthyroidism
    - Classically born premature
    - Intrauterine growth retardation
    - Goiter, exophthalmos, microcephaly
    - Irritable, hyperalert, with possible tachycardia, tachypnea, hyperthermia, hypertension

## Laboratory Studies

- Free or total $T_4$ and $T_3$ elevated
- TSH decreased
- Thyroid-stimulating immunoglobulin (TSI) and/or TBII positive
- Increased radioactive iodine uptake

## Treatment

### Medications
- Antithyroid medication
    - Propylthiouracil (PTU) delivered as twice or thrice daily dosing; side effects are agranulocytosis and liver dysfunction. Consider treating neonatal hyperthyroidism with PTU if the infant is symptomatic because of concerns for high-output cardiac dysfunction and/or premature suture closure.
    - Methimazole delivered as once daily dosing; do not use in women of childbearing age because of teratogenic nature.
- Symptomatic control with propranolol
- Radioactive iodine
- Thyroid storm: high-dose PTU, propranolol, and Lugol iodine if needed; antipyretics

### Surgery
- Subtotal thyroidectomy

# GOITER

- An enlargement in the thyroid gland

## Etiology

- Congenital
- Colloid goiter (prepubertal girls, euthyroid)
- Iodine deficiency
- Graves or Hashimoto disease
- Thyroiditis
- Multinodular (McCune-Albright syndrome)
- Thyroid tumor (rare in children, commonest papillary). It is important to rule out coexisting pathology such as multiple endocrine neoplasia syndrome before a surgical procedure.

## Diagnosis

- The child may be hypo-, hyper-, or euthyroid.
- Assess goiter for size and consistency. Determine whether it is diffuse or nodular.
- Additional investigations include thyroid ultrasound, neck CT, and fine needle aspiration of the gland.

## Treatment

- Monitor status regularly if the child is nonsymptomatic from the goiter.
- If goiter compromising airway or feeding, then consider surgical removal.
- Some endocrinologists prefer using thyroid medication in euthyroid patients to reduce the size of the goiter.

# SHORT STATURE

- Disturbances of growth are the most common presenting complaints in the pediatric endocrine clinic.
  - Fetal growth is dependent on maternal factors (placental sufficiency, maternal nutrition, etc.), insulin-like growth factor-2 (IGF-2) and insulin.
  - Growth in late infancy and childhood is dependent on growth hormone/IGF-1 axis and thyroid hormone. Growth is more rapid during infancy—up to 20 cm per year. It is common to see shifts in the growth curve in the first 18 months when children are adjusting to their genetic potential growth isopleth. During childhood, growth rate is fairly constant at approximately 2 inches (approximately 5 cm) per year.
  - Pubertal growth is dependent on sex hormones as well as growth hormone/IGF-1 axis and the thyroid gland. There is a mild deceleration in growth velocity before initiation of pubertal growth spurt.
- Abnormal growth and stature: criteria
  - Child's growth curve is crossing percentiles.
  - Child's growth rate is <2 inches or 5 cm per year.
  - Height is >2 standard deviations (SDs) (4 inches/10 cm) below from midparental height.
- If poor weight gain and lack of nutrition is the problem without affecting height velocity, it is unlikely to be an endocrine cause and patient may warrant a gastrointestinal evaluation instead.

## Etiology (Figure 14-3)

- Normal growth patterns that can look like a growth disorder
  - Genetic (familial) short stature. Children have normal growth velocity, normal timing of development and puberty, and bones fuse at the appropriate age. Height is short because of a short mother and/or a short father. Bone age (BA) = chronologic age (CA).
  - Constitutional delay of growth and puberty. Children have normal growth velocity, delayed timing of puberty, and delayed BA. There is a family history of late bloomers. Anticipate a less robust growth spurt.
- Primary growth failure
  - Chromosomal disorders such as Turner syndrome, Down syndrome, Noonan syndrome, Russell-Silver syndrome, Prader-Willi syndrome, and pseudohypoparathyroidism
  - Skeletal dysplasias such as hypochondroplasias, achondroplasias, osteogenesis imperfecta, and Albright hereditary osteodystrophy
- Secondary growth failure
  - Prenatal onset
    - Maternal hypertension, fetal alcohol syndrome, and congenital infections
    - Small for gestational age (SGA). Infants are born with weights below the 10th percentile for their gestational age. Russell-Silver syndrome is one of the many syndromes that includes SGA in the features.
  - Postnatal onset
    - Endocrine, such as hypothyroidism, growth hormone deficiency, growth hormone resistance (Laron dwarfism), and glucocorticoid excess
    - Nonendocrine, such as renal failure, renal tubular acidosis, malabsorption, cystic fibrosis, celiac disease, and Crohn disease

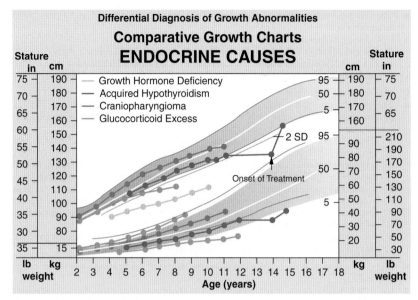

**Figure 14-3.** Endocrine causes of growth abnormalities.

## History

- Physical history
  - History of changes in growth pattern and onset of puberty
  - History of chronic illnesses
  - Prenatal exposures to toxins, drugs, or alcohol; use of other medications (e.g., steroids, psychostimulants)
  - History of prematurity; weight for gestational age and catch-up growth
- Social history
  - History of adoption and ethnic background
  - History of child abuse or neglect, which may give information supportive of psychosocial dwarfism
- Family history
  - History of pubertal development. Age of menarche in mother and age of physical changes or cessation of growth in father may give information that supports the diagnosis of constitutional growth delay.
  - Family history of chronic diseases (e.g., inflammatory bowel disease, neurofibromatosis, mental retardation and calcium problems, renal disease). The child's symptoms of these diseases are very important.

## Physical Examination

- Abnormal facial features, shortening of fourth or fifth metacarpals, cognitive impairment, and skin lesions may be suggestive of genetic disorders.
- Arm span and upper-to-lower segment (U/L). Determination of the arm span and U/L ratio (lower segment is the measurement from the symphysis pubis to the floor) is useful to determine the etiologies of short stature. Examples:
  - Short arm span or small legs and normal trunk (increased U/L ratio) may indicate skeletal dysplasia or hypothyroidism.
  - Long arms and decreased U/L ratio may indicate hypogonadism.
  - Arm span longer than height may also suggest abnormal spine growth.

- The U/L ratio varies with age and race: 1.7 at birth, 1.4 at 2 years, 1 at 10 years, ~0.9 at adulthood
- Calculating midparental height (in centimeters)
  - For girls: (Father's Height − 13 centimeters) ± (Mother's Height)/2
  - For boys: (Mother's Height ± 13 centimeters) ± (Father's Height)/2
  - Target height is midparental height ± 2 SD (1 SD = 5 cm)
- Measurement of growth
- The growth curve is the most valuable instrument for assessing the problem. The pattern of growth of a normal child is very consistent, and deviations in the process may warrant concern and further evaluation.
  - Obtain length up to age 2 and height onward. Note that at age 3, the height at 50th percentile is 95 cm and for length is 96.5 cm.
  - It is important to be consistent and systematic in the way height is obtained. Always measure it without shoes, and when plotting the patient in the growth curve, be as accurate as possible regarding the actual age of the child. Be sure to correct for genu recurvatum or leg length asymmetries when obtaining the measurements. Do not forget that pediatric patients do not shrink, so if unsure of your measurement, re-measure the patient again.
  - It is strongly recommended that you use the metric system. The tendency to round off numbers becomes problematic when an inch is the measure.
- BA: gives a level of bone maturation based on centers of ossification and closure of epiphyses.
- Up to a CA of 2 years, a hemiskeletal BA is more accurate; after that, obtain a left hand/wrist radiograph using the method of Greulich and Pyle.

## Laboratory Studies

- General screening tests: CBC with differential; BMP; urinalysis; bone age; $T_4$ and TSH; IGF-1 (>5 years of age)
- Specialized tests: karyotype; growth hormone stimulation test; dexamethasone suppression test
  - Growth hormone stimulation test
    - There is no gold standard test for the diagnosis of growth hormone deficiency.
    - Growth hormone stimulation tests are needed because of the pulsatile nature of growth hormone release. A growth hormone level by itself is meaningless in the evaluation of short stature. Provocative agents include clonidine, L-dopa, arginine, insulin, glucagon, and growth hormone–releasing hormone.
    - The tests should be performed by an endocrinologist.
    - Up to 25% of normal children fail any given stimulation test, so it is important to consider the rest of the clinical picture and document abnormal results using two different agents to classify a patient as growth hormone–deficient. It is considered a pass if the stimulation test has a peak growth hormone response >8 ng/mL.

## Treatment (Growth Hormone Therapy)

- Food and Drug Administration–approved indications for the use of growth hormone
  - Growth hormone deficiency
  - Turner syndrome
  - Renal insufficiency
  - Prader-Willi syndrome
  - SGA
  - Idiopathic short stature (predicted target height: girls: <4′11; boys: <5′3)
- Effectiveness: best response in the first year of therapy
- Administration and dosage
  - Give as a subcutaneous injection starting at 0.3 mg/kg/wk given 6–7 day/wk.
  - For patients with Turner syndrome, give 0.35 mg/kg/wk.

■ Cost: expensive
■ Adverse effects: slipped capital femoral epiphysis, glucose intolerance/diabetes, pseudo-tumor cerebri, scoliosis.

# PUBERTAL DEVELOPMENT

## Basics

### Definition
■ Puberty is the stage when primary and secondary sexual characteristics develop and growth is completed.
■ Pubertal changes are a consequence of increased gonadotropins and sex steroid secretion.
■ Skeletal age correlates better with pubertal events than CA (Table 14-8).
■ Sequence of puberty
  ▪ Girls. Typically the progression is breast development, initiation of growth spurt, pubic hair, and lastly, menarche (initiation of monthly menstrual periods).
  ▪ Boys. Typically the progression is testicular growth, followed by pubic hair development, and finally the peak growth spurt.

■ Time of puberty
  ▪ Girls
    • Mean age of onset: 9.5–10 years, although this can be as early as 6 years for African Americans and 7 years for Caucasians
    • Mean age of full pubertal breast development: 14 years
    • Mean age of menarche: 10–12 years.
    • Average duration of puberty: 3–4 years
  ▪ Boys
    • Mean age of onset: 10.5–12 years, although can be as early as 9 years
    • Average duration of puberty: 3.5 years

### Terminology for the Endocrine Changes During Puberty
■ Adrenarche: increased adrenal androgen that causes sexual hair and typically occurs at approximately the same time as puberty. However, in some disorders, this may occur prematurely, independent of puberty.
■ Gonadarche: increased gonadal activity resulting from a pubertal gonadotropin-releasing hormone (GnRH)–stimulated luteinizing hormone (LH) response or elevated estradiol
■ Pubarche: development of sexual hair
■ Thelarche: onset of breast development
■ Menarche: onset of menstrual periods
■ Pubertal gynecomastia: palpable or visible breast tissue in at least two thirds of boys during puberty. It may coincide with the onset of puberty and generally occurs before testosterone levels have reached adult levels. It lasts about 2 years.
■ Testicular enlargement

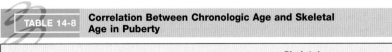

**TABLE 14-8   Correlation Between Chronologic Age and Skeletal Age in Puberty**

| Females | Chronologic age | Average skeletal age | Skeletal age occurs by in 95% of population |
| --- | --- | --- | --- |
| Breast Development | 10.8 ± 1.0 | 10.75 | 12.5 |
| Sexual Pubic Hair | 11.2 ± 1.1 | | |
| Menarche | 12.7 ± 1.0 | 13 | 14 |

## History

- Assess for the following:
  - Time of onset of pubertal changes such as presence of breasts, vaginal discharge, growth of pubic, axillary, or facial hair
  - Evidence of a growth spurt
  - Other signs and symptoms (neurologic) for CNS abnormalities, headaches, visual changes
- Medication or exposure history
- Ages at which parents underwent puberty; height of the biological parents

## Physical Examination

- It is important to determine the Tanner stage of the patient; these stages are used to grade pubertal progression, including breast development, testicular size, and pubic hair progression (see Appendix D). Breast and pubic hair progression is determined by a comparison method with the Tanner stages.
- The size of the testes is determined by using an orchidometer.
  - The Prader orchidometer consists of a set of ellipsoids encompassing the range of testicular volume from infancy to adulthood (1–25 mL) to use for direct comparison with the patient's testes.
  - A volume of 4 mL closely correlates with the onset of pubertal development. A volume of 4–6 mL corresponds to Tanner II, 8–10 mL to Tanner III, 12–15 mL to Tanner IV, and 20–25 mL to Tanner V.
- In girls, assess the vaginal mucosa for estrogen exposure (pink color, thickened mucosa, mucoid secretions).
- It is also very important to plot the patient's height and weight on a growth curve to determine any degree of growth acceleration and growth potential of the patient.

# PRECOCIOUS PUBERTY

- Classically, this is defined as the premature onset and rapid progression of sexual development (i.e., breast development, testicular enlargement), with concomitant pubertal levels of hormones and inappropriate acceleration of skeletal age.

## Etiology

- Central precocious puberty (CPP) (GnRH dependent)
  - Idiopathic (95% in girls)
  - CNS abnormalities (most common cause in males)
  - Lesion (e.g., hamartoma)
  - Disorder (e.g., cerebral palsy)
  - Neurofibromatosis
  - Obesity
- Peripheral-Precocious Pseudopuberty (PPP) (GnRH independent)
  - Congenital virilizing adrenal hyperplasia
  - McCune-Albright syndrome
  - Tumors (e.g., ovarian granulosa cell tumor, Leydig cell tumor, adrenal adenoma/adenocarcinoma, human chorionic gonadotropin-secreting tumor)
  - Ovarian cysts
  - Exogenous sex steroids (e.g., estrogen or testosterone cream, oral contraceptives)
  - Primary hypothyroidism
  - Familial testotoxicosis

## Diagnosis

### Initial Testing

- Gonadotropin elevation with LH predominance in the pubertal range is consistent with CPP.

- Plasma ultrasensitive estradiol levels and testosterone levels at time of obtaining gonadotropins, respectively, in girls and boys are helpful on making this diagnosis.
- A GnRH analogue stimulation test (Leuprolide) in which gonadotropins are measured at intervals following injection of GnRH can be used to diagnose CPP. If an LH peak of >8 IU/L is present, it is consistent with a pubertal response.
- Bone age will eventually show an acceleration.

*Imaging*
- Brain magnetic resonance imaging (MRI) should be performed in all boys with CPP or girls in which cause is unexplained.
- Pelvic ultrasound provides information on uterine and ovarian size and hormonal stimulation, as well as possible ovarian cyst or tumor.

## Treatment

- Treat the underlying cause if there is one (e.g., tumor, hypothyroidism, congenital adrenal hyperplasia).
- In other cases, GnRH therapy can be used to retard centrally mediated pubertal development, to avoid growth impairment, and to try to reach maximum growth potential.
- In conditions with autonomous gonadal steroid production, such as McCune-Albright syndrome or testotoxicosis, adjunct therapy with aromatase inhibitors, estrogen receptor antagonists, spironolactone, or ketoconazole has been used.

# PREMATURE ADRENARCHE

- The presence of adrenarche before age 9 for boys and 6 for girls.
- This can be differentiated from true puberty by the presence of adrenarche (sexual hair) without the presence of testicular enlargement or breast development.

## Etiology

- Idiopathic, benign (most common)
- True central precocious puberty
- Congenital adrenal hyperplasia
- Adrenal tumor

## Diagnosis

- Bone age
- 17-OHP level (to rule out CAH)
- Dehydroepiandrosterone sulfate (DHEAS) (to rule out adrenal tumor)

## Treatment

- Treatment is geared to treating the underlying disorder if present.
- If no underlying disorder is present, then reassurance is appropriate.

# DELAYED PUBERTY

- This is defined as lack of pubertal changes by age 12 in girls and 14 in boys.
- Patients should have an endocrine evaluation if >5 years have elapsed between the first signs of puberty and completion of genital growth in boys or menarche in girls (or if no menarche by 16 years).

## Etiology

- Delayed
  - Constitutional delay of growth and maturation (most common cause)
  - Hypothyroidism
  - Chronic illness and malnutrition

- Central (low gonadotropins)
  - Intracranial pathology: craniopharyngioma, prolactinoma, empty sella
  - Congenital conditions: genetic syndromes such as Kallmann syndrome (isolated gonadotropin deficiency with anosmia), Prader-Willi syndrome, Bardet-Biedl syndrome, CHARGE, septo-optic dysplasia
  - Acquired conditions: cranial radiation, autoimmune disease, sickle cell, hemosiderosis
- Gonadal (high gonadotropins)
  - Genetic syndromes: Turner syndrome, Klinefelter syndrome, androgen insensitivity, 5α-reductase deficiency, mixed gonadal dysgenesis, vanishing testis
  - Acquired conditions: autoimmune, mumps, orchitis, chemotherapy, surgery, gonadal torsion, radiation

## Diagnosis

- There is no reliable test to differentiate between those with normal late puberty (constitutional delay of growth and maturation) and those who have actual disorders preventing puberty.
- Therefore, all patients with no signs of puberty by 14 years of age, without a family history of late puberty, should have an evaluation, which should include:
  - Free $T_4$ and TSH (to rule out hypothyroidism)
  - LH and FSH (to rule out primary gonadal failure, if elevated have failure)
  - Smell test (to rule out Kallmann syndrome)
  - Head MRI (to rule out intracranial pathology)
  - Testosterone or estradiol level
  - Bone age
    - Prolactin (to rule out prolactinoma)

## Treatment

- Focus should be on treating the underlying cause first if one is identified.
- Treatment of primary gonadal failure as a cause of delayed puberty in males typically involves the administration of testosterone IM injections (100 mg) on a monthly basis, at gradually increasing doses or gradually increasing oral estrogen replacement for girls.

### Suggested Readings
Brook C. Clinical Paediatric Endocrinology. 3rd Ed. London: Blackwell Science, 1995.
Fisher DA. Clinical review 19: management of congenital hypothyroidism. J Clin Endocrinol Metab 1991;7:523–529.
Fisher DA. Thyroid Disorder in Childhood and Adolescence. In: Sperling M, ed. Pediatric Endocrinology. 2nd Ed. Philadelphia: WB Saunders, 2002:187–207.
Muglia L, et al. Disorder of the Posterior Pituitary. In: Sperling M, ed. Pediatric Endocrinology. Philadelphia: WB Saunders 2002: 289–321.
Pescovitz O, Eugster E. Pediatric Endocrinology: Mechanisms and Management. Philadelphia: Lippincott Williams & Wilkins March 2004, Chapter 27–30.
Sidwell R, et al. Endocrinology, growth and puberty. Concise Paediatr 2003;9:251–253.

## GASTROENTEROLOGIC DISEASES
### *William E. Bennett, Jr. and James P. Keating*

 **NEONATES AND INFANTS**

## VOMITING

### "Reflux" and Regurgitation

- Infants, physiologically, have frequent reflux of either food or acidic gastric contents into the esophagus.
- Gastroesophageal reflux disease (GERD) is uncommon.
- Physiologic reflux is often overtreated.
- Reflux usually occurs postprandially but can develop several hours later.

#### Clinical Presentation
- Symptoms and signs: crying, hoarseness, stridor, vomiting, poor weight gain, decreased appetite, back arching, apparent life-threatening events (ALTEs), and apnea have all been attributed to GERD by some authors. Pyrosis, dysphagia, and acid/water brash are classic symptoms of GERD in older children and adults.

#### Treatment
- pH monitoring is often used but is not effective in most cases.
- Surgical (fundoplication) and pharmacologic treatment ($H_1$ antagonists or proton pump inhibitors) may be necessary in extreme cases.

#### Special Considerations
- Vomiting is present in the majority of healthy infants and resolves during the first year of life. Therapy is not indicated.
- Physiologic reflux goes by many names among the lay public, such as infant reflux, possetting, and spitting.
  - Treatment with gastric acidity inhibitors (e.g., ranitidine, omeprazole) increases the risk of acute gastroenteritis and community-acquired pneumonia, and these drugs should be avoided.
  - Distinguishing this common, innocent process from pathologic vomiting is usually successfully done by the experienced mother or grandmother, supported as needed by the general pediatrician.
- If vomiting is associated with dehydration or slowed growth, the differential diagnosis includes pyloric stenosis, malrotation/volvulus, hyperammonemia, and increased intracranial pressure. Erosive esophagitis is rare in infancy unless a long-term nasogastric tube is in place or the infant has severe neurologic disease with dysphagia.
- There is no gold standard for the diagnosis of GERD in infants. The diagnosis of GERD, as reflected in the overuse of acid suppression medications in infants with infantile colic, infantile regurgitation, periodic breathing, and feeding problems, is often made in lieu of thoughtful assessment and reassurance.
- Infants are often subjected to a variety of tests, including upper gastrointestinal (GI) studies, pH probes or impedance studies, esophagoscopy and biopsy, and radiopharmaceutical-labeled milk studies, although none has proven utility.

## Malrotation/Volvulus

- Malrotation/midgut volvulus is incomplete rotation of the proximal small bowel during fetal development. This may result in midgut volvulus if it occurs about arterial supply of the small intestine.
- The condition may be subacute or chronic.
- See Chapter 9, Surgery for additional information.

*Epidemiology*
- Malrotation/volvulus is most common in infants <1 year of age (~75%).
- It can often present in the first week of life (~30%).
- It is more common if other GI malformations are present, such as duodenal or jejunal atresia. It is also more common in patients with Hirschsprung disease.

*Diagnosis*
- Symptoms and signs include acute bilious vomiting, abdominal distension and tenderness, and dilated small bowel loops.
- Abdominal examination may be normal when malrotation is intermittent.
- An upper GI series is commonly used.

*Treatment*
- Monitor for signs of perforation.
- Place Replogle tube to low intermittent suction.
- Use surgery (Ladd procedure), which is curative.

## Pyloric Stenosis

*Epidemiology and Etiology*
- Pyloric stenosis commonly occurs in infants >4 weeks and usually <2 months of age.
- The incidence of the condition is $\frac{1}{250} - \frac{1}{300}$.
- It is more common in boys (4:1 ratio); 25% of cases are first-born male children.
- It results from hypertrophy of the pylorus, causing delayed gastric emptying and eventually inability of food to enter the small intestine (see Chapter 9, Surgery for additional information).

*History and Physical Examination*
- Nonbilious projectile vomiting occurs after feeding.
- The infant is usually well appearing (although he or she can have poor growth or dehydration once severe).
- A pyloric mass (olive) may be palpated in the midepigastrium.

*Imaging*
- Pyloric ultrasound is the usual first test.
- A pylorus wall (one side) >3 mm with a length >14 mm is considered hypertrophic.

*Treatment*
- Measure electrolytes if the infant shows signs of dehydration.
- Rehydrate as appropriate.
- Use surgical myotomy, which is curative.

# CONSTIPATION

## Hirschsprung Disease

*Epidemiology and Etiology*
- Hirschsprung disease is more common in term infants. The incidence is approximately $\frac{1}{5000}$.

- Aganglionosis of a segment of colon results from incomplete migration of neural crest cells during embryogenesis.

### Clinical Presentation
- Delayed passage of meconium is characteristic; 99.5% of term infants have stool by 24 hours, 99.9% by 48 hours.
- Other symptoms and signs include vomiting, abdominal distension, and constipation outside of the newborn period.

### Laboratory Studies and Imaging
- Contrast enema shows a "transition zone"—a relative dilation of colon proximal to the rectum.
- Rectal suction biopsy establishes the diagnosis.
- Full-thickness biopsy required in some cases.

### Treatment
- Daily saline irrigations
- Surgical correction

## Constipation, Stool Holding, Soiling, and Encopresis

- Constipation is a variable combination of large, hard, painful, or infrequent bowel movements, often with fecal incontinence.

### Epidemiology and Etiology
- It occurs most commonly after 2 years of age.
- It is often behavioral in etiology and is associated with a cycle of painful defecation and stool withholding.
- Contrary to common belief, no evidence exists to show an association with oral iron supplementation.

### Diagnosis
- There is palpable stool on abdominal examination (scybala).
- Digital rectal examination reveals a mass of hard stool in the rectum.
- Fecal soiling is apparent on perianal skin.

### Treatment
- Encourage regular bowel movements.
- Use laxatives (magnesium citrate, polyethylene glycol [PEG]).
- Disimpaction may require use of a pediatric Fleet enema, although caution should be exercised in the use of repeated phosphate-containing enemas.
- Use complete evacuation with a PEG cleanout if these measures are ineffective.

# OTHER CONDITIONS

## Biliary Atresia

- This is atresia of the extrahepatic portion of the biliary tree.

### Epidemiology and Etiology
- The incidence of the condition is approximately $\frac{1}{15,000}$.
- Affected individuals are usually full-term infants, who present at 2–8 weeks (75%).
- The condition may be associated with situs inversus/asplenia
- Etiology is unknown, although an infectious etiology is suspected.

### Diagnosis
- Pale stools and jaundice
- Signs of cholestatic liver failure and cirrhosis, which are usually absent initially
- Conjugated hyperbilirubinemia

*Laboratory Studies and Imaging*
- Measure fractionated bilirubin, aspartate aminotransferase (AST), alanine aminotransferase (ALT), alkaline phosphatase, and gamma-glutamyl transferase (GGT).
- HIDA scan shows lack of excretion into bowel.

*Treatment*
- Therapy is surgical (Kasai portoenterostomy, transplantation), preferably before 2 months of age.

## Colic

- This is a syndrome of excessive infant irritability.
- It usually occurs in infants 2 weeks to 3 months of age, resolving before 3 months.

*History and Physical Examination*
- Paroxysmal crying (especially at night)
- Normal examination

*Treatment*
- No treatment is necessary.
- Simethicone is often given, but no evidence exists to support its use.
- Various methods of soothing are often used.

## Intussusception

- Intussusception is a telescoping of the bowel that results in progressive venous/lymphatic congestion and eventual arterial compromise, bowel ischemia, and obstruction.
- See Chapter 9, Surgery for additional information.

*Epidemiology and Etiology*
- It is most common in infants 4–12 months of age.
- It is most common at the ileocecal valve. It requires a "lead point," which is often the plentiful lymph tissue present in the terminal ileum.
- Enteric adenoviruses are often implicated.

*Clinical Presentation and Physical Examination*
- Symptoms and signs include colicky and intermittent abdominal pain, vomiting, and hematochezia or "currant jelly" stools.
- Palpable intussusceptum or distension is often present.

*Treatment*
- Surgical correction is necessary if the enema is not successful in reducing the intussusception.

## Meckel Diverticulum

- Meckel diverticulum is failure of the obliteration of the vitelline duct (which connects the midgut to the yolk sac) during embryogenesis, often with a heterotopic island of gastric mucosa, which leads to ulceration of the mucosa.

*Epidemiology*
- Fifty percent of cases occur in infants <2 years of age. The incidence of the condition is approximately 2%.
- Meckel diverticulum may cause obstruction if the diverticulum has a persistent attachment to portions of the small bowel or inverts and causes an intussusception.
- In older patients, it may cause diverticulitis.

*Clinical Presentation*
- Signs of acute blood loss such as tachycardia and shock may be present.
- Signs of obstruction or intussusception may be present.
- Painless bleeding is the most common sign.

*Laboratory Studies and Imaging*
- A Meckel scan may show uptake of radio-labeled technetium into the diverticulum if gastric mucosa is present but is commonly falsely negative.
- Obtain a complete blood count.

*Treatment*
- Transfuse if appropriate.
- Place Replogle to low intermittent suction if obstruction is suspected.
- Perform surgery (curative) with excision of the diverticulum, along with an adjacent segment of bowel.

#  ADOLESCENTS AND CHILDREN

## ABDOMINAL PAIN
- These problems typically present with pain alone.

### Benign Recurrent Abdominal Pain (BRAP)
*Epidemiology*
- BRAP is present in 10%–20% of school-aged children.
- This condition is more common in the evening, and it occurs intermittently, without associated symptoms such as diarrhea or vomiting.

*Diagnosis*
- Diagnosis is based on history and physical examination alone.
- No imaging is useful, although patients may have multiple diagnostic tests.

*Treatment*
- Reassurance is all that is necessary.

### Cholelithiasis/Biliary Colic
*Epidemiology*
- Rare in children compared with adults

*Clinical Presentation and History*
- Colicky pain in the right upper quadrant; worse after fatty meals
- Sometimes jaundice
- Often a family history

*Laboratory Studies and Imaging*
- Comprehensive metabolic profile plus fractionated bilirubin
- Ultrasound may show gallstones or a stone obstructing the common bile duct.

*Treatment*
- Surgery (cholelithiasis)
- Endoscopic retrograde cholangiopancreatography (ERCP) (choledocholithiasis)
- Antibiotics with Gram-negative coverage if obstruction is present
- Surgical consultation

### Peptic Ulcer Disease
*Etiology*
- Rare in children
- Two common causes:
  - *Helicobacter pylori* infection
  - "Stress ulcers" from severe illness, usually in the intensive care unit

*Clinical Presentation*
- Hematemesis, melena, and abdominal pain
- May be hemodynamically significant

*Laboratory Studies*
- Upper GI contrast study is occasionally helpful.
- Upper endoscopy is often useful.
- Rapid urease test and/or Steiner stain on antral biopsy is diagnostic for *Helicobacter*.

*Treatment*
- NPO
- Volume/hemodynamic support
- Proton pump inhibitor (PPI); continued for 1 month
- *H. pylori*: combination of PPI, amoxicillin, and clarithromycin for 2 weeks
- Severe bleeding
  - Octreotide drip sometimes effective
  - Surgical intervention for ongoing, hemodynamically significant bleed

## Pancreatitis

*Etiology (Children)*
- Trauma
- Idiopathic
- Drug
- Biliary
- Hereditary

*Clinical Presentation*
- Midepigastric abdominal pain, often radiating to the back.
- Vomiting

*Laboratory Studies and Imaging*
- Elevated amylase/lipase >3 times the upper limit of normal
- Abdominal computed tomography (CT) scan/abdominal ultrasound that shows peripancreatic fluid, pancreatic swelling or disruption, or pseudocyst

*Treatment*
- NPO; then once pain improved, advance diet
- Pain control: morphine preferable
- Serial amylase/lipase of little use
- Repeat imaging of little use unless symptoms recur

# DIARRHEA

## Infectious Enterocolitis

*Definition*
- Infection of the small or large intestine with a bacterial or protozoal pathogen
- Acute onset of cramping abdominal pain and bloody diarrhea

*Etiology*
- Five common bacteria
  - *Escherichia coli.* If *E. coli* serogroup H7:O157 is involved, patients may develop hemolytic uremic syndrome, characterized by hemolysis, thrombocytopenia, and acute renal failure.
  - *Salmonella*
  - *Shigella*

- *Yersinia*
- *Campylobacter*
- *Clostridium difficile*
- *Giardia lamblia*
- Amebiasis

### Diagnosis
- Stool culture
- Stool *Giardia* and *Cryptosporidium* antigens
- Stool *C. difficile* toxin
- Fecal leukocytes rarely of value
- Imaging studies of little value

### Treatment
- Rehydration
- Metronidazole for *C. difficile*
- Azithromycin for *Shigella*
- For others, antibiotics of little value

## Inflammatory Bowel Disease

- Chronic disease (weeks to months) characterized by abdominal pain, hematochezia, and diarrhea
- Composed of three types:
  - Crohn disease
  - Ulcerative colitis
  - Indeterminate colitis
- For the key differences between Crohn disease and ulcerative colitis, see Table 15-1.
- Unknown etiology

### Diagnosis
- Typical clinical pattern (see previous discussion)

**TABLE 15-1    Inflammatory Bowel Disease: Clinical Comparison**

|  | Crohn disease | Ulcerative colitis |
| --- | --- | --- |
| **Location** | Anywhere in gastrointestinal tract | Confined to colon |
| **Systemic versus local** | Systemic disease common<br>Anemia of chronic disease<br>Hypoalbuminemia<br>Weight loss | Systemic disease less common |
| **Complications** | Fistulae<br>Obstruction | Toxic megacolon |
| **Symptoms** | Pain and occasional hematochezia predominant symptoms | Pain and frequent bloody stools predominant symptoms |
| **Extraintestinal** | No primary sclerosing cholangitis<br>Mouth ulcers<br>Uveitis<br>Episcleritis<br>Arthritis<br>Erythema nodosum<br>Pyoderma gangrenosum | Similar to Crohn disease, with the addition of primary sclerosing cholangitis |

| TABLE 15-2 | Inflammatory Bowel Disease: Pathologic/Endoscopic Comparison | |
|---|---|---|
| | Crohn disease | Ulcerative colitis |
| Gross appearance | Skip lesions common | Contiguous involvement from rectum proximally |
| Histology | Granulomata frequently present<br>Transmural inflammation common<br>Fistulae common | No granulomata present<br>Only mucosa involved<br>Fistulae rare |

- Laboratory testing
  - Complete blood count: hepcidin-mediated anemia (more common in Crohn disease)
  - Hypoalbuminemia (more common in Crohn disease)
- Radiologic testing
  - Upper GI/small bowel follow-through, with possible stricture or edema of bowel wall
  - CT, with possible bowel wall thickening
- Endoscopy (Table 15-2)
  - Colonoscopy plus ileoscopy
  - Upper endoscopy if Crohn disease is suspected

*Treatment*
- Inducing remission: steroids
- Maintenance
  - 5-aminosalicylate (ASA) analogs: sulfasalazine, mesalamine
  - Other immune modulators: azathioprine, 6-mercaptopurine
- Refractory cases
  - Surgery
    - Crohn disease: resection of involved area
    - Ulcerative colitis: colectomy (curative)
  - Infliximab (Remicade) or adalimumab (Humira) (anti-TNF α-antibody)
  - Metronidazole: occasionally helpful in Crohn disease
  - Methotrexate

## Celiac Disease

- Autoinflammatory, lymphocytic infiltration of the small bowel with villous blunting and malabsorption
- A reaction to gluten, a protein in wheat
- Clinical presentation: abdominal pain, diarrhea, and slow growth

## Diagnosis

- Antitransglutaminase antibody (tTG) most sensitive and specific test
- Upper endoscopy with duodenal biopsies definitive

*Treatment*
- Gluten-free diet

# OTHER CONDITIONS

## Autoimmune Hepatitis (AIH)

- Progressive transaminitis, sometimes with cholestasis/jaundice

*Epidemiology*
- Occasional presentation with, or early progression to, cirrhosis
- Rare before 2–3 years of age
- Rare progression to liver failure

*Laboratory Studies and Imaging*
- AST/ALT and GGT, which confirm transaminitis
- Liver ultrasound to check for signs of portal hypertension
- AI hepatitis-specific tests:
  - Antismooth muscle antibody
  - Anti–liver-kidney microsomal antibody
  - Quantitative immunoglobulin G

*Treatment*
- Steroids for acute exacerbations
- Azathioprine, which is mainstay of maintenance
- Surveillance for signs of portal hypertension
- Liver transplant

## Foreign Bodies

*Epidemiology and Etiology*
- Patients: infants, toddlers, and the neurologically disabled
- Objects: coins, toys, food, and other small objects
- Locations: esophagus at the thoracic inlet, gastroesophageal junction, and the pylorus

*Diagnosis*
- Usually apparent on history
- If object is radiopaque, chest radiograph or abdominal radiograph is useful.

*Treatment*
- Esophageal: endoscopic removal within 24 hours (because of increased chance of perforation)
- Beyond gastroesophageal junction: expectant management is sufficient.
- Specific objects:
  - Multiple magnets: surgical removal
  - Disk batteries: consider surgical removal
  - Drug balloons: surgical removal
  - Sharp objects (e.g., needles): consider surgical removal

## Rectal Prolapse

*Etiology*
- Usually results from prolonged or repeated straining as well as severe diarrhea (*Shigella*, *E. coli* O157:H7)
- Occasionally results from rectal mass acting as a lead point (e.g., polyp)
- Other factor: cystic fibrosis (poor nutrition and chronic cough)
- Can be associated with obsessive-compulsive disorder or digitization of rectum

*Diagnosis*
- History and physical examination
- Digital rectal examination: feel for mass
- Sweat chloride test

*Treatment*
- Stool softener
- Removal of mass lead point if present
- Correction of underlying nutritional deficit if cystic fibrosis

## Short Bowel Syndrome

*Etiology*
- Originates with surgical resection of bowel, with decreased absorptive surface
- Occasionally resulting from atresias or other malformations

*Diagnosis*
Clinical presentation as basis of diagnosis; usually necrotizing enterocolitis in neonates

*Treatment*
- Slow introduction of predigested formula

## Superior Mesenteric Artery Syndrome

- Progressive bilious vomiting

*Etiology*
- Occurs after prolonged weight loss or body casting
- Loss of fat surrounding bifurcation of abdominal aorta/superior mesenteric artery (SMA)
- Subsequent squeezing of duodenum between descending aorta and SMA

*Diagnosis*
- Upper GI series, which shows proximal narrowing of third portion of the duodenum and to-and-fro movement of contrast

*Treatment*
- Duodenal feeding (with feeding tube past the point of obstruction)
- Sometimes total parenteral nutrition
- Regaining of weight, with resolution of obstruction

### Suggested Readings

Canani RB, et al. Therapy with gastric acidity inhibitors increases the risk of acute gastroenteritis and community-acquired pneumonia in children. Pediatrics 2006 May; 117(5):e817–820.

Crohn's and Colitis Foundation of America. www.ccfa.org.

Kleinman R, ed. American Academy of Pediatrics' Pediatric Nutrition Handbook. 5th Ed. Elk Grove Village, Ill: American Academy of Pediatrics, 2004.

Walker WA, ed. Pediatric Gastrointestinal Disease. 4th Ed. Hamilton, Ontario, Canada: BC Decker, 2004.

Zitelli B, Walker H. "Nutrition and Gastroenterology." Atlas of Pediatric Physical Diagnosis. 4th Ed. St. Louis: Mosby, 2002.

## DYSMORPHIC FEATURES AND MALFORMATIONS

### Definitions and Epidemiology

■ A *dysmorphic feature* is any alteration in the physical structure (morphology) of a person's anatomy.

■ A *malformation* is a specific type of dysmorphic feature in which an intrinsic (genetic) factor causes a structural abnormality.

■ Major malformations either require surgical intervention or have a significant impact on the patient's health.
  • Examples include craniosynostosis, global developmental delay/mental retardation, cleft lip and/or palate, congenital heart disease, and omphalocele.
  • They occur in up to 3% of all live births.

■ Minor malformations do not have a significant impact on the patient's health.
  • Examples include hypertelorism, ear pit or tag, smooth philtrum, transverse palmar crease, and mild soft tissue syndactyly.
  • They are not rare in the general population.

### Etiology

■ The pattern of dysmorphic features in a single individual may suggest a named genetic condition, such as up-slanting palpebral fissures, epicanthal folds, and a single palmar crease in individuals with Down syndrome.

■ There are also nongenetic causes for dysmorphic features. For example, the teratogenic effects of valproic acid can cause a constellation of facial features that resembles 22q11 deletion syndrome (velocardiofacial syndrome).

### Diagnosis and Evaluation

■ If a patient has at least two major or one major and two minor malformations, a karyotype is indicated. If the karyotype is normal, then chromosomal microarray analysis should be performed.

■ In a patient with two major or one major and two minor malformations, it is also necessary to consider the following studies to detect other occult anomalies:
  ■ Echocardiogram, abdominal ultrasound (with renal imaging), and neuroimaging study (magnetic resonance imaging [MRI])
  ■ Ophthalmologic examination and hearing screen (federally mandated newborn screening is sufficient in neonates or infants if there is no clinical concern for hearing loss)
  ■ Skeletal survey
  ■ Syndrome-specific testing directed by findings on examination, such as fluorescent in situ hybridization (FISH) for Williams syndrome if supravalvular aortic stenosis, developmental delay, and characteristic dysmorphic features are present

## NEWBORN SCREENING

■ The state mandated newborn screening test now evaluates for many disorders; information on which disorders are screened in each state is available at www.newbornscreening.info.

It is inappropriate to refer to newborn screening as "the PKU (phenylketonuria) test" because this is erroneous and misleading to families.

- For some disorders, the sensitivity relies on the infant eating protein, either breast milk or formula, before testing.
- If an infant is receiving total parenteral nutrition (TPN) at the time of testing, the amino acid analysis is uninterpretable and invalidates testing for certain disorders.
- If an infant has received a packed red blood cell transfusion before obtaining the newborn screening sample, the galactosemia and hemoglobinopathy assays are invalid.

- If a newborn screening result is abnormal, the report instructs the healthcare professional how to proceed given the severity of the abnormality and the likelihood that the patient is at risk.
  - The recommendation may be to send a repeat result or to refer the child to the appropriate specialist.
  - The American College of Medical Genetics ACTion sheets can be an invaluable resource to help primary care physicians follow up abnormal newborn screening results (see "Online Genetic Resources" section).

- For some disorders, a history of a normal newborn screening result should not preclude sending definitive testing if a specific disorder is clinically suspected.

# METABOLIC DECOMPENSATION AS A PRESENTATION OF INBORN ERRORS OF METABOLISM

## Clinical Presentation

- Children with an acute decompensation from an inborn metabolic disease may present with variable and nonspecific symptoms, such as mental status changes that range from fussiness to coma, poor feeding, vomiting, changes in breathing, abnormal movements, seizures, strokes, or liver failure. They may also have chronic conditions, including low tone, global developmental delay, mental retardation, autism, or cardiomyopathy.
- Children with an underlying metabolic disease and a superimposed acute metabolic stress, such as an infection or trauma, may present with more severe symptoms than expected from the acute stressor alone.
- Patients with an underlying metabolic disease may also experience difficulty recovering from surgery.
- Infants with bacterial sepsis may have an inborn metabolic illness as a predisposing factor, such as the increased incidence of *Escherichia coli* sepsis in patients with galactosemia. Also, a previously healthy neonate who presents with septic symptomatology but no fever or obvious source of infection should have a concurrent metabolic evaluation.

## Laboratory Studies

- To detect a wide range of metabolic disorders, several screening laboratory tests are recommended. If abnormalities are detected, then more definitive studies should be performed.
- For the highest yield, samples should be obtained during an acute illness. Tests to order include:
  - Blood tests: Accu-Chek, comprehensive metabolic panel, blood gas (arterial or capillary), ammonium, complete blood count (CBC) with differential, lactate and pyruvate, serum/plasma amino acids, acylcarnitine profile, quantitative carnitines, and save serum sample
  - Urine tests: urinalysis (including ketones), reducing substances, organic acids, and save urine sample
  - Cerebrospinal fluid (CSF) tests: routine studies (cell count, glucose, protein), lactate and pyruvate, amino acids, and save CSF sample
- Results of newborn screening tests should be verified.

## Treatment

- If the diagnosis of an inborn metabolic disease is considered, the patient should not receive enteral protein or TPN. Instead, the patient should receive 10% dextrose intravenous (IV) fluids at 1.5–2 times the maintenance rate.
- If a definitive diagnosis is made, then specific and directed therapy can be instituted.
- The appropriate management for an individual with a known metabolic disease depends on the underlying disorder.
  - Patients or their families should present a sick letter written by their geneticist with management instructions for their specific disorder.
  - Contact the geneticist on call for any patient who presents ill to the emergency department, is receiving sedation, or is undergoing a procedure.

## METABOLIC DISORDERS ASSOCIATED WITH METABOLIC ACIDOSIS

- Patients with acidosis secondary to a metabolic disorder may present with mild persistent acidosis or with severe acute acidosis.
  - The acidosis may be because of a buildup of lactate leading to a lactic acidosis or may be as a result of the accumulation of organic acids, such as propionic or methylmalonic acid.
  - Acidosis because of an inborn metabolic disease frequently causes a large anion gap (>25 mmol/L) during an acute illness.

### Laboratory Studies

- Several laboratory tests are recommended for a patient who has a metabolic acidosis, once the more common causes such as diarrhea and renal tubular acidosis have been ruled out.
  - Blood tests: comprehensive metabolic panel, amino acids, lactate and pyruvate, ammonium, acylcarnitine profile, quantitative carnitines, and blood gas (arterial or capillary). Consider uric acid and lipid profile.
  - Urine tests: urinalysis (including ketones) and organic acids

### Treatment

- If the diagnosis of an inborn metabolic disease is considered, the patient should not receive enteral protein or TPN.
- IV fluids containing 10% dextrose should be given at 1.5–2 times the maintenance rate.
- An individualized treatment plan can be created based on the results of the above evaluation and diagnosis.

## GENETIC DISORDERS PRESENTING WITH HYPERAMMONEMIA

### Clinical Presentation

- Table 16-1 includes selected clinical features characteristic of genetic conditions that present with an elevated ammonium level.

### Laboratory Studies

- An evaluation for hyperammonemia is warranted for ammonium >80 μmol/L in neonates or for ammonium >50 μmol/L in infants and children. A single elevated ammonium should be confirmed with a repeat sample.
- Ammonium levels should be drawn arterially or as a free-flowing venous sample, placed on wet ice, and processed immediately.

| TABLE 16-1 | Clinical Features of Selected Genetic Disorders Causing Elevated Ammonium Levels |
|---|---|
| **Disease** | **Selected clinical features** |
| Urea cycle defects | Acute onset of poor feeding, vomiting, altered mental status, which may progress to coma; respiratory alkalosis early in presentation, progressing to metabolic acidosis |
| Organic acidemias | Ketoacidosis with an increased anion gap (>25), hyperglycemia or hypoglycemia, may have hypocalcemia, neutropenia, or thrombocytopenia |
| Fatty acid oxidation disorders | Fasting hypoglycemia with relative hypoketosis, liver disease, cardiomyopathy, hypotonia, myopathy, hyperuricemia |
| Hyperammonemia, hyperornithinemia, homocitrullinuria (HHH) syndrome | Global developmental delay, seizures, periodic ataxia |
| Lysinuric protein intolerance (LPI) | Postprandial hyperammonemia (except breast milk), aversion to high-protein food, failure to thrive, moderate hepatosplenomegaly, hypotonia |
| Hyperinsulinism, hyperammonemia (HIHA) syndrome | Hypoglycemia (especially after protein meal), seizures, encephalopathy, global developmental delay |
| Transient hyperammonemia of the newborn | Prematurity, encephalopathy; usually self-limited, and full recovery expected |

## Evaluation

- Recommended laboratory tests for diagnostic evaluation include:
  - Blood tests: comprehensive metabolic panel, blood gas if acutely ill, serum/plasma amino acids, acylcarnitine profile, quantitative carnitines, lactate and pyruvate, and creatine kinase. Consider fasting glucose, insulin levels, and uric acid.
  - Urine tests: urinalysis (including ketones), urine organic acids, orotic acid, and urine amino acids

## Treatment

- The recommended specific treatment depends on the type of disorder. If the patient is acutely ill and the underlying diagnosis is unknown, eliminate oral and parenteral sources of protein and provide adequate fluid (1.5–2 times the maintenance rate) and calories (10% dextrose IV fluids, intralipids).
- After beginning the recommended evaluation for a child with hyperammonemia, the plan for further evaluation and management should be discussed with a geneticist. If the levels are significantly elevated and/or rising rapidly, ammonium scavenging drugs or dialysis may be indicated.

## GENETIC DISORDERS PRESENTING WITH INFANTILE HYPOTONIA

### Etiology

- Hypotonia is a nonspecific sign that may be caused by a wide variety of etiologies.

■ Dysfunction in any component of the central or peripheral nervous system can cause hypotonia, including diseases of the muscle, neuromuscular junction, nerves, spinal cord, brain stem, cerebellum, basal ganglia, and cerebrum. Central hypotonia with peripheral spastic hypertonia is highly suggestive of central nervous system (CNS) involvement.

## Clinical Presentation

■ Historical features supporting a genetic etiology include family history of neuromuscular disease, parental consanguinity, and a prior affected sibling. However, the absence of these features does not rule out a genetic cause.

■ Contractures in the newborn indicate prenatal onset but do not suggest a single, specific diagnosis.

■ Additional features that may indicate an underlying syndrome may not be present at a young age or may be difficult to appreciate in the neonate or infant.

■ Table 16-2, which is not comprehensive, applies to those children in whom the hypotonia is not secondary to a known feature, such as high phenobarbital levels or severe hypoxic ischemic injury.

## Laboratory Studies

■ Several tests are recommended in the evaluation of a child with hypotonia and concern for a genetic disorder.
  ■ Blood tests: methylation studies for Prader-Willi and Angelman syndromes, creatine kinase, lactate and pyruvate, serum/plasma amino acids, comprehensive metabolic panel, karyotype (if normal, perform chromosomal microarray analysis), very long-chain fatty acids quantification, *SMN* molecular analysis (if reflexes absent), and myotonic dystrophy molecular analysis. Consider leukocyte lysosomal enzyme panel.
  ■ Urine tests: organic acids. Consider mucopolysaccharidosis screen.
  ■ Other tests: electromyogram, nerve conduction studies, electrocardiogram, echocardiogram, brain MRI, and abdominal and pelvic ultrasound

## Treatment

■ Confirming a genetic diagnosis may affect the treatment regimen and allow parents to more fully understand the child's clinical course.

■ Treatment often involves physical therapy and providing methods that support the child, such as splints, braces, or assistive devices. In a few conditions, such as Pompe disease, enzyme replacement therapy is used to treat the underlying disorder and can improve all of the patient's symptoms.

# GENETIC DISORDERS ASSOCIATED WITH SEIZURES AND EPILEPSY

■ Individuals with medically intractable epilepsy, idiopathic seizures with dysmorphic features, or myoclonic epilepsy should have an evaluation for an underlying genetic disorder.

## Laboratory Studies and Imaging

■ Several laboratory tests are indicated for children with suspected genetic causes of epilepsy:
  ■ Blood tests: glucose, lactate and pyruvate, amino acids, karyotype, chromosomal microarray analysis (if karyotype is normal), and uric acid
  ■ Urine tests: organic acids, sulfite analysis, creatine metabolites, and purine and pyrimidine metabolites. Consider amino acids and consider mucopolysaccharide and oligosaccharide screen if consistent phenotype.
  ■ CSF: routine studies (cell count, glucose, protein), amino acids, lactate and pyruvate, neurotransmitter metabolites, and save CSF sample

| TABLE 16-2 | Clinical Features of Selected Genetic Disorders Manifested by Hypotonia |
|---|---|
| **Disorder** | **Selected features** |
| CNS malformations (including lissencephaly and holoprosencephaly) | Frequently associated with other neurologic findings, such as seizures |
| Congenital disorders of glycosylation (CDG) | Classic cases (type 1a): pontocerebellar atrophy, lipodystrophy, failure to thrive, strabismus, coagulopathy, transaminase elevations, and mental retardation |
| Mitochondrial cytopathies | Protean manifestations: skeletal myopathy, lactic acidosis, strokes, leukodystrophy, global developmental delay/mental retardation, movement disorders, vision impairment, hearing impairment, arrhythmias, cardiomyopathy, hepatocellular dysfunction, diabetes, other endocrinopathies, and short stature |
| Pompe disease (glycogen storage disease type II) | Severe cardiomyopathy with characteristic high-amplitude electrocardiographic changes |
| Prader-Willi syndrome | Neonates: feeding difficulty, profound hypotonia common; later features not present |
| | Children: aggressive food-seeking behavior leading to obesity, behavioral abnormalities, mental retardation, short stature, hypogonadism |
| Angelman syndrome | Happy disposition, severe learning disability, ataxia, absent speech, mental retardation, dysmorphic facial features, microcephaly; possibly hypopigmentation |
| Chromosomal disorders | May have dysmorphic features or other associated malformations |
| Congenital muscular dystrophies | Contractures, may have CNS abnormalities on brain MRI |
| Congenital myotonic dystrophy | Respiratory distress, feeding impairment, most with mental retardation and cardiomyopathy; mother usually affected |
| Down syndrome | Characteristic dysmorphic features, heart defect, can be difficult to detect in premature infants and neonates |
| Lysosomal storage disorders | Variable depending on subtype |
| | Leukodystrophies: brain MRI abnormalities |
| | Mucopolysaccharidoses: coarse features |
| Peroxisomal disorders | May have dysmorphic facial features, large fontanels, hepatocellular dysfunction, or seizures |
| Smith-Lemli-Opitz syndrome | Dysmorphic facial features, 2–3 toe syndactyly, liver disease, genitourinary malformations |
| Spinal muscular atrophy | Muscle weakness with relative sparing of facial musculature, absent reflexes, poor weight gain; scoliosis may develop |

CNS, central nervous system; MRI, magnetic resonance imaging.

## Additional Evaluation

- Gene testing is available for children with certain suspected conditions, such as Angelman syndrome (15q11–13 methylation analysis, *UBE3A* sequence analysis), Rett syndrome (*MeCP2* gene sequencing, *CDKL5* gene sequencing if *MeCP2* normal), tuberous sclerosis (*TSC1* and *TSC2* gene sequencing), or GLUT-1 transporter deficiency (*GLUT1* gene sequencing).
- A brain MRI is necessary in all patients with medically intractable epilepsy to detect a primary CNS malformation or features of a specific epilepsy syndrome, such as cortical tubers.
- An ophthalmology evaluation should also be considered because findings may suggest an underlying genetic disease.

## Treatment

- Refer to Chapter 19, Neurologic Diseases for specific information about seizure treatment.
- If a specific genetic diagnosis can be made, the treatment may be tailored to that disorder (e.g., a trial of vigabatrin in a patient with tuberous sclerosis).

# GENETIC DISORDERS PRESENTING WITH MENTAL RETARDATION OR GLOBAL DEVELOPMENTAL DELAY

## Definitions

- The term *mental retardation* applies to children with an IQ <70 as assessed on standardized testing and impaired activities of daily living.
  - A child must be physically and behaviorally capable of participating in the testing for the evaluation to be valid. Thus, the diagnosis of mental retardation is usually not made until a child is 4–6 years of age, unless a syndromic diagnosis is made in which all affected individuals have mental retardation (such as Down syndrome).
  - Approximately 70% of individuals with mental retardation have autism or autistic features.
- The term *developmental delay* is used for young children and infants who are not achieving their developmental milestones within the expected age range. The domains of development include expressive language, receptive language, gross motor, fine motor/problem solving, and social and adaptive skills.
  - If an individual is delayed in one of these domains, he or she has isolated delay in a single domain, and a genetic evaluation is not necessarily indicated.
  - If an individual is delayed in more than one domain, he or she has global developmental delay, and an evaluation for a genetic etiology should be strongly considered unless the cause of the delays is known (neonatal infection, trauma).
  - The degree of delay, or developmental quotient, is calculated by dividing the child's developmental age by the chronologic age. For example, if an 8-month-old infant is rolling, does not have a pincer grasp, and is not yet babbling, the developmental age is 4 months and the child has a developmental quotient of 50%. A developmental quotient can be calculated for each individual domain, and children commonly have variation across the domains. An individual has global developmental delay if he or she has a developmental quotient of 70% or less in two or more domains.
- Finally, the diagnosis of *psychomotor regression* is reserved for individuals who have lost developmental skills. The evaluation for psychomotor regression is beyond the scope of this chapter.

## Initial Evaluation

- In a child with developmental delay, it is essential to rule out a primary medical problem that could explain the delays. For example, any child with language delay should have an audiology evaluation to rule out hearing loss as the underlying pathology.

| TABLE 16-3 | Genetic Disorders Associated with Nonspecific Mental Retardation or Global Developmental Delay* | |
|---|---|---|
| **Disorder** | **Features** | **Tests** |
| Chromosomal anomaly | May have dysmorphic features or associated neurologic symptoms, such as hypotonia or seizures | Karyotype Chromosomal microarray analysis if karyotype normal |
| Congenital disorders of glycosylation (CDG) | Classic cases: pontocerebellar atrophy, lipodystrophy, strabismus, coagulopathy, and transaminase elevations | CDG screen |
| Fragile X syndrome | Facial dysmorphisms, postpubertal macro-orchidism, autism X-linked inheritance (females may be affected) | Fragile X mutation analysis (detects expansions and methylation status) |
| Metabolic disorders Aminoacidopathy Organic aciduria Mitochondrial cytopathy Creatine deficiency Purine or pyrimidine disorder | Possible history of intermittent metabolic decompensation and other associated features; possible isolated global developmental disorder or mental retardation | Serum/plasma amino acids Lactate and pyruvate Urine organic acids Urine creatine metabolites Urine purine and pyrimidine metabolites |
| Neuroimaging abnormality (hypoplasia, malformation, leukodystrophy) | Frequently associated with abnormal neurologic examination and/or seizures | Brain magnetic resonance imaging Consider genetic evaluation for detected abnormality |

*This table lists disorders in which the *only* symptom of a disorder may be mental retardation and/or global developmental delay.

- An ophthalmology examination may reveal retinal, corneal, or other abnormalities that could lead to a diagnosis even if there is no concern about visual acuity.
- Comorbid neurologic disorders (epilepsy, hypotonia) are not rare in individuals with mental retardation or global developmental delay, especially when the delay or cognitive impairment is severe.
- There are a myriad of genetic and nongenetic etiologies for global developmental delay and mental retardation. Given the large number of potential causes, the clinician should use the history, examination, and ancillary studies to narrow the scope of the evaluation. If a child has syndromic features suggestive of a specific, named genetic condition, then an appropriate evaluation for that syndrome is warranted.
- Table 16-3 addresses selected syndromes that may present with mental retardation and developmental delay in isolation, and Table 16-4 addresses those that routinely occur in conjunction with other syndromic features.

## Treatment

- Regardless of the etiology, it is important to emphasize that appropriate therapeutic interventions—physical, occupational, speech, and developmental therapies—should be provided to help the child maximize his or her potential.
- In the vast majority of patients, the identification of an underlying genetic etiology does not significantly alter the therapeutic interventions or symptomatic management that the child receives.

| TABLE 16-4 | Genetic Disorders with Mental Retardation or Global Developmental Delay* | |
|---|---|---|
| **Disorder** | **Selected features** | **Tests** |
| Alpha-thalassemia/mental retardation syndrome (ATR-X) | X-linked (predominately males affected) Poor growth, dysmorphic facial features, genital anomalies, most with evidence of alpha thalassemia (usually mild) | *ATRX* gene sequencing |
| Angelman syndrome | Happy disposition, ataxia, absent speech, mental retardation, dysmorphic facial features, microcephaly; possibly hypopigmentation | 15q11-13 methylation analysis (abnormal in ~80% of cases) *UBE3A* sequence analysis (abnormal in additional 10% of cases) (FISH or microarray analysis for deletion; detects only 70% of cases) |
| Down syndrome | Characteristic dysmorphic features, heart defect Can be difficult to detect in premature infants and neonates | Karyotype Aneuploidy screen |
| Prader-Willi syndrome | Neonates: feeding difficulty, profound hypotonia Children: aggressive food-seeking behavior leading to obesity, behavioral abnormalities, short stature, hypogonadism | 15q11-13 methylation analysis (abnormal in >99%) (FISH or microarray analysis for deletion detects only 70% of cases) |
| Rett syndrome | Females only Acquired microcephaly, developmental regression, hand wringing, autism, intermittent hyperventilation | *MeCP2* gene sequencing Consider *CDKL5* gene sequencing if *MeCP2* mutation analysis normal |
| Smith-Lemli-Opitz syndrome | Dysmorphic facial features, 2–3 toe syndactyly, liver disease, genitourinary malformations | 7-dehydrocholesterol (total cholesterol is not always low) |
| Smith-Magenis syndrome | Dysmorphic features, hearing loss, self-destructive behaviors | Karyotype or FISH/CMA with deletion of *17p11.2* |
| Sotos syndrome | Overgrowth (>97th percentile), dysmorphic facial features; possible seizures, kidney anomalies, scoliosis, slightly increased risk of malignancy | *NSD1* sequence/deletion analysis |
| Williams syndrome | Typical dysmorphic facies, supravalvular aortic stenosis, "cocktail party personality," hypercalcemia | FISH/CMA for deletion of 7q11.2 |

*This table lists disorders that have symptoms in conjunction with mental retardation/global developmental delay.
*CMA,* chromosomal microarray analysis; *FISH,* fluorescent in situ hybridization.

| TABLE 16-5 | Genetic Syndromes Associated with Cardiac Lesions |
|---|---|
| **Heart lesion** | **Syndrome** |
| Aortic stenosis | Pallister-Killian, Turner |
| Atrial septal defect | Holt-Oram, Pallister-Killian, Smith-Lemli-Opitz |
| Atrioventricular canal | Trisomy 21/18, heterotaxy syndromes, Ellis van Creveld, Smith-Lemli-Opitz |
| Bicuspid aortic valve | Turner, Williams |
| Cardiac rhabdomyomas | Tuberous sclerosis |
| Coarctation of the aorta | Turner, Noonan, Pallister-Killian, Alagille |
| Conotruncal defects | 22q11 deletion (velocardiofacial), CHARGE |
| Dextrocardia | Trisomy 13, heterotaxy syndromes |
| Double outlet right ventricle | Trisomy 18, heterotaxy syndromes, CHARGE |
| Hypoplastic left heart | Trisomy 18, Holt-Oram |
| Interrupted aortic arch | 22q11 deletion (velocardiofacial) |
| Muscular ventricular septal defect | Holt-Oram |
| Perimembranous ventricular septal defect | Trisomy 21/18, Pallister-Killian, Cornelia de Lange |
| Peripheral pulmonary artery stenosis | Williams, Alagille |
| Pulmonary valve stenosis | Noonan, Cornelia de Lange, Williams |
| Supravalvular aortic stenosis | Williams |
| Tetralogy of Fallot | 22q11 deletion (velocardiofacial), trisomy 21/13/18, CHARGE, Townes-Brocks |
| Total anomalous pulmonary venous return | Cat-Eye, Smith-Lemli-Opitz, heterotaxy syndromes |

## GENETIC DISORDERS ASSOCIATED WITH CONGENITAL HEART LESIONS

- Most congenital heart lesions are not pathognomonic for a particular syndrome, but they may provide a clue to the underlying genetic diagnosis. The cardiac lesion may be the only manifestation of a syndrome in some patients.

### Diagnosis and Evaluation

- Table 16-5 highlights characteristic cardiac lesions associated with a few syndromes, but it is not intended to be comprehensive. Additional information for specific syndromes is available online at Online Mendelian Inheritance in Man (see "Online Genetic Resources" section).
- Consider requesting a genetics consultation in the setting of congenital heart disease to assess for a possible syndrome.
- Karyotype analysis and FISH for 22q11 deletion should be strongly considered in any individual with a congenital heart lesion of unknown etiology.

## GENETIC DISORDERS ASSOCIATED WITH CARDIOMYOPATHY

- Metabolic cardiomyopathies affect the myocardium but do not cause structural anomalies.
  - When a cardiomyopathy is caused by an inborn metabolic disease, it may or may not have associated syndromic features.

- Many times the associated features, such as skeletal myopathy or hepatomegaly, may develop over time, and the absence of these features should not preclude an evaluation for a particular condition.
- If the patient has a cardiac biopsy, it may show evidence of intralysosomal storage of macromolecules (lysosomal storage disease), microvesicular lipid (fatty acid oxidation defect), or marked increase in the number of mitochondria (mitochondrial cytopathy).

## Laboratory Studies

- Blood tests recommended for children who present with cardiomyopathy include comprehensive metabolic panel, quantitative carnitines, acylcarnitine profile, ammonium, lactate, pyruvate, serum/plasma amino acids, creatine kinase, aldolase, lipid panel, uric acid, and Pompe enzyme analysis.

# GENETIC DISORDERS PRESENTING WITH HEPATIC SYMPTOMATOLOGY

- Patients with hepatic symptoms may present with conjugated or unconjugated hyperbilirubinemia, elevated liver enzymes, hepatomegaly, and/or synthetic dysfunction.

## Diagnosis and Evaluation

- In the conditions listed in Tables 16-6, 16-7, 16-8, and 16-9, the hepatic symptom or sign can be the most prominent presenting feature. These tables are not comprehensive because infectious etiologies, anatomic malformations, and exceedingly rare genetic conditions are not listed.

## Treatment

- Optimal treatment depends on the specific disorder.
- Therapy may include surgical correction, phototherapy, or restricting certain food in a child's diet (such as protein).

**TABLE 16-6** **Clinical Features and Recommended Tests for Genetic Disorders Presenting with Hepatomegaly**

| Disorder | Features | Tests |
|---|---|---|
| Glycogen storage diseases | Hypoglycemia, lactic acidemia, growth retardation, hyperlipidemia, hyperuricemia Individuals with glycogen storage disease type I: predisposition to hepatic adenomas | Uric acid Lactate/pyruvate Serum amino acids Lipid panel Liver biopsy for enzyme analysis |
| Lysosomal storage diseases | Variable depending on subtype Possible brain magnetic resonance imaging findings (leukodystrophy, atrophy) or coarse features (mucopolysaccharidoses) | Urine mucopolysaccharide screen Urine oligosaccharides Leukocyte lysosomal panel |

| TABLE 16-7 | Clinical Features and Recommended Tests for Genetic Disorders Presenting with Hepatic Dysfunction* | |
|---|---|---|
| **Disorder** | **Features** | **Tests** |
| Alagille syndrome | Characteristic facies, posterior embryotoxon and retinal pigmentary changes on ophthalmologic examination, and butterfly vertebrae | *JAG1* sequence analysis FISH for 20p12 microdeletion |
| Fructose 1,6 bisphosphatase deficiency | Hypoglycemia, lactic acidosis, mental status changes, and hypotonia Does not require exposure to oral fructose | Lactate and pyruvate Serum/plasma amino acids Uric acid Urine amino acids Enzyme analysis |
| Hemochromatosis, neonatal | Hypoglycemia, bleeding diathesis, and fatal liver and renal dysfunction | Alpha fetoprotein Ferritin Molecular etiology unknown |
| Hemochromatosis, juvenile | Hypogonadotropic hypogonadism, arthropathy, and cardiomyopathy | Ferritin DNA analysis of multiple genes |
| Hereditary fructose intolerance | Chronic diarrhea, poor weight gain, lactic acidosis, and diet history consistent with fructose intake (including some soy formulas, sugar water prepared with table sugar) | Enzyme analysis *ALDOB* mutation analysis |
| Fatty acid oxidation disorders • LCHAD • CPT1 deficiency | Hypoglycemia, skeletal myopathy, and cardiomyopathy | Acylcarnitine profile Quantitative carnitines Uric acid Ammonium Creatine kinase |
| Mitochondrial cytopathies | Protean manifestations: skeletal myopathy, lactic acidosis, strokes, leukodystrophy, global developmental delay/mental retardation, movement disorder, vision impairment, hearing impairment, arrhythmias, cardiomyopathy, hepatocellular dysfunction, diabetes, other endocrinopathies, and short stature | Lactate and pyruvate in blood and cerebrospinal fluid Amino acids Organic acids Acylcarnitine profile Muscle biopsy with enzyme analysis mtDNA sequencing Limited nuclear DNA sequencing |
| Wilson disease | Progressive neurologic findings, psychiatric disturbance, renal tubular dysfunction, mild or acute hemolysis, and Kayser-Fleischer ring in cornea | Ceruloplasmin Serum copper *ATP7B* mutation analysis |

*Hepatic dysfunction refers to elevated liver enzymes, with or without synthetic dysfunction, which may progress to cirrhosis.
*CPT1*, carnitine palmitoyl transferase 1; *LCHAD*, long-chain 3-hydroxyacyl coenzyme A dehydrogenase

**TABLE 16-8** Clinical Features and Recommended Tests for Genetic Disorders Presenting with Unconjugated Hyperbilirubinemia

| Disorder | Features | Tests |
|---|---|---|
| Crigler-Najjar type I | Severe lifelong jaundice, with high risk of kernicterus<br>No hemolysis or significant hepatocellular dysfunction | UGT1A1 enzyme assay in liver |
| Gilbert syndrome | Chronic mild fluctuating unconjugated hyperbilirubinemia<br>No hemolysis or hepatocellular dysfunction | UGT1A1 targeted mutation analysis |
| Glucose-6-phosphate dehydrogenase (G6PD) deficiency | Hemolytic anemia, frequently precipitated by illness or oxidizing drugs | Quantitative G6PD analysis |
| Pyruvate kinase deficiency | Hemolytic anemia of variable severity | Pyruvate kinase isozyme analysis |

**TABLE 16-9** Clinical Features and Recommended Tests for Genetic Syndromes Presenting with Conjugated Hyperbilirubinemia

| | | |
|---|---|---|
| $\alpha_1$-Antitrypsin deficiency | Poor weight gain; possible cirrhosis, portal hypertension, and ascites<br>Pulmonary manifestations rare in pediatric patients | Protease inhibitor phenotyping<br>DNA mutation analysis |
| Bile acid metabolism defects | Hepatosplenomegaly, steatorrhea with fat-soluble vitamin deficiency leading to coagulopathy and rickets | Plasma and urine bile acids<br>Enzyme assays in fibroblasts |
| Cerebrotendinous xanthomatosis | Persistent diarrhea, cataracts, tendon xanthomas (adolescence or later), and neurologic symptoms (spasticity, ataxia, psychiatric problems) | Cholestanol level |
| Congenital disorders of glycosylation (CDG) | Type Ia (classic symptoms): ponto-cerebellar atrophy, lipodystrophy, strabismus, coagulopathy, and benign elevation of liver enzymes<br>Type Ib: chronic diarrhea, failure to thrive, protein-losing enteropathy, hypotonia, bleeding tendency | CDG screen/carbohydrate deficient transferrin |
| Cystic fibrosis | Pancreatic insufficiency, pulmonary disease, meconium ileus, and infertility | Sweat analysis<br>CFTR common mutation panel and full sequence analysis |
| Galactosemia | Hyperbilirubinemia, hypoglycemia, bleeding diathesis, edema, ascites, and cataracts | Galactose-1-phosphate level<br>Galactose-1-phosphate uridyltransferase (GALT) enzyme activity<br>*GALT* DNA analysis |
| Fatty acid oxidation disorders<br>• LCHAD | May present acutely with Reye-like syndrome, or with cardiomyopathy, skeletal myopathy, and hypoketotic hypoglycemia | Acylcarnitine profile<br>*HADHA* mutation analysis |

(continued)

| TABLE 16-9 | Clinical Features and Recommended Tests for Genetic Syndromes Presenting with Conjugated Hyperbilirubinemia (*Continued*) | |
|---|---|---|
| Niemann Pick type C | Neonates: hydrops or ascites, liver failure, and respiratory failure<br>Infants/children: neurologic manifestations such as global developmental delay, ataxia, gaze palsy, dementia, dystonia, and seizures<br>Adults: neurologic manifestations such as dementia or psychiatric symptoms | Fibroblast enzyme analysis and filipin staining |
| Peroxisomal disorders | Possible dysmorphic facial features, large fontanels, feeding difficulties, hypotonia, and seizures | VLCFA |
| Progressive familial intrahepatic cholestasis | Growth failure, progressive liver disease<br>May initially have relapsing/remitting course | DNA sequencing for some subtypes |
| Smith-Lemli-Opitz syndrome | Dysmorphic features, 2-3 toe syndactyly, polydactyly, heart defects, hypoplastic lungs, abnormal genitalia, renal anomalies, mental retardation, and seizures | Cholesterol level<br>7-dehydrocholesterol<br>*DHCR7* mutation analysis |
| Tyrosinemia type 1 (hepatorenal) | Rapidly progressing acute hepatic failure<br>Anorexia, irritability, hypotonia, severe anemia, thrombocytopenia, and renal tubular acidosis | Serum amino acids<br>Urine organic acids (for succinylacetone)<br>Serum succinylacetone<br>Prothrombin time/partial thromboplastin time<br>Alpha-fetoprotein |

*LCHAD*, long-chain 3-hydroxyacyl coenzyme A dehydrogenase; *VLCFA*, very long-chain fatty acids.

# ONLINE GENETIC RESOURCES

## GeneTests

http://www.genetests.org

GeneTests functions to identify diagnostic and research laboratories offering genetic testing, genetic clinics, reviews for healthcare professionals, and resources for patients and their families. This Web site also contains GeneReviews, which provides clinical information on selected genetic diseases including presentation, diagnosis, and suggested management. The number of reviews is limited, and there are no reviews of complex traits, such as hypertension. Some general reviews, such as an overview of ataxia, are available.

## Online Mendelian Inheritance in Man (OMIM)

http://www.ncbi.nlm.nih.gov/sites/entrez?db=OMIM

OMIM is an annotated bibliography of the vast majority of publications on genetic conditions and the genetic contribution to disease. The database can be searched by disease name, gene, or phenotype. Information on the main page is a cumulative list of data reported in the literature. The clinical synopsis tab on the left (in the blue area) links to an outline of disease-specific features.

## American Academy of Pediatrics (AAP) Committee on Genetics

http://www.aap.org/visit/cmte18.htm

The AAP has published management guidelines for a number of relatively common genetic syndromes for the general practitioner. These guidelines include salient features on physical examination, screening parameters, and anticipatory guidance by age for the particular disorder. Because the field of genetics is rapidly changing, these publications may become outdated relatively soon after publication and should not be relied on as the sole tool for the management of patients.

## American College of Medical Genetics (ACMG) Newborn Screening ACTion (ACT) Sheets

http://www.acmg.net/ Selected Resources: reference materials

The ACT sheets and the accompanying algorithms are intended to help guide the general practitioner in evaluating abnormal newborn screening results. These sheets provide a brief synopsis of the disorder being screened and guide the physician through the appropriate follow up procedures. Nonetheless, it is strongly recommended that general practitioners also contact the appropriate subspecialist for assistance.

### Suggested Readings

Clarke JTR. A Clinical Guide to Inherited Metabolic Diseases. Cambridge, UK: Cambridge University Press, 2006.

Fernandes J, Saudubray JM, van den Berghe G, et al., eds. Inborn Metabolic Diseases: Diagnosis and Treatment. Heidelberg Wurzburg, Germany: Springer Medizin Verlag, 2006.

Gorlin RJ, Cohen MM, Hennekam RCM. Syndromes of the Head and Neck (Oxford Monographs on Medical Genetics). New York: Oxford University Press, 2001.

Rimoin DL, Connor JM, Pyeritz RE. Emery and Rimoin's Principles and Practice of Medical Genetics. 5th Ed. New York: Churchill Livingstone, 2006.

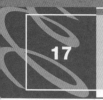

# HEMATOLOGY AND ONCOLOGY
*Aarati Rao and David B. Wilson*

## FEVER AND NEUTROPENIA

### General Principles

- Absolute risk of infection increases when the absolute neutrophil count (ANC) is $<1,000/mm^3$ and increases dramatically when it is $<500/mm^3$.
- ANC $<1,500/mm^3$ is defined as neutropenia.
  - Congenital neutropenia: cyclic neutropenia, reticular dysgenesis, chronic benign neutropenia, Shwachman Diamond syndrome, Fanconi anemia
  - Acquired neutropenia: malignancies such as leukemia, lymphoma, chemotherapy, radiation, aplastic anemia, infections (viral, bacterial sepsis), autoimmune or alloimmune neutropenia, and hypersplenism
- Most common organisms are *Streptococcus* spp., *Staphylococcus epidermidis, Pseudomonas aeruginosa, Escherichia coli, Klebsiella pneumoniae, Staphylococcus aureus*, methicillin-resistant *S. aureus, Enterococcus faecalis, Campylobacter jejuni, Candida albicans*, and vancomycin-resistant enterococcus.
- Time to defervescence in cancer patients with fever and neutropenia is 2–7 days (mean of 5 days); thus continuation of antibiotics for a minimum of 7 days (and ANC $>500/mm^3$ for 72 hours) is often considered—even in patients with no isolated organism(s).
- Only 30% of patients have positive blood cultures.
- Fever is $>38.3°C$.

### Diagnosis

- Obtain blood cultures (from each lumen of venous access device if more than one is present; peripheral cultures are not necessary up front; q24h is usually sufficient).
- Obtain urine culture if the patient has symptoms or hematuria (also send urine specimen for BK virus and cytomegalovirus [CMV] viral polymerase chain reaction [PCR] if hematuria is present).

### Treatment

- Usually, continue trimethoprim-sulfamethoxazole (TMP-SMX) prophylaxis, but discontinue other oral antibiotics (e.g., ciprofloxacin).
- Initially, use cefepime 150 mg/kg/day q8h. Alternate lumens with a double-lumen Broviac catheter.
  - Add vancomycin 15 mg/kg q8h (adjust dose per renal function) after 48 hours for persistent fever.
  - Alternatively, add vancomycin up front for unstable patients, patients with acute myeloid leukemia (AML) on chemotherapy (at risk for α-streptococcal sepsis), signs of catheter infection, signs of sinus infection (consider fungal coverage), cutaneous breakdown, or prior gram-positive infection.
- If fever lasts for $>5$ days, add amphotericin B lipid complex 5 mg/kg once a day (may give voriconazole in place of amphotericin).
- Continue broad antibiotic coverage until the patient is no longer febrile and neutropenic (or the ANC is rising).

- For patients allergic to penicillin/cephalosporins, use up-front therapy with vancomycin and ciprofloxacin (consider age). Alternatives include ticarcillin/clavulanate (Timentin), imipenem, or aztreonam and vancomycin.
- For signs of sepsis (e.g., hypotension) and for double coverage of Gram-negative infections/suspected infections until susceptibilities are known, use gentamicin/tobramycin.
- Evaluate patients with tachypnea, low oxygen saturation, and fever for *Pneumocystis jirovecii* infection.
    - Lung signs may be minimal; a chest radiograph may often show diffuse interstitial disease.
    - Definitive testing includes bronchoalveolar lavage with sputum sent for silver staining along with all other cultures, and until proven otherwise, these patients benefit from steroid pulses and high-dose TMP-SMX.

# TRANSFUSION PRINCIPLES

## Packed Red Blood Cells

- Generally, for weight <20 kg, give one-half unit of packed red blood cells (PRBCs); for weight >20 kg, give one unit.
- For hemoglobin (Hb) ≤7 g/dL, typically give 10–20 mL/kg PRBCs over 2 to 4 hours.
- Irradiated cellular components are necessary for patients in the neonatal intensive care unit (NICU), fetuses, oncology patients, patients with an immunodeficiency (congenital or acquired), solid-organ transplant recipients (before and after), bone marrow transplant (BMT) recipients, patients receiving immunosuppressive chemotherapy or radiation, and patients receiving directed donor blood.
    - Allogeneic BMT patients and BMT candidates require irradiated, leukocyte-poor, CMV-negative PRBCs. CMV-seropositive patients can receive PRBCs that have not been screened for CMV (i.e., CMV-indeterminate).
    - Solid-organ, autologous BMT patients receive leukocyte-poor, CMV-indeterminate PRBCs.
    - Patients with sickle cell anemia receive leukocyte-poor, Sickledex-negative, and minor antigen-compatible (if available) PRBCs.

## Transfusion Reactions

- Allergic reactions (bronchospasm, urticaria, hypotension)
    - **Stop infusion** and administer antihistamines, glucocorticoids, or epinephrine
        - Diphenhydramine: treatment of pruritus and hives: 1 mg/kg
        - Epinephrine (for severe reactions, such as bronchospasm, hypotension, shock): 0.1–0.4 mg subcutaneous (SC)/IV
        - Fluids: for hypotension
        - Narcotics for rigors: 0.1 mg/kg of intravenous (IV) morphine or 0.5–1 mg/kg of meperidine
        - Acetaminophen: 15 mg/kg oral dose for fever
        - Glucocorticoids for moderate to severe reactions, such as urticaria, fever, chills, diaphoresis, and pallor): 50–100 mg of hydrocortisone (or comparable dose of methylprednisolone)
- Febrile nonhemolytic reactions (fever, chills, diaphoresis)
    - **Stop infusion**; send sample of blood from patient for Coombs testing; treat with acetaminophen, antihistamines, and narcotics (for rigor); glucocorticoids may help
- Acute hemolytic reaction (primarily from ABO incompatibility; fever, chills, diaphoresis, abdominal pain, hypotension, hemoglobinuria)
    - **Stop infusion**; send patient's blood sample and transfusion bag to blood bank to ensure correct type and crossmatch; IV fluids for hypotension and to ensure adequate urinary output (may need mannitol for diuresis)
- Delayed transfusion reaction (occurs 3–10 days after transfusion; unexplained anemia, hyperbilirubinemia, abdominal pain)
    - Confirm with Coombs test.

## Platelets

- General guidelines: give one-half unit of single-donor (SD) platelets to patients who weigh <20 kg and one unit to patients who weigh >20 kg; this dosing minimizes the amount of wasted platelets.
- Transfuse for platelets ≤10,000/mm$^3$ (in the setting of decreased production; that is, not necessary in idiopathic thrombocytopenic purpura [ITP]); typically give 10–20 mL/kg.
- Allogeneic BMT patients and BMT candidates require SD, irradiated, CMV-negative (unless known to be CMV-positive), leukocyte-poor platelets.
- Solid-organ, autologous BMT patients receive leukocyte-poor, irradiated, CMV-indeterminate platelets.
- Causes for poor response are fever, sepsis, amphotericin administration, splenomegaly, allo-antibodies, blood loss, hemolytic uremic syndrome, thrombotic thrombocytopenic purpura, and necrotizing enterocolitis.
  - To determine the effectiveness of the transfusion, obtain platelet counts at 1 hour and 24 hour posttransfusion.

## Fresh Frozen Plasma (FFP)

- Fresh frozen plasma (FFP) may be needed for patients with disseminated intravascular coagulation (DIC).
- FFP contains clotting factors, immunoglobulin, and albumin; it does not need to be screened for CMV.
- Typical dose is 10–20 mL/kg (may also require parental vitamin K).

## Cryoprecipitate

- This may be needed for patients with DIC who have hypofibrinogenemia (enriched in fibrinogen, von Willebrand factor [vWF], and other high-molecular weight factors).
- One unit is 10–15 mL; dose is approximately 1 U/5 kg.

# ONCOLOGIC EMERGENCIES

## Superior Vena Cava Syndrome/Superior Mediastinal Syndrome

- Rule out infection, malignancy, and iatrogenic conditions.
- Symptoms include cough, hoarseness, dyspnea, orthopnea, and chest pain.
- Signs are upper body or facial swelling; plethora and cyanosis of the face, neck, and upper esophagus; diaphoresis; wheezing; and stridor.
- Differential diagnosis for mediastinal masses in the posterior mediastinum includes neuroblastoma, paraganglionic masses, and primitive neuroectodermal tumor (PNET); and for those in the anterior/superior mediastinum, T-lymphoma, teratoma, thymoma, and thyroid masses.
- Because of risks of anesthesia, the diagnosis should be established using the least invasive means possible.
  - Check serum α-fetoprotein and human chorionic gonadotropin to differentiate germ-cell tumors from lymphomas.
  - Use spiral computed tomography (CT) to differentiate calcification in neuroblastoma.
  - Use peripheral smear in the case of lymphoblastic lymphomas.
- Treatment
  - High risk
    - Empiric therapy (prednisone 40 mg/m$^2$/day divided four times a day; radiographic therapy: 100–200 cGy b.i.d.) should be given.
    - After the patient has been stabilized, the lesion should be biopsied.
  - Low-risk: biopsy, then treatment
    - Symptomatic patients should be monitored in the intensive care unit (ICU).

## Pleural/Pericardial Effusion

- Thoracentesis: send for protein content, specific gravity, cell count, lactate, dehydrogenase (LDH), cytology, culture, and other biologic/immunologic assays.
- Tamponade: chest radiograph shows water bag cardiac shadow; electrocardiogram (ECG) shows low-voltage QRS.
- Treatment
  - Treat the underlying etiology.
  - Pericardiocentesis may relieve cardiac symptoms.

## Massive Hemoptysis

- Most common cause is invasive pulmonary aspergillosis (incidence with hemoptysis is 2%–26%).
- Diagnosis involves chest radiography and chest CT.
- Treatment involves lying on same side as hemorrhage to prevent collection in the normal lung, correction of low platelets, transfusion of PRBCs to maintain normal Hb, and volume resuscitation.

## Gastric/Duodenal Ulcer (Stress, Cushing Ulcer)

- Children taking high-dose glucocorticoids should always be on histamine blockers or proton pump inhibitors.
- For bleeding, correct low platelets/coagulation abnormalities.

## Neutropenic Enterocolitis (Typhilitis)

- Mortality is high.
- Clinical picture involves acute abdomen or paralytic ileus.
- Signs and symptoms are abdominal pain in setting of severe neutropenia, often with fever.
- The condition usually follows cytotoxic chemotherapy; CT and ultrasound are more sensitive than plain films.
- Treatment
  - Broad-spectrum antibiotics cover Gram-negative enterics and anaerobes.
  - Bowel rest/decompression is necessary.
  - Granulocyte colony-stimulating factor (G-CSF) should be given; transfusion of irradiated granulocytes may be considered.
  - Surgical intervention is reserved for patients with bowel perforation or other dire complications.

## Hemorrhagic Cystitis

- History of blood in urine (microscopic more common than macroscopic)
  - Usually painless
  - History of cyclophosphamide or ifosfamide therapy
  - BK virus or adenovirus in BMT patients
- Diagnosis: urinalysis, ultrasound (boggy, edematous bladder wall), cystoscopy
- Treatment
  - Stopping radiation treatment/chemotherapy
  - Hydration
  - Transfusion; correction of low platelets and coagulopathy
  - Removal of clots by catheter or cystoscope; bladder irrigation with cold saline
- Prevention: vigorous hydration during and after treatment, IV and/or oral mercaptoethane sulfonate (Mesna)

## Altered Consciousness

### Etiology (most common to least common)
- Metastatic disease, sepsis/DIC, primary central nervous system (CNS) fungal/bacterial, metabolic abnormality, viral encephalitis, leukoencephalopathy, intracranial hemorrhage,

cerebrovascular accident (CVA), oversedation, hypercalcemia (see later discussion), hyperammonemia because of hepatic dysfunction
- Chemotherapy-induced
  - Ifosfamide: acute somnolence, neurologic deterioration, coma (worse in poor renal clearance that leads to build up of toxic metabolite chloroacetaldehyde)
  - Others: carmustine, cisplatin, thiotepa, high-dose cytarabine (Ara-C), amphotericin, interleukin-2, trans-retinoic acid

*Treatment (increased intracranial pressure)*
- Hyperventilation (to $PaCO_2$ of 20–25 mm Hg)
- IV dexamethasone (1–2 mg/kg)
- Mannitol (20% solution at 1.25–2 g/kg)

## Cerebrovascular Accident (Stroke)

*Etiology*
- Among hematology-oncology patients, the most common cause of cerebrovascular accident (CVA) is sickle cell anemia.
- Patients may have infarcts or reversible posterior leukoencephalopathy syndrome (see "Sickle Cell Disease" section).
- Hyperdynamic blood flow and altered vascular architecture in the area of the circle of Willis predisposes to RBC sludging and strokes.
- Other causes of stroke in hematology are cerebral arterial/venous thrombosis as a result of inherited thrombophilic states, intracranial hemorrhage, chemotherapy-related (L-asparaginase), sepsis/DIC, and radiation therapy–induced vascular occlusions.

*Diagnosis and Treatment*
- Stabilize, and then evaluate with CT or magnetic resonance imaging (MRI); the study may need to be repeated in 7–10 days to evaluate full extent.
- Give corticosteroids, mannitol, fresh-frozen plasma (± antithrombin III concentrate in patients with L-asparaginase-induced CVA), and platelets.

## Seizures

*Etiology*
- Metastatic disease, CVA, infections, chemotherapy (VCR, intrathecal methotrexate, cisplatin, ara-C), syndrome of inappropriate secretion of antidiuretic hormone/hyponatremia

*Diagnosis*
- CT with and without contrast plus MRI, followed by cerebrospinal fluid (CSF) analysis
- Basic metabolic panel and antiseizure medicine serum levels

*Treatment*
- Address underlying problem (e.g., infection)
- Consider anticonvulsants (use first three for their rapid onset of seconds to minutes)
  - Lorazepam (Ativan): 0.05–0.1 mg/kg IV over 2 minutes. Watch for respiratory depression/ hypotension.
  - Diazepam (Valium): 0.1–0.3 mg/kg (max 10 mg) at 1 mg/min (maximum of three doses); rectal form available. Duration is short. Watch for respiratory depression/ hypotension.
  - Fosphenytoin: loading dose of 15–20 mg/kg of phenytoin equivalent at 100–150 mg/min; maintenance is approximately 6–8 mg/kg/day q12h (level required is 10–20 mg/L). Watch for cardiac depression.
  - Phenobarbital: 20 mg/kg IV or IM (max 150 mg or 40 mg/kg); maintenance is approximately 5 mg/kg/day (serum level required is 15–40 mg/L). Watch for respiratory depression—long half-life/delayed effect (consider pentobarbital).

## Spinal Cord Compression

- Symptoms
  - Back pain (local or radicular) occurs in 80% of cases, with local tenderness in 80–90%.
  - Any patient with cancer and back pain should be considered to have this until proven otherwise.
- Evaluation
- Spine radiographs (although condition is seen in <50%), bone scan, and MRI (with and without gadolinium) is necessary.
- If patients are not ambulatory, they should undergo emergent MRI (or myelography).
- Treatment: Dexamethasone bolus dose of 1–2 mg/kg IV immediately, followed by MRI

## Hyperleukocytosis

- White blood cell (WBC) count >100,000/mm$^3$
- Clinical presentation: signs of hypoxia, dyspnea, blurred vision, agitation, confusion, stupor, cyanosis
- Treatment: hydration, alkalinization, allopurinol or urate oxidase (rasburicase), leukapheresis, platelet transfusion if <20,000/mm$^3$. Use PRBCs with caution (keep Hb <10 g/dL to minimize viscosity)
- Complications: death, CNS hemorrhage, thrombosis, pulmonary leukostasis, metabolic derangements (hyperkalemia, hypocalcemia/hyperphosphatemia), renal failure, gastrointestinal hemorrhage

## Tumor Lysis Syndrome

- Triad: hyperuricemia, hyperkalemia, and hyperphosphatemia (resulting in secondary renal failure and symptomatic hypocalcemia)
- May trigger DIC, especially in patients with high tumor burdens
- Risk factors: bulky abdominal tumors (e.g., Burkitt lymphoma), hyperleukocytosis, increased uric acid and LDH levels, poor urinary output
- Laboratory studies: CBC, serum electrolytes, calcium, phosphorus, uric acid, urinalysis, LDH, prothrombin time/partial thromboplastin time (PT/PTT; consider fibrinogen/fibrin degradation product [FDP])
- Imaging: ECG if potassium >7 mEq/L, ultrasound to rule out kidney infiltrations or ureteral obstruction
- Treatment
  - Hydration: $D_5W$ + $NaHCO_3$ 40 mEq/L at 3,000 mL/m$^2$/day. Avoid potassium in IV fluid.
  - Allopurinol: 10 mg/kg/day or 300 mg/m$^2$/day (divided t.i.d.), or urate oxidase (rasburicase) 0.15 mg/kg/dose IV qday.
  - Urate oxidase (rasburicase): test for glucose-6-phosphate dehydrogenase (G6PD) deficiency first in males of African or Mediterranean descent.
  - Monitor metabolites; perform serum electrolytes, phosphorus, calcium, uric acid, urinalysis, DIC profile if needed.
  - If potassium is >6 mEq/L, uric acid is >10 mg/dL, serum creatinine is >10 times normal, serum phosphate is >10 mg/dL, or hypocalcemia is symptomatic, use dialysis and chemotherapy.
  - If uric acid is <7 mg/dL, specific gravity is <1.010, and urine pH is 7–7.5, give chemotherapy and then discontinue $NaHCO_3$; monitor metabolites q4–6h.
  - For hyperkalemia, stop all potassium infusion, Kayexalate (1 g/kg PO with 50% sorbitol), calcium gluconate (100–200 mg/kg/dose; for cardioprotection only), insulin (0.1 unit/kg + 2 mL/kg of 25% glucose), and albuterol nebulizer therapy for temporary palliation.

## Hypercalcemia

- Effects
  - Anorexia, nausea, vomiting, polyuria, diarrhea leading to dehydration, leading to gastrointestinal/renal impairment, leading to a rise in calcium
  - Results: lethargy, depression, hypotonia, stupor, coma, bradycardia, and nocturia
- Risk factors: paraneoplastic syndrome and hyperleukocytosis
- Treatment: Note that a serum calcium level <14 mg/dL may respond to loop diuretics alone (see later discussion)
  - Pamidronate (considered first-line therapy)
    - <12 mg/dL: 30 mg
    - >12 mg/dL: 40 mg over 4 hours
    - >18 mg/dL: 90 mg over 24 hours (wait 7 days for second txt; repeat q2–8wk); monitor for hypocalcemia.
  - Hydration with normal saline (three times maintenance) and loop diuretics (2–3 mg/kg qs q2h)
  - Glucocorticoids (1.5–2 mg/kg/day of prednisone): requires 2–3 days to work

# BONE MARROW TRANSPLANT ISSUES

- Note: in addition, see prior sections for relevant issues: infection, fluid, and blood component therapy.

## Veno-occlusive Disease of the Liver (Sinusoidal Obstructive Syndrome)

- Most common life-threatening complication related to BMT
- Capillary endothelial inflammation leading to third spacing of fluids
- Syndrome
  - Usually occurs in first 30 days post-BMT; maximum risk is first 10 days post transplant
  - Clinical presentation
    - Hepatomegaly or right upper quadrant pain
    - Jaundice (usually hyperbilirubinemia without any other liver function abnormalities until end-stage)
    - Ascites/weight gain
    - Platelet consumption
- Risk factors: preexisting hepatitis, antibiotic usage before treatment (vancomycin, acyclovir), age >15 years, CMV-seropositive, female sex, pretreatment radiation to abdomen, intensive conditioning [single-dose total body irradiation (TBI), use of busulfan], and second BMT
- Treatment
  - Therapy is mainly supportive.
  - However, encouraging results have been reported with defibrotide, a single-stranded polydeoxyribonucleotide with antithrombotic properties.

## Fluid Management

- All BMT patients are fluid restricted starting 12–24 hours infusion of stem cells at $1,500/m^2$/day.
- This is continued until engraftment occurs.

## Infection

- The threshold for suspecting infection in children undergoing transplant is very low. Any change in clinical status should alert a resident to the possibility of infection.
- Prophylactic antibiotics may be used when ANC is <500/mm$^3$.
- Consider the addition of vancomycin and amphotericin, respectively, at 24 hours and 48 hours of continued fevers.

- Drug interaction of antifungals such as voriconazole with immunosuppressants such as cyclosporine A should be considered when adding medications.

## Vaccination

- Vaccinations are resumed in BMT recipients 1 year posttransplant.
- Patients should avoid all family members who have received a live virus vaccine for 4 weeks.

## Graft-versus-Host Disease

- Graft-versus-host disease (GVHD) is seen only in recipients of allogeneic transplants.
- Acute: usually 20–100 days after BMT
    - Symptoms: dermatitis (rash on palms, soles, face/neck/upper torso), hepatitis, colitis (diarrhea)
    - Treatment: glucocorticoids, cyclosporine A (target range of 250–350 ng/mL), tacrolimus (target range of 8–12 ng/mL)
- Chronic: usually 150 or more days after BMT
    - Sicca syndrome with thickened skin, lichen planus, papules, cholestatic jaundice, scleroderma-like skin, and eye and gastrointestinal lesions
    - Treatment: glucocorticoids, cyclosporine A, azathioprine, mycophenolate, thalidomide, psoralen ultraviolet A (PUVA) [skin], hydroxychloroquine, pentostatins

# ACUTE LYMPHOBLASTIC LEUKEMIA

## Epidemiology

- Acute lymphoblastic leukemia (ALL) is the most common cancer in pediatrics.
- Risk assessment: age <1 year and >10 years, male sex, WBC >100,000/mm$^3$, CNS disease, unfavorable cytogenetics, pretreatment with steroids

## Clinical Presentation

- ALL presents as increased or decreased WBC with low platelet and/or hemoglobin (two or more cell lines affected)
- Symptoms are low-grade unexplained fever, mucosal bleeds, and bone pain. On exam child may have pallor and petechiae, generalized lymphadenopathy, hepatomegaly, and/or splenomegaly. Retinal hemorrhage or leukemic infiltrates may be seen on funduscopy.

## Classification

- Types of ALL are differentiated by surface markers.
- Pre-B ALL is the most common and has CD19 and 20+, with CALLA+.
- Others are T cell, which has CD4 and CD8+, with TdT+, and Burkitt or mature B cell, which has surface immunoglobulin and CD20+.
- Presence of trisomy +4, +10, +17 or t(12;21)(p13;q22) in the leukemia cells confers a favorable prognosis.
- Presence of the Philadelphia chromosome [t(9;22)(q34;q11)] or translocations involving the mixed lineage leukemia (MLL) gene on 11q23 confers a poor prognosis.

## Treatment

- Therapy is usually a 28-day induction with three or four drugs depending on risk of patient.
    - Common drugs used in induction: prednisone, vincristine, and asparaginase.
    - Adriamycin or daunorubicin is added for four-drug induction therapy.
- If child is in remission at end of induction, they receive consolidation therapy for approximately 24 weeks. Consolidation therapy is to ensure that bone marrow is rid of any

residual leukemia cells. Drugs used for consolidation therapy include vincristine, methotrexate as key drugs with or without 6-mercaptopurine (6-MP), and others.
- Maintenance therapy of approximately 130 weeks follows consolidation and typically involves oral 6-MP with weekly methotrexate and intrathecal methotrexate once every 12 weeks.
- Children with CNS leukemia receive additional intrathecal therapy and occasionally radiation therapy.

## Complications (addressed in the remainder of the sections)

- Bleeding and anemia, leading to cardiac failure; treat with platelet and PRBC transfusion as needed, and ensure adequate renal output.
- Tumor lysis syndrome
- Fever and neutropenia following start of induction therapy, infection
- Hypercalcemia/hypocalcemia
- Cranial nerve involvement/stroke
- Nausea and vomiting: treat with ondansetron (Zofran; 0.15 mg/kg/dose q8h), metoclopramide (Reglan) with diphenhydramine (Benadryl; 1 mg/kg/day), or lorazepam (Ativan; 0.5 mg/m$^2$/day). Other commonly used antiemetics are promethazine (Phenergan), granisetron (Kytril), aprepitant (Emend), and dronabinol (Marinol).

## ACUTE MYELOBLASTIC LEUKEMIA

- Acute myeloblastic leukemia (AML) has a poor prognosis compared with ALL.
- AML may be classified according to surface markers (Table 17-1).
- Cytogenetics
- Presence of t(8;21)(q22;q22) or inversion of chromosome 16 confers a favorable prognosis
  - Presence of t(15;17)(q22;q21), which is characteristic of acute promyelocytic leukemia (APL), confers a favorable prognosis.
  - Presence of monosomy 5, monosomy 7, or 11q23 abnormalities confers a worse prognosis.

- More prolonged and severe neutropenia than with ALL. Patients have high risk of Gram-positive sepsis, such as α-streptococcal and staphylococcal infections.
- Treatment
  - Therapy involves shorter duration (approximately 6 months) but more intense chemotherapy compared with ALL.
  - Various therapy combinations exist. The mainstays of treatment are anthracyclines (e.g., daunomycin or idarubicin) and Ara-C.
  - Induction recovery and clinical remission is followed with two courses of consolidation therapy.

**TABLE 17-1** Surface Markers for Acute Myeloblastic Leukemia

| Marker | M1/M2 | M3 | M4/M5 | M6 | M7 |
|---|---|---|---|---|---|
| CD11b | | + | ++ | | |
| CD13 | | + | ++ | + | + |
| CD14 | | | ++ | | |
| CD15 | + | ++ | ++ | | |
| CD33 | ++ | ++ | ++ | ++ | ++ |
| CD34 | ++ | + | + | + | + |
| CD41 | | | | | ++ |
| CD42 | | | | | ++ |

- In children with poor response to induction, siblings are tested for human leukocyte antigen (HLA) matching for potential reinduction of child with high-dose chemotherapy and matched sibling allogeneic BMT.
  - Patients with no matched siblings are usually offered chemotherapy only.
  - Matched, unrelated donor transplant is considered at the time of second relapse, or in the case of resistant leukemias because of the risks associated with unrelated donor transplant.

# NON-HODGKIN'S LYMPHOMA

- Non-Hodgkin's lymphoma (NHL) encompasses >12 neoplasms.
- It is the most frequent malignancy in children with AIDS; thus HIV screening should be performed in all children with NHL.
- Lineage category information is presented in Table 17-2.

## Clinical Presentation and Classification

- Low grade: painless, diffuse peripheral lymphadenopathy (LAD), mainly in older adults
- Intermediate grade
  - Painless peripheral LAD, although localized extranodal disease is also common (e.g., GI and bone)
  - Median age is 55 years, but this type of NHL is also common in children and young adults.
- High grade
  - Lymphoblastic lymphoma is a disease of children and young adults. Approximately two thirds of patients are male, and most (50%–75%) have mediastinal involvement at presentation (manifesting as: shortness of breath, dyspnea, wheezing, stridor, dysphagia, and head/neck swelling).

**TABLE 17-2    Classification of Non-Hodgkin's Lymphoma**

| Lineages (immunophenotype/genotype) | Median survival (yr) |
|---|---|
| B Lineage (nodal) | |
| Low-grade: | |
| Small lymphocytic | 5.5–6 |
| Lymphoplasmacytic/lymphoplasmacytoid | 4 |
| Follicular small cleaved cell | 6.5–7 |
| Follicular mixed small cleaved/large cell | 4.5–5 |
| Intermediate-grade: | |
| Follicular large cell | 2.5–3 |
| Diffuse small cleaved/mixed small and large | 3–4 |
| Intermediate lymphocytic/mantle cell | 3–5 |
| High-grade: | |
| Diffuse large cell lymphoma | 1–2 |
| Immunoblastic | 0.5–1.5 |
| Small non-cleaved cell | 0.5–1 |
| T Lineage: | |
| Lymphoblastic | 0.5–2 |
| Peripheral T-cell lymphoma | 1–2 |
| Primary extranodal lymphoma (classified by site; most are B-cell and MALT lineages) | |

- Small non-cleaved cell lymphoma (SNCCL)/Burkitt/non-Burkitt: usually a childhood disease but with a second peak after 50 years of age
  - Burkitt commonly presents in the abdomen and GI tract (~80%).
  - Non-Burkitt presents in the bone marrow and with peripheral LAD.
  - Presentation in the right lower quadrant is common and can be confused with appendicitis.

## Staging Studies

- Essential: physical examination, CBC, serum electrolytes with liver function studies, LDH, uric acid, chest radiograph, chest CT (if chest radiograph is abnormal), abdominal CT (or abdominal ultrasound), bilateral bone marrow aspiration/biopsy, CSF analysis, gallium scan
- Suggested: bone scan, MRI for bone marrow involvement, positron emission tomography (PET) scan

## Treatment

- Treatment of NHL is dependent on pathologic subtype and stage.
- Therapy of Burkitt is usually short (around 4–6 months), whereas T-cell lymphomas require treatment for a longer duration period, with emphasis on CNS prophylaxis.
  - Resistant Burkitt may benefit by addition of rituximab (anti-CD20) to the therapeutic protocol.
  - Patients with Burkitt lymphoma are at high risk for tumor lysis syndrome (see previous discussion).

# HODGKIN'S DISEASE

## Definition

- Hodgkin's disease (HD) is a lymphoma with pleomorphic lymphocytic infiltrate.
- Reed-Sternberg (RS) cells are multinucleated giant cells and are considered to be the malignant cells of HD.

## Epidemiology

- Most cases outside of the United States, but only approximately one third of cases in the United States, are associated with Epstein-Barr virus (EBV) in RS cells.
- Distribution is bimodal, with early peak in the mid-late 20s and a second peak after 50 years of age.

## Clinical Presentation

- Usually painless adenopathy (common in the supraclavicular/cervical areas; usually firm; usually spreads contiguously)
- Many patients: some degree of mediastinal involvement (approximately two thirds)
- Systemic symptoms in some patients, whereas others are asymptomatic ("A" after stage designation denotes "asymptomatic" and "B" denote presence of B symptoms)
  - B symptoms: presence of fever >38°C for 3 consecutive days, night sweats, or unexplained weight loss of 10% or more in the 6 months preceding admission
  - Cough (need to fully assess airway before procedures)
- Generalized pruritus, ethyl alcohol–induced pain in lymph nodes (rare, but pathognomonic), primary subdiaphragmatic disease (rare; approximately 3%)

## Diagnosis

- Physical examination and determination of history for B symptoms; measurement of lymph nodes

- CBC (autoimmune thrombocytopenia and autoimmune hemolytic anemia are commonly associated), LDH, ESR, and uric acid (more commonly elevated in NHL); renal and hepatic function tests
- Neck/chest/abdomen/pelvic CT, gallium scan, bone scan (for those with bone pain or elevated alkaline phosphatase); PET scan (more commonly used)
- Bilateral bone marrow aspirate and biopsy (not just aspirate; performed usually just in patients with stage III-IV or with B symptoms, or at relapse)

## Treatment

- Therapy commonly involves cycles of Adriamycin, bleomycin, vinblastine, dactinomycin (ABVD) every 2 weeks.
- However, other chemotherapy combinations may be used (e.g., COMP, ESHAP).

# WILMS/RENAL TUMORS

- Clinical syndromes associated with Wilms (listed in order of frequency of Wilms tumor); 10% of Wilms tumors are associated with malformation syndromes.
    - Denys-Drash syndrome (>90%): intersex disorders, nephropathy, mutation in 11p13 region
    - Sporadic aniridia (33%): absence of the iris (11p13 region → *Pax6* gene)
    - WAGR syndrome (>30%): **W**ilms tumor, **A**niridia, **G**enitourinary anomalies, mental **R**etardation; 11p13 region deletion (*WT1* suppressor gene product and *Pax6* gene)
    - Beckwith-Wiedemann syndrome (BWS): approximately 5%)
        - Macroglossia, organomegaly, midline abdominal defects (e.g., omphalocele, umbilical hernia, divarication of recti); gigantism, neonatal hypoglycemia, and ear pits or grooves.
        - Duplication of paternal allele/LOH/LOI at 11p15 (including involvement of *IGF2, H19*, and *LIT1* genes); bilateral Wilms tumor in approximately 20% of patients, who are also at increased risk for metachronous recurrence
    - Hemihypertrophy (approximately 5%): asymmetric overgrowth syndrome; may be a clinical variant of BWS as a result of incomplete penetrance of *LIT1* epigenetic mutations
- Primary presentation: abdominal mass, usually not crossing midline (neuroblastoma often crosses midline)
- Histology (embryonal vs. anaplastic) and staging of tumor: important in deciding chemotherapy and radiation therapy

# NEUROBLASTOMA

- Age at presentation: 75% of cases present before 5 years of age, and 97% are diagnosed before 10 years of age (peak is 2–4 years).

## Clinical Presentation

- Palpable abdominal mass, bone pain from metastases, and mass effects from the tumor or metastases (e.g., proptosis and periorbital ecchymosis from retrobulbar mets, skin nodules-blueberry muffin rash, hypertension)
- Other symptoms: fever, anemia, diarrhea, Horner syndrome, cerebellar ataxia, opsoclonus/myoclonus
- Metastatic disease: metastatic disease in approximately 70% of patients at presentation (majority are N-myc amplified).

## Diagnosis

- Investigations needed before treatment: bilateral bone marrow aspiration/biopsy, bone scan, CT scans, chest radiograph, urine vanillylmandelic acid (VMA) and homovanillic acid (HVA), LDH, histologic examination of palpable lymph nodes, and MIBG scan

- Considerations: chest CT if positive chest radiograph or bone scan, pelvic CT if notable extension, CT/MRI of other metastatic sites, and a skeletal survey

## Treatment

- The choice of therapy depends on patient age, tumor staging, and other factors.
- Treatment may entail chemotherapy, surgical excision, radiation therapy, and autologous BMT.

# OSTEOSARCOMA

## Epidemiology

- This disease occurs primarily in adolescents and young adults, with approximately 50% of cases in the bones around the knee.
- Approximately 80% of patients with apparently localized tumors have disease recurrence if treated only with surgical excision, indicating that the majority of patients have disseminated disease at presentation.
- Peak incidence is in the second decade of life, during the adolescent growth spurt.

## Clinical Presentation

- Most patients present with pain over the involved area (usually for many months).
- From 15%–20% of patients have detectable metastatic disease at presentation (poor prognosis), of which >85% are pulmonary metastases.

## Imaging

- Results are highly variable, with no pathognomonic radiologic features.
- Common presentations include periosteal new bone formation (lifting of cortex forming of Codman triangle), soft tissue masses, invariable involvement of the metaphyseal portion (<10% involve the diaphysis), ossification in the soft tissue in a radial or "sunburst" pattern, osteosclerotic (~45%), osteolytic (~30%), and mixed sclerotic/osteolytic (~25%).
- MRI is invaluable to assess the intraosseous extent of the tumor and distinction of muscle groups/fat, joints, and neurovascular structures.
- Bone scan is important to examine extent of primary tumor and for metastases.
- Chest radiograph/CT is important because the lung is the first metastatic site in approximately 90% of cases.

## Treatment

- Primary management is surgical excision with wide margins because of the unresponsiveness to radiation.
- Neo-adjuvant chemotherapy is usually given presurgery and postsurgery
- Follow-up is needed for at least 5 years after therapy.
  - Chest radiography should be performed every 3 months for 2 years, with decreased frequency thereafter.
  - Chest CT should be performed every 4–6 months for the first 2 years.
  - Evaluation of the primary site should also be examined at intervals, determined by the orthopedic surgeon.

# RHABDOMYOSARCOMA

- Soft tissue malignancy of skeletal muscle origin

## Clinical Presentation

- The most common primary sites for rhabdomyosarcoma to arise include the head and neck (e.g., parameningeal, orbit, pharyngeal), genitourinary tract, and the extremities.

- Other sites include the trunk, intrathoracic, and gastrointestinal tract (liver, biliary, and perianal/anal).

## Treatment

- Surgery: complete resection with negative margins (basic principle)
- Chemotherapy: for all patients (extent/duration depends on risk factor analysis)
- Radiation therapy: effective for microscopic and gross residual disease following initial surgical resection or chemotherapy

# EWING SARCOMAS

- Ewing sarcoma refers to tumors of either bone (Ewing tumor of bone) or soft tissue (extraosseous Ewing; "classic Ewing") origin. It is derived from primitive pluripotent cells of neural crest origin (postganglionic parasympathetic autonomic nervous system).
- PNET is considered to be a more differentiated form of this entity and can occur as a primary tumor of bone or soft tissue.
- Clinical presentation
  - Symptoms include pain, palpable mass, pathologic fracture, and fever.
  - These have often been present for months.

## Diagnosis

- Imaging: radiograph of bone (usually destructive lesion of the diaphysis with cortex erosion and multilaminar periosteal reaction; [i.e. "onion peel"]), MRI of primary tumor (better than CT), bone scan, chest CT for lung metastases, and chest radiograph
- Laboratory studies: LDH, urine VMA/HVA (to distinguish from neuroblastoma), and bilateral bone marrow aspiration/biopsy
- Treatment: requires combination chemotherapy, in addition to radiation therapy and possible surgery

# RETINOBLASTOMA

## Hereditary Variant

- Positive family history is found in 6%–10% of patients; however, 30%–40% of "sporadic" cases may be hereditary.
- Mean age at diagnosis is 14–15 months.
- Disease is usually bilateral/multifocal, with a high risk of developing secondary nonocular tumors such as osteosarcoma.
- Second primary tumors develop, usually distant to the first tumor, which contrasts with the past belief that they occur in the radiation field of the first tumor.
- Treatment is a combination of cryotherapy and chemotherapy.
- Genetic counseling of parents and child (regarding risk to progeny) important.

## Nonhereditary Variant

- Negative family history
- Mean age at diagnosis is 23–27 months.
- Disease is always unilateral/unifocal.
  - Note that 15% of patients with unilateral tumors may have hereditary disease.
  - There is no increased risk of secondary nonocular tumors.

# SICKLE CELL DISEASE

- Sickle cell anemia (Hb SS), sickle cell disease (Hb SC, Hb $S\beta^{\circ}$-thalassemia, Hb $S\beta^{+}$-thalassemia, sickle trait HbAS)

## Etiology

- Abnormal hemoglobin (sickle hemoglobin) produced as a consequence of amino acid glutamine substitution for valine in the globin gene.
- The abnormal hemoglobin affects red blood cell (RBC) rheology and deformability in the small capillaries of the body.
- Recurrent damage of the RBC shortens the lifespan to an average of 20 days (normal 120 days) and hence chronic anemia.
- Splenic hypofunction is noted consequent to recurrent vaso-occlusive episodes in the splenic sinusoids.
- There is increased susceptibility to encapsulated organisms (*Streptococcus* spp., pneumococcus, *Salmonella*, and *Meningococcus*).
- Penicillin prophylaxis is given to prevent infection and continued ideally until the child is around 8 weeks of life.

## Febrile Illness in Child With HbSS

- Temperature: >38.5°C (101.3°F)

### Outpatient Management

- History and physical examination: vital signs (with $O_2$ saturation), pallor, evidence of infection, cardiopulmonary status, spleen size (vs. normal baseline), neurology examination
- Laboratory studies and imaging
  - CBC with differential, reticulocyte count (to exclude aplastic crisis because of parvovirus B19), blood culture, urinalysis and urine culture (if indicated), CSF analysis (if indicated), type and cross if pallor/acute splenomegaly/respiratory or neurologic symptoms
  - Chest radiograph (especially if symptoms of cough, history of acute chest syndrome (ACS), toxic appearance, $O_2$ saturation <92% or <4% of baseline, or febrile)
- Treatment
  - While waiting for laboratory results (but after obtaining the blood culture), start IV ceftriaxone (50–75 mg/kg, 2 g max).
    - Observe 1 hour after ceftriaxone administration with repeat vital signs and assessment.
    - Substitute clindamycin (10 mg/kg, 600 mg max dose) for those with cephalosporin allergy.
  - If necessary, change the antibiotic to cefotaxime in cases of suspected drug-induced hemolytic anemia or cholestasis and cholecystitis
  - The presence of a focus of infection (e.g., otitis media) does *not* alter urgency of administration of parental antibiotics
  - Give acetaminophen (Tylenol) 15 mg/kg (if not given in last 4 hours). Avoid ibuprofen if contraindicated (e.g., gastritis, renal impairment, ulcers)
- Admission considerations
  - Ill appearance
  - Most infants <3 years of age with Hb SS or Sβ°-thalassemia
  - Most infants with previous episodes of bacteremia/sepsis
  - Postsplenectomy
  - Most infants with temperature >40°C (104°F), WBC >30,000/mm$^3$ or <5,000/mm$^3$, and/or platelets <100,000/mm$^3$ (except in patients with Hb SC, longstanding splenomegaly, and thrombocytopenia)
  - Evidence of severe pain, aplastic crisis (reticulocyte count <5% in Hb SS or <2% in Hb SC), splenic sequestration, ACS stroke, or priapism
  - No hematology visit within past 12 months regardless of age (indication of poor compliance)
  - Oxygen saturation <92% on room air or 4% difference from baseline
  - Hb <5 g/dL, or ≥2 g/dL below baseline (particularly Hb SC disease)

## Inpatient Management

- Laboratory studies and imaging
  - Order CBC with differential and reticulocyte count (both daily until improving), chest radiograph, blood culture, urinalysis, and urine culture.
  - Consider lumbar puncture (LP), liver function tests, and DIC screen (especially with signs of encephalopathy).
  - Consider abdominal ultrasound.
  - Order amylase/lipase for upper quadrant/severe abdominal pain (rule out cholelithiasis, cholecystitis, and pancreatitis).
  - Type and cross if Hb is 1–2 g/dL below baseline or if evidence of ACS (positive chest radiograph infiltrate and fever)—remember to request, if available, minor antigen-matched blood.
  - Consider orthopedic consult to rule out osteomyelitis or septic arthritis.
- Monitoring
  - Order vital signs q4h, daily input and output, and pulse oximetry for severe illness or respiratory symptoms/$O_2$ saturation <92% on room air or 4% less than baseline.
  - Consider cardiac monitoring/ICU for signs of cardiovascular instability.
- Fluids
  - Give $D5_{1/4}NS$ or $D5_{1/2}NS$ at 1,500 mL/m$^2$/day
  - Avoid excess fluids.
- Treatment
  - Antibiotics
    - Give ceftriaxone 50 mg/kg IV q12h or cefotaxime 50 mg/kg IV q8h.
    - Substitute clindamycin 10 mg/kg IV q6h for patients with known or suspected cephalosporin allergy.
    - Add azithromycin (despite age) 10 mg/kg for 1 day, followed by 5 mg/kg daily for 4 days if patient has chest radiograph infiltrate with fever, or fever with respiratory symptoms.
    - Consider vancomycin 15 mg/kg IV q8h for severe illness or suspected CNS infection.
    - Discontinue prophylactic penicillin while giving broad-spectrum antibiotics.
  - Pain medications
    - Acetaminophen 15 mg/kg q4h
    - Possible addition of ibuprofen 10 mg/kg q6h if no contraindication (e.g., gastritis, renal impairment, coagulopathy, ulcer)
  - $O_2$ to keep saturation ≥92% *or* at patient's baseline value ($SpO_2$ often does not correlate with $PO_2$ and central $SaO_2$)
  - Investigate causes (e.g., repeat CXR) for any new or increasing $O_2$ requirement.
  - Avoid excess $O_2$ (exacerbates anemia and suppresses reticulocytosis).

## Current Management of Acute Chest Syndrome

- Consult hematology and oncology.
- ACS is a constellation of chest pain, fever, and new infiltrate on chest radiograph. There may or may not be increased oxygen requirement in a child with sickle cell disease.
- Type and screen patients with new chest radiograph infiltrate in anticipation for probable simple transfusion and/or exchange; consider type and cross for severe illness or Hb <1 g/dL below baseline (request minor antigen-matched if available, sickle-negative/leukocyte-poor)
- Monitoring should include vital signs with blood pressure q2–4h, continuous pulse oximetry, and input and outputs.
- Laboratory studies include daily CBC with differential and reticulocyte counts (may require more frequent CBCs with reticulocytes to monitor Hb level), blood gas for severe illness, serum electrolytes with liver function studies, and fractionated bilirubin for severe illness (rule out multiorgan failure syndrome).

- Treatment
    - Give IV fluids for maintenance ($1,500$ mL/m$^2$/day) or for euvolemia.
    - Begin on double antibiotic coverage (cefotaxime/ceftriaxone or azithromycin/erythromycin). Substitute clindamycin for cefotaxime/ceftriaxone in cephalosporin-allergic patients.
    - Begin incentive spirometry (q2h while awake)—write this as an order.
    - Provide adequate pain control (see previous discussion) with bowel regimen (high-fiber stool softener: Dulcolax or lactulose, plenty of oral fluids).
    - Consider scheduled albuterol—especially if patient has history of asthma/reactive airway disease or wheezing on examination (a trial is often indicated)
    - Glucocorticoids (prednisone) at 2 mg/kg/day in divided dose for 5 days
    - Give supplemental $O_2$ to keep saturation $\geq 92\%$ or at baseline (watch carefully for increased $O_2$ requirement that is a signal of poor $O_2$ delivery and the need for probable transfusion).

- **Watch carefully!** ACS is the most common cause of death in sickle cell disease, with a mortality rate of 1–4%.

## Acute Splenic Sequestration

- Consult hematology and oncology.
- Acute illness with Hb of 2 g/dL or more below patient's baseline with acutely enlarging spleen.
    - Mild to moderate thrombocytopenia is often present.
    - Reticulocytosis usually occurs (consider aplastic crisis if reticulocyte count decreased).
- Consider ICU for observation/requirement for partial exchange. Type and cross "stat" (consider minor antigen-matched PRBCs if time permits).
- Monitoring
    - Vital signs with blood pressure q2h
    - Pulse oximetry
    - Daily CBC with differential and reticulocyte count
    - Serial abdominal/cardiovascular examinations q2-4h, cardiorespiratory monitor
- Fluids: D5$_{1/4}$NS or D5$_{1/2}$NS at $1,500$/m$^2$/day (more if dehydrated, fever)
- Incentive spirometry
- Treatment
    - PRBC transfusion of 10 mL/kg for Hb <4–5 g/dL and/or signs of cardiovascular compromise. In severe cases, urgent initiation of transfusion before inpatient admission may be life saving.
    - Antibiotics if febrile (acute splenic sequestration)
    - $O_2$ to keep saturation $\geq 92\%$ or at patient's baseline
    - Pain
        - Acetaminophen 15mg/kg PO q4h
        - Possible addition of ibuprofen 10 mg/kg PO q6h if no contraindication (e.g., gastritis, renal impairment, coagulopathy, ulcer)

## Aplastic Crisis

- Consult hematology and oncology.
- Acute illness associated with hemoglobin below patient's baseline with substantially decreased reticulocyte count (often <1%)—most are because of parvovirus B19 infection.
- Treatment
    - Contact/respiratory isolation if aplastic crisis is suspected.
    - Daily CBC with differential and reticulocyte count; parvovirus B19 PCR or titers; consider blood culture, urinalysis, and urine culture if febrile (also CSF)
    - Type and cross (consider minor antigen-matched blood and sickle-negative/leukocyte-poor)

- PRBC transfusions for symptomatic anemia or Hb <5 g/dL with no evidence of erythroid recovery
  - Repeat transfusion if necessary.
  - Avoid transfusion of Hb >10 g/dL.

## Acute Stroke

- Stroke or a neurologic event occurs in 7%–11% of patients with Hb SS.
- Consult hematology, oncology, and neurology.
- Consider ICU and/or cardiorespiratory monitoring until stable or first 24 hours; order neurology checks q2h and monitor blood pressure.
- Laboratory studies and imaging
  - CBC with differential, reticulocyte count, RBC minor antigen phenotype, blood and urine cultures if febrile, type and screen, and daily serum electrolytes
  - Possible coagulation workup and lumbar puncture/CSF analysis
  - MRI and magnetic resonance angiography; if not immediately available, CT *without* contrast to exclude intracranial hemorrhage
- Fluids: D5$_{1/4}$NS or D5$_{1/2}$NS at 1,500 mL/m$^2$/day (caution with fluid overload)
- Rule out reversible posterior leukoencephalopathy syndrome (RPLS) (because the treatment is different)
- Treatment
  - Seizure therapy if needed
  - Steroids if signs of increased intracranial pressure
  - Erythrocytapheresis/partial exchange to maintain Hb of 10 g/dL should be considered for patients with Hb <6–7 g/dL (do not transfuse Hb >10 g/dL)
  - Simple transfusion with PRBCs to Hb of 10 g/dL may be considered as an alternative to partial exchange for stable patients with Hb <6–7 g/dL (do not transfuse Hb >10 g/dL).
  - Antibiotics if there is fever or suspected CNS infection (see previous discussion)

## Immunizations and Prophylactic Medications

- Pneumococcal prophylaxis:
  - Dosage
    - Children <3 years of age: penicillin VK 125 mg PO b.i.d.
    - Children >3 years of age: penicillin VK 250 mg PO b.i.d.
- Folic acid
  - 400 μg to 1 mg PO four times a day for children with significant hemolysis (e.g., Hb SS, Sβ° thalassemia)
  - Bone marrow RBC turnover of 5–6 times normal

## Pain/Vaso-occlusive Crises

- Physical examination
  - Always consider other etiologies other than sickling for pain (e.g., cholecystitis, appendicitis, trauma), and compare with prior pain/vaso-occlusive crises.
  - Examine for hydration, evidence of infection, pallor, spleen size, and penis.
  - Conduct a neurologic examination.
- Laboratory studies and imaging
  - CBC with differential and reticulocyte count (both daily until improving)
  - Chest radiograph
  - Type and cross if Hb is 1–2 g/dL below baseline or if evidence of ACS (positive chest radiograph infiltrate and fever)—remember to request, if available, minor antigen-matched blood.
  - Possible abdominal ultrasound and amylase/lipase for upper quadrant/severe abdominal pain (rule out cholelithiasis, cholecystitis, pancreatitis)
- Fluids: 10 mL/kg bolus over 1h of IV fluids to start, then at 1,500 mL/m$^2$/day (higher if dehydrated).

- Mild-moderate pain
  - Give acetaminophen/codeine (codeine at 1 mg/kg) PO, and then q4h; if inadequate relief in 30 minutes, use morphine or alternatives discussed later.
  - Consider ibuprofen or nonsteroidal anti-inflammatory drugs.
    - If no contraindications, use acetaminophen 15 mg/kg q4h.
    - Add ibuprofen 10 mg/kg q6h if no contraindication (e.g., gastritis, renal impairment, coagulopathy, ulcer).
- Moderate-severe pain
  - Consider morphine or other alternative analgesics below.
  - Morphine (discuss with pediatric hematologist)
    - Start at 0.05–0.15 mg/kg q2h and titrate (many patients require *a lot more*).
      - Ensure continuous pulse oximetry and consider cardiorespiratory monitoring.
      - Reassess pain q 15–30 minutes.
    - In most cases, as-needed analgesic orders are **not** appropriate.
    - If pain relief is obtained with 1 or 2 doses of morphine, consider acetaminophen/codeine (1 mg/kg based on codeine) or other oral narcotics as outpatient therapy.
    - Always start the oral medications an hour before stopping the IV morphine to allow their action to start before turning off the IV medications.
    - For itching associated with morphine drips, add nalbuphine hydrochloride (Nubain) to infusion therapy if necessary. Dose titration is according to dose of morphine used.
    - Add stool softeners to regimen of patients on morphine infusion to avoid constipation.
  - Other drugs to relieve pain
    - Hydromorphone (Dilaudid) at 0.015–0.02 mg/kg IV q3–4h
    - Ketorolac 0.5 mg/kg (30 mg max) IV q6–8h in addition to opioid (do not use with ibuprofen)
- Priapism: vaso-occlusive crisis in the cavernous sinus of penis, leading to prolonged and persistent erection in young adolescent males
  - Treat pain as previously. Oral Sudafed (antihistamine) 1 mg/kg may be added.
  - Consult urology for cavernous sinus irrigation.
  - Monitor Hb/Hct and transfuse if Hb <7 g/dL.

# ANEMIAS

- These are a decrease in the oxygen carrying capacity of RBCs consequent to decreased production of Hb, increased destruction of RBC, or abnormal Hb.
- Classification is based on extrinsic destruction, RBC membrane disorders, and intrinsic (abnormal Hb or enzyme) abnormalities of the RBC (Figure 17-1).

## Diagnosis

- History: past medical history; dietary history (including both mother and newborn; iron deficiency anemia in term infants is rarely seen before 6 months); neonatal history (history of hyperbilirubinemia suggests congenital hemolytic anemia, such as hereditary spherocytosis (HS), hereditary elliptocytosis (HE), G6PD deficiency); trauma/blood loss; history of transfusions, medications, or illness (e.g., infections such as hepatitis-induced aplastic anemia); family history (anemia, jaundice, gallstones, splenomegaly, surgeries, transfusions)
- Other factors: gender (consider X-linked diseases, such as G6PD deficiency, race (Hb S, C, β-thalassemia, in blacks/Mediterraneans; and α-thalassemia in blacks/Asians)

## Laboratory Studies

- Initial tests: CBC, reticulocyte count, evaluation of smear, Coombs test, creatinine level
- Other tests after initial evaluation: hemoglobin electrophoresis, infectious workup, osmotic fragility, G6PD test, bone marrow aspiration/biopsy, Heinz bodies, hemoglobin stability (others: bilirubin panel, LDH, serum haptoglobin, serum $B_{12}$, RBC folate, serum ferritin, iron, total iron-binding capacity, circulating transferrin receptor, serum lead, RBC zinc protoporphyrin, RBC enzyme panel, membrane protein studies)

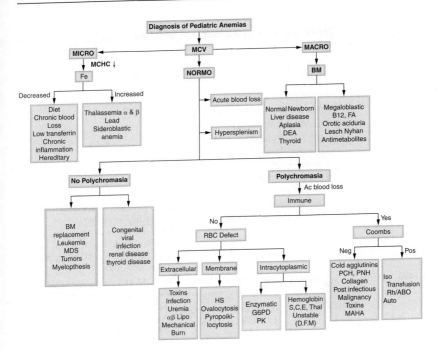

**Figure 17-1.** Diagnosis of pediatric anemias.

## Treatment

- Treat etiology (e.g., iron supplementation in iron deficiency anemia (6 mg/kg/day) for 3 months after Hb normalizes).
- For G6PD, avoid oxidant drugs or exposure.
- For thalassemia, use chronic transfusion therapy or hematopoietic stem cell transplant.
- For aplastic anemia, use hematopoietic stem cell transplant or immunosuppression.
- Sickle cell anemia (see previous discussion)

# LEAD POISONING

- This is also known as plumbism.
- The source of lead may be lead-based paints, toys, or home-glazed pottery.

## Clinical Presentation

- Onset is insidious, with nonspecific symptoms, such as vague abdominal pain, weakness, weight loss, vomiting, ataxia, constipation, and personality changes. In severe cases, there may be convulsions, encephalopathy, or coma.
- Pica or abnormal eating habits may be observed.

## Diagnosis (Table 17-3)

- Blood lead levels are used to assess severity of exposure.
- A CBC and ferritin are necessary to assess anemia (microcytic slightly hypochromic anemia).
- Abnormal levels in asymptomatic patients should be repeated to exclude laboratory error.
- An abdominal radiograph may show lead particles in the gut.
- An LP may be needed in the presence of neurologic symptoms.

| TABLE 17-3 | Treatment of Lead Poisoning in Children | |
|---|---|---|

| Blood level (μg/dL) | Action | Treatment |
|---|---|---|
| 0–9 | No immediate concern | None |
| 10–14 | Environmental survey | None |
| 15–19 | Educational intervention, periodic monitoring | None |
| ≤30 | Education, removal of lead source | None |
| 29–45 | Medical attention, removal of lead source | CaNaEDTA (3–5 days) |
| 45–69 | Medical attention, removal of lead source | Wait 10 days and retest; if completely controlled, then: oral succimer 10 mg/kg q8h for 5 days, then q12h for 14 days (remeasure at 10 days); repeat cycles until ≤30 |
| ≥70 | Emergency hospitalization | CaNaEDTA and dimercaprol (BAL): start with BAL at 50 mg/m² IM q4h (300 mg/day); start EDTA 4 hr later—preferably by continuous infusion; discontinue BAL on day 3 if level ≤50; continue EDTA for 5 days, then repeat level in 2 days; repeat as needed (only EDTA if ≤50) |

CaNaEDTA: 1,000 mg/m² IV.
*Source:* American Academy of Pediatrics, Committee on Environmental Health: Lead exposure in children: prevention, detection, and management. Pediatrics 2005;116:1036–1046.

## Treatment

- Asymptomatic children (see Table 17-3)
    - Succimer (an oral chelator) should be started at 10 mg/kg (350 mg/m²) every 8 hours for 5 days, then every 12 hours for 14 days.
    - Lead level may rebound after stopping succimer transiently.
    - Another course may be repeated in 2 weeks.
- Symptomatic children
    - Gastrointestinal decontamination: maintain diuresis ($D_{10}W$ or D5 $_{0.2}$NS—keep urine output at 350–500 mL/m²/day)
    - Encephalopathy: control convulsions (diazepam 0.15 mg/kg; repeat as needed q20-30 min)
    - BAL (dimercaprol) (75 mg/m², 450 mg/day) and calcium edetate (CaEDTA) (continue both for 5 days, interrupt for 2 days, and then retest and repeat as needed).
        - No encephalopathy: maintain diuresis ($D_{10}W$ or D5 $_{0.2}$NS with urine output at 35–500 mL/m²/day), treat with BAL (75 mg/m²) and CaEDTA (continue both for 3 days; if ≤50 μg/dL, continue with CaEDTA for 5 days; and repeat)

## WORKUP FOR BLEEDING

- Screening tests: CBC with platelet count, platelet function analysis (PFA-100), Protime (PT), activated partial thromboplastin time (aPTT), thrombin time (TT), fibrinogen level, FDPs

**TABLE 17-4**   Abnormal Screening Tests in Various Hemorrhagic Disorders

| Disorder | Platelet count | PFA-100 | aPTT | PT | TT | Fibrinogen |
|---|---|---|---|---|---|---|
| Thrombocytopenia | X | | | | | |
| Platelet dysfunction | | X | | | | |
| Hemophilia | | | X | | | |
| Factor VII deficiency | | | | X | | |
| Dysfibrinogenemia | | | | | X | |
| Hypofibrinogenemia | | | | | | X |
| DIC | X | | X | X | X | X |

- Abnormal platelet number: immune thrombocytopenic purpura (ITP), bone marrow suppression/replacement (rule out drug role), bone marrow hypoplasia, von Willebrand disease (vWD) type IIb
- Normal platelet number, but abnormal PT or PTT: factor deficiency (Table 17-4) normal platelet number and PT/PTT, abnormal PFA-100: platelet dysfunction (acquired, congenital, such as gray platelet syndrome)
- Abnormal platelet morphology ± abnormal number: platelet aggregation disorder (Table 17-5)
- Abnormal platelets, PT, aPTT, TT: possibly DIC, liver disease, dysfibrinogenemia
- Normal platelets, PT, aPTT: possibly FXIII, $\alpha_2$-antiplasmin
- Abnormal PT or PTT: consider mixing studies.
  - Normal control plasma is added to a patient's plasma and incubated.
  - Correction of prolonged PT or PTT suggests deficiency of coagulation factor.
  - Noncorrection of PT or PTT suggests the presence of inhibitors to coagulation.
- Abnormal PT corrected with mixing studies: possible factor VII, V, or prothrombin deficiency
- Prolonged PTT corrected with mixing studies: possible factor VIII or IX deficiency (commonly) or XII or XIII deficiency (rare)

# DISSEMINATED INTRAVASCULAR COAGULATION

- Generalized dysregulation with activation of coagulation and fibrin, as well as fibrinolysis. Thus, patients may experience bleeding, thrombosis, or both, or none.
- DIC is triggered by exposure of tissue factor on tissue (subendothelium, brain, placenta, activated endothelial cells, monocytes)

**TABLE 17-5**   Platelet Aggregation Responses in Inherited Platelet Function Disorders

| | Storage pool disease | Glanzmann thrombasthenia | Bernard Soulier disease |
|---|---|---|---|
| Collagen | ↓ | ↓↓ | N |
| ADP | ↓ | ↓↓ | N |
| Epinephrine | ↓ | ↓↓ | N |
| Arachidonic acid | N | ↓↓ | N |
| Ristocetin | N | N | ↓↓ |

- PT and PTT are prolonged; fibrinogen is <100 mg/dL; platelet count is low; D-dimer is >2 μg/mL (commonly positive in infants without DIC); clotting factors II, V, VIII, antithrombin III, and protein C are usually low; and microangiopathic hemolytic anemia on peripheral smear.
- Treatment
  - Treat the underlying cause.
  - Give FFP, cryoprecipitates, and platelet transfusions. See above sections for doses (heparin therapy has shown no benefit).
- General guidelines
  - Keep platelets >50,000/mm³.
  - Keep fibrinogen >100 mg/dL.
  - Keep PT/PTT within normal range for age.

## HEMOPHILIA

- Factor VIII deficiency (hemophilia A)
  - Laboratory studies show normal bleeding time; normal PT; prolonged aPTT; and a PTT that corrects with 50:50 mixing.
  - An infant with factor VIII deficiency must be evaluated for vWD (neonates have higher von Willebrand factor [vWF] levels, and only severely affected ones might show bleeding problems).
  - Treatment
    - Each unit of factor VIII/kg raises blood factor activity level approximately 2%.
    - Limited oral bleeding: aminocaproic acid (Amicar) 100 mg/kg PO q6h (antifibrinolytic agent); never used in cases of joint bleeds or hematuria
    - Mild to moderate bleeding: factor VIII 25–30 U/kg IV and/or desmopressin (DDAVP) 0.3 μg/kg IV (DDAVP nasal spray—150 μg/spray: <50 kg: 1 spray, >50 kg: 1 spray each nostril) in patients who respond
    - Severe, life threatening: factor VIII 50 U/kg IV, followed by repeated infusions of 20–25 U/kg IV ql2h
    - Surgical patients: 50 U/kg IV; usually requires repeat administration q 6–12h for a total of 10–14 days or until healed
    - Joint bleeds: factor VIII 40 U/kg on day 1, followed by 20 U/kg on day 2 and day 4
- Factor IX deficiency (hemophilia B; Christmas disease)
  - Laboratory studies: normal bleeding time, normal PT, prolonged aPTT, normal TT, PTT corrects with 50:50 mix
  - Treatment
    - Each unit of factor per kilogram raises blood factor activity level approximately 1%.
    - Limited oral bleeding: aminocaproic acid (Amicar) 100 mg/kg PO q6h
    - Mild to moderate bleeding: factor IX 30 U/kg IV
    - Severe, life threatening: factor IX 80 U/kg, followed by 40 U/kg q24h (note longer half-life)
- Factor XI deficiency (hemophilia C)
  - Rare autosomal recessive disorder (Ashkenazi Jews, Noonan syndrome)
  - Treatment: fresh frozen plasma
- Factor XIII deficiency
  - Autosomal recessive inheritance
  - Often presents with umbilical cord bleeding (80% with homozygous deficiency) and intracranial hemorrhage (33%)
  - Diagnosis: urea solubility test; assessment of clot stability in 5 M urea
  - Treatment: cryoprecipitate

## VON WILLEBRAND DISEASE

- Autosomal dominant inheritance
  - Presents as recurrent epistaxis
  - Varying severity

- Laboratory studies: PFA-100, PTT, von Willebrand factor (vWF) antigen and ristocetin cofactor activity, and vWF multimer levels and factor VIII levels
- Types
- Type 1 (70%–80%)
  - Reduced antigen and ristocetin cofactor activity
  - Possibly low factor VIII concentration but normal vWB multimers
  - Treatment: DDAVP (0.3 µg/kg IV or 150 µg/nostril q 12–24 h) and/or factor VIII/vWF concentrate (e.g., Humate-P, Alphanate)
- Type 2A (10%–12%)
  - Small multimers, reduced multimers but normal factor VIII
  - Severe deficiency of cofactor activity
  - Reduced vWB antigen
  - Treatment: factor VIII/vWF concentrate
- Type 2B (3%–5%)
  - Abnormal vWF antigen that spontaneously binds to platelets and increases clearance; possibly low vWF antigen
  - Possibly ristocetin cofactor activity; low multimers; and normal factor VIII
  - Increased ristocetin-induced platelet aggregation
  - Treatment: factor VIII/vWF concentrate
- Type 2N (1%–2%)
  - No binding of vWF to factor VIII leading to accelerated clearance of factor VIII
  - Low vWF antigen, ristocetin cofactor, and factor VIII levels; normal multimer levels
- Types 2M and 3: rarely seen. Consult a hematologist.

## THROMBOCYTOPENIAS

### Etiology

- In newborns
  - Decreased production of platelets
  - Thrombocytopenia with absent radii (TAR), Wiskott-Aldrich syndrome, or osteopetrosis
  - Increased destruction of platelets
  - Immune-mediated: neonatal alloimmune thrombocytopenia, maternal ITP, maternal systemic lupus erythematosus (SLE), maternal hyperthyroidism, maternal drugs, maternal preeclampsia, neonatal alloimmune thrombocytopenia
  - Nonimmune-mediated (probably related to DIC): asphyxia, aspiration, necrotizing enterocolitis, hemangiomas (Kasabach-Merritt syndrome), thrombosis, respiratory distress syndrome, hemolytic uremic syndrome, heart disease (congenital/acquired)
  - Unknown: hyperbilirubinemia, phototherapy, polycythemia, Rh disease, congenital thrombotic thrombocytopenic purpura, total parenteral nutrition (TPN), inborn errors
  - Hypersplenism
  - Fatty acid–induced thrombocytopenia

- In older children
  - Decreased production: amegakaryocytic thrombocytopenia, myelodysplasia, aplastic anemia, leukemia
  - Increased destruction: ITP, DIC, sepsis, HUS, hypersplenism, drugs

## IDIOPATHIC (IMMUNE) THROMBOCYTOPENIC PURPURA

- Peak age of diagnosis of acute ITP is 2–4 years of age. However, any child can develop ITP; those <1 year or >10 years are more likely to develop chronic ITP, possibly in conjunction with other immune disorders (e.g., SLE).
- Acute ITP occurs in approximately 90% of cases and is self-limited disease, typically resolving in 6 months—irrespective of whether therapy is given.

- The child is clinically well, with petechiae and a palpable spleen in approximately 10% of cases.
- Treatment
    - This may include observation alone, anti-D globulin (WinRho) 50–75 µg/kg/dose (used in Rh+ patients only), intravenous immune globulin 1 g/kg, or prednisone 2–4 mg/kg/day.
    - In case of intracranial hemorrhage, emergent splenectomy may be life saving. Platelet infusion is generally not recommended.
    - Thrombocytopenia lasting >6 months is considered chronic. Monoclonal antibodies to CD20 present on B lymphocytes (Rituximab) at 375 mg/m$^2$/wk for 4 weeks or splenectomy may be used in treatment of severe thrombocytopenia in chronic ITP.

## THROMBOCYTOSIS

- Platelets are acute phase reactants.
- Most cases of thrombocytosis are secondary (e.g., acute infection, asplenia).
- Primary thrombocytosis (e.g., essential thrombocytosis) is rare in pediatric populations.

## HYPERCOAGULOPATHY

- Spontaneous clots in veins and arteries may arise in children with cancer, congenital heart disease, infection, sepsis, nephrotic syndrome, following surgery or TPN, obesity, SLE, liver disease, or sickle cell disease.
- Laboratory studies include CBC, PT, PTT, antithrombin III levels, proteins C and S, factor V Leiden, prothrombin gene 20210 mutation studies, factor VIII level, and lipoprotein A levels. Homocysteine levels are rarely tested.
- Clots are managed with low-molecular-weight heparin (LMW heparin) at 1mg/kg SC q12h. When LMW heparin is used prophylactically to avoid clots in postoperative or high-risk patients, the anti-Xa level desired is 0.3–0.5 U/mL.
- Activated factor Xa levels should be checked 4 hours following the 4th dose for therapeutics; the desired therapeutic level is 0.5–1 U/mL.
- Tissue plasminogen activator, which converts plasminogen to plasmin, may be used to dissolve central line clots. Use may lead to higher chances of bleeding.

## CAUSES OF LYMPHADENOPATHY

- Infection
    - Bacterial: *Streptococcus, Staphylococcus,* mycobacteriosis, brucellosis, tularemia, *Bartonella,* tuberculosis, and syphilis
    - Viral: EBV, CMV, HIV, and rubella
    - Fungal: histoplasmosis and coccidiomycosis
    - Protozoal: toxoplasmosis and malaria
- Autoimmune disease: rheumatoid arthritis, SLE, serum sickness, and autoimmune hemolytic anemia
- Storage disease: Niemann-Pick and Gaucher diseases
- Drug reactions: phenytoin and others
- Malignancy: lymphoma, leukemia, metastatic (rhabdomyosarcoma, neuroblastoma, thyroid, carcinomas), and histiocytosis (Langerhans cell and malignant histiocytosis)
- Others: sarcoidosis, Kawasaki disease, cat-scratch disease

### Suggested Readings

2008 Drug Topics Red Book, 112th Ed. Medical Economics.
Lanzkowsky P. Pediatric Hematology and Oncology. 4th Ed. Burlington, Mass; San Diego: Elsevier Academic Press, 2005.
Nathan D, Orkin S, Look T, et al. Nathan and Oski's Hematology of Infancy and Childhood, 6th Ed. Philadelphia: WB Saunders, 2003.
Pizzo P, Poplack D. Principles and Practice of Pediatric Oncology, 3rd Ed. Philadelphia: Lippincott-Raven Publishers, 1997.

# CONGENITAL INFECTIONS

## Toxoplasmosis

### Epidemiology and Etiology

- Congenital infection occurs when the organism crosses the placenta and invades fetal tissue.
  - The incidence of congenital toxoplasmosis is $1/1,000$–$1/10,000$ live births in the United States.
  - The disease severity is worse with a first- or second-trimester infection, but transmission is more likely if the infection occurs during the third trimester of pregnancy.
- The causative agent is *Toxoplasma gondii.*
- Maternal infection is acquired by eating cysts in undercooked or raw meat; receiving blood products, bone marrow, or an organ from a donor with latent infection; or from inadvertent ingestion of cysts in contaminated cat litter.
- Evaluation of the infant with suspected toxoplasmosis should include ophthalmologic, neurologic, and auditory examinations.

### Clinical Presentation

- The large majority (70%–90%) of infants are asymptomatic at birth.
- Symptomatic infants may exhibit hepatosplenomegaly, jaundice, lymphadenopathy, thrombocytopenia, rash and meningoencephalitis with hydrocephalus, seizures, calcifications, chorioretinitis, microphthalmia, and microcephaly. Late sequelae include chorioretinitis leading to visual impairment, as well as learning disabilities, mental retardation, and hearing loss.

### Laboratory Studies and Imaging

- Postnatal diagnosis includes the following:
  - Detection of *Toxoplasma* DNA in blood or cerebrospinal fluid (CSF) by polymerase chain reaction (PCR)
  - *Toxoplasma*-specific immunoglobulin M (IgM) and IgA
  - *Toxoplasma*-specific IgG persisting beyond 1 year
- In cases of suspected toxoplasmosis, head imaging is necessary.

### Treatment and Prevention

- Treatment for symptomatic and asymptomatic infants with congenital disease is pyrimethamine and sulfadiazine for a prolonged period.
- Pregnant women should wash fruits and vegetables well, avoid undercooked meat, and avoid contact with cat feces.
- Spiramycin may be given to pregnant women with primary *Toxoplasma* infection to prevent fetal transmission (treatment will not alter outcome if transmission has already occurred).

## Rubella

- Congenital infection occurs through maternal viremia with placental seeding leading to fetal infection.
- Infection occurring during the first 8 weeks of gestation carries the worst prognosis.

*Clinical Presentation*
- More than half of all infected infants are asymptomatic at birth but may develop symptoms within the first 5 years of life.
- The most common abnormalities are patent ductus arteriosus or peripheral pulmonary artery stenosis, cataracts, retinopathy, congenital glaucoma, or sensorineural hearing loss, as well as mental retardation, behavioral problems, or meningoencephalitis.
- Other manifestations include radiolucent bone disease, "blueberry muffin" lesions (because of extramedullary hematopoiesis), growth retardation, hepatosplenomegaly, and thrombocytopenia.

*Laboratory Studies*
- **One** of the following:
  - Viral isolation from nasopharyngeal secretions, throat, blood, urine, CSF, or stool
  - Persistent or increasing rubella-specific IgG or rubella-specific IgM antibody in the infant

*Treatment and Prevention*
- There is no specific treatment for rubella.
- Prevention involves immunization of all susceptible women before pregnancy, with postpartum immunization of nonimmune women.

## Cytomegalovirus

- Cytomegalovirus (CMV) is the most common congenital infection, occurring in 1%–2% of all live births.
- The virus establishes a chronic infection in the central nervous system (CNS), eyes, cranial nerve VIII, and liver.
- CMV is transmitted transplacentally after maternal primary infection or reactivation of infection. The greatest risk of congenital infection with symptomatic disease occurs after maternal primary infection. CMV can also be transmitted postnatally through contact with cervical secretions or breast milk and occasionally by contact with saliva or urine.

*Clinical Presentation*
- Most infants (85%–90%) are asymptomatic at birth. (From 7%–15% may develop hearing loss or learning disabilities later.)
- A few infants (5%) are severely affected, with intrauterine growth retardation, jaundice, purpura, hepatosplenomegaly, microcephaly, CNS sequelae, periventricular calcifications, chorioretinitis, and sensorineural hearing loss.

*Laboratory Studies*
- Isolation of virus from the infant's urine obtained within 3 weeks of birth
- Blood viral culture and blood CMV PCR (available at some centers)

*Treatment*
- There is no approved antiviral agent for congenital CMV.
- The use of ganciclovir is controversial but may be considered in life-threatening or vision-threatening disease.

## Herpes Simplex Virus

- See "Herpes Simplex Virus" discussion.

## Human Immunodeficiency Virus

- See "Human Immunodeficiency Virus" discussion.

## Syphilis

- Congenital syphilis is primarily transmitted transplacentally and less commonly intrapartum.

■ Transmission may occur with maternal primary, secondary, or early latent disease, but it is greatest with maternal primary or secondary syphilis.

*Clinical Presentation*
■ Syphilis may result in stillbirth, hydrops fetalis, or prematurity.
■ Infants symptomatic at birth may present with a rash or mucocutaneous lesions, lymphadenopathy, hepatosplenomegaly, hemolytic anemia, thrombocytopenia, osteochondritis, and rhinitis (snuffles).
■ Late manifestations may involve the skin, eyes, ears, teeth, bones, or CNS.

*Laboratory Studies and Imaging*
■ Quantitative nontreponemal test (RPR); confirmation of positive results with a specific treponemal antibody test (Table 18-1)
■ CSF evaluation: cell count, protein, and Venereal Disease Research Laboratory test
■ Long bone radiographs for evidence of osteochondritis

**TABLE 18-1    Guide for Interpretation of Syphilis Serologic Test Results of Mothers and Their Infants**

| Nontreponemal test result (e.g., VDRL, RPR, ART) | | Treponemal test result (e.g., TP-PA, FTA-ABS) | | Interpretation* |
|---|---|---|---|---|
| Mother | Infant | Mother | Infant | |
| − | − | − | − | No syphilis or incubating syphilis in the mother or infant or prozone phenomenon |
| + | + | − | − | No syphilis in mother (false-positive result of nontreponemal test with passive transfer to infant) |
| + | + or − | + | + | Maternal syphilis with possible infant infection; mother treated for syphilis during pregnancy; or mother with latent syphilis and possible infant infection[†] |
| + | + | + | + | Recent or previous syphilis in the mother; possible infant infection |
| − | − | + | + | Mother successfully treated for syphilis before or early in pregnancy; or mother with Lyme disease, yaws, or pinta (i.e., false-positive serologic test result); infant syphilis unlikely |

VDRL indicates Venereal Disease Research Laboratory; *RPR,* rapid plasma reagin; *ART,* automated reagin test; *TP-PA, Treponema pallidum* particle agglutination test; *FTA-ABS,* fluorescent treponemal antibody absorption; +, reactive; −, nonreactive.
*This table is a guide and not a definitive interpretation of serologic test results for syphilis in mothers and their newborn infants. Maternal history is the most important aspect for interpretation of test results. Factors that should be considered include timing of maternal infection, nature and timing of maternal treatment, quantitative maternal and infant titers, and serial determination of nontreponemal test titers in both mother and infant.
[†]Mothers with latent syphilis may have nonreactive nontreponemal test results.
Adapted from American Academy of Pediatrics. Syphilis. In: Pickering LK, Baker CJ, Long SS, et al., eds. Red book: 2006 Report of the Committee on Infectious Diseases. 27th Ed. Elk Grove Village, Ill: American Academy of Pediatrics, 2006:631–644.

*Treatment and Prevention*
- Administration of aqueous crystalline penicillin G intravenously is effective.
- Prevention is through serological screening of pregnant women and treatment of infected women during pregnancy with penicillin G. Infected women with a penicillin allergy should be desensitized and given penicillin G, because it is the only documented effective therapy for treating both the mother and the fetus.

## Varicella-Zoster Virus

- Congenital infection of varicella-zoster virus (VZV) occurs via transplacental transmission during maternal viremia.
- Congenital varicella syndrome occurs in 0.4%–2.2% of infants born to infected mothers and is most common when the maternal infection occurs in the first 20 weeks of gestation.

*Clinical Presentation*
- Abnormalities include limb atrophy, scarring of the extremities, CNS, and eye manifestations.
- Neonatal chickenpox is because of maternal infection during the last several weeks of pregnancy.

*Laboratory Tests and Imaging (Table 18-2)*

*Treatment and Prevention*
- Treatment with acyclovir is usually not indicated.
- Infants born to mothers who develop clinical varicella infection between 5 days before and 2 days after delivery should receive immune globulin.
    - Although varicella zoster immune globulin (VZIG) is no longer manufactured, an investigational product, VariZIG (Cangene Corporation, Winnipeg, Canada) is available under an investigational new drug expanded access protocol for the following patients (provided significant exposure has occurred):
        - Immunocompromised children (including those infected with HIV) without history of varicella or varicella immunization
        - Immunocompromised adolescents and adults known to be susceptible
        - Susceptible pregnant women. If VariZIG is not available, clinicians may choose to administer intravenous immune globulin (IVIG) or closely monitor the woman for signs and symptoms of varicella and institute treatment with acyclovir if disease develops.

| TABLE 18-2 | Diagnostic Approach to the Newborn With Suspected Congenital Varicella Infection |
|---|---|

| Nonspecific tests | Specific tests |
|---|---|
| Complete blood count | Viral culture: |
| Lumbar puncture |   Oropharynx, urine, rectum |
| Long bone radiograph |   Optional: cerebrospinal fluid, conjunctiva |
| Head computed tomography | Smears-skin lesions: |
| Ophthalmologic evaluation |   Fluorescent antibody stain |
| Audiology evaluation |   Darkfield examination |
|  |   Tzanck smear |
|  | Serology: |
|  |   Rubella |
|  |   *Toxoplasma gondii* |
|  |   Syphilis |
|  |   Hepatitis B |

Adapted from Alpert G, Plotkin SA. A practical guide to the diagnosis of congenital infections in the newborn infant. Pediatr Clin N Amer 1986;33:465–479.

- Newborn infants whose mothers had the onset of chickenpox within 5 days before delivery or within 48 h after delivery
- Hospitalized premature infants (>28 wk of gestation) whose mothers lack a reliable history of chickenpox or serologic evidence of protection against varicella
- Hospitalized premature infants (<28 wk of gestation or <1,000 g birth weight), regardless of maternal history of varicella or varicella-zoster virus serostatus

■ VariZIG may be obtained through FFE Enterprises (800-843-7477). If VariZIG is not available, IVIG is recommended.

■ Susceptible women should be vaccinated before pregnancy.

## APPROACH TO THE FEBRILE NEONATE

■ Fever in infants <2 months of age is defined as a temperature equal to or >38°C, equal to two standard deviations above the average temperature of well children, 37°C.

■ Infants with fever present a challenge and deserve special consideration. Infants lack a fully developed immune system, are exposed to a unique group of bacterial pathogens, and often do not localize a source of infection.

■ Many studies have tried to devise screening tools to identify febrile infants most likely to have a serious bacterial infection, with varying criteria, and varying results. See Table 18-3, which is one institution's approach to the well-appearing febrile neonate. Remember that although guidelines and flow charts may be useful in managing certain classes of patients, diagnostic testing and management decisions should always incorporate clinical judgment.

■ Although some clinicians would obtain a chest radiograph for all febrile neonates, others consider this examination only in infants with tachypnea, nasal flaring, retractions, grunting, crackles, rhonchi, wheezing, cough, or rhinitis.

■ Indications for herpes simplex virus (HSV) testing and empiric acyclovir therapy in neonates with fever:
  ▪ There are no published criteria to apply in deciding which febrile neonates should be evaluated and treated empirically for HSV infection. Decisions may be guided by maternal history, physical findings (e.g., skin lesions), presenting symptoms (e.g., seizures), or local practice patterns.
  ▪ Consultation with an infectious diseases specialist may be warranted.

## HERPES SIMPLEX VIRUS

### Neonatal Herpes Simplex Virus Infection

#### Epidemiology and Etiology

■ HSV infects 33%–50% of exposed infants born vaginally to mothers with primary genital infections. The risk of transmission to an infant born to a mother with HSV reactivation is much lower (0%–5%). >75% of infants who acquire perinatal HSV are born to women without signs or symptoms of HSV infection before or during pregnancy.

■ Postnatal transmission may occur from a caregiver with oral or hand lesions.

■ Approximately 75% of neonatal infections are a result of HSV-2.

#### Clinical Presentation

■ Neonatal HSV infections typically present between 5 and 21 days of age, and they have three types of manifestations.

■ Only one-third of infants with localized CNS disease or disseminated disease have visible skin lesions.
  ▪ Disseminated disease: 25% of all cases
    - Onset during first week of life
    - Involves multiple organs, predominantly the liver and lungs; may include CNS involvement
    - Signs and symptoms: sepsis, liver dysfunction, coagulopathy, and respiratory distress

| TABLE 18-3 | Approach to the Febrile Neonate | |
|---|---|---|
| Age | Evaluation* | Management |
| 0–28 days | 1. Detailed history and complete physical examination<br>2. Laboratory evaluation for sepsis:<br>• Blood: CBC with differential and culture<br>• Urine: catheterized urinalysis and culture<br>• CSF: cell count, protein, glucose, and culture<br>• Chest radiograph (if indicated)<br>• Stool for heme test and culture (if indicated)<br>• Consider herpes simplex virus and enteroviral polymerase chain reaction for CSF | 1. Admit for IV/IM antibiotics until culture results available:<br>**Ampicillin:** Age <1 week, 100 mg/kg/dose q12h<br>Age >1 week, 50 mg/kg/dose q6h<br>**Plus cefotaxime:** <1 week, 50 mg/kg/dose q8h<br>1–4 weeks, 50 mg/kg/dose q6h<br>**Or plus gentamicin:** 5 mg/kg/day q24h<br>2. If herpes is suspected, add **acyclovir:** 20 mg/kg/dose q8h |
| 29–60 days | 1. Detailed history and complete physical examination<br>2. Laboratory evaluation for sepsis: Same as 0–28 days<br>3. Determine if patient is low-risk for serious bacterial infection by meeting *all* of the following criteria:<br>• Nontoxic appearance<br>• No focus of infection on examination (except otitis media)<br>• No known immunodeficiency<br>• WBC count <15,000/mm³<br>• Band-to-neutrophil ratio <0.2<br>• Normal urinalysis<br>• CSF <8 WBC/mm³, negative Gram's stain, normal glucose or protein<br>• Normal chest radiograph (if performed) | 1. If toxic-appearing or high-risk, hospitalize for IV/IM antibiotics until culture results available:<br>**Ampicillin:** 50 mg/kg/dose q6h<br>**Plus cefotaxime:** 50 mg/kg/dose q6h (meningitis dose)<br>(Or plus gentamicin 2.5 mg/kg/dose q8h if meningitis is not suspected)<br>2. If low-risk, choose option after discussion with attending and/or primary care provider:<br>50 mg/kg ceftriaxone IM and reexamine in 24 and 48 hours (Must have LP)<br>OR<br>No antibiotics and reexamine in 24 and 48 hours |
| 61–90 days | 1. Detailed history and complete physical examination<br>2. Limited laboratory evaluation for sepsis:<br>• Blood: CBC with differential and culture<br>• Urine: catheterized urinalysis and culture<br>• LP if clinical concern for meningitis<br>• Chest radiograph (if indicated)<br>• Stool for heme test and culture (if indicated) | 1. If toxic-appearing, hospitalize for IV/IM antibiotics until culture results available:<br>**Ceftriaxone:** 50 mg/kg/dose q12h<br>2. If nontoxic appearing:<br>No antibiotics and reexamine in 24 and 48 hours |

*CBC*, complete blood count; *LP*, lumbar puncture; *WBC*, white blood cell; *CSF*, cerebrospinal fluid
*Evaluation may also include studies for other (e.g., viral) infections as dictated by clinical signs and symptoms and by seasonal and geographic patterns.
Table courtesy of Dr. Kristine Williams.

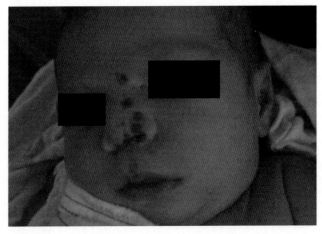

**Figure 18-1.** Lesions in a neonate with herpes simplex virus (HSV) skin, eye, and mucous membrane (SEM) disease. Photo by Indi Trehan, MD.

- Disease limited to the skin, eye, mucous membranes (SEM) (Figure 18-1): 40% of all cases
  - Onset at 1–2 weeks of age
  - Signs and symptoms: skin or mucosal lesions and keratitis
  - Progresses to more severe disease if not treated
- CNS disease: 35% of all cases
  - Onset at 2–3 weeks of age
  - Signs and symptoms: lethargy, irritability, fever, and seizures

### Laboratory Studies
- HSV DNA can be detected by PCR from CSF, blood, or swabs of skin lesions or mucosal surfaces. These tests are highly sensitive and specific when performed by experienced laboratories.

### Treatment
- IV acyclovir should be given 60 mg/kg/day divided every 8 hours, typically for 14 days (SEM disease) or 21 days (disseminated and CNS disease).
  - Acyclovir can cause neutropenia and renal toxicity.
  - Thus, the white blood cell (WBC) count should be monitored 1–2 times per week during course of therapy, and vigorous hydration and monitoring of renal function is required.
- Infants with CNS disease should have a lumbar puncture (LP) repeated at the end of therapy to confirm clearance of the virus by PCR.

### Prevention
- Delivery by caesarean section should be performed before rupture of membranes if the mother has clinical evidence of an active genital herpes infection.
- Neonates exposed to HSV at delivery should be carefully monitored for evidence of HSV infection. Most experts do not currently recommend prophylactic antiviral therapy in these infants. However, if signs of HSV infection develop, appropriate testing should be initiated and the infant should be treated promptly with IV acyclovir.

## Herpes Simplex Virus Encephalitis

### Clinical Presentation
- Signs and symptoms include fever, seizures, altered mental status, personality changes, and focal neurologic findings.
- Onset is acute.
- Untreated disease progresses to coma and death.

### Laboratory Studies
- CSF reveals elevated WBC ($25$–$1,000$/mm$^3$) with a predominance of lymphocytes.
- Erythrocytes are present in the CSF in 50% of cases.
- HSV (usually HSV-1) can be detected in CSF by PCR.

### Imaging
- Electroencephalography reveals a specific pattern of periodic lateralizing epileptiform discharges (PLEDs).
- Magnetic resonance imaging (MRI) is significantly more sensitive than computed tomography in HSV encephalitis. Typical MRI findings include abnormal edema or hemorrhagic necrosis involving the white matter of the temporal lobe region (Figure 18-2).

### Treatment
- IV acyclovir should be given 60 mg/kg/day divided every 8 hours, typically for 21 days.

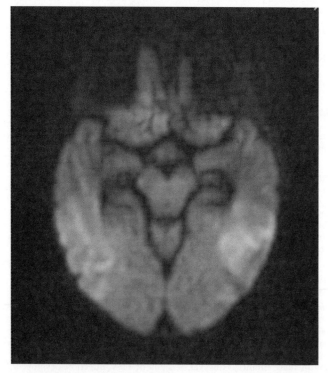

**Figure 18-2.** Temporal lobe white matter changes in a magnetic resonance image of a patient with herpes simplex virus encephalitis.

# MENINGITIS

## Clinical Presentation

■ Young infants may only present with fever or temperature instability, irritability, somnolence, poor feeding, vomiting, and seizures.

■ Older children may experience fever, headache, neck pain or stiffness, nausea and vomiting, photophobia, and irritability.

■ Syndrome of inappropriate antidiuretic hormone secretion (SIADH) occurs in 30%–60% of children with bacterial meningitis.
  ▪ The treating clinician must monitor the patient's weight, strict fluid intake and output, and urine specific gravity.
  ▪ Urine and serum osmolalities can be obtained to diagnose SIADH.

## Physical Examination

■ In infants, examination may reveal a bulging fontanel.

■ Common physical findings include lethargy, somnolence, meningismus, rash (including petechiae and/or purpura), and hemodynamic instability.

■ Seizures can occur in 20%–30% of patients within the first 3 days of their meningitis course, usually resulting from inflammation. In many children, fever may persist for 5 days after the initiation of appropriate antibiotic therapy.

## Laboratory Studies

■ The diagnosis is made on the basis of CSF findings after LP. CSF findings in meningitis are presented in Table 18-4.

■ In the event of a traumatic LP, some clinicians use a correction factor to help discern which patients are unlikely to have meningitis and thus do not need to be admitted to the hospital.

**TABLE 18-4  Cerebrospinal Fluid Parameters in Suspected Meningitis**

| | Leukocytes/ mm$^3$ | Neutrophils (%) | Glucose (mg/dL) | Protein (mg/dL) | Erythrocytes/ mm$^3$ |
|---|---|---|---|---|---|
| Normal children | 0–6 | 0 | 40–80 | 20–30 | 0–2 |
| Normal newborn | 0–30 | 2–3 | 32–121 | 19–149 | 0–2 |
| Bacterial meningitis | >1,000 | >50 | <30 | >100 | 0–10 |
| Viral meningitis | 100–500 | <40 | >30 | 50–100 | 0–2 |
| Herpes meningitis | 10–1,000 | <50 | >30 | >75 | 10–500 |
| Tuberculous meningitis | 10–500 | Polymorphonuclear neutrophils may predominate early but typically there is a lymphocytic predominance | 20–40 | >400 | — |

Adapted from Wubbel L, McCracken GH Jr. Management of bacterial meningitis: 1998. Pediatr Rev 1998;19:78–84; Jacobs RF, Starke JR. Mycobacterium tuberculosis. In: Long SS, Pickering LK, Prober CG, eds. Principles and Practice of Pediatric Infectious Diseases. 2nd Ed. New York: Churchill Livingstone, 2003:796.

| TABLE 18-5 | Common Etiologies and Empiric Antibiotics for Meningitis | |
|---|---|---|
| **Age group** | **Common organisms** | **Suggested empiric therapy** |
| 0–3 mo | Group B *Streptococcus*<br>*Escherichia coli*<br>*Listeria monocytogenes*<br>Viruses (HSV, enterovirus) | 0–1 month: Ampicillin PLUS gentamicin or cefotaxime/ceftriaxone<br>1–3 months: cefotaxime or ceftriaxone; acyclovir if HSV is suspected |
| 3 mo to 18 yr | *Streptococcus pneumoniae*<br>*Neisseria meningitidis*<br>Tuberculosis<br>Viruses (enterovirus, HSV, HHV 6) | Cefotaxime or ceftriaxone; vancomycin should be added unless specific diagnosis of *N. meningitidis* infection is clear; acyclovir if HSV encephalitis is suspected |
| Immunocompromised | *S. pneumoniae*<br>*N. meningitidis*<br>Fungi (*Aspergillus, Cryptococcus*)<br>Viruses<br>*Toxoplasma gondii*<br>Tuberculosis | |

*HSV,* herpes simplex virus; *HHV,* human herpes virus.
Note: *Haemophilus influenzae* is no longer a common pathogen where the Hib conjugate vaccine is routinely administered.
Adapted from Wubbel L, McCracken GH Jr. Management of bacterial meningitis: 1998. Pediatr Rev 1998;19:78–84.

- A recent study found that a CSF WBC:red blood cell (RBC) ratio of ≤1:100 (0.01) and an observed-to-predicted CSF WBC count ratio of ≤0.01 have a high positive predictive value for predicting the absence of meningitis, where CSF predicted WBC count = CSF RBC × (peripheral blood WBC/peripheral blood RBC).
- However, such ratios must be interpreted in the context of other parameters, including the CSF WBC differential, glucose, and Gram's stain, as well as the patient's clinical appearance.

### Treatment
- Give empiric antibiotic therapy as presented in Table 18-5.
- Duration of therapy varies with etiology, as shown in Table 18-6.
- Corticosteroids have been administered to patients with bacterial meningitis with the purpose of decreasing inflammation and thus decreasing the risk of hearing loss. However, conflicting literature exists regarding the benefit of corticosteroids in improving neurologic sequelae or reducing hearing loss.
  - Current American Academy of Pediatrics (AAP) guidelines state that dexamethasone should be recommended in conjunction with antibiotics for children with *H. influenzae* type b meningitis. The AAP guidelines state that dexamethasone therapy should be considered for infants and children with pneumococcal meningitis who are at least 6 weeks of age.
  - If dexamethasone is used, it should be given before or concurrently with the first antibiotic dose.

### Follow-Up
- Considerations for repeat lumbar puncture include the following:
  - Meningitis caused by resistant strains of *Streptococcus pneumoniae*
  - Meningitis caused by Gram-negative bacilli
  - Lack of clinical improvement 24–36 hours after the start of therapy

| TABLE 18-6 | Duration of Antibiotic Therapy Based for Children With Meningitis* |
|---|---|

| Etiology | Typical length of therapy |
|---|---|
| Herpes simplex virus | 21 days |
| *Neisseria meningitidis* | 5–7 days |
| *Haemophilus influenzae* | 10 days |
| *Streptococcus pneumoniae* | 10–14 days |
| Enteric Gram-negative bacilli | 21 days or longer after cerebrospinal fluid sterilization |
| Group B *Streptococcus* or *Listeria monocytogenes* | 14 days or longer |

*The length of therapy should be considered on an individual basis. Patients with complications such as brain abscess, subdural empyema, delayed cerebrospinal fluid sterilization, or prolonged fever may need extended therapy.
Adapted from Wubbel L, McCracken GH Jr. Management of Bacterial Meningitis: 1998. Pediatr Rev 1998;19:78–84; Long SS, Dowell SF. Principles of anti-infective therapy. In: Long SS, Pickering LK, and Prober CG, eds. Principles and Practice of Pediatric Infectious Diseases. 2nd Ed. New York: Churchill Livingstone, 2003:1427.

- Prolonged (>5 days) or secondary fever
- Recurrent meningitis
- Immunocompromised host

- All children with bacterial meningitis require a hearing evaluation at the end of therapy. Sensorineural hearing loss occurs in approximately 30% of children with pneumococcal meningitis as well as in 5%–10% of children with meningococcal and *H. influenzae* meningitis.

# INFECTIOUS MONONUCLEOSIS

### Epidemiology and Etiology
- Infectious mononucleosis is most commonly caused by Epstein-Barr virus (EBV) and is transmitted via close personal contact or sharing of eating and drinking utensils.
- Other causes of infectious mononucleosis-like illness include CMV, toxoplasmosis, HIV, rubella, hepatitis A virus, human herpes virus-6 (HHV-6), and adenovirus.

### Clinical Presentation
- Signs and symptoms include fever, exudative pharyngitis, headache, generalized lymphadenopathy, malaise, and hepatosplenomegaly. A morbilliform rash may occur in patients treated with penicillin antibiotics, especially ampicillin.
- Symptoms typically last 1 week to 1 month in duration, and fatigue may persist for several months.
- Unusual complications include CNS manifestations (aseptic meningitis, encephalitis, Guillain-Barré syndrome, cranial or peripheral neuropathies), splenic rupture, thrombocytopenia, agranulocytosis, hemolytic anemia, hemophagocytic syndrome, orchitis, and myocarditis.

### Laboratory Studies
- Although the heterophil antibody test (Monospot) is often negative in children <4 years of age, it can identify 90%–98% of cases in older children and adults.
  - Diagnosis also may be made via EBV antibody tests, including IgM and IgG to the viral capsid antigen (VCA), antibody to the early antigen (EA) complex diffuse component, and antibody to the EBV-associated nuclear antigen (EBNA).

| TABLE 18-7 | Serum Epstein-Barr Virus (EBV) Antibodies in EBV Infection | | |
| --- | --- | --- | --- |
| Infection | VCA IgG | VCA IgM | EBNA |
| No previous infection | − | − | − |
| Acute infection | + | + | − |
| Recent infection | + | +/− | +/− |
| Past infection | + | − | + |

*EBNA*, EBV nuclear antigen; *Ig*, immunoglobulin; *VCA*, viral capsid antigen (e.g., VCA IgG, IgG class antibody to VCA).
Adapted from American Academy of Pediatrics. Epstein-Barr virus infection. In: Pickering LK, Baker CJ, Long SS, et al., eds. Red book: 2006 Report of the Committee on Infectious Diseases. 27th Ed. Elk Grove Village, Ill: American Academy of Pediatrics, 2006:286–288.

- All antibody tests may be negative in patients presenting in their first days of illness.
- Some laboratories may also perform blood EBV PCR, which has been reported to be 75% sensitive and 98% specific during acute mononucleosis, with a negative predictive value of 87.7%.
- Table 18-7 presents information about the presence of EBV antibodies in infectious mononucleosis.

■ Patients with active infection may exhibit elevated serum transaminases.
■ A rise in the proportion of atypical lymphocytes in the peripheral smear, often >10%, usually occurs during the second week of illness. However, this finding is less common in young children.

### *Treatment*
■ Supportive care is appropriate.
■ Corticosteroids may be used in patients with marked tonsillar inflammation with impending airway obstruction, massive splenomegaly, myocarditis, hemolytic anemia, aplastic anemia, hemophagocytic syndrome, or neurologic disease.
■ Patients should avoid contact sports until fully recovered and the spleen is no longer palpable.

## CHILDHOOD RASHES

### The Numbered Exanthems
■ For further information, see Table 18-8.

### Erythema Multiforme
■ A benign, self-limited entity consisting of acute, fixed, erythematous macules that develop into papules and target lesions in which the central portion of the lesion becomes dusky or necrotic surrounded by concentric rings of erythema. These target lesions may coalesce to form plaques.
■ In many cases a definite cause is not identified. The most common infectious causes are HSV, *Mycoplasma pneumoniae*, and group A *Streptococcus*.
■ The initial surrounding blanching erythema may resemble hives or insect bites. Lesions in different stages can be seen at the same time. With resolution of the lesions, scaling, desquamation, hyperpigmentation, or hypopigmentation may occur.
■ The rash is usually symmetric and involves the hands, mouth, face, palms, soles, and extensor surfaces of the extremities. It may also affect the conjunctiva, genital tract, or upper airway.

**TABLE 18-8** The Numbered Exanthems of Childhood

| Entity | Etiology | Clinical manifestations | Rash |
|---|---|---|---|
| First disease: Measles (Rubeola) | Paramyxovirus | Prodrome: 2–4 day with high fever, cough, coryza, and conjunctivitis | Koplik spots: 1–3 mm elevations may appear on the buccal mucosa; can be white, blue, or gray in color with an erythematous base. About 48 hours later, a maculopapular, erythematous, blanching rash erupts, starting on the head and spreading inferiorly; the rash may become confluent but spares the palms and soles (Figure 18-5). After 2–3 days the rash begins to fade and the patient experiences desquamation. |
| Second disease: Scarlet fever | *Streptococcus pyogenes* pyrogenic exotoxin A | Sudden onset of fever and sore throat accompanied by malaise, headache, abdominal pain, and nausea and vomiting | Fine, diffuse, blanching red rash, which feels like sandpaper. The rash begins on the face and within 24 hours becomes generalized. The skin folds of the flexor surfaces exhibit intensified erythema, a sign known as "Pastia lines." Desquamation occurs 1 week after the onset of the rash, starting on the face and progressing inferiorly. |
| Third disease: Rubella (German measles) | Rubivirus | Prodrome: Tender lymphadenopathy with mild catarrhal symptoms and fever, eye pain, arthralgia, sore throat, and nausea and vomiting | 1–4 mm erythematous blanching macules begin on the face and spread to the trunk and extremities. The rash then fades to a nonblanching brownish color in the order of its appearance, which is followed by desquamation. |
| Fourth disease: Filatov-Dukes disease | This term is no longer used, but the entity was initially thought to be a "scarlet fever variety" of rubella. More recently it is thought to be consistent with staphylococcal exotoxin disease (e.g., staphylococcal scalded skin syndrome) | | |
| Fifth disease: Erythema infectiosum | Parvovirus B19 | Prodrome: low-grade fever, headache, malaise, and coryza. These symptoms may be accompanied by pharyngitis, myalgias, arthralgias, arthritis, cough, conjunctivitis, nausea, and diarrhea. | Abrupt onset of facial erythema, giving the appearance of "slapped cheeks" with circumoral pallor. This is followed by the development of a lacy, erythematous rash on the trunk and extremities. The rash may be exacerbated by hot baths, emotion, sunlight, or exercise. |

*(continued)*

**TABLE 18-8** The Numbered Exanthems of Childhood *(Continued)*

| Entity | Etiology | Clinical manifestations | Rash |
|--------|----------|-------------------------|------|
| Sixth disease: Roseola infantum (Exanthem subitum) | HHV-6 and HHV-7 | Intermittent high fevers for 1–8 days accompanied by mild upper respiratory symptoms, adenopathy, and vomiting and diarrhea. Occasionally, the child may have neurologic symptoms including a bulging anterior fontanel, seizures, or encephalopathy. On physical exam, the child may have pharyngitis or inflamed tympanic membranes. | Within 2 days after defervescence, the rash develops, consisting of 2–3 mm rose-colored blanching macules and papules surrounded by a white halo, which begin on the trunk and spread to the face, neck, and extremities. |

*HHV,* human herpes virus.
*Sources:* Wolfrey JD, et al. Pediatric exanthems. Clin Fam Pract 2003;5:557–588; Tanz RR, Shulman ST. Pharyngitis. In: Long SS, Pickering LK, and Prober CG, eds. Principles and Practice of Pediatric Infectious Diseases. 2nd Ed. New York: Churchill Livingstone, 2003:180–181; Maldonado YA. Rubella virus. In: Long SS, Pickering LK, and Prober CG, eds. Principles and Practice of Pediatric Infectious Diseases. 2nd Ed. New York: Churchill Livingstone, 2003:1123–1129; Weisse ME. The fourth disease, 1900–2000. Lancet 2001;357:299–301.

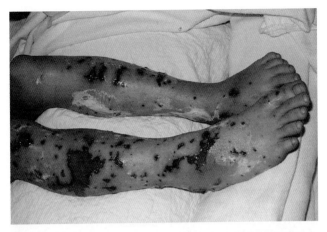

**Figure 18-3.** Purpuric lesions in a patient with meningococcemia. Photo by David A. Hunstad, MD.

## Petechial Eruptions

■ Petechial rashes necessitate prompt evaluation to exclude severe, life-threatening illness.
■ The most common infectious causes of petechiae are:
  ▪ Meningococcemia (*Neisseria meningitidis*) (Figure 18-3)
    • Prodrome: cough, headache, sore throat, nausea, and vomiting
    • Acute illness: petechial rash, high spiking fevers, tachypnea, tachycardia, and hypotension
  ▪ Other bacterial causes: *Rickettsia rickettsii* (Rocky Mountain spotted fever) (Figure 18-4), *R. prowazekii* (endemic typhus), *N. gonorrhoeae*, *Pseudomonas aeruginosa*, *Streptococcus pyogenes*, and *Capnocytophaga canimorsus*

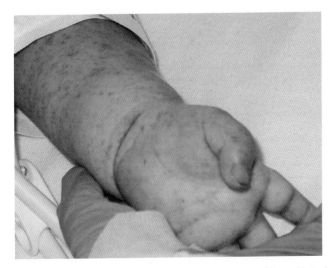

**Figure 18-4.** Petechial rash in a patient with Rocky Mountain spotted fever. Photo by Celeste Morley, MD, PhD.

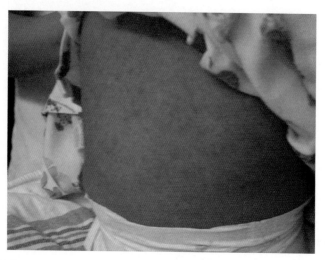

**Figure 18-5.** Erythematous rash caused by measles. Photo by Stephanie A. Fritz, MD.

- Viral causes: enteroviruses (especially coxsackievirus A4, A9, B2-B5 and echovirus 3, 4, 7, 9, 18), EBV, CMV, parvovirus B19, hepatitis virus B and C, rubeola virus (typical and atypical measles), and viral hemorrhagic fevers caused by arboviruses and arenaviruses

## TUBERCULOSIS

*Clinical Presentation*
- Although *Mycobacterium tuberculosis* infection (tuberculosis [TB]) is often asymptomatic in children and adolescents, patients may have fever, growth delay or weight loss, cough, sputum production, night sweats, and/or chills.
- Extrapulmonary manifestations include meningitis and involvement of the middle ear, mastoid, lymph nodes, bones, joints, and skin.
- Tuberculous infection of the vertebrae (known as Pott disease) manifests as low-grade fever, irritability and restlessness, refusal to walk, and back pain without significant tenderness.
- High-risk populations include immigrants from high-prevalence regions, homeless people, and residents of correctional facilities.

*Laboratory Studies*
- Diagnosis is established by acid-fast stain and culture from specimens of gastric aspirates, sputum, bronchial washings, pleural fluid, CSF, urine, or other body fluids, or biopsy specimens. The best specimen from young children is three consecutive early-morning gastric aspirates.
- The purified protein derivative (PPD) skin test becomes positive within 2–12 weeks of initial infection (Table 18-9).
- Interpretation of PPD in recipients of the bacille Calmette-Guérin (BCG) vaccine should generally be the same as for people who have not received BCG. TB should be suspected in any symptomatic patient with a positive PPD, regardless of BCG immunization. If the PPD is positive in a person who has received the BCG vaccine, consider the following factors:
  - Time since BCG immunization
  - Number of doses of BCG received

| TABLE 18-9 | Definitions of Positive Tuberculin Skin Test Results in Infants, Children, and Adolescents* |
|---|---|

**Induration ≥5 mm**

Children in close contact with known or suspected contagious cases of TB.

Children suspected to have TB:
- Findings on chest radiograph consistent with active or previously active TB
- Clinical evidence of TB[†]

Children receiving immunosuppressive therapy[‡] or with immunosuppressive conditions, including HIV infection

**Induration ≥10 mm**

Children at increased risk of disseminated TB:
- Those <4 years of age
- Those with other medical conditions, including Hodgkin's disease, lymphoma, diabetes mellitus, chronic renal failure, or malnutrition

Children with increased exposure to TB:
- Those born, or whose parents were born, in high-prevalence regions of the world
- Those frequently exposed to adults who are HIV infected, homeless, users of illicit drugs, residents of nursing homes, incarcerated or institutionalized, or migrant farm workers
- Those who travel to high-prevalence regions of the world

**Induration ≥15 mm**

Children 4 years of age or older without any factors for TB

TB, tuberculosis.
*These definitions apply regardless of previous bacille Calmette-Guérin (BCG) immunization; erythema at tuberculin skin test (TST) site does not indicate a positive test result. TSTs should be read at 48–72 hours after placement.
[†]Evidence by physical examination or laboratory assessment that would include TB in the working differential diagnosis (e.g., meningitis).
[‡]This includes immunosuppressive doses of corticosteroids.
Adapted from American Academy of Pediatrics. Tuberculosis. In: Pickering LK, Baker CJ, Long SS, et al., eds. Red book: 2006 Report of the Committee on Infectious Diseases. 27th Ed. Elk Grove Village, Ill: American Academy of Pediatrics, 2006:678–698.

- Prevalence of TB in the country of origin
- Contacts in the United States
- Radiographic findings

### Imaging
- A chest radiograph may demonstrate hilar, subcarinal, or mediastinal lymphadenopathy; pleural effusion; segmental lobar atelectasis or infiltrate; cavitary lesion; or miliary disease.

### Treatment
- Initial therapy for active pulmonary TB (Table 18-10)
  - Two months of daily isoniazid, rifampin, and pyrazinamide, followed by 4 months of isoniazid and rifampin is appropriate.
  - If drug resistance is suspected, ethambutol or streptomycin should be added until drug susceptibilities are determined.
  - Consultation with local health officials is recommended.
- Isolation
  - Most children with TB are not contagious and require only standard precautions. (Children are considered contagious when they have cavitary or extensive pulmonary

| TABLE 18-10 | Recommended Treatment Regimens for Drug-Susceptible Tuberculosis in Infants, Children, and Adolescents | |
|---|---|---|
| **Infection or disease category** | **Regimen** | **Remarks** |
| **Latent tuberculosis (TB) infection** (positive TST result, no disease) | | |
| **Isoniazid-susceptible TB** | 9 mo of isoniazid, once a day | If daily therapy is not possible, DOT twice a week can be used for 9 mo. |
| **Isoniazid-resistant TB** | 6 mo of rifampin, once a day | If daily therapy is not possible, DOT twice a week can be used for 6 mo. |
| **Isoniazid-rifampin resistant TB*** | Consult a TB specialist | |
| **Pulmonary and extrapulmonary TB (except meningitis)** | Drug-susceptible *Mycobacterium tuberculosis:* 2 mo of isoniazid, rifampin, and pyrazinamide daily, followed by 4 mo of isoniazid and rifampin[†] by DOT[‡] Drug-susceptible *Mycobacterium bovis:* 9–12 mo of isoniazid and rifampin | If possible drug resistance is a concern, another drug (ethambutol or an aminoglycoside) is added to the initial three-drug therapy until drug susceptibilities are determined. DOT is highly desirable. If hilar adenopathy only, a 6 mo course of isoniazid and rifampin is sufficient. Drugs can be given 2 or 3 times/wk under DOT in the initial phase if nonadherence is likely. |
| **Meningitis** | 2 mo of isoniazid, rifampin, pyrazinamide, and an aminoglycoside or ethionamide, once a day, followed by 7–10 mo of isoniazid and rifampin, once a day or twice a week (9–12 mo total) for drug-susceptible *M. tuberculosis.* At least 12 mo of therapy without pyrazinamide for drug-susceptible *M. bovis.* | A fourth drug, such as an aminoglycoside, is given with initial therapy until drug susceptibility is known. For patients who may have acquired tuberculosis in geographic areas where resistance to streptomycin is common, kanamycin, amikacin, or capreomycin can be used instead of streptomycin |

TST indicates tuberculin skin test; *DOT,* directly observed therapy.
*Duration of therapy is longer for human immunodeficiency virus-infected people, and additional drugs may be indicated.
[†]Medications should be administered daily for the first 2 weeks to 2 months of treatment and then can be administered 2–3 times per week by DOT.
[‡]If initial chest radiograph shows cavitary lesions and sputum after 2 months of therapy remains positive, duration of therapy is extended to 9 months.
Adapted from American Academy of Pediatrics. Tuberculosis. In: Pickering LK, Baker CJ, Long SS, et al., eds. Red book: 2006 Report of the Committee on Infectious Diseases. 27th Ed. Elk Grove Village, Ill: American Academy of Pediatrics, 2006:678–698.

TB, positive sputum acid-fast bacilli smears, laryngeal involvement, or suspected congenital TB.)
■ However, adult household members (if infected) may be contagious; therefore, inpatient children with TB should be placed in a negative-pressure isolation room, and appropriate particulate respirator masks should be worn by hospital personnel.

# HEPATITIS

## Hepatitis A Virus (HAV)

### Epidemiology and Etiology
■ Mode of transmission: fecal-oral
■ Common sources of infection:
   ■ Close personal contact with a person infected with HAV
   ■ Child care centers
   ■ International travel
   ■ Recognized foodborne or waterborne outbreak
   ■ Male homosexual activity
   ■ IV drug use

### Clinical Presentation
■ Acute, self-limited illness associated with fever, malaise, jaundice, anorexia, and nausea
■ May be asymptomatic in young children

### Laboratory Studies
■ HAV-specific total immunoglobulin and HAV IgM antibody

### Treatment and Prevention
■ Supportive care is appropriate.
■ IVIG may be effective in preventing symptomatic infection if given within 2 weeks of exposure.
■ Hepatitis A vaccine is available for all children ≥1 year of age. Preexposure prophylaxis with immunoglobulin should be considered for unvaccinated travelers to countries where HAV is prevalent and for children <1 year who cannot receive vaccine.

## Hepatitis B Virus (HBV)

### Epidemiology and Etiology
■ Mode of transmission: blood or body fluids
■ Groups at highest risk:
   ■ IV drug users
   ■ People with multiple heterosexual partners
   ■ Young men who have sex with men
■ Other groups at risk:
   ■ People with occupational exposure to blood or body fluids
   ■ Staff of institutions and nonresidential child care programs for the developmentally disabled
   ■ Sexual or household contacts of people with an acute or chronic HBV infection

### Clinical Presentation
■ Ranges from a subacute illness with nonspecific symptoms such as anorexia, malaise, and nausea, to clinical hepatitis with jaundice, to fulminant fatal hepatitis

### Laboratory Studies
■ Chronic HBV infection is defined as the presence of hepatitis B surface antigen (HBsAg) for at least 6 months or by the presence of HBsAg in a person testing negative for the IgM antibody to hepatitis B core antigen (anti-HBc) (Table 18-11).

| TABLE 18-11 | Diagnostic Tests for Hepatitis B Virus (HBV) Antigens and Antibodies | |
| --- | --- | --- |
| Factor to be tested | HBV antigen or antibody | Use |
| Hepatitis B surface antigen (HBsAg) | HBsAg | Detection of acutely or chronically infected people; antigen used in hepatitis B vaccine |
| Anti-HBs | Antibody to HBsAg | Identification of people who have resolved infections with HBV; determination of immunity after immunization |
| Hepatitis B early antigen (HBeAg) | HBeAg | Identification of people at increased risk of transmitting HBV |
| Anti-HBe | Antibody to HBeAg | Identification of infected people with lower risk of transmitting HBV |
| Anti-HBc | Antibody to hepatitis B core antigen (HBcAg)* | Identification of people with acute, resolved, or chronic HBV infection (not present after immunization) |
| IgM anti-HBc | IgM antibody to HBcAg | Identification of people with acute or recent HBV infections (including HBsAg-negative people during the "window" phase of infection) |

*IgM,* immunoglobulin M.
*No test is available commercially to measure hepatitis B core antigen (HBcAg).
Adapted from American Academy of Pediatrics. Hepatitis B. In: Pickering LK, Baker CJ, Long SS, et al., eds. Red book: 2006 Report of the Committee on Infectious Diseases. 27th Ed. Elk Grove Village, Ill: American Academy of Pediatrics, 2006:335–355.

- >90% of perinatal infections lead to chronic HBV, whereas only 6%–10% of acutely infected older children develop chronic HBV infection.

### Treatment and Prevention
- There is no specific treatment for acute HBV infection.
  - Interferon-α therapy may lead to long-term remission.
  - Lamivudine may be used in children >2 years of age with chronic hepatitis B virus infection
- Recombinant HBV vaccine is recommended for all infants. Postexposure prophylaxis is available.
- Breastfeeding of infants by HBsAg-positive mothers poses no additional risk of HBV acquisition.

## Hepatitis C Virus (HCV)

### Epidemiology and Etiology
- Mode of transmission: parenteral exposure to blood of HCV-infected people
- Groups at highest risk:
  - IV drug users
  - Hemophiliacs who received clotting factors before 1987
  - Patients on dialysis
  - People who engage in high-risk sexual behaviors
  - Healthcare professionals because of sporadic percutaneous exposures
- Perinatal transmission

- Maternal coinfection with HIV has been associated with an increased risk of perinatal transmission of HCV. Approximately 2%–12% of children born to women with HCV infection acquire HCV.
- Method of delivery does not appear to affect vertical transmission rate.
- Recommended testing for infants born to mothers with HCV infection includes HCV PCR at 6–8 weeks of life; it should be repeated at 6 months.
- HCV transmission through breastfeeding has not been demonstrated and thus maternal HCV infection is not a contraindication to breastfeeding. However, mothers should refrain from breastfeeding if the nipples are cracked or bleeding.

### Clinical Presentation
- Most infections are asymptomatic. Jaundice occurs in <20% of patients.
- Persistent infection with HCV occurs in 50%–60% of infected children.

### Laboratory Studies
- Anti-HCV Ig can be detected within 15 weeks after exposure and within 5–6 weeks of the onset of hepatitis.
- Reverse transcription-PCR can detect HCV RNA within 1–2 weeks after exposure to the virus.

### Treatment
- The combination of interferon-α-2b and ribavirin has been approved by the U.S. Food and Drug Administration for children 3–17 years of age.

## Hepatitis D Virus (HDV)

- HDV requires the presence of HBV (acute or chronic disease) to cause hepatitis. Infection with HDV may exacerbate an asymptomatic or mild HBV infection to a more severe or rapidly progressive disease.
- HDV is acquired via the same routes as HBV, and HDV may cause coinfection with HBV or superinfection of an established HBV infection.
- Hepatitis B vaccine protects against HDV infection, as HDV can only be transmitted in the presence of HBV infection.

## Hepatitis E Virus (HEV)

- Transmission is via the fecal-oral route, and outbreaks are often associated with contaminated water.
- Infection with HEV leads to an acute illness with fever, jaundice, anorexia, abdominal pain, malaise, and arthralgia.
- Pregnant women infected with HEV have a high mortality rate.

## Hepatitis G Virus (HGV)

- Transmission is via contact with infected blood or body fluids.
- HGV does not seem to be a cause of acute, fulminant, or chronic liver disease, although it may cause chronic infection and viremia.

# HUMAN IMMUNODEFICIENCY VIRUS (HIV)

## Maternal Infection

- Risk factors for perinatal HIV transmission
  - High maternal viral load
  - Rupture of membranes >4 hours
  - Vaginal delivery
  - Breastfeeding

*Treatment*

■ Intrapartum management

  ■ The mother should receive IV zidovudine (AZT) 2 mg/kg during the first hour of labor and then 1 mg/kg per hour until delivery; AZT should be stopped when the infant is born.

  ■ When possible, invasive procedures (e.g., fetal scalp monitor, artificially rupturing membranes, vacuum, forceps, or episiotomy) should be avoided.

  ■ A caesarean section is recommended for women with an HIV viral load ≥1,000 copies/mL.

  ■ Because HIV can be transmitted through breast milk, breastfeeding should be avoided where alternative formulas are readily available.

■ Management of the HIV-exposed newborn

  ■ Obtain complete blood count with differential, RPR, HIV DNA PCR, and urine CMV culture.

  ■ Administer AZT within the first 2 hours of life and continue as follows:

    • Term infant: 2 mg/kg/dose PO q6h for 6 weeks; if the infant cannot take medication by mouth, give 1.5 mg/kg/dose intravenously q6h.

    • Premature infant (<35 weeks gestational age): 2 mg/kg/dose PO q12h or 1.5 mg/kg/dose IV q12h. After 2 weeks, if ≥30 weeks gestational age: 2 mg/kg/dose PO q8h. After 4 weeks, if infant is <30 weeks gestational age: 2 mg/kg/dose PO q8h.

■ Other medications (e.g., didanosine and/or nevirapine) may be added in some cases. Because of resistance and other factors, the newborn's antiviral regimen should be considered on an individual basis and discussed with an infectious diseases specialist.

■ Suggested follow-up for the uncomplicated HIV-exposed infant (Table 18-12).

■ It is important to be aware of common and/or severe side effects associated with antiretroviral agents (Table 18-13). Contact the child's HIV specialist if the patient is having an associated adverse effect. Gastrointestinal symptoms are very common, especially in the first month of therapy. Hepatotoxicity and osteoporosis can be caused by all classes of antiretroviral agents.

| TABLE 18-12 | Suggested Follow-Up in an Uncomplicated HIV in an Exposed Infant | | | |
|---|---|---|---|---|
| Age of visit | ELISA | PCR | Complete blood count with differential | Medications |
| Outpatient 2–4 wk | | | | AZT 2 mg/kg/dose orally q6h |
| 6 wk | | | X | Discontinue AZT; Start trimethoprim/ sulfamethoxazole (TMP/ SMX) at 150 mg/m$^2$ divided twice a day |
| 4 mo | | DNA | | Discontinue TMP/SMX if the DNA PCR is negative |
| 6 mo | | RNA | | |
| 12 mo | X | | X | (Should also check lead and serum IgG levels) |
| 18 mo (if ELISA is positive at 12 mo visit) | X | | | Discharge from clinic if ELISA is negative |

*ELISA*, enzyme-linked immunosorbent assay; *PCR*, polymerase chain reaction.

| TABLE 18-13 | Side Effects of Drugs Used in the Treatment of HIV |
|---|---|
| **Class/Drug** | **Side effects** |
| Nucleoside/Nucleotide Reverse Transcriptase Inhibitors (NRTIs) | Lipodystrophy (fat atrophy), severe lactic acidosis, hepatic microvascular steatosis |
| Zidovudine (AZT; Retrovir) | Anemia, pancytopenia |
| Didanosine (ddI; Videx) | Neuropathy, pancreatitis |
| Zalcitabine (Hivid) | Neuropathy, pancreatitis |
| Stavudine (D4T; Zerit) | Neuropathy, pancreatitis |
| Lamivudine (3TC: Epivir) | |
| Abacavir (Ziagen) | Multisystem hypersensitivity reaction, including fever, rash (maculopapular or urticarial), GI symptoms (abdominal pain, nausea, vomiting, diarrhea), malaise and fatigue, arthralgias, cough, sore throat, and dyspnea. Patients may have an elevated CPK or transaminases and lymphopenia. This reaction most frequently occurs in the first 6 weeks of therapy and requires immediate withdrawal of the drug; do not rechallenge. |
| Tenofovir (Viread) | |
| Emtricitabine (Emtriva) | |
| Nonnucleoside Reverse Transcriptase Inhibitors (NNRTIs) | Hepatotoxicity |
| Nevirapine (Viramune) | Hypersensitivity reaction including fever; erythematous, maculopapular rash (with or without pruritus) on the face, trunk, and extremities; arthralgias; and myalgias. Severe hepatotoxicity may also occur. This reaction most commonly occurs in the first 6 weeks of treatment. The drug should be discontinued if rash is accompanied by fever, blisters, mucous membrane involvement, conjunctivitis, edema, arthralgias, or malaise. |
| Delavirdine (Rescriptor) | |
| Efavirenz (Sustiva) | |
| Protease Inhibitors (PIs) | Hyperlipidemia, fat accumulation, insulin resistance, hepatotoxicity |
| Saquinavir (Fortovase, Invirase) | |
| Indinavir (Crixivan) | |
| Ritonavir (Norvir) | |
| Nelfinavir (Viracept) | |
| Amprenavir (Agenerase) | |
| Lopinavir (Kaletra) | |
| Atazanavir (Reyataz) | |
| Fosamprenavir (Lexiva) | |
| Entry (Fusion) Inhibitor | |
| Enfuvirtide (T-20, Fuzeon) | |
| Combination Agents | |
| Lamivudine + Zidovudine (Combivir) | |
| Abacavir + Lamivudine (Epzicom) | |
| Emtricitabine + Tenofovir (Truvada) | |
| Abacavir + Lamivudine + Zidovudine (Trizivir) | |

## Occupational Exposure

- Risk factors for HIV transmission after a needlestick injury include:
  - High viral inoculum (i.e., high viral load in source patient)
  - Large volume of blood (from a large diameter needle)
  - Deep puncture wound

- Occupational exposures to blood or other bodily fluids should be managed according to local institutional policy and in consultation with the designated occupational health official. In general, postexposure prophylaxis is most effective when started within 1–2 hours of the exposure.
- A healthcare worker with a percutaneous or mucous membrane exposure to blood or bloody secretions from an HIV positive patient should be evaluated immediately after the exposure.
- A baseline HIV antibody test (enzyme-linked immunosorbent assay [ELISA]) should be obtained. The exposed individual should be retested 4–6 weeks, 12 weeks, and 6 months after the exposure to determine whether transmission has occurred.
- The individual should be prescribed a 4-week regimen of two drugs:
  - Zidovudine + lamivudine OR
  - Stavudine + lamivudine OR
  - Stavudine + didanosine

- A third antiretroviral drug should be considered for high-risk exposures.

## INFECTIONS ASSOCIATED WITH ANIMALS

- Common pathogenetic organisms in bite wounds
  - Human: *Streptococcus* species, *Staphylococcus aureus*, *Eikenella corrodens*, anaerobes
  - Dog or cat: *Pasteurella* species, *S. aureus*, *Moraxella* species, *Streptococcus* species, *Neisseria* species, *Corynebacterium* species, *Capnocytophaga canimorsus* (especially in splenectomized patients), anaerobes
  - Reptile: enteric Gram-negative bacteria, anaerobes

- A 2- to 3-day course of prophylactic antibiotics (e.g., amoxicillin-clavulanate) should be considered for "high-risk" injuries such as cat and human bites, hand and foot wounds, bites to the face, genital area, or joints, puncture wounds, wounds >12 hours old, or wounds in immunocompromised and asplenic people. When culture results become available, antibiotic therapy may then be tailored to the infecting agent.

### Rabies

*Epidemiology*
- Animals most commonly associated with the transmission of rabies infection include bats, skunks, raccoons, and foxes.
- Rabies is rarely or never transmitted by squirrels, chipmunks, rats, mice, guinea pigs, gerbils, hamsters, or rabbits.

*Clinical Presentation*
- Prodromal phase (2–10 days): fever, headache, photophobia, anorexia, sore throat, musculoskeletal pain, itching, pain, and tingling at the site of the bite
- Acute neurologic phase (2–30 days): delirium, paralysis, hydrophobia, coma, and respiratory arrest

*Laboratory Studies*
- The virus may be isolated from the saliva, and viral nucleic acid may be detected in infected tissues.
- Antibody may be detected in the serum or CSF.

■ Diagnosis may also be based on fluorescent microscopy on a skin biopsy specimen from the nape of the neck.

*Treatment*
■ Scratches or bites should be thoroughly irrigated with soap and water.
■ Postexposure prophylaxis should ideally be given within 24 hours of the exposure.
  ▪ Rabies vaccine is given intramuscularly (1.0 mL) in the deltoid area or anterolateral aspect of the thigh, on day 0 and repeated on days 3, 7, 14, and 28.
  ▪ Rabies immune globulin (RIG) should be given concurrently with the first dose of vaccine. The recommended dose is 20 IU/kg; as much of the dose as possible should be used to infiltrate the wound and the remainder should be given intramuscularly.
  ▪ Rabies vaccine should not be administered in the same part of the body used to administer RIG.
■ If a bat is discovered in a room with a sleeping, intoxicated, or very young person, rabies prophylaxis is recommended even if the person does not recall a bite.
■ Domesticated animals that are captured should be observed closely by local animal control officials for 10 days for evidence of rabies. No case of human rabies has been attributed when an animal remained healthy throughout this confinement period.
■ Wild animals should be immediately euthanized for examination of the brain by local health officials.

## Cat-Scratch Disease

*Epidemiology and Etiology*
■ Cats are the common reservoir for this infection, and children are often infected by kittens through scratches, licks, and bites.
■ The causal bacterium is *Bartonella henselae*.

*Clinical Presentation*
■ Regional lymphadenopathy (usually involving the nodes that drain the site of inoculation) (Figure 18-6) is accompanied by fever and mild systemic symptoms including malaise, anorexia, and headache.

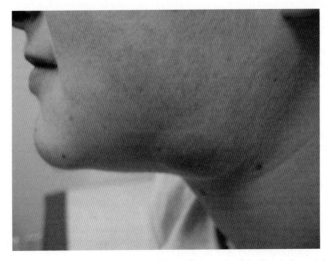

**Figure 18-6.** Lymphadenopathy caused by *Bartonella henselae* infection (cat scratch disease). Photo by Celeste Morley, MD, PhD.

- The most commonly affected lymph nodes include the axillary, cervical, epitrochlear, and inguinal lymph nodes.
- The skin overlying the affected lymph nodes is usually warm, erythematous, and indurated. Cat-scratch disease is a common cause of fever of unknown origin in children.

- Other manifestations include Parinaud oculoglandular syndrome (inoculation of the conjunctiva results in preauricular or submandibular lymphadenopathy), encephalopathy/encephalitis, aseptic meningitis, granulomatous disease of the liver and spleen, endocarditis, neuroretinitis, osteolytic lesions, hepatitis, pneumonia, thrombocytopenic purpura, and erythema nodosum.

### Laboratory Studies
- PCR and the indirect immunofluorescence antibody assay for detection of serum antibodies are available in some laboratories.

### Treatment
- Localized adenopathy is usually self-limited, resolving spontaneously in 2–4 months. Antimicrobial therapy may hasten recovery and is recommended uniformly for immunocompromised patients. Effective agents include azithromycin, doxycycline, trimethoprim-sulfamethoxazole, ciprofloxacin, and rifampin.
- Systemic *Bartonella* syndromes should be managed in conjunction with an infectious diseases specialist.

## Q Fever

### Epidemiology and Etiology
- Transmission is effected by inhaled aerosols during the birth of domesticated mammals, including sheep, goats, and cows.
- *Coxiella burnetii* is the causal agent.

### Clinical Presentation
- Acute infection follows initial exposure and results in fever, chills, cough, headache, anorexia, pneumonia, and hepatitis. Meningoencephalitis and myocarditis occur rarely. The illness typically lasts 1–4 weeks and resolves gradually.
- Chronic infection occurs years after exposure and manifests as endocarditis in patients with underlying heart disease or prosthetic valves, vascular aneurysms, or vascular grafts.
- Q fever during pregnancy is associated with miscarriage, premature birth, and low–birth-weight.

### Laboratory Studies
- *C. burnetii* may be detected via culture from a clinical specimen or PCR.
- Alternatively, one may demonstrate a four-fold change in *C. burnetii* antibody, between specimens obtained 2–3 weeks apart, by complement fixation, immunofluorescence antibody test, ELISA, or positive immunostaining of the organism in tissue (e.g., heart valve).

### Treatment
- Doxycycline is the drug of choice.
- However, a fluoroquinolone may also be used.

## Brucellosis

### Epidemiology and Etiology
- Humans become infected by direct contact with infected animals or their carcasses or by ingesting unpasteurized milk or milk products. Inoculation may occur through cuts and abrasions in the skin, through inhalation of contaminated aerosols, through contact with conjunctival mucosa, and through oral ingestion.
- Causal agents are *Brucella* species: *Brucella abortus*, *Brucella melitensis*, *Brucella suis*, and *Brucella canis*.

*Clinical Presentation*
- In children, brucellosis is usually a mild, self-limiting disease.
- However, infections with the species *Brucella melitensis* can be severe and manifest as fever, night sweats, headache, abdominal pain, weakness, malaise, arthralgias, myalgias, anorexia, and weight loss.

*Laboratory Studies*
- *Brucella* may be grown in culture from blood, bone marrow, or other tissues (cultures should be incubated a minimum of 4 weeks if brucellosis is suspected).
- The diagnosis may also be made by serologic testing (serum agglutination test) with a four-fold increase in antibody titers collected at least 2 weeks apart.

*Treatment*
- Administer oral doxycycline or tetracycline in older patients for 4–6 weeks.
- Use trimethoprim-sulfamethoxazole in younger children.

## Psittacosis

*Epidemiology and Etiology*
- Birds are the major reservoir, and the organism is transmitted in fecal dust or secretions.
- The causal agent is *Chlamydophila* (formerly *Chlamydia) psittaci.*

*Clinical Presentation*
- Signs and symptoms include fever, chills, nonproductive cough, sore throat, headache, and malaise.
- Extensive interstitial pneumonia may develop.
- Rare complications include pericarditis, myocarditis, endocarditis, superficial thrombophlebitis, hepatitis, and encephalopathy.

*Laboratory Studies*
- A four-fold increase in antibody titer by complement fixation testing from specimens collected 2–3 weeks apart is consistent with the diagnosis of psittacosis.
- Some laboratories offer immunofluorescence or PCR.

*Treatment*
- Tetracyclines are the drug of choice, but erythromycin, azithromycin, and clarithromycin are also effective.
- Patients should be treated for 10–14 days after defervescence.

## Rat-Bite Fever

*Epidemiology and Etiology*
- The causal agent, *Streptobacillus moniliformis,* is part of the normal oral flora in rats and can be excreted in rat urine. (The disease is also caused by *Spirillum minus* in Asia.)
- Rat-bite fever may also be transmitted by squirrels, mice, gerbils, cats, and weasels, by ingestion of contaminated milk or food, or through contact with an infected animal.

*Clinical Presentation*
- The disease involves the abrupt onset of fever, chills, maculopapular or petechial rash located predominantly on the extremities (including the palms and soles), myalgias, vomiting, headache, and adenopathy.
- This course may be followed by migratory polyarthritis or arthralgia.

*Laboratory Studies*
- *S. moniliformis* can be isolated from blood, material from bite lesions, abscess aspirates, or joint fluid; laboratory personnel should be notified that this organism is suspected.
- Giemsa or Wright stain should also be performed on blood specimens.

*Treatment*
- Penicillin G procaine is the drug of choice.
  - Alternatively, ampicillin, cefuroxime, or cefotaxime may be used.
  - Doxycycline or streptomycin may be used in patients with a penicillin allergy.
- Without treatment, the course relapses within 3 weeks. Complications include soft-tissue and solid organ abscesses, pneumonia, endocarditis, myocarditis, and meningitis.

## Leptospirosis

*Epidemiology and Etiology*
- The causal organism, *Leptospira,* is excreted by animals in urine, amniotic fluid, or placenta and remains viable in the water or soil for weeks to months. Contact of abraded skin or mucosal surfaces with contaminated water, soil, or animal matter facilitates human infection.
- Thus, outbreaks of disease have been associated with recreational wading, swimming, or boating in contaminated water.

*Clinical Presentation*
- An acute febrile illness may be accompanied by generalized vasculitis.
- The onset of infection is characterized by fever, chills, transient rash, nausea, vomiting, and headache.
- Other notable features include conjunctivitis without discharge and myalgias in the lumbar region and lower leg.
- Severe illness occurs in 10% of patients infected, which includes jaundice, renal dysfunction, cardiac arrhythmias, hemorrhagic pneumonitis, or circulatory failure.

*Laboratory Studies*
- The organism may be recovered from blood, urine, or CSF; laboratory personnel should be notified that *Leptospira* infection is suspected.
- Serologic antibody testing, immunohistochemistry, and PCR are available in some laboratories.

*Treatment*
- Patients with severe illness requiring hospitalization should be treated with intravenous penicillin G.
- Mild infections may be treated with doxycycline or amoxicillin for children <8 years.

## Yersiniosis

*Epidemiology and Etiology*
- The principal reservoir is swine and thus infection likely occurs by ingesting contaminated food, including raw or undercooked pork products, unpasteurized milk, contaminated water, or contact with animals. Infants may be infected by caregivers who handle raw pork intestines (chitterlings).
- The causal pathogen is *Yersinia enterocolitica.*

*Clinical Presentation*
- The most common finding in young children is enterocolitis with fever and diarrhea in which the stool contains mucus, blood, and leukocytes.
- Older children and young adults may present with a pseudoappendicitis syndrome including fever, right lower quadrant tenderness, and leukocytosis.

*Laboratory Studies*
- The organism can be cultured from the stool during the first two weeks of illness.

*Treatment*
- Antibiotic therapy decreases the duration of fecal excretion of the organism. Isolates are commonly susceptible to aminoglycosides, cefotaxime, trimethoprim-sulfamethoxazole, fluoroquinolones, and tetracycline or doxycycline.

■ It is not clear whether antibiotics are beneficial for patients with enterocolitis, mesenteric adenitis, or pseudoappendicitis syndrome.

## TICKBORNE INFECTIONS

■ Prevention of tickborne diseases involves the following:
  ▪ Avoid tick-infested areas (woodlands).
  ▪ If entering a tick-infested area, wear light-colored clothing that covers the arms, legs, and other exposed areas.
  ▪ Use tick and insect repellent. The best, all-purpose insect repellent is N,N-diethyl-m-toluamide (DEET). In repellents, DEET concentrations between 10% and 30% can be safely used on children's skin. DEET is not recommended for children under 2 months of age.
  ▪ After possible tick exposure, inspect children's clothing and bodies (especially hairy regions of the body, including the head and neck, where ticks often attach).

■ For additional details about specific tickborne diseases and their treatment, see Table 18-14.

## INFECTIOUS DISEASE AND THE INTERNATIONALLY ADOPTED CHILD

■ Each year, families in the United States adopt >20,000 children from other countries. These children deserve special consideration because many come from countries with limited resources with less than optimal living conditions and may have unknown medical histories.

■ Several screening tests should be performed in internationally adopted children (Table 18-15). In addition, children with serologic evidence of syphilis should undergo radiologic evaluation and lumbar puncture. Other tests that may be indicated include lead level, urinalysis, thyroid-stimulating hormone and thyroxine, alanine transferase and aspartate transferase, bilirubin, and alkaline phosphatase, as well as vision and hearing screening and developmental testing.

■ Common skin infections in international adoptees include impetigo, molluscum contagiosum, and scabies.

### Immunizations

■ Many foreign adoptees have deficient immunizations or may have inaccurate or incomplete or missing preadoption immunization records. To address these issues, antibody levels may be measured to verify immunity or the series of immunizations may be repeated.

■ The recommended immunization protocol for these children is presented in Table 18-16.

### Intestinal Parasites

■ Parasites and other intestinal pathogens are common in children immigrating from or returning from travel to foreign countries.

■ Such children who are symptomatic (e.g., signs of gastroenteritis or malnutrition) should have the following testing performed:
  ▪ Three specimens should be tested for ova and parasites.
  ▪ One specimen should be tested specifically for *Giardia lamblia* and *Cryptosporidium parvum* antigens.

■ In addition, children with active diarrhea (especially those with bloody stools) should have the stool cultured for *Salmonella*, *Shigella*, *Campylobacter*, and *E. coli* O157:H7. Stool assays for *Shiga* toxins (produced by O157:H7 and other serotypes of diarrheagenic *E. coli*) should be performed.

■ Many intestinal parasites are not considered pathogens. However, their presence suggests that the patient may also be infected with other, pathogenic parasites. Examples of

*(text continues on p. 306)*

**TABLE 18-14  Description and Treatment of Tickborne Diseases**

| Disease | Organism | Geographic distribution | Reservoir | Common presenting symptoms | Rash | Initial laboratory findings and diagnostic tests | Treatment |
|---|---|---|---|---|---|---|---|
| Lyme disease | *Borrelia burgdorferi* | Northeastern and midwestern parts of the United States, plus states on the west coast | Migratory birds | Fever, chills, headache, myalgias, arthralgias Complications: carditis and neurologic manifestations (cranial nerve palsy, meningitis) Sequelae of late disease: chronic arthritis, subacute encephalopathy, optic neuritis | Erythema migrans (Figure 18-7) | ELISA: if positive, confirm by Western blot | Doxycycline* or amoxicillin; IV ceftriaxone |
| Tularemia | *Francisella tularensis* | Southern, southeastern, and midwestern United States | Rabbits, dogs, rodents | Dependent on route of acquisition Fever, chills, adenopathy, headache, fatigue, cough, pharyngitis, myalgias, vomiting, abdominal pain, diarrhea, skin ulcers, pneumonia | | Normal or slightly elevated white blood cell count and ESR Serology can confirm by 1–2 weeks | Gentamicin, streptomycin, doxycycline,* or fluoroquinolones |

| | | | | | | | |
|---|---|---|---|---|---|---|---|
| Rocky Mountain spotted fever | *Rickettsia rickettsii* | Southeastern and midwestern United States | Dogs, cats, rodents, rabbits | Abrupt onset of fever, headache, myalgias, malaise, and vomiting<br>Severe disease: possibly heart (myocarditis, arrhythmias, CHF), lungs (pneumonitis, edema, ARDS), central nervous system (meningismus, altered mental status, ataxia, seizures) | Begins as blanching red macules that evolve into petechiae<br>Rash starting on wrists and ankles and spreading to extremities and trunk; includes palms and soles (see Figure 18-5); involves skin necrosis in severe disease | Leukopenia, thrombocytopenia, elevated transaminases, bilirubin, and blood urea nitrogen; hyponatremia.<br>Possible to make diagnosis with acute and convalescent serology or skin biopsy | Doxycycline* |
| Ehrlichiosis | Human monocytic ehrlichiosis (HME): *Ehrlichia chaffeensis* and *Ehrlichia ewingii*<br>Human granulocytic ehrlichiosis (HGE) (also known as *Anaplasma*): *Ehrlichia phagocytophila* and *Ehrlichia equi* | Southern, southeastern, and midwestern United States | Dogs, rodents | Fever, chills, myalgias, headache, vomiting, anorexia, hepatosplenomegaly | Petechiae or erythematous maculopapular lesions involving trunk and sparing hands and feet | Leukopenia, thrombocytopenia, anemia, elevated transaminases, cerebrospinal fluid abnormalities (lymphocytic pleocytosis, elevated protein)<br>Wright stain of blood smear: possible morulae<br>Serology can confirm at 1–2 weeks<br>Blood PCR very sensitive | Doxycycline* |

*(continued)*

**TABLE 18-14** Description and Treatment of Tickborne Diseases *(Continued)*

| Disease | Organism | Geographic distribution | Reservoir | Common presenting symptoms | Rash | Initial laboratory findings and diagnostic tests | Treatment |
|---|---|---|---|---|---|---|---|
| Relapsing fever | *Borrelia recurrentis* (epidemic relapsing fever: louseborne and tickborne), *Borrelia hermsii* and *Borrelia turicatae* (endemic relapsing fever: tickborne), and other *Borrelia* species | Louseborne: *B. recurrentis*: Africa; Tickborne: *B. hermsii*: Western mountainous areas; *B. turicatae*: Texas | *B. recurrentis*: no animal reservoir *B. hermsii* and *B. turicatae*: rodents | Sudden onset of high fever, sweats, chills, headache, arthralgias, myalgias, and weakness Possible complications: cough, pleuritic pain, pneumonitis, myocarditis, meningitis, hepatosplenomegaly, jaundice, epistaxis, and iridocyclitis Initial febrile episode lasts 3–7 days and is followed by afebrile period lasting days to weeks, which is then followed by one or more relapses | Possible transient maculopapular rash of trunk and petechiae of skin and mucous membranes | Specimens can be sent to Division of Vector-Borne Infectious Diseases, CDC, Fort Collins, Colo, for laboratory testing | Penicillin or doxycycline* or erythromycin |

| Babesiosis | Babesia microti, Babesia divergens, Babesia bovis | Coastal areas and islands of Connecticut, Massachusetts, Rhode Island, and New York | Rodents | Malaria-like illness with high fever, weakness, headache, myalgias, nausea, vomiting, arthralgia, weight loss, cough, dyspnea, renal failure  Complications: renal failure, ARDS, CHF, disseminated intravascular coagulation, hypotension and shock, and myocardial infarction | Rash is uncommon | Mild to severe hemolytic anemia; slightly decreased leukocyte count  Diagnosis is usually based on typical blood smear morphology; Giemsa or Wright-stained smear demonstrates intraerythrocytic parasites | Quinine plus clindamycin or atovaquone plus azithromycin |

ELISA, enzyme-linked immunosorbent assay; CHF, congestive heart failure; ESR, erythrocyte sedimentation rate; ARDS, acute respiratory distress syndrome; PCR, polymerase chain reaction; CDC, Centers for Disease Control and Prevention.
*Although doxycycline is not recommended for children under 8 years of age because of associated dental staining, short courses have been safely used.
Adapted from Jacobs RF. Tick exposure and related infections. Pediatr Infect Dis J 1988;7(612–614); Gayle A, Ringdahl E. Tick-borne diseases. Am Fam Physician. 2001;64:461–466.

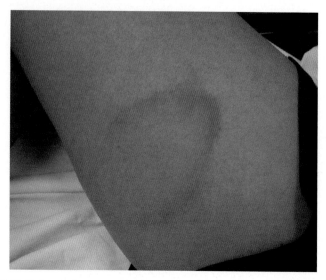

**Figure 18-7.** Erythema migrans in a patient with Lyme disease. Photo by Indi Trehan, MD.

these nonpathogenic parasites include *Trichomonas hominis*, *Endolimax nana*, *Entamoeba coli*, and *Entamoeba dispar*.

■ Treatment for pathogenic intestinal parasites is presented in Table 18-17.

## OTHER CHILDHOOD INFECTIONS

■ Other common childhood infections are described in Table 18-18.

|  TABLE 18-15 | Screening Tests for Infectious Diseases in Internationally Adopted Children |
|---|---|

| |
|---|
| Hepatitis B virus serologic testing: |
|    Hepatitis B surface antigen (HBsAg) |
|    Hepatitis B surface antibody (anti-HBs) |
|    Hepatitis B core antibody (anti-HBc) |
| Hepatitis C virus serologic testing (see text) |
| Syphilis serologic testing |
|    Nontreponemal test (RPR, VDRL, ART) |
|    Treponemal test (MHA-TP, FTA-ABS) |
| Human immunodeficiency virus 1 and 2 serologic testing |
| Complete blood cell count with red blood cell indices |
| Stool examination for ova and parasites (3 specimens) |
| Stool examination for *Giardia lamblia* and *Cryptosporidium* antigen (1 specimen) |
| Tuberculin skin test |

RPR indicates rapid plasma reagin; *VDRL*, Venereal Disease Research Laboratory; *ART*, automated reagin test; *MHA-TP*, microhemagglutination test for *Treponema pallidum*; *FTA-ABS*, fluorescent treponemal antibody absorption.
Adapted from American Academy of Pediatrics. In: Pickering LK, Baker CJ, Long SS, et al., eds., Red book: 2006 Report of the Committee on Infectious Diseases. 27th Ed. Elk Grove Village, Ill: American Academy of Pediatrics, 2006:182–188.

| TABLE 18-16 | Approaches to the Evaluation and Immunization of Internationally Adopted Children | |
|---|---|---|
| **Vaccine** | **Recommended approach** | **Alternative approach** |
| Hepatitis B | Perform hepatitis B panel | — |
| Diphtheria and tetanus toxoids (DTaP, DT, Td) | Immunize with diphtheria and tetanus-containing vaccine as appropriate for age; Serologic testing for antitoxoid antibodies 4 wk after dose 1 if severe local reaction occurs | Children whose records indicate receipt of ≥3 doses: serologic testing for antitoxoid antibody to diphtheria and tetanus toxins before administering additional doses or administer a single booster dose of diphtheria and tetanus-containing vaccine, followed by serologic testing after 1 month for antitoxoid antibody to diphtheria and tetanus toxins with reimmunization as appropriate |
| *Haemophilus influenzae* type b (Hib) | Age-appropriate immunization | — |
| Pertussis (DTaP) | No serologic test routinely available. May use antibodies to diphtheria or tetanus toxoids as a marker of receipt of diphtheria, tetanus, and pertussis-containing vaccine | — |
| Poliovirus | Immunize with inactivated poliovirus vaccine (IPV) | Serologic testing for neutralizing antibody to poliovirus types 1, 2, and 3 or administer single dose of IPV, followed by serologic testing for neutralizing antibody to poliovirus types 1, 2, and 3 |
| Measles-mumps-rubella (MMR) | Immunize with MMR vaccine or obtain measles antibody and if positive, give MMR vaccine for mumps and rubella protection | Serologic testing for immunoglobulin G (IgG) antibody to vaccine viruses indicated by immunization record |
| Varicella | Age-appropriate immunization of children who lack reliable history of previous varicella disease or serologic evidence of protection | — |
| Pneumococcal | Age-appropriate immunization | — |

Adapted from American Academy of Pediatrics. In: Pickering LK, Baker CJ, Long SS, et al., eds. Red book: 2006 Report of the Committee on Infectious Diseases. 27th Ed. Elk Grove Village, Ill: American Academy of Pediatrics; 2006:182–188.

**TABLE 18-17** Treatment of Commonly Identified Intestinal Parasites in International Adoptees

| Parasite | Treatment of choice |
|---|---|
| Giardia lamblia | Metronidazole |
| Hymenolepis species (dwarf tapeworm) | Praziquantel |
| Taenia species (beef and pork tapeworms) | Praziquantel |
| Ascaris lumbricoides (roundworm) | Albendazole or mebendazole or pyrantel pamoate |
| Trichuris trichiura (whipworm) | Albendazole or mebendazole |
| Strongyloides stercoralis | Ivermectin |
| Entamoeba histolytica | Asymptomatic: Iodoquinol or paromomycin, or diloxanide furoate Intestinal or extraintestinal disease: Metronidazole or tinidazole followed by iodoquinol or paromomycin |
| Hookworm | Albendazole or mebendazole or pyrantel pamoate |

Adapted from American Academy of Pediatrics. Drugs for parasitic infections. In: Pickering LK, Baker CJ, Long SS, et al., eds. Red book: 2006 Report of the Committee on Infectious Diseases. 27th Ed. Elk Grove Village, Ill: American Academy of Pediatrics, 2006:791–817.

**TABLE 18-18** Other Common Childhood Infections

| Infection | Common etiologies | Initial therapy* |
|---|---|---|
| **Acute otitis media or sinusitis** | Viruses Streptococcus pneumoniae Haemophilus influenzae Moraxella catarrhalis | Consider no antibiotics if age >2 yr and afebrile; amoxicillin (high dose) or amoxicillin-clavulanate (high dose) or cefdinir or cefpodoxime or cefuroxime |
| **Skin and soft tissue infection** | Staphylococcus aureus (including MRSA) Group A streptococci | Dependent on local resistance patterns and severity of infection, but might include dicloxacillin, cephalexin, clindamycin, trimethoprim-sulfamethoxazole, oxacillin, or vancomycin |
| **Osteomyelitis** | Newborn (age <4 mo): S. aureus Gram-negative bacilli Group B streptococci Children: S. aureus, group A streptococcus, Gram-negative bacilli Young children: consider Kingella kingae | If MRSA is likely: vancomycin **plus** third-generation cephalosporin If MRSA is unlikely: oxacillin or nafcillin **plus** third-generation cephalosporin If MRSA is likely: vancomycin If MRSA is unlikely: nafcillin or oxacillin Add third-generation cephalosporin if Gram-negative bacilli are present on Gram's stain |

*(continued)*

| TABLE 18-18 | Other Common Childhood Infections *(Continued)* |  |
|---|---|---|
| **Infection** | **Common etiologies** | **Initial therapy*** |
| **Septic arthritis** | Neonate (age <3 mo):<br>S. aureus<br>Enterobacteriaceae<br>Group B streptococci<br>Children:<br>S. aureus<br>Streptococcus pyogenes<br>S. pneumoniae<br>H. influenzae<br>Gram-negative bacilli<br>Neisseria gonorrhoeae<br>Neisseria meningitidis | If MRSA is likely: vancomycin plus third-generation cephalosporin<br>If MRSA is unlikely: oxacillin or nafcillin plus third-generation cephalosporin<br>Vancomycin plus third-generation cephalosporin until culture results are available |
| **Lower respiratory tract infection/ pneumonia** | Neonate (age <1 month):<br>Group B streptococci, respiratory viruses, enteric Gram-negative organisms, S. aureus<br>Listeria monocytogenes<br>Chlamydia trachomatis<br>Age 1–3 mo:<br>RSV, parainfluenza, Bordetella pertussis, S. pneumoniae, S. aureus<br>C. trachomatis<br>Age 4 mo to 5 yr:<br>RSV and other respiratory viruses, S. pneumoniae, H. influenzae, mycoplasma, S. aureus<br><br>Age 5–15 yr:<br>S. pneumoniae, respiratory viruses<br>Mycoplasma pneumoniae<br>Chlamydophila pneumoniae | Cefotaxime; consider adding vancomycin for severe disease or if S. aureus or resistant S. pneumoniae is suspected<br><br>Ampicillin<br>Erythromycin or azithromycin<br>Cefotaxime; consider adding vancomycin for severe disease<br><br><br>Erythromycin or azithromycin<br>Cefotaxime or ceftriaxone; consider adding vancomycin for severe disease or if S. aureus or resistant S. pneumoniae is suspected<br><br>Cefotaxime or ceftriaxone; consider adding vancomycin for severe disease or if S. aureus or resistant S. pneumoniae is suspected<br>Erythromycin or azithromycin<br>Erythromycin, azithromycin, or clarithromycin; also a tetracycline or fluoroquinolone |
| **Endocarditis** | Viridans streptococci<br>Streptococcus bovis<br>Enterococci<br>S. aureus<br>Coagulase-negative staphylococci | Treatment dependent on blood culture results and nature of affected valve; refer to the American Heart Association Scientific Statement on Infective Endocarditis for specific treatment regimens |
| **Urinary tract infection** | Enterobacteriaceae (Escherichia coli)<br>Staphylococcus saprophyticus<br>Enterococci | Amoxicillin, trimethoprim-sulfamethoxazole, cefpodoxime, cefixime |
| **Tinea capitis** | Trichophyton tonsurans<br>Microsporum canis | Terbinafine or griseofulvin |

*(continued)*

| TABLE 18-18 | Other Common Childhood Infections *(Continued)* | |
|---|---|---|
| **Lymphadenitis** | Cervical: group A streptococcus, oral streptococci, *S. aureus,* anaerobes | Dicloxacillin, cephalexin, clindamycin, oxacillin |
| | Nontuberculous mycobacteria | Clarithromycin, ethambutol |
| | Tularemia | Gentamicin, streptomycin, fluoroquinolones, doxycycline |
| | *Bartonella henselae* | Azithromycin, rifampin, trimethoprim-sulfamethoxazole |
| | Inguinal: as above, plus herpes simplex virus | Consider acyclovir |
| **Conjunctivitis** | Ophthalmia neonatorum Onset on day 1 of life: chemical irritation because of silver nitrate prophylaxis | None |
| | Onset 2–4 day of age: *N. gonorrhoeae* | Ceftriaxone |
| | Onset 3–7 day of age: *C. trachomatis* | Erythromycin syrup |
| | Onset 2–16 day of age: herpes simplex virus | Consider IV acyclovir |
| | Viral: adenovirus | None |
| | Suppurative conjunctivitis nongonococcal, nonchlamydial: *S. aureus, S. pneumoniae, H. influenzae* | Topical gatifloxacin, levofloxacin, moxifloxacin, or polymyxin B plus trimethoprim solution |

*Should be modified when culture results are available.
*MRSA,* methicillin-resistant *Staphylococcus aureus; RSV,* respiratory syncytial virus.

**Suggested Readings**
Alpert G, Plotkin SA. A practical guide to the diagnosis of congenital infections in the newborn infant. Pediatr Clin North Am 1986;33:465–479.

American Academy of Pediatrics. Cytomegalovirus infection. In: Pickering LK, Baker CJ, Long SS, et al., eds. Red book: 2006 Report of the Committee on Infectious Diseases. 27th ed. Elk Grove Village, Ill: American Academy of Pediatrics; 2006:273–277.

American Academy of Pediatrics. Epstein-Barr virus infection. In: Pickering LK, Baker CJ, Long SS, et al., eds. Red book: 2006 Report of the Committee on Infectious Diseases. 27th Ed. Elk Grove Village, Ill: American Academy of Pediatrics, 2006:286–288.

American Academy of Pediatrics. Hepatitis A. In: Pickering LK, Baker CJ, Long SS, et al., eds. Red book: 2006 Report of the Committee on Infectious Diseases. 27th Ed. Elk Grove Village, Ill: American Academy of Pediatrics, 2006:326–335.

American Academy of Pediatrics. Hepatitis B. In: Pickering LK, Baker CJ, Long SS, et al., eds. Red book: 2006 Report of the Committee on Infectious Diseases. 27th Ed. Elk Grove Village, Ill: American Academy of Pediatrics, 2006:335–355.

American Academy of Pediatrics. Hepatitis C. In: Pickering LK, Baker CJ, Long SS, et al., eds. Red book: 2006 Report of the Committee on Infectious Diseases. 27th Ed. Elk Grove Village, Ill: American Academy of Pediatrics, 2006:355–359.

American Academy of Pediatrics. Hepatitis D. In: Pickering LK, Baker CJ, Long SS, et al., eds. Red book: 2006 Report of the Committee on Infectious Diseases. 27th Ed. Elk Grove Village, Ill: American Academy of Pediatrics, 2006:359–360.

American Academy of Pediatrics. Hepatitis E. In: Pickering LK, Baker CJ, Long SS, et al., eds. Red book: 2006 Report of the Committee on Infectious Diseases. 27th Ed. Elk Grove Village, Ill: American Academy of Pediatrics, 2006:360–361.

American Academy of Pediatrics. Hepatitis G. In: Pickering LK, ed. Redbook: 2003 Report of the Committee on Infectious Diseases. 26th Ed. Elk Grove Village, Ill: American Academy of Pediatrics, 2003:343.

American Academy of Pediatrics. Pneumococcal infections. In: Pickering LK, Baker CJ, Long SS, et al., eds. Red book: 2006 Report of the Committee on Infectious Diseases. 27th Ed. Elk Grove Village, Ill: American Academy of Pediatrics, 2006:530.

American Academy of Pediatrics. Rubella. In: Pickering LK, Baker CJ, Long SS, et al., eds. Red book: 2006 Report of the Committee on Infectious Diseases. 27th Ed. Elk Grove Village, Ill: American Academy of Pediatrics, 2006:574–579.

American Academy of Pediatrics. Syphilis. In: Pickering LK, Baker CJ, Long SS, et al., eds. Red book: 2006 Report of the Committee on Infectious Diseases. 27th Ed. Elk Grove Village, Ill: American Academy of Pediatrics, 2006:631–644.

American Academy of Pediatrics. *Toxoplasma gondii* infections. In: Pickering LK, Baker CJ, Long SS, et al., eds. Red book: 2006 Report of the Committee on Infectious Diseases. 27th Ed. Elk Grove Village, Ill: American Academy of Pediatrics; 2006:666–671.

American Academy of Pediatrics. Tuberculosis. In: Pickering LK, Baker CJ, Long SS, et al., eds. Red book: 2006 Report of the Committee on Infectious Diseases. 27th Ed. Elk Grove Village, Ill: American Academy of Pediatrics, 2006:678–698.

American Academy of Pediatrics. Varicella-zoster infections. In: Pickering LK, Baker CJ, Long SS, et al., eds. Red book: 2006 Report of the Committee on Infectious Diseases. 27th Ed. Elk Grove Village, Ill: American Academy of Pediatrics, 2006:711–725.

Anonymous. A new product (VariZIG) for postexposure prophylaxis of varicella available under an investigation new drug application expanded access protocol. MMWR 2006; 55:209–210.

Avner JR, Baker MD. Management of fever in infants and children. Emerg Med Clin North Am 2002;20:49–67.

Bartlet JG, Gallant JE. 2004 Medical Management of HIV Infection. Baltimore: Johns Hopkins Medicine Health Publishing Business Group, 2004:89–101, 128–129, and 243–244.

Byington CL, et al. Serious bacterial infections in febrile infants 1–90 days old with and without viral infection. Pediatrics 2004;113:1662–1665.

Cardo DM, Culver DH, Ciesielski CA, et al. A case-control study of HIV seroconversion in healthcare workers after percutaneous exposure. Centers for Disease Control and Prevention Needlestick Surveillance Group. N Engl J Med 1997;337:1485–1490.

Centers for Disease Control and Prevention. Updated U.S. Public Health Service guidelines for the management of occupational exposures to HBV, HCV, and HIV and recommendations for postexposure prophylaxis. MMWR 2001;50(RR-11):[1–42].

Darmstadt GL. Purpura. In: Long SS, Pickering LK, and Prober CG, eds. Principles and Practice of Pediatric Infectious Diseases. 2nd Ed. New York: Churchill Livingstone, 2003:437–440.

Feigin RD. Use of corticosteroids in bacterial meningitis. Pediatr Infect Dis J 2004;23: 355–357.

Fleisher GR, et al. Limitations of available tests for diagnosis of infectious mononucleosis. J Clin Microbiol 1983;17:619–624.

Hunstad DA. Bacterial meningitis in children. Pediatr Case Rev 2002;2:195–208.

Hupertz V, Wyllie R. Perinatal hepatitis C infection. Pediatr Infect Dis J 2003;22:369–371.

Jacobs RF, Starke JR. Mycobacterium tuberculosis. In: Long SS, Pickering LK, Prober CG, eds. Principles and Practice of Pediatric Infectious Diseases. 2nd Ed. New York: Churchill Livingstone, 2003:791–807.

Katz BZ. Epstein-Barr Virus (Mononucleosis and lymphoproliferative disorders). In: Long SS, Pickering LK, Prober CG, eds. Principles and Practice of Pediatric Infectious Diseases. 2nd Ed. New York: Churchill Livingstone, 2003:1059–1068.

Koelfen W, Freund M, Guckel F, et al. MRI of encephalitis in children: comparison of CT and MRI in the acute stage with long-term follow-up. Neuroradiology 1996;38:73–79.

King SM, et al. Evaluation and treatment of the human immunodeficiency virus-1-exposed infant. Pediatrics 2004;114:497–505.

Lin TY, Nelson JD, McCracken GH Jr. Fever during treatment for bacterial meningitis. Pediatr Infect Dis J 1984;3:319–322.

Long SS, Dowell SF. Principles of anti-infective therapy. In: Long SS, Pickering LK, Prober CG, eds. Principles and Practice of Pediatric Infectious Diseases. 2nd Ed. New York: Churchill Livingstone, 2003:1427.

Maldonado YA. Rubella virus. In: Long SS, Pickering LK, and Prober CG, eds. Principles and Practice of Pediatric Infectious Diseases. 2nd Ed. New York: Churchill Livingstone, 2003:1123–1129.

Mazor SS, et al. Interpretation of traumatic lumbar punctures: who can go home? Pediatrics 2003;111:525–528.

McKinnon Jr. HD, Howard T. Evaluating the febrile patient with a rash. Am Fam Physician 2000;62:804–816.

Pitetti RD, et al. Clinical evaluation of a quantitative real time polymerase chain reaction assay for diagnosis of primary Epstein-Barr virus infection in children. Pediatr Infect Dis J 2003;22:736–739.

Ramilo O. Global impact of the HIV/AIDS pandemic. 26th Annual National Pediatric Infectious Disease Seminar, San Francisco, April 20, 2006.

Tanz RR, Shulman ST. Pharyngitis. In: Long SS, Pickering LK, Prober CG, eds. Principles and Practice of Pediatric Infectious Diseases. 2nd Ed. New York: Churchill Livingstone, 2003:180–181.

The International Perinatal HIV Group: The mode of delivery and the risk of vertical transmission of human immunodeficiency virus type 1. N Engl J Med 1999;40:977–987.

Waggoner-Fountain LA, Grossman LB. Herpes simplex virus. Pediatr Rev 2004;25:86–93.

Prober CG. Perinatal HSV infections. 26th Annual National Pediatric Infectious Disease Seminar, San Francisco, April 19, 2006.

Weisse ME. The fourth disease, 1900-2000. Lancet. 2001;357:299–301.

Wolfrey JD, et al. Pediatric exanthems. Clin Fam Pract 2003;5:557–588.

Wubbel L, McCracken GH Jr. Management of bacterial meningitis: 1998. Pediatr Rev 1998;19:78–84.

**Other Resources:**

American Academy of Pediatrics. Bite wounds. In: Pickering LK, Baker CJ, Long SS, et al., eds. Red book: 2006 Report of the Committee on Infectious Diseases. 27th Ed. Elk Grove Village, Ill: American Academy of Pediatrics, 2006:191–195.

American Academy of Pediatrics. Borrelia infections. In: Pickering LK, Baker CJ, Long SS, et al., eds. Red book: 2006 Report of the Committee on Infectious Diseases. 27th Ed. Elk Grove Village, Ill: American Academy of Pediatrics, 2006:233–235.

American Academy of Pediatrics. Brucellosis. In: Pickering LK, Baker CJ, Long SS, et al., eds. Red book: 2006 Report of the Committee on Infectious Diseases. 27th Ed. Elk Grove Village, Ill: American Academy of Pediatrics, 2006:235–237.

American Academy of Pediatrics. Cat-scratch disease. In: Pickering LK, Baker CJ, Long SS, et al., eds. Red book: 2006 Report of the Committee on Infectious Diseases. 27th Ed. Elk Grove Village, Ill: American Academy of Pediatrics, 2006:246–248.

American Academy of Pediatrics. Chlamydial infections. In: Pickering LK, Baker CJ, Long SS, et al., eds. Red book: 2006 Report of the Committee on Infectious Diseases. 27th Ed. Elk Grove Village, Ill: American Academy of Pediatrics, 2006:251–252.

American Academy of Pediatrics. Drugs for parasitic infections. In: Pickering LK, Baker CJ, Long SS, et al., eds. Red book: 2006 Report of the Committee on Infectious Diseases. 27th Ed. Elk Grove Village, Ill: American Academy of Pediatrics, 2006:791–817.

American Academy of Pediatrics. Leptospirosis. In: Pickering LK, Baker CJ, Long SS, et al., eds. Red book: 2006 Report of the Committee on Infectious Diseases. 27th Ed. Elk Grove Village, Ill: American Academy of Pediatrics, 2006:424–426.

American Academy of Pediatrics. Medical evaluation of internationally adopted children In: Pickering LK, Baker CJ, Long SS, et al., eds. Red book: 2006 Report of the

Committee on Infectious Diseases. 27th Ed. Elk Grove Village, Ill: American Academy of Pediatrics, 2006:185.

American Academy of Pediatrics. Prevention of tickborne infections. In: Pickering LK, Baker CJ, Long SS, et al., eds. Red book: 2006 Report of the Committee on Infectious Diseases. 27th Ed. Elk Grove Village, Ill: American Academy of Pediatrics, 2006: 195–197.

American Academy of Pediatrics. Q fever. In: Pickering LK, Baker CJ, Long SS, et al., eds. Red book: 2006 Report of the Committee on Infectious Diseases. 27th Ed. Elk Grove Village, Ill: American Academy of Pediatrics, 2006:550–552.

American Academy of Pediatrics. Rabies. In: Pickering LK, Baker CJ, Long SS, et al., eds. Red book: 2006 Report of the Committee on Infectious Diseases. 27th Ed. Elk Grove Village, Ill: American Academy of Pediatrics, 2006:552–559.

American Academy of Pediatrics. Rat-bite fever. Medical evaluation of internationally adopted children for infectious diseases. In: Pickering LK, Baker CJ, Long SS, et al., eds. Red book: 2006 Report of the Committee on Infectious Diseases. 27th Ed. Elk Grove Village, Ill: American Academy of Pediatrics, 2006:559–560.

American Academy of Pediatrics. Yersinia enterocolitica and Yersinia pseudotuberculosis infections. In: Pickering LK, Baker CJ, Long SS, et al., eds. Red book: 2006 Report of the Committee on Infectious Diseases. 27th Ed. Elk Grove Village, Ill: American Academy of Pediatrics, 2006:732–734.

American Academy of Pediatrics. West Nile virus information. Available at: www.aap.org/family/wnv-jun03.htm. Accessed on June 6, 2006.

American Academy of Pediatrics. Medical evaluation of internationally adopted children for infectious diseases. In: Pickering LK, Baker CJ, Long SS, et al., eds. Red book: 2006 Report of the Committee on Infectious Diseases. 27th Ed. Elk Grove Village, Ill: American Academy of Pediatrics, 2006:182–188.

Baddour LM, et al. Infective endocarditis. Diagnosis, antimicrobial therapy, and management of complications. Circulation 2005;e394–434 (available at www.circulationaha.org).

Bregstein J, et al. Emergency medicine. In: Polin RA, Ditmar MF, eds. Pediatric Secrets. 4th Ed. Philadelphia: Elsevier Mosby, 2005:146.

Gayle A, Ringdahl E. Tick-borne diseases. Am Fam Physician 2001;64:461–466.

Gilbert DN, Moellering RC, Eliopoulos GM, et al., eds. Sanford Guide to Antimicrobial Therapy, 36th Ed. Sperryville, Va: Antimicrobial Therapy, Inc, 2006.

Hebert AA, Carlton S. Getting bugs to bug off: a review of insect repellents. Contemp Pediatr 1998;15:85–92.

Hostetter MK. Infectious diseases in internationally adopted children: the past five years. Pediatr Infect Dis J 1998;17:515–518.

Jacobs RF. Tick exposure and related infections. Pediatr Infect Dis J 1988;7:612–614.

Litwin CM. Pet-transmitted infections: diagnosis by microbiologic and immunologic methods. Pediatr Infect Dis J 2003;22:768–777.

Miller LC. International adoption: infectious diseases issues. Clin Infect Dis 2005;40:286–293.

Mylonakis E. When to suspect and how to monitor babesiosis. Am Fam Physician 2001;63:1969–1974.

National HIV/AIDS Clinician's Consulting Center at 888-448-4911 www.hopkins-hivguide.org

Prober CG. Viral infections of the central nervous system. 26th Annual National Pediatric Infectious Disease Seminar, San Francisco, April 20, 2006.

Razzaq S, Schutze GE. Rocky Mountain spotted fever: a physician's challenge. Pediatr Rev 2005;26:125–129.

Talan DA, et al. Bacteriologic analysis of infected dog and cat bites. NEJM 1999; 340:85–92.

# NEUROLOGIC DISEASES
*Amit Malhotra and Christina A. Gurnett*

## NEUROLOGIC EXAMINATION

Although this section is not exhaustive, helpful points are outlined.

### Head Circumference

- Always document in children <2 years of age and in those whom you are seeing for the first time. The rule of 3s and 9s (birth: 35 cm; 3 months: 40 cm; 9 months, 45 cm; 3 years, 50 cm; 9 years to adult, 55 cm) is helpful to remember approximate occipitofrontal circumference (OFC) appropriate for age.
- Document parental OFCs if there is a concern for macrocephaly or microcephaly; benign familial macrocephaly is a leading cause of macrocephaly.

### General Examination

- Be sure to assess the following: vital signs, including respiratory pattern; dysmorphic features, including ambiguous genitalia; the pulmonary, cardiac, and gastrointestinal systems; cutaneous manifestations (look for such features such as café au lait macules, neurofibromas, ash leaf spots, hypomelanotic macules, whorled lines); and extremities.

### Cranial Nerves

- Olfactory: use nonnoxious stimuli, such as coffee or vanilla.
  - Performance is mandatory in cases of facial trauma.
- Optic nerve
  - Pupillary examination (use actual size and change [i.e., 4/4 down to 2/2 brisk])
  - Funduscopic examination—evaluate for:
    - Papilledema (takes approximately 24 hours to develop)
    - Hemorrhage (most sensitive clinical indicator of subarachnoid hemorrhage, easier to demonstrate with pupillary dilation)
    - Venous pulsations (present when intracranial pressure [ICP] is below 180 mm; note that approximately 20% of normal people do not have venous pulsations)
  - Visual fields, visual acuity: this helps differentiate between optic neuritis and papilledema because there is little change in fields or acuity with papilledema.
  - Relative afferent pupillary defect: this is brought out by the swinging flashlight test, which documents abnormality in afferent arc of pupillary light response proximal to dorsal midbrain (i.e., lesion in the macula, retina, optic nerve or tract, brainstem; it is generally not seen with cataracts).
  - Red reflex: hold the ophthalmoscope at arm's length in a darkened room and examine for equivalence in color, intensity, clarity, and absence of opacities or white spots; it will be lighter than usual in pigmented individuals or absent in retinoblastoma. If abnormal, examine dilated pupils or refer to ophthalmology.
- Cranial nerves (CNs III, IV, and VI)
  - Extraocular movements: using H-shaped path to isolate muscles, pay particular attention to nystagmus (end-gaze nystagmus that extinguishes is normal, most often indicative of myopia), CN VI (lateral rectus) and CN III palsy (affecting pupil) are often early signs of increased ICP

- Conjugate gaze: examine whether light reflects identically from each iris; does alternating cover test uncover a latent esophoria (inward deviation) or exophoria (outward)?
- Facial nerve (CN VII): assess facial symmetry; distinguish between upper motor neuron (UMN) and lower motor neuron (LMN) disease (i.e., if the whole face is weak then it is likely LMN, but if only the lower face is weak, then it is UMN because of bilateral cortical input to the forehead).
- Hearing: test with Weber and Rinne.
- CN IX and X: determine any changes in voice and gag reflex.
- CN XI: test shoulder elevation and head rotation.
- CN XII: check tongue movements and look for atrophy or fasciculations.

## Motor Examination

- Assess muscle bulk, tone (appendicular and axial), and strength graded on the Medical Research Council (MRC) scale (0–no contraction, 1–contraction but no movement across joint, 2–movement across joint without gravity, 3–movement against gravity but not resistance, 4–movement against some resistance but not against examiner's full force, 5–examiner cannot overcome patient force).
- Assess adventitial movements (e.g., tics, chorea).

## Sensory Examination

- Check four modalities (temperature/pinprick, vibration, light touch, joint position sense).
- Try to determine if deficits correlate with regions controlled by the nerve, plexus, root, cord, or cerebral cortex.

## Deep Tendon Reflexes

- Perform after the motor and sensory examinations because it relies on information gleaned from the motor and sensory exams (i.e., evidence of myopathy, neuropathy, weakness).
- Grade it on an MRC scale (0–no reflex, which occurs faster in neuropathy compared with myopathy; 1–trace reflex; 2–normal reflex; 3–hyperreflexia, although not always pathologic; 4–hyperreflexia with clonus or spread that is always pathologic).
- Perform special reflexes such as jaw jerk, trapezius, pectoralis, suprapatellar, abdominal, cremasteric, and ankle clonus as needed.

## Coordination

- This is sometimes difficult to test in children, so look for velocity and accuracy on reaching for objects as a surrogate.
- Formally use rebound, finger-nose-finger, mirror, and heel-shin-heel movements.

## Gait

- Assess multiple parts of the neuraxis.
- Look for stance, arm swing, evidence of hemiparesis with circumduction, weakness with heel or toe walking, and ataxia with tandem.

## Coma Examination

- This portion of the examination is critical in patients with an altered level of consciousness.
- Mental status. Document response to commands, regard, and speech.
- Respiratory pattern. If intubated, determine whether the patient is breathing at a rate above that set by the ventilator.
- Pupillary reactivity
  - Document size and reactivity; it may be necessary to use an otoscope to see poorly reactive pupils.

- Response is resistant to metabolic disturbance with the following exceptions:
  - Opiates: pinpoint but may be fixed and dilated
  - Anticholinergics: pinpoint
  - Cholinergics or barbiturates: fixed and dilated
  - Hypoxia or hypothermia: fixed and dilated
- Extraocular movements
  - Cold water calorics (20 mL in each ear) to activate the vestibulo-ocular reflex. The Doll's examination may be substituted if the cervical spine is stable.
  - Be sure there is no wax in the ears and that the tympanic membrane is intact.
- Corneal reflex: tests afferent CN V and efferent CN VII
- Facial grimace to noxious stimuli: nail bed pressure, nostril swab, or mandibular pull are preferable to sternal rub.
- Cough/gag reflex
- Response to pain
  - Check for purposeful withdrawal, triple flexion (stereotyped response), decerebrate (extensor) or decorticate (flexor) posturing, or no response.
  - Look for asymmetries.
- Adventitial movements: note any tremor, myoclonus, or other involuntary movements.
- Stretch reflexes and Babinski reflex
  - Hyperreflexia often indicates structural lesion, whereas hyporeflexia often indicates metabolic or spinal cord injury (acutely). However, uremia, hypo/hyperglycemia, and hepatic coma may give focal signs with hyperreflexia.
  - Look for asymmetries.

# INTRACRANIAL HYPERTENSION (INCREASED INTRACRANIAL PRESSURE)

## Clinical Signs and Symptoms

- Bulging fontanel in infants
- Decreased mental status
- Early morning headache and nausea
- Emesis without nausea
- Cushing response (increased blood pressure, decreased pulse, irregular respirations, late finding)
- Meningismus
- Asymmetric or sluggish pupillary response
- Absent venous pulsations
- Papilledema
- Retinal/subhyaloid hemorrhages
- Extraocular nerve palsies, such as CN VI palsy or setting-sun sign with paralysis of upgaze

## Treatment

- Consult with neurology and neurosurgery.
- Do not lower blood pressure acutely (central perfusion pressure = mean arterial pressure–intracranial pressure).
- Elevate the head of the bed 30°.
- Order a "stat" head computed tomography (CT) scan.
- Check electrolytes, complete blood count (CBC), and "stat" glucose.
- Use a cardiac monitor.
- Avoid hyposmolar intravenous (IV) solutions (use normal saline, avoid anything else, even in infants).

- Use acute management hyperventilation ($PCO_2$: 30–35 mm Hg) as a temporizing measure.
- Mannitol works for vasogenic edema (i.e., tumor) but not well for cytotoxic edema (i.e., stroke); hypertonic saline may be considered.
- Treat hyperthermia aggressively with antipyretics, and closely monitor blood glucose.
- Order a lumbar puncture (LP) if indicated (e.g., pseudotumor cerebri, meningitis) [post–head CT in most cases].

## SPINAL CORD COMPRESSION

- Consider extensive differential diagnosis (trauma, tumor, transverse myelitis, infarct, vascular malformation, epidural abscess or hematoma, infection, disk protrusion, atlantoaxial subluxation).

### Symptoms

- Back pain (focal tenderness—most sensitive indicator)
- Lower extremity and/or upper extremity weakness depending on location of lesion
- Paresthesias or numbness
- Constipation or incontinence
- Change in urinary function

### Early Signs

- Sensory level (best obtained over the back using pinprick; remember that the lesion is at the level of the lesion or above)
- Weakness variably
- Decreased tone
- Position or vibration loss in feet
- Changes in deep tendon reflexes (decreased early, specifically in spinal shock)
- Changes in sphincter tone

### Late Signs

- Hyperreflexia with extensor plantar responses (below the level of the lesion)
- Increased tone
- Weakness variably
- Loss of anal sphincter tone, loss of bulbocavernous reflex, absent abdominal reflexes, or absent or reduced cremasteric reflex
- Urinary retention

### Treatment

- Remember that cord compression (myelopathy) is an emergency.
- Immobilize neck (cervical collar).
- Stabilize airway but avoid hyperextension of neck.
- Consider plain films of spine.
- If symptoms and signs are acute in onset (<3 days) or rapidly progressive, obtain a "stat" magnetic resonance imaging (MRI) of spine.
- Insert a Foley catheter.
- Consult trauma/neurosurgery if needed (e.g., trauma, epidural abscess, mass).
- Give methylprednisolone within 8 hours of injury: 30 mg/kg load over first 15–30 min followed by 5.4 mg/kg/hr for next 23 hours.
  - Be aware that steroids may make diagnosis more difficult, but do not delay for this reason.
  - Be aware that no children were included in the initial study and that use remains somewhat controversial.

# ACUTE WEAKNESS

## Methods of Characterizing Weakness

- Consider region (hemiplegia, diplegia, quadriplegia, facial involvement).
- Consider time course (acute, subacute, or chronic).
- Attempt to localize (central nervous system, spinal cord, nerve, neuromuscular junction, muscle).
- Determine origin of weakness.
  - UMN signs are hyperreflexia, spasticity, and Babinski sign; weakness may be more prominent in the upper extremity extensors and lower extremity flexors.
  - LMN signs are hyporeflexia, hypotonicity, fasciculations, weakness, and atrophy.
- Ataxia is primarily cerebellar but can also originate from hemispheric lesions.
- Further consider systemic disease, especially sickle cell, cardiac defects, and coagulopathies.
- History of trauma should prompt consideration of bleeding and arterial dissection.

## Features Helpful for Localization

- Central nervous system
  - Hemiplegia typical in middle cerebral artery infarct (arm > face = leg)
  - Bilateral cortical involvement nearly always depresses mental status
  - "Neighborhood" signs (e.g., CN involvement) nearly always present with UMN signs indicative of brainstem injury. Remember a Bell palsy results in weakness in the ipsilateral entire half of the face, and weakness without facial involvement should prompt consideration of the brainstem and spinal cord.
- Spinal cord: back or neck pain, sensory level, or bowel or bladder changes
  - Corticospinal tract involvement results in UMN signs below the lesion (may not be present in acute injury).
  - Anterior horn cell or nerve root involvement results in LMN signs.
- Neuropathy: weakness is greater distal than proximal, and areflexia is more likely than in myopathy.
- Neuromuscular junction: often facial involvement with bulbar symptoms, history of fatigability, and evidence of muscle fatigue on examination. Tensilon testing is rarely used.
- Myopathy: flaccid weakness, proximal greater than distal, depressed or absent reflexes; may have elevation of serum creatine kinase, hypertrophy, or myotonia

## Differential Diagnosis Based on Localization

- Central nervous system: stroke, metabolic abnormality, hypoxic ischemic injury (i.e., watershed involving bilateral hemispheres), infection, demyelinating disease, reversible posterior leukoencephalopathy, complicated/hemiplegic migraine, alternating hemiplegia of childhood
- Spinal cord: trauma, tumor, transverse myelitis, demyelinating disease, stroke, vascular malformation, epidural abscess or hematoma, infection (i.e., enteroviral infection such as poliomyelitis), disk protrusion, atlantoaxial subluxation (see section on spinal cord compression)
- Radiculopathy/neuropathy: Guillain-Barré syndrome, acute intermittent porphyria, heavy metal intoxication, drugs, Bell palsy, nerve impingement, Wegner, Churg-Strauss, vasculitis
- Neuromuscular junction: myasthenia gravis, botulism, tick paralysis
- Myopathy: polymyositis, dermatomyositis, rhabdomyolysis (multiple causes, often viral and drugs), periodic paralysis

## Diagnosis

- All cases: a thorough neurologic examination and complete systemic examination guides workup and treatment.

- Central nervous system and spinal cord
    - MRI is best, although CT is most expedient and should be used when MRI is not immediately available.
    - Remember that diagnosis of subarachnoid hemorrhage may require LP, because 5%–10% of cases are missed on CT scan. If an infarct is seen, a complete metabolic, hematologic, and cardiac workup is generally undertaken.
- Neuropathy: nerve conduction studies, electromyography (EMG), LP to evaluate for albuminocytologic dissociation in Guillain-Barré syndrome, peripheral neuropathy antibody panel, nerve biopsy
- Neuromuscular junction: repetitive nerve stimulation studies, EMG, acetylcholine receptor antibodies, Tensilon test (generally discouraged), or trial of anticholinesterase inhibitor
- Myopathy: serum creatine kinase, nerve conduction studies, EMG, muscle biopsy

## Selected Disorders

### Stroke
- This diagnosis should be considered in any acute neurologic condition. In neonates, any change in neurologic function should prompt a consideration of infarct.
- Approximately 8 per 100,000 children per year are affected.
- Causes are numerous, but general categories to consider include trauma, arteriopathies, vasospasm, vasculitis, systemic vascular disease, hematologic disorders including neoplasia, prothrombotic states both acquired and congenital, metabolic disorders including mitochondrial and Fabry disease, and congenital and acquired heart disease.
- Caution: up to 15% of children with known congenital cardiac defects and stroke also have other definable risk factors such as a prothrombotic state. So, the workup of a stroke in a child with congenital cardiac disease should include a search for other causes.
- The most common presentation involves motor weakness, but a stroke can include loss of any other neurologic function, including sensory abilities, language, or vision.
- There is typically a loss of function, not a gain. However, up to 48% of strokes present with seizures.
- Diagnosis is clinical. However, MRI with diffusion sequences and magnetic resonance angiography to evaluate for dissection or vasculopathy is often revealing.
- Optimal **treatment** continues to evolve.
    - Consider admission to an intensive care unit (ICU), permissive hypertension that allows blood pressure to be moderately elevated early after acute stroke, prevention of hypoglycemia, aggressive treatment of fevers, use of isotonic fluids (to prevent worsening of cerebral edema), and close monitoring.
    - There are no randomized controlled trials in children regarding anticoagulation or antiplatelet therapy. However, neonates with stroke have low risk of recurrence; hence, aspirin is not routinely recommended. Older children have a recurrence risk of 7%–20%, so aspirin should be considered.
    - More aggressive therapy such as anticoagulation and endovascular procedures is more controversial.

### Guillain-Barré Syndrome
- Also called acute inflammatory demyelinating polyradiculoneuropathy
- An antecedent viral infection (Epstein-Barr virus [EBV], cytomegalovirus [CMV], *Campylobacter jejuni*) occurs in many cases.
- Hallmark features include ascending weakness and areflexia.
- Symmetric weakness reaches its nadir by 2 weeks in 50% of patients.
- Autonomic dysfunction is common.
- Pain, extreme enough to mimic encephalopathy, can be a significant part of the presentation in young children.
- Diagnosis is suggested by the following:
    - Cerebrospinal fluid (CSF) albuminocytologic dissociation (protein value elevated, cell count typically normal)

- Nerve conduction studies may demonstrate either axonal or demyelinating neuropathy, although these changes may take between 1 and 2 weeks to develop. (Axonal has a worse prognosis for recovery.)
- Serum for EBV and CMV antibodies
- Loose stools for culture (for *C. jejuni*)
- Serum for peripheral neuropathy antibody panel (before giving intravenous immune globulin [IVIG])

- Treatment is recommended for patients too weak to ambulate independently.
- Treatment of choice: IVIG
  - Pretreat with acetaminophen and diphenhydramine.
  - IVIG may cause anaphylaxis in individuals with immunoglobulin A (IgA) deficiency. Consider sending Ig levels before treatment.
  - Plasma exchange is also effective.

- Intubation may be necessary for respiratory weakness. Follow respiratory function closely with forced vital capacity (FVC) and negative inspiratory function (NIF), particularly during the first few days of illness when weakness may progress most rapidly. Intubation may be necessary if FVC falls to 50% of normal or if NIF is low.
- Monitor for vasomotor instability (i.e., labile blood pressures), but treat cautiously.

### Botulism
- The infantile form results from ingestion and colonization of *Clostridium botulinum*, whereas all others result from ingestion of the toxin produced by this organism.
- Diplopia, dysarthria, dysphagia, and vertigo may be associated with flaccid weakness. Ophthalmoplegia may spare pupils.
- Repetitive nerve stimulation gives incremental response but is not always present.
- Treatment consists of supportive care, and in select cases botulism immune globulin may be used.

### Tick Paralysis
- The cause of this disease is toxin exuded from a tick.
- Ocular and pupillary abnormalities are common. Areflexia may also occur.
- This disorder is differentiated from Guillain-Barré syndrome by descending rather than ascending paralysis.
- Treatment requires removal of the tick.
- Assisted ventilation is frequently necessary in cases of respiratory paralysis.

### Transverse Myelitis
- Sudden demyelination of spinal cord (often thoracic) with maximal weakness within days is characteristic. In addition to weakness, sensory deficits, areflexia or hyperreflexia, and bowel and bladder involvement are typically present.
- The disease may be asymmetric and painful.
- In adolescents consider multiple sclerosis, but there are many causes, including infectious/parainfectious (especially mycoplasma), vascular, and autoimmune.
- An MRI may show area of demyelination. An LP may show elevated CSF protein.
- Treatment involves IV methylprednisolone followed by oral steroid taper and supportive care.

## THE HYPOTONIC INFANT

- Recall that tone increases with gestational age (before 28 weeks gestation, extremities held in extension; by term all held in flexion).

### Localizing the Lesion

- Central nervous system: often with depressed mental status, poor initial feeding, UMN findings such as weakness, hyperreflexia, developing spasticity, differential involvement of axial and appendicular muscle, seizures (common)

■ Spinal cord: UMN or LMN findings; with anterior horn cell involvement, fasciculations, atrophy, mental status preserved. In a hypotonic, weak infant with a smile and good interaction, consider spinal cord involvement.
■ Neuropathy: LMN findings
■ Neuromuscular junction: facial involvement common, fatigability, and poor feeding
■ Myopathy: diffuse weakness that may involve face, atrophy

## Differential Diagnosis Based on Localization

■ Central nervous system: hypoxic-ischemic encephalopathy, kernicterus, hypothyroidism, central nervous system (CNS) malformation, congenital infection, metabolic abnormality, mitochondrial disorder, chromosomal abnormality (i.e., trisomy 21), Angelman syndrome, Prader-Willi syndrome
■ Spinal cord: spinal muscular atrophy (anterior horn cell)
■ Neuropathy: congenital demyelinating neuropathy
■ Neuromuscular junction: botulism, familial neonatal myasthenia, congenital myasthenic syndrome
■ Myopathy: congenital muscular dystrophy, congenital myopathy, myotonic dystrophy

## Diagnosis

■ Central nervous system: MRI brain, chromosomes, serum lactate, pyruvate, methylation studies for Prader-Willi and Angelman syndromes, thyroid-stimulating hormone, and free thyroxine
■ Spinal cord: SMN gene test, MRI of spine, EMG/nerve conduction study
■ Neuropathy: nerve conduction studies, EMG
■ Neuromuscular junction: repetitive nerve stimulation, acetylcholine receptor antibodies, trial of anticholinesterase inhibitor
■ Myopathy: serum creatine kinase, nerve conduction studies, EMG, muscle biopsy, gene test for Duchenne muscular dystrophy, myotonic dystrophy, or other specific muscle disorder

## Specific Disorders

### Spinal Muscular Atrophy
■ Condition involves progressive loss of anterior horn cells in spinal cord and brainstem.
■ Type is based on maximal ability.
  ■ Type I: unable to ever sit independently (present earlier in infancy)
  ■ Type II: unable to stand or walk
  ■ Type III: able to stand

■ Characteristic signs are fasciculations of tongue, fine hand tremor, generalized hypotonia, and bright alert infant with relative preservation of facial strength.
■ The course is complicated by poor feeding and respiratory weakness, with death typically by 2 years of age.
■ Diagnosis is made by test for deletions in SMN gene.
■ Treatment is supportive, although there is suggestion that valproate (Depakote) may be helpful.

### Familial Infantile Myasthenia
■ Inherited defect of synaptic transmission
■ Not associated with acetylcholine receptor antibodies
■ Characterized by respiratory insufficiency and feeding difficulty
■ Diagnosed by specialized nerve conduction study testing and by response to acetylcholinesterase inhibitor

### Transitory Neonatal Myasthenia
■ Observed in 10%–15% of infants of mothers with myasthenia
■ Characterized by generalized hypotonia and feeding difficulties
■ Diagnosed by identification of acetylcholine receptor antibodies and response to acetylcholinesterase inhibitor

- Treatment
  - Exchange transfusion or if severe, supportive care
  - Resolves over time

*Prader-Willi Syndrome*
- Characterized by hypotonia, hypogonadism, feeding problems in infancy (followed by obesity in adulthood)
- Diagnosed by study of chromosome 15 for both deletion and methylation status. Methylation studies must be considered because 5%–10% of cases may result from uniparental disomy from the father.

*Myotonic Dystrophy*
- This results from amplification of trinucleotide repeat with anticipation.
- Mothers of severely affected infants generally have myotonia (prolonged muscle relaxation), abnormal facies, and cataracts.
- Infants have hypotonia and generalized weakness (often affecting respiratory and swallowing ability in severely affected infants).
- Diagnosis is by EMG showing myotonia and a gene test for expansion of trinucleotide repeats.

## PAROXYSMAL DISORDERS ("SPELLS")

- Consider evaluating for the most life-threatening causes (i.e., cardiac) first. History is the most helpful diagnostic tool. Think about getting a videotape of the events, with electroencephalogram (EEG) if possible.
- Differential diagnosis (extensive)
  - Cardiac arrhythmias, apnea, syncope, transient ischemic attack/cerebral hypoperfusion
  - Seizure
  - Jitteriness, startle responses, breath-holding spell
  - Night terrors, narcolepsy-cataplexy, benign nocturnal myoclonus
  - Paroxysmal dystonias, dyskinetic syndromes, tic disorder (Tourette syndrome), stereotypies
  - Migraine or migraine variant (cyclic vomiting, basilar migraine), benign paroxysmal vertigo

## HEADACHE/MIGRAINE

### Definition

- There are multiple types of headache, of which migraine is one. The most important factor in treatment is appropriate diagnosis. One would not want to erroneously diagnose a headache associated with subarachnoid hemorrhage a migraine.
- The criteria for the diagnosis of pediatric migraine without aura is the occurrence of five attacks fulfilling the following features:
  - Headache attack lasting 1–72 hours
  - Headache has at least two of the following four features:
    - Either bilateral or unilateral (frontal/temporal) location
    - Pulsating quality
    - Moderate to severe intensity
    - Aggravated by routine physical activities
  - At least one of the following accompanies headache:
    - Nausea and/or vomiting
    - Photophobia and phonophobia (may be inferred from their behavior)

### History and Physical Examination

- Palpate the head: look for evidence of trauma, pain over temporal artery, cutaneous allodynia, temporomandibular joint dysfunction.

- CNs: mainly eye and funduscopic examination—look for ocular palsies, papilledema, hemorrhage, optic pallor, and visual field cut.
- Motor and sensory: any deficits?
- Cerebellar: ataxia can be an important clue to basilar migraine or stroke.
- Warning flags: repetitive worsening headaches, "worst headache of my life," hypertension, temporal artery tenderness, papilledema, retinal hemorrhages, any focal deficit, or alternating consciousness

## Treatment

- In pediatrics, most headaches can be controlled with nonsteroidal anti-inflammatory drugs (NSAIDs), but be aware of NSAID overuse induced headaches and chronic daily headaches. These require a different treatment plan than that outlined below.
- In the emergency department, after thorough assessment, we recommend IV fluids, IV NSAIDs (ketorolac [Toradol]) as first-line treatment. Some authors advocate use of antiemetics such as metoclopramide (Reglan), although rates of dystonic reaction can reach 25%.
- If the first-line therapy fails or the patient is triptan-naive, has no contraindications to triptan use (i.e., hypertension, focal deficit, sickle cell), and does not already have cutaneous allodynia, we use a short-acting triptan.
- If the patient has already taken a triptan that day, has cutaneous allodynia, has a contraindication, or is many hours into the headache, then opioids tend to work better.
- If opioids or triptans fail, then the patient will likely need to be admitted for IV therapy with either dihydroergotamine (DHE), valproic acid, or steroids, depending on patient characteristics. Dosing for these is variable, but ranges are DHE 0.2–1 mg t.i.d., valproic acid 15–18 mg/kg/day t.i.d., and IV methylprednisone 0.5–2 mg/kg/day.
- Remember to get a urine human chorionic gonadotropin in all women because all of these medications except opioids are relatively contraindicated in pregnancy.

# SEIZURES

## Definition and Classification

- Seizure occurs with excessive electrical discharge of cerebral neurons, manifested as transient impairment of function of the region(s) that are involved—motor, sensory, cognitive (language), visual, and/or auditory.
- Many disorders can mimic seizures (see "Paroxysmal Disorders" section). A history of early clinical features and any focal features (i.e., head or eye deviation, dystonic posturing of limbs, automatisms) should be obtained from observers.
- Seizure classification according to clinical type (Table 19-1)

## Etiology

- Most often seizures are idiopathic; genetic; related to a syndrome, drug overdose, trauma, hemorrhage, tumor, or infection; a medication side effect; or metabolic (see Chapter 16, Genetic Diseases for further information).
- In a patient with known epilepsy, the cause is often noncompliance or missed doses of antiepileptic medication, concurrent illness, sleep deprivation, or an unknown factor, but if he or she is febrile, serious infection must be excluded.

## Treatment

- Management of first-time afebrile seizure
  - Clinical laboratory studies: $Ca^{2+}$, $Mg^{2+}$, phosphorus, and glucose are not typically indicated but may be necessary in some situations.
  - EEG is useful to help diagnosis and to classify seizure type (focal discharges versus generalized). Note that a normal EEG does not rule out seizures or epilepsy.
  - Brain MRI should be considered for any focal seizure but is not indicated for true generalized seizures.

| TABLE 19–1 | Classification of Seizures By Clinical Type |
|---|---|

Partial (focal) seizures
  Simple partial seizures (consciousness not impaired)
    With motor symptoms
    With somatosensory or special sensory symptoms (tingling, flashes, buzzing)
    With autonomic symptoms or signs (e.g., epigastric sensation, piloerection, mydriasis)
    With psychic symptoms (e.g., fear, déjà-vu)
  Complex partial seizures (impairment of consciousness and often automatisms)
    Unimpaired consciousness onset followed by impairment of consciousness
    Impaired consciousness at onset
  Partial onset with secondary generalization
    Simple partial seizures evolving to generalized seizures
    Complex partial seizures evolving to generalized seizures
    Simple partial seizures evolving to complex partial and further evolving to generalized seizures
Generalized seizures (convulsive or nonconvulsive)
  Absence seizures (impairment of consciousness alone or with mild clonic, atonic, or tonic component and automatisms).
  Myoclonic
  Clonic
  Tonic
  Tonic-clonic
  Atonic

*Source:* Commission on Classification and Terminology of the International League against Epilepsy. Proposal for revised clinical and electroencephalographic classification of epileptic seizures. Epilepsia 1981;22(4):489–501.

- If the seizure stops spontaneously after 5 minutes or less, await EEG, MRI, and laboratory studies before determining treatment. If no cause is found, most first seizures are not treated with antiepileptic medication. Recall that epilepsy is defined as two or more unprovoked seizures and that most neurologists will not commit a patient to antiepileptic medication for one isolated seizure.
- Consider rectal diazepam (Diastat) for home use for any child with history of status epilepticus.
- Seizure precautions: no swimming except with supervision in clean pool, encourage showers instead of baths, no activities involving heights or open fires, and no driving until seizure-free for at least 6 months (this varies state to state)

# FEBRILE SEIZURES

## Definitions

- Febrile seizures are seizures occurring in children >1 month of age and are associated with febrile illness not caused by an infection of the CNS. Seizures do not meet criteria for other acute symptomatic seizures. Patients have no previous neonatal seizures or previous unprovoked seizures.
- **Simple febrile seizures** are generalized in onset, are <10–15 minutes, *and* do not recur within 24 hours. They constitute 85% of all febrile seizures.
- **Complex febrile seizures** are focal in nature, last >10–15 minutes, *or* recur within 24 hours.

## Epidemiology

- The most common age for febrile seizures is 6 months to 3 years; they are rare after 6 years of age.

- Overall risk in children is 2%–5%; if parent or sibling has had febrile seizures, the risk is 10%–20%.
- The seizures may occur early in illness as a temperature rises or even before a fever/illness is recognized.
- Risk of febrile seizure recurrence is 25%–30%. Risk factors for recurrence:
    - First febrile seizure before 1 year
    - Febrile seizures following low-grade fevers
    - Family history of febrile seizures
    - Day care attendance
    - Epilepsy in first-degree relatives, complex febrile seizures, or neurodevelopmental abnormalities
- Risk of epilepsy later in life after febrile seizure (overall 2%–4%). Risk factors for eventual epilepsy:
    - Complex febrile seizures (raise recurrence risk two-fold)
    - Neurodevelopmental abnormalities, including abnormal examination
    - Afebrile seizures in first-degree relatives
    - Recurrent febrile seizures

## Treatment

- Management of first febrile seizure
    - If seizure lasts >5 minutes, treat as status epilepticus (see later discussion).
    - Recommend LP for all infants <1 year of age. Strongly consider LP for infants 12–18 months (neurologists typically recommend LP for every first febrile seizure under age 18 months because meningeal signs are unreliable at <18–24 months of age) and for any child with meningeal signs (neck stiffness, Kernig sign).
    - Consider brain MRI (nonurgent) for child with seizures with focal features.
    - Consider laboratory blood tests based on clinical discretion (i.e., CBC, $Mg^{2+}$, phosphorus, $Ca^{2+}$, electrolytes).
    - EEG is not routinely recommended.
- Prophylactic treatment is not typically recommended because most febrile seizures are self-limited and medications are not without risks. If an antiepileptic agent is selected, valproate and phenobarbital are effective; phenytoin, carbamazepine, and antipyretics are ineffective.
- Rectal diazepam should be prescribed for children with history of prolonged or multiple seizures so that it may be given acutely for seizures lasting >5 minutes.

# STATUS EPILEPTICUS

## General Principles

- Although defined as any seizure (or group of seizures without recovery to baseline) lasting >30 minutes, pharmacologic treatment of seizures is typically required for any seizure >5 minutes in duration.
- Status epilepticus is an **emergency**. All medications are more effective when used early. Order the next anticipated medication immediately after giving the first.
- Prognosis is generally related to underlying medical diagnosis. Overall mortality is 1%–3%.

## Treatment

- First 5 minutes
    - Airway, breathing, circulation, or ABCs (turn to side, do not place anything in mouth, oxygen mask often placed but typically unnecessary)
    - Establish IV access (but also consider intraocular, rectal, and intrabuccal routes as alternatives)
    - Check glucose, electrolytes, $Mg^{2+}$, $PO_4$, $Ca^{2+}$, antiepileptic drug levels

- Administer IV lorazepam (0.05–0.1 mg/kg; maximum dose 4–6 mg) or IV diazepam (0.1–0.3 mg/kg) from minute 2–5. Doses may be given up to 3 times separated by 2 minutes each.
- If the IV route is unavailable, give rectal diazepam (age 1–5 years: 0.5 mg/kg; 6–11 years: 0.3 mg/kg; $12^+$ years: 0.2 mg/kg). This takes approximately 10–15 minutes to achieve effective blood levels, so do not redose before 15 minutes.
- 6–15 minutes
  - Administer long-acting antiepileptic drug (fosphenytoin 20 mg/kg at maximum rate 150 mg/min or phenobarbital 20 mg/kg).
  - Reexamine patient, follow blood pressure.

- 16–30 minutes
  - If seizure continues 15–20 minutes after completing long-acting antiepileptic drug load, give additional 10 mg/kg fosphenytoin *or* 10 mg/kg phenobarbital.
  - If seizure has clinically stopped, consider possibility of nonconvulsive status if patient is not waking or arousable.

- After 30 minutes
  - Arrange an ICU bed.
  - Consider intubation and central lines.
  - Order a "stat" EEG.
  - Consider probable treatment with pentobarbital or other agent to induce pharmacologic coma.

- Treatment notes:
  - If the patient known to have juvenile myoclonic epilepsy (JME), do not give fosphenytoin. Consider IV valproate (Depacon) after initial benzodiazepine. Also, if seizures worsen after fosphenytoin, consider JME and switch to either valproate or phenobarbital.
  - Refractory status typically has an underlying etiology that needs to be addressed; look for abnormal electrolytes, infection, hemorrhage, stroke, genetic or metabolic syndrome, rarely pseudoseizures.

# GROWTH AND DEVELOPMENT ISSUES

## Primitive Reflexes

- Palmar grasp: present from birth to 2–4 months
  - Plantar grasp: present birth until 8 months
  - Moro: birth until 4–6 months
  - Tonic neck: birth until able to roll over (3–6 months)
  - Galant (ipsilateral trunk curvature with stroking along spine): birth until 2–3 months

## Growth Goals in the Newborn

- Infants may lose weight (5%–10% of birth weight) during the first week of life.
  - Preterm infants: ↑ weight >15 g/kg/day, length 0.8–1.1 cm/wk, and OFC 0.5–0.8 cm/wk (first month of life)
  - Full-term infants: ↑ weight 20–30 g/day, length 0.66 cm/wk, and OFC 0.33 cm/wk (first month)

## Growth

- OFC: should increase 2 cm/mo from 0–3 months, then 1 cm/mo from 3–6 months, and then 0.5 cm/mo until 1 year. OFC should increase by 2 cm from 1–2 years.
- Weight: should increase approximately 30 gm/day for the first 3 months. Birth weight should double by 5 months and triple by 1 year. Until puberty, the usual gain after 2 years is 5 lb/year.

- Height: should increase by 50% in the first year and double by 4 years. Until the adolescent growth spurt, the annual increase in height is 5 cm/year.
- Dentition: central incisors at 6 months, lateral incisors at 8 months, first molars at 14 months, canines at 19 months, and second molars at 24 months

## Development

- Although it is important during routine well-child checkups to evaluate development closely, you usually are not able to do this on a busy ward rotation.
- Lists of what constitutes normal development are extensive (Table 19-2). Using this table, you can focus on assessing some developmental skills during an admission history and physical.

| TABLE 19-2 | Normal Developmental Skills According to Age | | |
|---|---|---|---|
| Age | Gross motor | Fine motor | Cognitive and languages |
| 1 mo | Head up while prone | Hands fisted | Fixes and follows |
| 2 mo | Chest up in prone | Hands unfisted 50% of the time, grasps rattle placed in hand | Regards speaker, social smile, coos |
| 4 mo | Up on hands in prone, rolls front to back, no head lag | Reaches for and retains objects in hand, hand to midline | Orients to voice, laughs, vocalizes when speaker stops talking |
| 6 mo | Sits with support, rolls back to front | Transfers hand-hand | Discriminates strangers, consonant babbling |
| 7 mo | Sits without support, supports weight while standing, beginning commando crawl | | Mimics speaker's voice |
| 9 mo | Sits well, pulls to stand, creeps on hands and knees | Brings two toys together, finger feeds | Peek-a-boo, uncovers hidden objects, says "dada" and "mama," indiscriminately explores by poking, understands "no," orients to name |
| 12 mo | Cruises, walks with support, may take independent steps | Pincer grasp—objects held between fingertips | Follows command with gesture, immature jargoning, says "dada/mama" appropriately |
| 15 mo | Walks alone, creeps up stairs | Builds tower of two cubes, imitates scribble | Follows simple commands, names one object, says "no" meaningfully, points to one or two body parts |

*(continued)*

| TABLE 19-2 | Normal Developmental Skills According to Age *(Continued)* |
|---|---|

| Age | Gross motor | Fine motor | Cognitive and languages |
|---|---|---|---|
| 18 mo | Throws ball while standing, walks up stairs with hand held, sits in chair | Builds tower of three to four cubes, initiates scribbling | Points to three body parts and to self, 10–25 words |
| 24 mo | Jumps in place, kicks ball, throws overhand, walks up and down stairs holding rail | Imitates vertical stroke, builds tower of six cubes | Follows two-step commands, 50+ words, refers to self by name, two word phrases, uses pronouns, points to six body parts |
| 3 yr | Pedals a tricycle, alternates feet ascending stairs | Builds tower of nine cubes, independent eating, copies circle | Gives full name, knows age and sex, counts to three, recognizes colors, toilet trained |
| 4 yr | Alternates feet descending stairs, hops on one foot | Builds tower of 10 cubes, able to cut and paste, copies a cross | Uses "I" correctly, dresses and undresses self with supervision, knows colors |
| 5 yr | Skips, walks on tiptoes | Copies a triangle | Identifies coins, names four to five colors, can tell age and birthday |
| 6 yr | Tandem walk | Tie shoes, comb hair | Knows left vs right, days of the week, own telephone number |
| 7 yr | Rides bicycle | Bathe alone | Tells time to the half hour |
| 8 yr | Reverse tandem walk | | Tells time within 5 minutes, knows the months of the year |

## Suggested Readings

AAN Practice Parameter. First afebrile seizure. Neurology 2000;55:616–623.

Adams C. Neonatal hypotonia. In: Bernard Maria, ed. Current Management in Child Neurology. Canada: BC Decker Inc: 455–460.

Knudsen FU. Febrile seizures: treatment and prognosis. Epilepsia 2000 Jan;41(1):2–9.

Larsen G, Goldstein B. Increased intracranial pressure, Peds Rev 1999;20(7):234.

Mitchell WG. Status epilepticus and acute serial seizures in children. J Child Neurol 2002 Jan;17 Suppl 1:S36–43.

Practice Parameter. Febrile seizure. Pediatrics 1996;97(5):769–773.

Proctor MR. Spinal cord injury. Crit Care Med 2002 Nov;30(11 Suppl):S489–499.

deVeber G, Arterial ischemic strokes in infants and children: an overview of current approaches. Semin Thromb Hemost 2003 Dec;29(6):567–573.

## CROUP OR VIRAL LARYNGOTRACHEOBRONCHITIS

### Definition and Epidemiology

- Croup or viral laryngotracheobronchitis is an acute inflammation of the entire airway, mainly in the glottis and subglottic area, resulting in airway narrowing, obstruction, and voice loss. Therefore, it has generally been described as a triad of hoarse voice, harsh barking cough, and inspiratory stridor.
- Typically, the condition affects younger children (6–36 months), with a peak incidence at 2 years of age. It is the most common cause of acute upper airway obstruction in young children; a reported 3% of children experience it before 6 years of age.
- Seasonal outbreaks have been described in the fall and winter, although it may occur year round in some areas.
- Males are more often affected than females.

### Etiology and Pathophysiology

- Viral infection is the predominant etiology; parainfluenza (types 1, 2, and 3) is the most common agent. Other common viral agents are respiratory syncytial virus (RSV) and influenza. Less commonly encountered viruses include adenovirus, rhinovirus, enterovirus, and measles virus.
- *Mycoplasma pneumoniae* is one of the few bacterial microorganisms that has been reported as an etiologic agent.
- In children, the larynx is very narrow and is comprised by the rigid ring of the cricoid cartilage; therefore, a viral infection causing inflammation of this area leads to airway edema and subsequent obstruction. This obstruction results in the classic symptoms of stridor and cough.

### Clinical Presentation

- Croup usually presents initially with a coryzal prodrome (1–4 days).
- Common symptoms include clear rhinorrhea, low-grade temperature, and mild tachypnea followed by barking cough, hoarseness, and stridor.
- Obstructive symptoms occur most commonly at night.
- Severity of airway narrowing may be determined by the presence of stridor at rest, tachypnea, retractions, tracheal tug, cyanosis, and pallor, as well as decreased breath sounds, which indicate critical narrowing.

### Diagnosis

- The diagnosis is clinical.
- Radiography of the neck is not necessary but may show the typical "steeple sign" or subglottic narrowing. Radiographic appearance does not correlate with disease severity.
- Radiographs should be obtained if there is concern about the diagnosis, and they may distinguish croup from other causes of upper airway obstruction such as epiglottitis.
- Oxygen saturations and arterial blood gases should be obtained if hypoxemia, which may be indicated by restlessness, altered mental status, and cyanosis, is a concern.

- The differential diagnosis includes epiglottitis (but the patient is usually toxic-appearing), spasmodic croup (no viral prodrome and mostly in atopic children), bacterial tracheitis, laryngitis, foreign body, and laryngospasm.

## Treatment

- A few clinical scoring systems that guide assessment and management have been described in the literature. The most commonly used is the Westley score system, which is described below:
  - Scores are given based on the presence of stridor (none 0, when agitated 1, at rest 2), retractions (none 0, mild 1, moderate 2, severe 3), level of air entry (normal 0, decreased 1, markedly decreased 2), and cyanosis in room air (none 0, with agitation 4, at rest 5), and level of consciousness (normal 0, disoriented 5).
  - Mild croup is described as scores 1–2, moderate croup as scores 3–8, and severe croup as scores >8, with consideration of pharmacologic therapy and hospitalization in moderate and severe cases.
- In general, management of patients without signs of severe airway narrowing or stridor at rest may be managed on an outpatient basis after appropriate observation. Parents should be reassured and instructed about signs of worsening respiratory distress.
- Management strategies include use of cool-mist vaporizer, avoidance of cold air exposure when riding in a motor vehicle, and use of steam inhalation, although these methods are anecdotal and have not proved beneficial during several studies.
- General supportive measures such as increased fluid intake, decreased handling, and careful observation are usually recommended.
- For children with evidence of stridor at rest and/or signs of moderate to severe airway compromise, pharmacologic therapy is beneficial.
  - Nebulized racemic epinephrine acts by reducing vascular permeability of the airway epithelium; therefore, diminishing airway edema and improving airway caliber by decreasing resistance to airflow.
  - It should be administered at doses of 0.25–0.5 mL along with humidified oxygen as needed. If no response is elicited after the first treatment, the dose may be repeated.
  - The patient may return to pretreatment state 30–60 minutes after a dose, and therefore they should be observed for at least 2 hours.
- Systemic corticosteroids are effective in reducing symptoms within 6 hours and for at least 12 hours after initial treatment.
  - Dexamethasone 0.6 mg/kg/dose IM, IV, PO is the glucocorticoid most commonly used, but prednisolone 1–2 mg/kg/dose PO has also been described.
  - Studies comparing nebulized corticosteroids and systemic corticosteroids have proven the nebulized agents to be inferior.

# EPIGLOTTITIS

## Definition and Epidemiology

- Epiglottitis is an acute infectious supraglottic obstruction that may rapidly lead to life-threatening airway obstruction. It is a true pediatric emergency.
- It may affect children of all ages, with a peak about 3–6 years of age, although its incidence has declined significantly since *Haemophilus influenzae* type B immunization was enforced in 1998.

## Etiology and Pathophysiology

- Causative agents in the postvaccine era include group A *Streptococcus, Staphylococcus, Candida albicans*, and *Pneumococcus*. Infections with *H. influenzae* type B are still reported.

■ Direct invasion by the inciting agent causes inflammation of the epiglottis, aryepiglottic folds, ventricular bands, and arytenoids. Subsequently, there is accumulation of inflammatory cells and edema fluid where the stratified squamous epithelium is loosely adherent to the anterior surface and the superior third of the posterior portion of the epiglottis.

■ Diffuse infiltration with polymorphonuclear leukocytes, hemorrhage, edema, and fibrin deposition occurs. Microabscesses may form. As the edema increases, the epiglottis curls posteriorly and inferiorly. This causes airway obstruction.

■ Inspiration tends to draw the inflamed supraglottic ring into the laryngeal inlet.

## Clinical Presentation

■ Epiglottitis is a rapidly progressing illness in previously healthy individuals. Patients are usually anxious, toxic-appearing, and assume the classic "tripod position" (forward-leaning posture with bracing arms and extension of the neck that allows for maximal air entry).

■ Other symptoms typically present are high fever, muffled or absent voice ("hot potato"), sore throat, drooling, inspiratory stridor, dysphagia, protruded jaw, and extended neck.

## Diagnosis

■ Presumptive diagnosis should be made on clinical grounds.

■ If patient is in little distress, and the diagnosis is unclear, a lateral neck radiograph may be obtained, which shows the classical thumbprint sign that represents a swollen epiglottis and aryepiglottic folds. Radiographs can be normal in 20% of the patients.

■ The definitive diagnosis requires direct visualization of a red swollen epiglottis under laryngoscopy, but this examination should be attempted only in a controlled setting in collaboration with an anesthesiologist and an otolaryngologist.

■ The differential diagnosis includes foreign body aspiration, anaphylactic reaction, angioneurotic edema, caustic ingestion, thermal injury, inhalation injury, and laryngotracheobronchial and retropharyngeal infection.

## Treatment

■ Airway stabilization and maintenance must be performed quickly and early in the course.

■ Oxygen should be administered at the minimal sign of distress.

■ Stimulation and patient disturbance should be minimized to avoid complete obstruction.

■ An artificial airway should be available next to the patient, and it should always be ready for use.

■ After appropriate management of the airway has been established, antibiotic therapy should be initiated. Therapy of choice is broad-spectrum intravenous (IV) antibiotics against β-lactamase-producing pathogens.

■ Although IV steroids are frequently administered for the management of airway inflammation, no controlled studies exist to justify this approach.

# BACTERIAL TRACHEITIS

## Definition and Epidemiology

■ This acute bacterial infection of the trachea often also involves the larynx and bronchi. It has been called bacterial laryngotracheobronchitis and pseudomembranous croup.

■ A cause of acute airway obstruction, this condition may potentially be life threatening.

■ Most patients are <3 years of age (usually 3 months to 2 years), although older children may be affected. There are no clear sex differences in incidence or severity.

■ There seems to be no seasonal preferences.

### Etiology and Pathophysiology

- The most common cause is *Staphylococcus aureus*, but other encountered agents are *H. influenzae*, *S. pneumoniae*, and *Moraxella catarrhalis*. Anaerobic organisms have also been reported.
- Invasion of opportunistic bacterial organisms, often following an upper airway viral infection, causes subglottic edema with ulcerations, copious and purulent secretions, and pseudomembrane formation.

### Clinical Presentation

- The typical presentation involves a history of an upper respiratory infection (URI) for approximately 3 days characterized by a low-grade fever and a "brassy" cough. The illness then evolves rapidly with high fever and onset of stridor, resulting in progressive deterioration and development of acute respiratory distress.
- Patients generally appear toxic.
- There is also evidence of purulent airway secretions.

### Diagnosis

- Diagnosis is clinical with classical signs of epiglottitis and croup absent. Direct visualization of the trachea via laryngoscopy demonstrates thick, abundant, and purulent secretions.
- The differential diagnosis includes epiglottitis (although no dysphagia or drooling, and patient may lie flat), croup (although voice is normal and there is a lack of a barky cough), and laryngeal and retropharyngeal abscess.

### Treatment

- Management of the airway is critical with intubation, and assisted ventilation should be strongly considered.
- There is no proven role for bronchodilators or corticosteroids.
- Antimicrobial therapy should be immediately instituted. Choice of therapy includes broad-spectrum antibiotics with antistaphylococcal activity.

## FOREIGN BODY ASPIRATION

### Definition and Epidemiology

- This accidental ingestion occurs commonly in children <5 years of age but has been described at any age.
- Younger children are typically at higher risk because of oral exploration and immaturity of their swallowing functions.
- This situation may be life threatening; it is the leading cause of accidental death by ingestion in younger children.

### Etiology and Pathophysiology

- Ingestion of food and toy parts are aspirated into the airways, causing choking.
  - A foreign body can be localized in the larynx, trachea, or bronchi.
  - Impaction of the larynx is particularly dangerous, although most particles travel well into the airways and lodge in the intrathoracic area.
- The foreign particle provokes localized airway inflammation with mucosal edema, inflammation, and development of granulation tissue. Atelectasis of the area involved and empyema may occur.

### Clinical Presentation

- In general, following a witnessed aspiration or choking episode, patients develop a loud persistent cough along with gagging and stridor. However, the symptoms manifested are largely dependent on the localization of the particle, its size, and its composition.

- Foreign bodies in the larynx may cause hoarseness, aphonia, croupy cough, odynophagia, wheezing, and difficulty breathing, depending on the degree of obstruction.
- Foreign bodies in the trachea can cause what has been described as an audible slap, a palpable thud, and wheezing.
- Foreign bodies in the bronchus usually are manifested by coughing and wheezing.
- Regardless of the position of the foreign body, if the event is unwitnessed and the particle remains lodged in the airway for a prolonged period of time, the patient usually develops a chronic cough with or without wheeze that is often treated as asthma.
- Hemoptysis may be a sign of airway injury.
- There is no fever associated such as in acute infectious airway obstruction.
- Position of the patient has no effect on the degree of airway obstruction, as in epiglottitis.
- Asymmetric findings on chest auscultation may provide a diagnostic clue but should not serve as an exclusion criterion.

### Diagnosis

- A history of the choking event sometimes can be elicited from parents. The diagnosis should also be entertained when a child exhibits unexplained symptoms that fail to respond to standard medical treatment, such as treatment for asthma or antibiotic therapy for a suspected pneumonia.
- Radiography of the upper airway and the chest can be useful to confirm aspiration of a radiopaque particle, but negative, this should not exclude the possibility of foreign body aspiration.
- Inspiratory and expiratory chest films may show a "ball-valve" effect or persistent inflation of the area suspected to be lodging the particle. Other radiographic findings may include persistent unilateral infiltrates or atelectasis.
- If suspicion is high, referral for laryngoscopy and rigid bronchoscopy is often the only method of visualizing (and removing) the foreign body.
- The differential diagnosis includes epiglottitis, viral laryngotracheobronchitis, bacterial tracheitis, asthma, pneumonia, airway malacia, and psychogenic cough.

### Treatment

- Management usually involves removal of the foreign body via bronchoscopy (typically rigid) for appropriate control of the airway.
- There is no established role for antibiotic or corticosteroid use.
- If the particle remains in the airway for a prolonged period of time, potential complications may arise, including bronchial stenosis, distal bronchiectasis, tracheoesophageal fistula, abscess formation, and airway lacerations or perforation.

## BRONCHIOLITIS

### Definition and Epidemiology

- Bronchiolitis is an acute infectious disease of the lower respiratory tract, specifically the small passages in the lungs (bronchioles), usually caused by a viral infection.
- It is usually most prominent during winter and early spring, with annual epidemics in temperate climates. However, sporadic infections can occur year round.
- It accounts for 100,000 hospitalizations per year and about $300 million in healthcare costs per year.
- It occurs in the first 2 years of life (0–24 months) and it peaks at 6 months of age (2–8 months). It is more common in male infants (1.5:1), bottlefed infants, infants living in crowded conditions, and infants with cigarette-smoking mothers.

### Etiology

- Etiology is predominantly viral. The most common source of the virus is a family member with a URI.

- The most common viral agents are:
  - RSV (most common cause [85%])
  - RSV is spread primarily by direct contact (safe >6 feet away). Large droplets survive up to 6 hours on surfaces, and up to 30 minutes in the hands. Therefore, frequent handwashing is essential for infection control. Virus shedding occurs for approximately 3–8 days, but in young infants shedding may last 3–4 weeks.
  - This infection is the leading cause of infant hospitalization and the leading cause of lower respiratory tract infection in infants and small children, with two thirds of the infants infected in their first year and universal infection by 2 years of age. The mortality rate from RSV infection may be as high as 5% in high-risk patients.
  - Reinfection is common because infection does not provide long-lasting immunity.
- Parainfluenza virus (second most common cause)
  - This virus is unstable in the environment, but spread occurs from respiratory secretions.
  - Four serotypes exist. Type 1 (5%–12%) and type 2 (1%–5%) are responsible for outbreaks in the fall, and type 3 (8%–15%) occurs predominantly in the spring to fall. Type 4 is isolated infrequently.
- Adenovirus (causes 3%–10% of cases)
  - Survival outside of the body is prolonged, and transmission can occur via direct contact, the fecal-oral route, and occasionally water. Shedding can occur for months or years.
  - Infection is endemic in all seasons.
  - Type 4 is responsible for acute respiratory distress.
- Influenza (causes 5%–8% of cases). Infection occurs in epidemics during the winter to spring.
- Rhinovirus (causes 3%–8% of the cases)
  - Transmission is by aerosol or direct contact.
  - The infection is endemic in all seasons.
  - Most cases are mild and self-limited, but shedding may last up to 3–4 weeks (peak, 2–7 days).
- *M. pneumoniae* (causes 1%–7% of cases). Infection is endemic in all seasons.
- Enterovirus (causes 1%–5% of cases). Infection usually occurs during the summer to fall.
- Human metapneumovirus (unknown frequency in the United States)
  - Recovered during the winter season
  - Pathophysiology that seems to parallel that of RSV

## Pathophysiology

- Disease occurs by invasion of the smaller bronchioles by the viral particles followed by viral colonization and replication. This causes necrosis of ciliated cells and proliferation of nonciliated cells, causing impaired clearance of secretions, submucosal edema, and congestion, which results in plugging of bronchioles (mucus and debris) and peripheral airway narrowing. The increased respiratory effort is secondary to inflammatory obstruction of the small airways (bronchioles) because of edema.
- These changes are indicated by increased functional residual capacity, decreased compliance, increased airway resistance, and increased physiologic dead space with increased shunt. Therefore, a ventilation-perfusion mismatch with impaired gas exchange occurs, resulting in hypoxia and $CO_2$ retention.
- Infants are particularly more susceptible to severe disease. Their airways are easily plugged by mucus or inflammatory debris because their collateral pathways of ventilation (pores of Cohn and Lambert) are less well developed, have more mucous glands, and are more collapsible in response to pressure changes.

## Clinical Presentation

- Usually, there is a history of exposure to URI within 1 week of onset of illness.
- First symptoms are usually a mild URI (1–4 days), decreased oral intake, and fever with gradual development of respiratory distress. If RSV is the etiology, symptoms usually peak at approximately the fifth day of illness.

- Patients develop a paroxysmal wheezy cough and dyspnea. In mild cases, symptoms last for approximately 1–3 days. Severe cases have a protracted course.
- Pertinent physical examination findings include tachypnea (60–80 breaths/min), hyperexpanded chest, nasal flaring, use of accessory muscles, widespread fine crackles, prolonged expiration, diffuse wheezes, and decreased breath sounds.

## Diagnosis

- Diagnosis is based on clinical presentation.
- Aids to confirm diagnosis and predict the course of the illness include nasopharyngeal swab for viral culture, rapid RSV test (enzyme-linked immunosorbent assay and direct fluorescent antibody), and serology for viral antibodies.
- Routine radiographs are not recommended but may be helpful if suspicious of bacterial pneumonia.
    - Radiographic findings may include hyperinflation, increased anteroposterior chest diameter, peribronchial thickening, diffuse interstitial infiltrates, and atelectasis.
    - There is no correlation between radiographic findings and severity of illness. Ten percent of chest radiographs are normal.
- Complete blood tests and electrolytes are nonspecific and therefore not routinely recommended unless there is suspicion of sepsis or dehydration.
- Pulse oximetry is recommended to assess the degree of hypoxia and response to oxygen.
- Arterial oxygen saturation while feeding has been described as the single best objective predictor of severe disease in the literature. Blood gas sampling is recommended in severe respiratory disease to assess possible impending respiratory failure.
- The differential diagnosis includes asthma, cystic fibrosis, myocarditis, congestive heart failure, foreign body or aspiration of food, pertussis, organophosphate poisoning, bacterial bronchopneumonia, *Mycoplasma* or *Chlamydia* infection, and anatomic abnormality.

## Treatment

- Many therapeutic methods have been described, although most are anecdotal and unproved. In general, the most important foundation for treatment is supportive care, careful monitoring, and minimal handling.
- Hospitalization. Consider admission to the hospital if there is apnea, resting respiratory rate >70 breaths/min, decreased arterial oxygen saturation (<95%), atelectasis on chest radiograph, or ill appearance. Hospitalization may also be appropriate for infants <2–3 months of age or those born at <34–37 weeks gestation; those with a history of chronic lung disease, heart disease, or immunodeficiency; and those with a history of poor feeding.
    - About 2%–7% of infants with severe disease progress to respiratory failure and require intubation. Indications for intubation include severe respiratory distress, apnea, hypoxia or hypercapnia, lethargy, poor perfusion, and metabolic acidosis.
- Nonpharmacologic methods
    - Positioning. Usually it is recommended that the patient be positioned at a sitting angle of 30–40°, with slight head and chest elevation.
    - Assessment of hydration
    - Cool, humidified oxygen supplementation via nasal prongs or face mask and blowby oxygen if agitation is present
- Pharmacologic methods
    - Bronchodilators (albuterol, levalbuterol, racemic epinephrine, ipratropium bromide)
        - Their use is controversial.
        - There has been no significant decrease in hospitalization rate demonstrated with the use of bronchodilator therapy, although some studies have shown improvement in clinical scores such as decreased respiratory rate and increased arterial oxygen saturation. Racemic epinephrine, and potentially albuterol, has been shown to be superior to placebo.
    - Glucocorticoids
        - Use is also controversial.
        - Dexamethasone has shown no beneficial effect in various studies.

- Antibiotics
  - Secondary bacterial infection is uncommon; therefore, routine use of antibiotics is rarely indicated.
  - Use should be considered in persistently febrile young children because there have been some reports in the literature of bacteremia, UTI, and bacterial otitis media in children with bronchiolitis.
- Antivirals
  - Use is controversial.
  - Consider inhaled ribavirin in high-risk infants. Ribavirin has virostatic activity; it interferes with messenger RNA and prevents replication of the virus. The American Academy of Pediatrics recommends its use based on an individual basis in patients with specific conditions such as complicated congenital heart disease, cystic fibrosis, chronic lung disease, underlying immunosuppression, and severe illness, as well as in patients <6 weeks of age.

## Prevention

- Most important method of prevention: frequent handwashing, along with hospital control measures (isolation), and patient education
- Pharmacologic methods
  - RSV intravenous immune globulin (RSV-IVIG)
    - IV RSV-IVIG is used to minimize or prevent morbidity in a select population, usually <24 months with bronchopulmonary dysplasia and premature birth (<35 weeks). The dose is 15 mL/kg IV or 750 mg/kg IV given in five sequential monthly doses beginning before onset of RSV season (November).
    - If RSV-IVIG is given, the mumps-measles-rubella and varicella vaccines should be delayed for 9 months after the last dose.
    - RSV-IVIG is contraindicated in cyanotic congenital heart disease.
  - Palivizumab
    - This agent is recommended in:
      - Children <2 years of age with chronic lung disease who have required therapy for RSV within the previous 6 months
      - Infants born <32 weeks estimated gestational age (EGA)
      - Infants born <28 weeks EGA for the first 12 months of life
      - Infants born between 29 and 32 weeks EGA up to 6 months of age
      - Infants born between 32 and 35 weeks EGA if more than two risk factors are present, such as day care, school-aged siblings, exposure to environmental air pollutants, congenital airway anomalies, severe neuromuscular disease, and/or age <6 months at RSV season
      - Infants <12 months of age with congenital heart disease at risk for severe disease, those receiving medication to control congestive heart failure, as well as those with moderate to severe pulmonary hypertension and cyanotic heart disease
    - Prophylaxis should be initiated before the onset of the RSV season (beginning of November), and it should be terminated at the end of RSV season (beginning of March). Healthcare practitioners should individualize the season according to their area.
    - Palivizumab does not interfere with responses to vaccines.

# CYSTIC FIBROSIS

## Epidemiology

- Cystic fibrosis (CF) is the most common life-shortening genetic disorder in the white population, with an estimated mean survival age of 33.4 years in the United States. The estimated incidence in the U.S. white population ranges from 1:1,900–1:3,700.
- CF occurs more often in northern Europeans and Ashkenazi Jews than in American whites. It is also present, but less frequent, in African Americans (1:15,000), Hispanics (1:9,000), and Asians (1:32,000).

## Pathophysiology

- CF is an autosomal recessive disorder caused by mutations of both alleles of the CF gene (chromosome 7), resulting in abnormalities in the production of gene product CF transmembrane conductance regulator (CFTR).
    - The most common mutation is a three-base pair deletion that encodes for phenylalanine at position 508 of the CF gene, or ΔF508, and this accounts for 70% of the mutations in whites.
    - CFTR allows chloride to be transported out of the cell to the epithelial surface and determine hydration of the mucous gel. Inadequate hydration of the gel is believed to cause inspissated secretions and organ damage. It affects the lungs, sinuses, liver, pancreas, and genitourinary tract. In the lungs it impairs ciliary clearance, promoting bacterial infection, which accounts for most of the morbidity and mortality of the disease.
- The major colonizing microorganisms are *S. aureus, H. influenzae,* and *Escherichia coli* early in the disease; then *Pseudomonas aeruginosa, Stenotrophomonas maltophilia, Achromobacter xylosoxidans;* and finally *Burkholderia cepacia* complex later in the disease. In this later complex, *Burkholderia cenocepacia* (genomovar III) accounts for increased morbidity and mortality in the CF population.

## Clinical Presentation

- The most common clinical manifestations involve the gastrointestinal and respiratory tract.
    - Gastrointestinal manifestations usually are evident early in life, with meconium ileus occurring in 10% of the neonates. Other common gastrointestinal manifestations include failure to thrive, steatorrhea, obstructive jaundice, rectal prolapse, and hypoproteinemia.
    - Respiratory manifestations become evident during the first years of life with recurrent respiratory tract infections (pneumonia, chronic sinusitis), cough, and wheezing that may be misinterpreted as asthma.
- Other clinical signs and symptoms that should prompt evaluation for CF include delayed passage of meconium (>24–48 hours after birth), meconium plug syndrome, prolonged cholestasis, distal intestinal obstruction, recurrent or chronic pancreatitis, nasal polyps, chronic sinusitis, allergic bronchopulmonary aspergillosis, *Pseudomonas* bronchitis, spontaneous pneumothorax, hyponatremic dehydration, hypochloremic metabolic alkalosis, obstructive azoospermia (congenital bilateral absence of the vas deferens), hypertrophic osteoarthropathy, and digital clubbing.
- A CF pulmonary exacerbation is defined inconsistently in the literature, but in general it is characterized by all or some of the following: increased cough, fever, changes in spirometry (change in $FEV_1$ >10%), change in activity level, decreased appetite, weight loss, new findings on chest radiograph (increased mucous plugging or new infiltrates), new adventitious sounds on auscultation (new rales), change in respiratory rate, exercise intolerance, school or work absenteeism, increased sputum production, and hemoptysis.

## Diagnosis

- The diagnosis of CF is made on the basis of two positive sweat chloride tests using pilocarpine iontophoresis (60 mmol/L) along with classic clinical findings and a history of CF in an immediate family member.
    - False-positive sweat test results are uncommon but may occur in the presence of adrenal insufficiency, nephrogenic diabetes insipidus, type I glycogen storage disease, hypothyroidism, hypoparathyroidism, familial cholestasis, and malnutrition.
- Additional diagnostic tests include neonatal screening with increased circulating levels of immunoreactive trypsinogen, genotyping for CFTR mutations (two mutations confirm the diagnosis), nasal potential difference testing, a computed tomography scan of sinuses demonstrating pansinusitis, 24-hour fecal fat measurement looking for signs of pancreatic insufficiency, and ultrasound to assess absence of the vas deferens in males.

# Treatment

- Treatment goals. These include to delay or prevent lung disease, to promote good nutrition and growth, and to treat complications.
- Maintenance treatment for patients with classic CF
  - Airway clearance. Daily airway clearance is one of the most important methods of prevention of respiratory tract infections.
    - There are many different methods, including manual chest physiotherapy, postural drainage, autogenic drainage, high-frequency chest oscillation vests, and manual percussion therapy.
    - Adjunctive therapies include the Flutter valve and Acapella device.
    - The use of a specific method is mostly dependent on patient preferences; no studies demonstrate superiority of one method over another.
  - Optimization of nutrition. Nutritional failure has been proven to be closely related to increased morbidity and frequency of pulmonary exacerbations. Therefore, it is important to maintain adequate nutrition via encouragement of a high-calorie and high-protein diet.
    - For patients who are not able to achieve appropriate oral caloric intake, a feeding gastrostomy tube may be an option.
  - Pancreatic enzyme supplementation. Patients with the pancreatic-insufficient form of CF manifest signs of malabsorption. Pancreatic enzyme supplementation is key for these patients.
  - Usual dose ranges from 1,500–2,500 U of lipase per kilogram of patient's weight per meal.
  - Dosing is usually started at the lowest level and titrated up as needed, and it should not exceed 2,500 U/kg/meal because high doses have been associated with chronic intestinal strictures.
  - Lipid-soluble vitamin supplementation (vitamins A, D, E, and K). Lipid-soluble vitamins are not well absorbed in patients with pancreatic insufficiency.
  - Antimicrobials. Chronic antimicrobial therapy is frequently used in patients with increased morbidity from colonizing microorganisms to attempt prevention of pulmonary exacerbation. These are commonly used against methicillin-resistant *S. aureus,* methicillin-sensitive *S. aureus* (Panton-Valentine leukocidin-positive), *Pseudomonas,* and *Aspergillus.* In particular, chronic azithromycin therapy has proven beneficial in terms of its immunomodulatory effects; it interferes with *Pseudomonas* biofilm formation in the CF airways.
  - Anti-inflammatory drugs. Oral glucocorticoid therapy and nonsteroidal anti-inflammatory drugs such as ibuprofen have proven benefits for some patients; however, the side effects of long-term therapy should be weighed against the benefits.
- Therapy for a pulmonary exacerbation
  - This should always include intensive chest physiotherapy 3–4 times a day along with good nutritional support. Outpatient antibiotic therapy should always be attempted first if there are no signs of respiratory distress or decompensation. Choice of therapy should be based on previous sputum cultures.
  - The duration of therapy depends on clinical improvement but is generally between 2–3 weeks.
    - If there is failure to improve clinically while on outpatient therapy, the patient should be admitted to initiate IV antibiotic therapy for a total of 2–4 weeks.
    - All patients should be hospitalized in separate rooms with strict isolation measures as needed for resistant organisms.
    - The duration of admission depends on the severity of the patient's illness and clinical judgment (clinical improvement, improvement in spirometry, easiness of completing IV treatment at home).
- Special considerations
  - Allergic bronchopulmonary aspergillosis (ABPA)
    - ABPA is an exaggerated immunologic response in the lungs against Aspergillus that results in signs of airway obstruction. It occurs in 6%–25% of patients with CF.

- Criteria for diagnosis include positive skin prick testing against *Aspergillus*, along with detection of specific *Aspergillus* anti-IgG and anti-IgE in serum. Radiographic evidence of central bronchiectasis is suggestive of the diagnosis.
- Treatment includes oral corticosteroids and antifungals such as itraconazole.

■ Cystic fibrosis–related diabetes mellitus (CFRD)
- CFRD is caused by destruction of pancreatic islet cells and resultant insulin deficiency. Patients with CF should undergo frequent (annual) oral glucose tolerance tests to screen for evidence of CFRD.
- Treatment is generally managed by a pediatric endocrinologist. It frequently involves administration of insulin and carbohydrate counting without compromising lipid intake and high caloric necessities.

■ Lung transplantation
- The most common cause of death related to CF is advanced lung disease, and for these patients, lung transplantation may be the only alternative to prolong survival.
- The most commonly used model for survival was published by Kerem, et al., and describes high mortality risk for patients with an $FEV_1$ <30% of predicted, hypercarbia (>50 mm Hg), hypoxemia (<55 mm Hg), young age, female gender, and nutritional failure. These patients should be referred for evaluation of lung transplantation.

## Suggested Readings

Behrman R. Nelson Textbook of Pediatrics, 17th Ed. Philadelphia: WB Saunders, 2004.

Colin AA, et al. Cystic fibrosis. Pediatr Rev 1994;5:192–200.

Dayan P, et al. Controversies in the management of children with bronchiolitis. Clin Pediatr Emerg Med 2004;5:41–53.

Eckel HE, Widemann B, Damm M, et al. Airway endoscopy in the diagnosis and treatment of bacterial tracheitis in children. Int J Pediatr Otorhinolaryngol 1993;27:147–157.

Ferkol TW, et al. Cystic fibrosis pulmonary exacerbations. J Pediatr 2006;259–264.

Fitzgerald DA. The assessment and management of croup. Paediatr Respir Rev 2006;7(1): 73–81.

Gibson RL, et al. Pathophysiology and management of pulmonary infections in cystic fibrosis. AJRCCM 2003;168:918–951.

Hammer J. Acquired upper airway obstruction. Paediatr Respir Rev 2004;5(1):25–33.

Knutson D. Viral croup. Am Fam Physician 2004;69(3):535–540.

Kerem E, et al. Prediction of mortality in patients with cystic fibrosis. N Engl J Med 1992; 326(18):1187–1191.

Rafei K, et al. Airway infectious disease emergencies. Pediatr Clin North Am 2006;53(2): 215–242.

Stern RC. The diagnosis of cystic fibrosis. N Engl J Med 1997;336:487–491.

Stevens DA, et al. Allergic bronchopulmonary Aspergillosis in cystic fibrosis—state of the art: Cystic Fibrosis Foundation Consensus Conference. Clin Infect Dis 2003;37(Suppl 3):S225–S264.

Taussig L. Pediatric Respiratory Medicine, 1st Ed. Philadelphia: Mosby, 1999.

Wainwright C, et al. A multicenter, randomized, double-blind controlled trial of nebulized epinephrine in infants with acute bronchiolitis. N Engl J Med 2003;349:27–35.

Westley CR, et al. Nebulised racemic epinephrine by IPPB for the treatment of croup: A double-blind study. Am J Dis Child 1978;132:484–487.

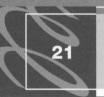

# RADIOLOGIC CONCERNS

**21**

### Keith A. Kronemer and William H. McAlister

## ORDERING A RADIOLOGY EXAMINATION

- Certain imaging procedures may be requested depending on the clinical condition of the patient (Tables 21-1 and 21-2). Recommendations for imaging may represent either optimal selection (based on availability) or complementary examinations that build on each other.
- The radiologist may customize the examination or even suggest a different one to answer the specific clinical question. Key information should be provided:
  - Radiologic procedure requested
  - Specific clinical question or clinical situation
    - Gastrointestinal (GI) conditions (see Table 21-1)
    - All other conditions (see Table 21-2)
  - Relevant medical diagnoses and surgeries
    - Cancer patients: last chemotherapy or radiation therapy
  - Allergy to iodinated intravenous (IV) contrast
  - Renal function (serum creatinine) if IV contrast is to be used
  - IV access (location and gauge)
  - Patient factors: stability (examination at bedside or in radiology department), nothing by mouth (NPO) status, mechanical ventilation, cooperativeness, and need for sedation

### Safety Considerations

- Monitored conscious sedation with agents such as IV pentobarbital, midazolam (Versed), or propofol are appropriate for young patients who cannot stay still, for uncooperative patients, and for potentially painful procedures.
- Have patients NPO when ordering any sedated examination, intravenous pyelography (IVP), computed tomography (CT) that involves IV contrast, or a GI fluoroscopic examination.

### Radiation Considerations

- Radiography, fluoroscopy, and CT expose the patient to ionizing radiation, whereas ultrasound and magnetic resonance imaging (MRI) do not.
- At children's hospitals and imaging centers, radiation doses can be, and often are, significantly reduced.

### Gastrointestinal Contrast Considerations

- The radiologist chooses between barium and water-soluble contrast.
  - Barium is usually the GI contrast of choice but should not be used if a leak is suspected or surgery is imminent because it can cause peritonitis or mediastinitis. Also, barium can limit future abdominal CT imaging because of scatter artifact from retained material.
  - Water-soluble contrast (Hypaque, Gastroview) is used when barium is contraindicated. Its advantage over barium is that it reabsorbs from body cavities, but the disadvantage is that image quality is poorer.
    - It is hyperosmolar; although this causes fluid shifts into the GI tract, this is usually tolerated by the patient.

| TABLE 21-1 | Gastrointestinal Conditions: Recommended Imaging |
|---|---|

| Condition | Imaging used |
|---|---|
| Necrotizing enterocolitis | Serial abdominal radiographs every 4–6 hours may demonstrate pneumatosis, free peritoneal air, and portal vein gas. See text for additional information. |
| Intussusception | Obstructive series may be useful in suggesting (mass effect) or excluding (air or stool in right colon and terminal ileum). Ultrasound may help establish the diagnosis. See text for additional information. |
| Malrotation | Obstructive series is usually normal; upper gastrointestinal (GI) study is required. Urgent imaging is appropriate. |
| Appendicitis | Abdominal radiographs are often nonspecific, although occasionally appendicoliths may be seen. Ultrasound is imaging study of choice in young, thin children. Computed tomography (CT) is study of choice in older children with moderate body fat. Use of oral, rectal, and intravenous (IV) contrast may vary. |
| Question of bowel perforation | Obstructive series may show free air. CT may be useful in demonstrating small amounts of free air and suggesting a cause. |
| Pyloric stenosis | Ultrasound directly shows the thickened pyloric muscle. Upper GI examination is comparable. |
| Esophageal atresia/ tracheoesophageal fistula | Chest and abdominal radiographs may suggest diagnosis (coiled proximal nasogastric tube with or without abdominal gas). Upper GI is study of choice for looking for "H-type" fistula. |
| Duodenal atresia | Abdominal radiograph is diagnostic (distended stomach and proximal duodenum with an otherwise gasless abdomen). |
| Meckel diverticulum | Often difficult to diagnose. Nuclear medicine "Meckel scan" may demonstrate (approximately 80%–90% sensitivity and 90%–95% specificity) if there is gastric mucosa. CT with oral and IV contrast may demonstrate diverticulum if inflamed. |
| Biliary atresia | Ultrasound is useful to access for presence of the gallbladder and its size as well as to exclude biliary obstruction from choledochal cysts. HIDA scan is useful in evaluating biliary function. |
| Ascites | Ultrasound can diagnose and localize for drainage. |

- It should not be used when large volume aspiration is a possibility. In the lungs, it causes pulmonary edema.
■ Dilute injectable low osmolar contrast (Omnipaque, Optiray) may be used orally in infants when the risk of aspiration is high.

## Intravenous Contrast Considerations

■ The radiologist helps determine appropriateness based on such factors as clinical indications and renal function.
■ Contrast power injectors provide optimal imaging for all CT scans, except for head CT scans, but these require a 22-gauge or larger needle, and preferably antecubital IV access. Hand IV lines and central lines must be injected by hand, which leads to suboptimal vessel opacification.

| TABLE 21-2 | Selected Nongastrointestinal Conditions: Recommended Imaging |
|---|---|
| **Condition** | **Imaging used** |
| Stridor/croup | Soft tissue neck and chest radiographs are useful. |
| Pleural effusion | Frontal and lateral chest radiographs may be sufficient. Decubitus radiographs may demonstrate fluid mobility. Use ultrasound if they are inconclusive or localization for drainage is required. Use computed tomography (CT) with contrast if there is concern for empyema, loculated fluid, or necrotizing pneumonia. |
| Pulmonary embolism | CT with pulmonary embolism protocol is necessary, which requires excellent intravenous (IV) access for contrast. If such CT is not available, nuclear ventilation-perfusion scan is good but less specific option. |
| Orbital cellulitis | Orbital CT with IV contrast is useful. |
| Abdominal trauma | CT with IV contrast is study of choice. |
| Thoracic trauma | CT with IV contrast is study of choice. In patients with minor trauma, chest radiographs may be useful. |
| Head trauma, epidural/ subdural hematoma | CT with and without IV contrast is used, with magnetic resonance imaging (MRI) if CT is inconclusive. |
| Stroke | CT without IV contrast is used to evaluate for bleeding and edema, MRI without contrast and magnetic resonance arteriogram for suspected hemorrhagic etiology, and for patient with sickle cell disease. |
| Extremity deep vein thrombosis | Use venous ultrasound with Doppler. |
| Ventriculoperitoneal shunt malfunction | Shunt series (radiographs of skull, chest, and abdomen) to access for discontinuity is useful, with noncontrast head CT to evaluate hydrocephalus. |
| Retropharyngeal abscess | Soft tissue neck radiographs for initial evaluation. If inconclusive or needs further characterization, use CT neck with IV contrast. |
| Cervical spine trauma | Anteroposterior (AP) and lateral cervical spine radiographs (also odontoid view in children >age 6 years) are useful, with CT if there is still question of fracture. If there is concern for ligamentous injury, flexion and extension lateral radiographs or MRI without contrast are necessary. |
| Scoliosis | Use scoliosis survey (AP total spine radiograph), adding lateral view if significant scoliosis, lordosis, or kyphosis. |
| Developmental dysplasia of the hip | Imaging is not preferable until patient is at least age 2 wk; earlier imaging is often inconclusive because of transient ligamentous laxity as a result of maternal hormones. Ultrasound is study of choice until age 6 mo. AP radiograph of the pelvis after age 6 mo is useful unless condition has teratogenic cause. |
| Pyelonephritis | Use ultrasound for evaluation of acute pyelonephritis or complications of pyelonephritis, such as perinephric abscess or pyonephrosis. Contrast CT, DMSA scans, and MRI are excellent for this diagnosis. Consider voiding cystourethrogram for evaluation of vesicoureteral reflux once infection has resolved. |
| Ovarian torsion | Surgical or gynecologic evaluation is very useful before imaging. Use pelvic ultrasound with Doppler. |
| Testicular torsion | Recommend urologic evaluation before imaging. Use scrotal ultrasound. |

- Contrast is relatively contraindicated in patients with sickle cell crisis, acute renal failure, or prior anaphylactic allergic reaction to contrast.
- Patients with histories of less severe contrast reactions may have IV contrast if premedicated.
  - Lacking high-quality randomized clinical trials, premedication regimens vary. The authors use prednisone 1 mg/kg PO 20, 14, 8, and 2 hours before the scan. In addition, an antihistamine 2 hours before the scan is given.
  - Dose and drug are age dependent.
    - Neonate: diphenhydramine (Benadryl) not recommended; consider hydroxyzine (Atarax) 10 mg
    - 2–5 years: diphenhydramine 6.25 mg
    - 6–12 years: diphenhydramine 12.5–25 mg
    - >12 years: diphenhydramine 25–50 mg

## Magnetic Resonance Imaging Considerations

- Contraindications to MRI include presence of programmable implanted devices (e.g., pacemakers, cochlear implants), MRI-noncompatible aneurysm clips, and metallic fragments in the eye. Compatibility must also be considered for other implants, prostheses, metal objects, and some dark tattoos.
- Closed loop wires have a tendency to heat up during the examination. Skin staples are usually tolerated if they are taped securely.
- Some stents, filters, coils, and prosthetic valves require 6–8 weeks to allow tissue ingrowth before an MRI may be performed.
- Patients usually must lie flat for 30–90 minutes, are relatively unmonitored, and must be cooperative enough to lie still (or be sedated). Consider claustrophobia as a limitation.

# CHEST RADIOGRAPHY

- Check for infiltrates, thickened bronchial walls, pulmonary edema, increased or decreased pulmonary vascularity, pleural effusions, pneumothorax, heart size, midline trachea, rib fractures, and septal lines (Kerley B lines). Figure 21-1A shows a normal chest radiograph.
- Check aeration. Flattened or inverted diaphragm on lateral view suggests air trapping. Figure 21-1B shows a normal lateral chest radiograph.
- Check for anomalies. Check on which side (left or right) the cardiac apex, aortic arch, stomach bubble, and liver shadow appears.

## Evaluating for Infiltrates

- Check for subtle infiltrates behind the diaphragm and heart on the frontal view. Normally, the borders of heart and diaphragm are sharp, and the right and left heart shadows should be similar in density. Right middle lobe and lingular infiltrates project over heart on lateral.
- Infiltrates are present if the lung projecting over the spine does not become increasingly dark inferiorly; however, note normal posterior lower lobe vessels are often mistaken for infiltrates.
- The normal thymus, which can be large and triangular in young children, is sometimes confused for upper lobe infiltrates.
- Classic appearances of common entities
  - Viral pneumonia: hyperinflation, perihilar infiltrates, and thickened bronchial walls (Figure 21-2)
  - Bacterial pneumonia: focal infiltrates, especially lobar consolidation, parapneumonic pleural fluid
  - Atelectasis: linear opacities and volume loss
- Often the appearance of viral or bacterial infiltrates and atelectasis is similar, especially in infants.

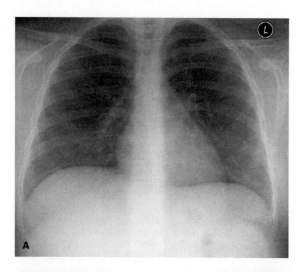

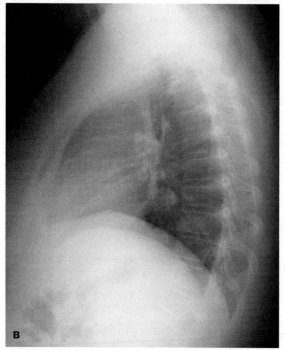

**Figure 21-1.** Normal chest. Frontal **(A)** and lateral **(B)** views of the chest demonstrate a normal cardiac contour, clear lungs, and normal thorax.

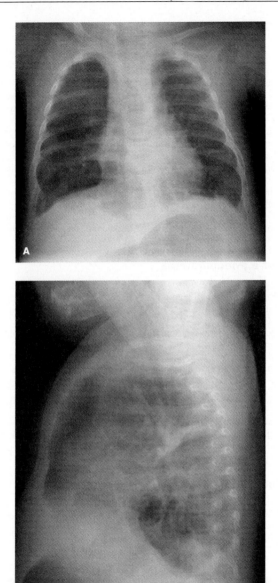

**Figure 21-2.** Viral disease. Frontal **(A)** and lateral **(B)** views of the chest show hyperinflation with perihilar infiltrates and peribronchial cuffing consistent with reactive airways disease.

## Evaluating Chest Radiographs from the Neonatal Intensive Care Unit

■ Check every line and tube position.
■ Check for pneumothorax.
■ Check for classic appearances of common entities.
  ■ Transient tachypnea of the newborn: streaky densities extending from the hilar areas that tend to resolve in a few days, fluid in the minor fissure usually with normal lung volumes
  ■ Hyaline membrane disease: diffuse ground glass or finely granular appearance, small lung volumes and typically no pleural effusions in a premature neonate. With worsening opacification, consider patent ductus arteriosus or fluid overload. When on a ventilator, the neonate may progress to pulmonary interstitial emphysema or bronchopulmonary dysplasia.
  ■ Meconium aspiration pneumonia: usually in term or post-term newborns; hyperinflated lungs with patchy, coarse infiltrates
  ■ Neonatal pneumonia: variable appearance, including asymmetric infiltrates, often with pleural effusions; can simulate hyaline membrane disease. Group B streptococcus is a common pathogen.

### Checking for a Pneumothorax

■ Look for classic appearance, with a thin sharp line representing pleural surface, no vessels in pleura, and air beyond pleura (air is dark, lucent). A small left pneumothorax is visible in Figure 21-3A, and a large right pneumothorax is seen in Figure 21-3B.
■ Other signs to look for are:
  ■ Deep sulcus sign: lateral costophrenic angle deepened with increased lucency (basilar pneumothorax)
  ■ Increased lucency over one lung (anterior pneumothorax)
  ■ Increased sharpness of cardiomediastinal border (medial pneumothorax)
■ If uncertain, request an upright or expiratory examination in cooperative patients and a lateral decubitus (opposite side down) view in uncooperative or intubated patients.
■ Tension pneumothorax is suggested by mediastinal shift away from pneumothorax or hemidiaphragm depressed on side of pneumothorax. These radiographic findings of tension may not be seen with positive end-expiratory pressure ventilation or diseased noncompliant lungs.

### Checking for a Foreign Body

■ In young children, aspirated foreign bodies most often cause ipsilateral air trapping and hyperinflation. Thus to evaluate for radiolucent foreign bodies, expiratory or lateral decubitus chest radiographs may be helpful.
■ Real-time fluoroscopy may be performed if radiographs are equivocal.

## CHEST COMPUTED TOMOGRAPHY AND MAGNETIC RESONANCE IMAGING

■ Noncontrast CT is adequate for evaluating peripheral pulmonary nodules and mild lung parenchymal disease.
■ IV contrast optimizes evaluation of patients with more extensive pneumonias, pleural versus parenchymal disease, masses in the lungs or mediastinum, chest trauma, and complex pulmonary infiltrates. Its use in the question of pulmonary embolism is increasing.
■ High-resolution CT imaging may be performed to further characterize lung parenchymal disease.
■ MRI is used most in evaluating the heart and great vessels.

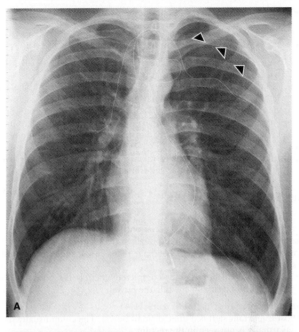

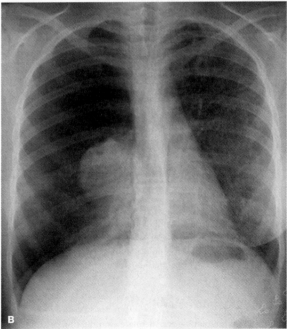

**Figure 21-3.** Pneumothorax. Two chest radiographs on different patients demonstrate a small left pneumothorax **(A)** and a large right pneumothorax **(B)**. A sharp pleural line (arrowheads) with absent pulmonary markings beyond is seen. The large right pneumothorax **(B)** also shown near total collapse of the right lung with mild mediastinal shift to the left from a tension pneumothorax. The left lung has patchy infiltrates and bronchiectasis associated with cystic fibrosis.

# ABDOMINAL RADIOGRAPHY

- Abdomen 1 view: synonymous with kidneys, ureters, and bladder (KUB), abdominal flat plate (AFP), and supine abdomen radiograph
- Abdomen 2 view: synonymous with obstructive series (two views; supine and either upright or left lateral decubitus); may include an upright chest view
    - The supine radiograph is used to evaluate bowel gas pattern and abnormal calcifications (e.g., renal calculi, gallstones, and appendicoliths). The upright or left lateral decubitus views allow an evaluation for pneumoperitoneum and gas-fluid levels.
    - Decubitus radiographs are usually taken in young children, whereas erect radiographs are usually taken in older children.

## Evaluating Bowel Gas Pattern

- Normal bowel gas pattern
    - Typically this includes nondilated colon with stool and gas, gas in the rectum, a few loops of nondilated gas-filled small bowel, and a gastric bubble.
    - Crying infants often swallow air and have many loops of gas filled nondilated proximal small bowel loops.
    - Remember that small bowel folds completely encircle the bowel and that colonic folds (haustra) only partially encircle the bowel.
- Complete small bowel obstruction (Figure 21-4)
    - The most important sign is a dilated small bowel. The colon usually has little or no gas. Gas usually is not seen in the rectum.
    - The more loops of dilated small bowel, the more distal the obstruction.
- Partial or early small bowel obstruction
    - The small bowel is dilated.
    - Some gas and stool are still seen in the colon and rectum.
- Ileus
    - The small and large bowels are dilated, with the large bowel dilated more prominently than the small bowel.
    - The patient may be postoperative.
- Intussusception: small bowel obstruction pattern; may be a nonspecific bowel gas pattern
    - Classic sign of a soft tissue mass in the right upper quadrant
    - Ultrasound can be used to confirm the diagnosis.
    - An air-soluble or water-soluble enema may be used for diagnosis and treatment.
- Necrotizing enterocolitis. Look for pneumatosis in the bowel wall (Figure 21-5). Also look for portal venous gas (Figure 21-6) and pneumoperitoneum (Figure 21-7). The bowel may be dilated.
- Nonspecific bowel gas pattern: not normal but not clearly obstructed
    - There are usually a few loops of mildly dilated small bowel or a gasless abdomen.
    - This may be seen in many abdominal diseases such as gastroenteritis or pancreatitis.
- Remember, if dilated bowel loops are fluid-filled, they may not be appreciated. Hence, a paucity of bowel gas may suggest a small bowel obstruction in the appropriate clinical setting.

## Evaluating a Pneumoperitoneum

- Upright view: subdiaphragmatic gas. Adequate examination must include a portion of the chest.
- Left lateral decubitus view (see Figures 21-5 and 21-7B): gas between liver and body wall. Adequate examinations must include the entire right hemidiaphragm.
- Supine view (often subtle). Findings include sharp appearance of inferior liver edge; increased lucency, especially over liver; falciform ligament outlined by air; visible inner and outer margins of bowel wall; and air not conforming to typical bowel appearance such as in the subhepatic space or other atypical locations.

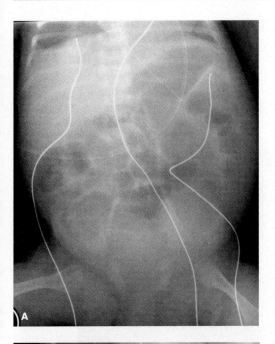

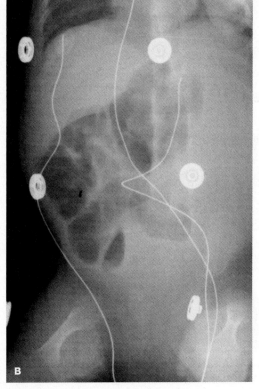

**Figure 21-4.** Small bowel obstruction. Frontal **(A)** and left lateral decubitus **(B)** views of the abdomen show multiple dilated bowel loops with a gasless rectosigmoid and right colon. The decubitus view shows scattered small bowel air fluid levels in a pattern typical of distal small bowel obstruction.

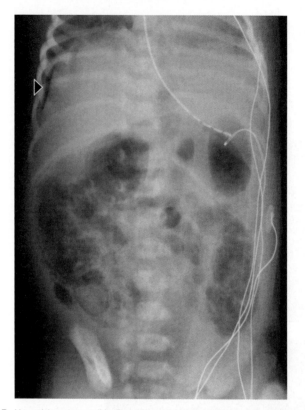

**Figure 21-5.** Necrotizing enterocolitis. Decubitus view of the abdomen shows linear pneumatosis in the right colon with air tracking within the bowel wall. A more bubbly appearance is seen to the pneumatosis in the left colon. The patient also has a small pneumoperitoneum (arrowhead) and portal venous gas.

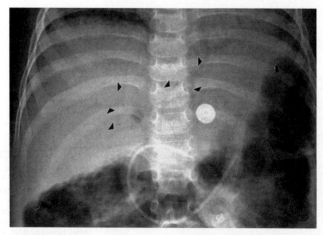

**Figure 21-6.** Necrotizing enterocolitis. Portal venous gas. Detail view of the upper abdomen shows the branching linear lucencies (arrowheads) in the liver because of portal venous gas.

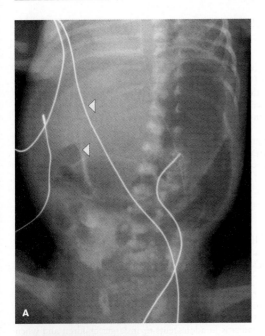

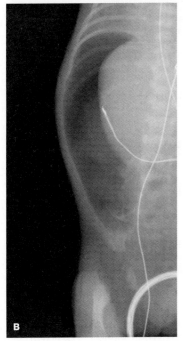

**Figure 21-7.** Pneumoperitoneum. Frontal view **(A)** of the abdomen shows a large amount of air outside the confines of bowel. The falciform ligament (arrowheads) is visualized since it is outlined by air. Left lateral decubitus (left side down) view **(B)** of the abdomen shows peritoneal air lateral to edge of liver. Peritoneal air also demarcates the outer border of the bowel wall in the loop of bowel inferior to the liver.

## Evaluating Abdominal Radiographs from the Neonatal Intensive Care Unit

- Check all line positions.
  - Umbilical arterial catheter: courses caudally from umbilicus to internal iliac arteries and then cranially to aorta. There are two preferred positions:
    - Between middescending thoracic aorta (below ductus arteriosus) and above vertebral body T10 (above celiac artery; usually T7-T9)
    - At the level of vertebral body L3 or L4 (below renal arteries and above aortic bifurcation)
    - Umbilical venous catheter: courses from umbilicus cranially through umbilical vein to ductus venosus to intrahepatic inferior vena cava. The preferred position is at the inferior vena cava/right atrial junction. Check for malpositioned catheters.

# ABDOMINAL IMAGING

- Abdominal ultrasound
  - Assesses abdominal organs: liver, gallbladder, bile ducts, pancreas, spleen, and kidney; sensitive for gallstones; unable to assess gas-filled structures such as intestines
  - Can be performed at patient's bedside; keep patient NPO
- Abdominal/pelvic CT
  - Evaluates abdominal solid organs, intestines, mesentery, and retroperitoneum very well; may be used in diagnosing bowel obstruction. Ultrasound may be better for characterizing adnexal and uterine pathology.
  - Preferred for evaluating appendicitis in adolescents or in larger children and when ultrasound is equivocal
  - Typically performed with oral and IV contrast
    - Without oral contrast, differentiation of small bowel from masses or fluid collections may be more difficult.
    - Without IV contrast, evaluation of solid abdominal organs and vessels is limited. Keep patient NPO.
- Abdominal/pelvic MRI
  - Usually reserved for characterizing atypical lesions seen by other imaging
  - May be used to characterize pancreatic and biliary ductal anatomy

# GASTROINTESTINAL FLUOROSCOPIC EXAMINATIONS

- Fluoroscopic examinations can be performed with barium or water-soluble contrast (Gastroview, Hypaque).
- Examinations involve radiologist at patient's side performing the procedure.
- Patient should be NPO.

## Speech Swallow Study

- Multiple food and liquid consistencies given with real-time fluoroscopic evaluation to assess which food types can be tolerated without aspiration
- Performed in conjunction with trained speech therapist

## Barium Swallow/Upper Gastrointestinal Examination

- This procedure is used to assess the pharynx, esophagus, stomach, and duodenum. Upper gastrointestinal (UGI) is the examination of choice to evaluate for malrotation and midgut volvulus (additional small bowel follow-through is generally not needed).
- When evaluating for hypertrophic pyloric stenosis (HPS), UGI can find other GI pathology if HPS not present, such as malrotation. Ultrasound is also a first-line option for HPS.

### Small Bowel Follow-Through

- This procedure is used to evaluate the small intestines. It is usually performed in conjunction with a UGI examination.
  - Conditions assessed usually include Crohn disease, strictures, masses, and sometimes obstruction.
  - Small bowel obstruction can usually be diagnosed by plain radiographs of the abdomen.
- Administered oral contrast is fluoroscopically evaluated periodically as peristalsis carries the contrast through the entire small intestines.

### Contrast Enema

- This procedure is used to evaluate the colon for strictures, obstruction, masses, and fistulas.
  - This is the examination of choice for intussusception, Hirschsprung disease, meconium ileus, or any suspected distal bowel obstruction.
  - With intussusception, therapeutic reduction (with air or water-soluble contrast) may be performed.
- Therapeutic reductions carry a small risk of perforation, so IV access and a surgical consult before examination are necessary. Active colitis is a relative contraindication to an enema.

## GENITOURINARY IMAGING

### Voiding Cystourethrogram (VCUG)

- After the bladder is catheterized, fluoroscopy is performed during bladder filling and with spontaneous or voluntary voiding.
- A VCUG can grade vesicoureteral reflex and diagnose obstructions including posterior urethral valves or bladder dyssynergia. Urine must be clear of infection.

### Ultrasound

- Renal ultrasound
  - This procedure is used to evaluate for age-appropriate kidney size, solid masses, cysts, and hydronephrosis, scarring, stones, and diseases that alter renal echogenicity.
  - CT is more sensitive for small solid masses and tiny calculi.
- Scrotal ultrasound
  - This is the examination of choice to assess for testicular or scrotal pathology, including testicular torsion, trauma, masses, and infection.
  - Doppler evaluation is performed to assess blood flow.
- Pelvic ultrasound
  - This is the examination of choice for ovarian and uterine pathology.
  - Pediatric pelvic ultrasound is performed transabdominally. A full bladder is required.
    - Doppler evaluation is performed to assess blood flow.
    - Common indications include pelvic pain, ovarian torsion, tubo-ovarian abscess, pregnancy, ectopic pregnancy, adnexal masses, and uterine bleeding.

### Genitourinary Computed Tomography and Magnetic Resonance Imaging

- Stone protocols are performed without oral or IV contrast to assess for renal and ureteral calculi and associated obstruction.
- Contrast CT is used to evaluate possible masses, pyelonephritis, obstruction, and anomalies of the genitourinary tract.
- MRI is increasingly used to diagnose tumors, pyelonephritis, masses, and function.

## Intravenous Pyelography

- Intravenous pyelography (IVP) consists of a series of abdominal radiographs taken after administering IV contrast.
- IVP is usually reserved for problem solving of urinary tract abnormalities diagnosed by other imaging.

# EXTREMITY IMAGING

- Bones are generally evaluated with plain radiographs.
- CT provides excellent bone detail and some soft tissue detail.
- Ultrasound and MRI can be used for better soft tissue differentiation.
- In a skeletal survey, radiographs of the skull, chest, abdomen, and extremities are performed for indications such as child abuse, skeletal dysplasias, and occasionally histiocytosis X.
- Hip ultrasound is usually performed for two different reasons in two different populations:
  - To assess for dislocation (developmental dysplasia of the hip) in children <6 months of age
  - To check for effusion in older children in whom developmental dysplasia of the hip is clinically suspected
- Bone age is one of two methods chosen by radiologists to assess if skeletal age is advanced or delayed relative to chronological age.
  - A single left hand radiograph is compared with an atlas of normal standard examples.
  - Multiple radiographs of one side of patient are taken to count ossification centers throughout the skeleton; this is more accurate in patients <2 years of age.

# NEUROIMAGING

- Neonatal head ultrasound: used to assess for hemorrhage, hydrocephalus, periventricular leukomalacia, large arterial-venous shunts, developmental anomalies of the brain, extraaxial fluid collections, and gross brain maturity
- Head CT (Figures 21-8, 21-9, and 21-10)
  - After the neonatal period, noncontrast head CT is the usual screening procedure, including for hematomas and trauma.
  - Contrast may be used to assess for tumors, but MRI is preferred for greater sensitivity.
- MRI: used to evaluate seizures, tumors, congenital anomalies, and strokes, as well as to further characterize CT findings. The indications keep increasing (Figures 21-11 and 21-12).
- Cerebral magnetic resonance arteriogram: screening examination for cerebral arterial pathology
- Spine CT: excellent for evaluating injury after plain radiographs as well as for assessing tumors, infections, and congenital vertebral deformities
- Spine MRI: excellent for overall spine imaging, including spinal cord, intervertebral disks, and subarachnoid and epidural pathology. MRI is the examination of choice for tumors, tumor extension into spinal canal such as neuroblastoma, congenital anomalies, and epidural abscesses.
- Positron emission tomography (PET)/CT is primarily used for tumor detection and surveillance and to locate seizure foci.

# NUCLEAR MEDICINE

- Nuclear medicine examinations can provide functional information that other imaging modalities cannot. However, anatomic detail is usually much less than with other imaging modalities.
- Some nuclear medicine examinations can be performed portably.
- Bone scan

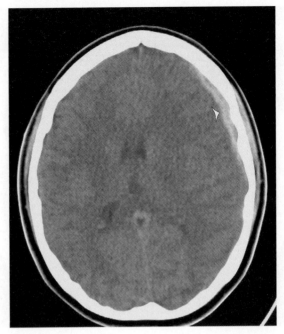

**Figure 21-8.** Computed tomography of subdural hematoma. Crescentic high attenuation blood along the frontoparietal region on this computed tomography slice (arrowhead). Note the mass effect with subtle bowing of the falx. Subdural bleeds result from venous tears on the subdural space. The bleeding follows the dura and crosses sutures.

- This scan is more sensitive than a radiograph but less specific for bone pathology. MRI is also excellent for bone pathology and is far more specific.
- The radiologist helps determine which of the two types of bone scans is more appropriate.
  - Three-phase bone scan consists of blood flow, immediate uptake, and delay retention (about 2–4 hours after injection) imaging of a technetium-radiolabeled agent injected intravenously. The imaging of the first two phases is limited to the primary region of concern. Delayed imaging is often of the whole body. Usual indication is osteomyelitis (which can be multifocal in children via hematogenous spread) or occult fracture.
  - Delayed whole-body imaging only: usually for skeletal metastasis survey or follow-up
- Renal scan
  - A technetium-radiolabeled agent is injected intravenously, and the kidneys are imaged.
  - Purposes are to assess the relative contribution of function of each kidney and to assess for urinary obstruction. Furosemide (Lasix) is helpful in diagnosing obstruction.
- Hydroxy iminodiacetic acid (HIDA) scan
  - A technetium-radiolabeled agent is excreted into the biliary system.
  - Some radiologists administer phenobarbital for a few days before imaging to improve sensitivity for biliary atresia. Patients should be kept NPO.
  - HIDA scans are useful for differentiating congenital biliary atresia from neonatal hepatitis and for diagnosis of acute or chronic cholecystitis.

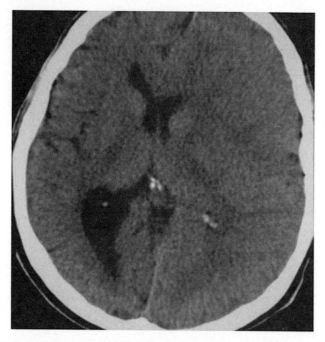

**Figure 21-9.** Isointense subdural hematoma. The natural course of a subdural hematoma is to go from acute high attenuation density blood to chronic lower attenuation cerebrospinal fluid density. When subacute, the subdural hematoma may be isointense to the surrounding gray matter, and it is recognized by its mass effect and effacement of sulcal markings.

- Tagged red cell scan for GI bleeding
  - Technetium-radiolabeled (tagged) red blood cells are injected intravenously to evaluate for bleeding over 60–90 minutes of imaging.
  - The patient must be actively bleeding to obtain a positive result.
  - Because GI bleeding is episodic, evacuation of bloody stools does not directly correlate with the timing of active bleeding.
- Meckel scan
  - A technetium-radiolabeled compound is injected intravenously, and the abdomen is imaged.
  - This is a highly specific examination for Meckel diverticulum containing ectopic gastric mucosa.
  - It does not require active bleeding.
- Lung scan
  - Usually a two-part examination
    - Ventilation imaging with inhaled xenon gas or technetium-radiolabeled particles
    - Perfusion imaging with technetium-labeled intravenously injected particles, which are trapped in small arterial branches
  - Used to evaluate for pulmonary embolism and lung transplantation surveillance. CT is being used more often for pulmonary embolism.
- PET/CT is primarily used for tumor detection and surveillance, and to locate seizure foci.

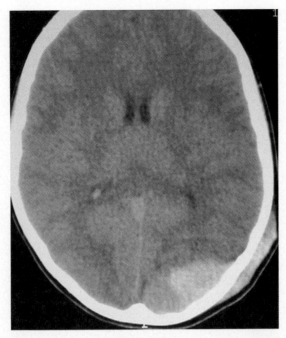

**Figure 21-10.** Epidural hematoma. The lenticular high attenuation focus in the left occipital region represents an epidural hematoma. Epidural hematomas typically result from arterial bleeds and are frequently associated with fractures. They are limited by the suture and typically convex in appearance. This patient also has a subgaleal hematoma adjacent to the outer table of the left calvarium.

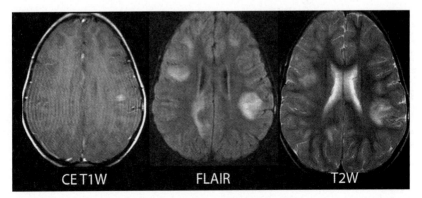

**Figure 21-11.** Acute disseminated encephalomyelitis (ADEM). Magnetic resonance imaging demonstrates multifocal signal changes throughout the white matter in this 5-year-old who presented 1 week following an upper respiratory infection. ADEM is an autoimmune demyelinating inflammatory disease seen rarely following immunizations or upper respiratory infection.

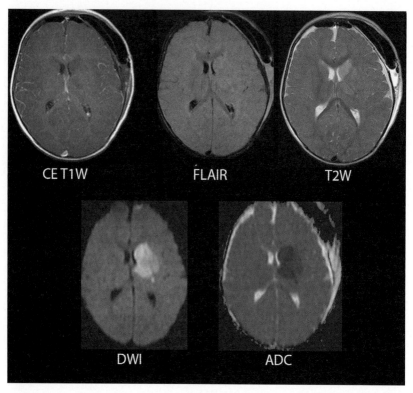

**Figure 21-12.** Acute infarct. Magnetic resonance imaging scans from a postoperative patient (note the subgaleal air and fluid over the left frontoparietal region) demonstrate changes typical of an acute infarct. T1-, FLAIR, and T2-weighted images demonstrate subtle mass effect with decreased signal seen on the T1-weighted image as well as an increased T2-weighted signal. Diffusion-weighted image (DWI) and apparent diffusion coefficient map (ADC) are more sensitive to acute ischemia.

**Suggested Readings**

Burton EM, Brody AS, eds. Essentials of Pediatric Radiology. New York: Thieme, 1999.

Donnelly LF, ed. Diagnostic Imaging Pediatrics, 1st Ed. Salt Lake City: Amirsys, 2005.

Hilton SvW, Edwards DK, eds. Practical Pediatric Radiology, 2nd Ed. Philadelphia: WB Saunders, 1994.

Seibert JJ, James CA, eds. Pediatric Radiology Case Base. New York: Thieme, 1998.

Slovis TL, ed. Caffey's Pediatric Diagnostic Imaging, 11th ed. Philadelphia: Mosby Elsevier, 2008.

Swischuk LE, ed. Imaging of the Newborn, Infant, and Young Child, 5th ed. Baltimore: Lippincott Williams & Wilkins, 2003.

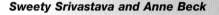

## RENAL DISEASES
*Sweety Srivastava and Anne Beck*

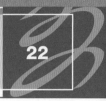

**22**

## RENAL FUNCTION AND URINE STUDIES

- Three essential attributes of renal function:
  - Glomerular ultrafiltration
  - Tubular absorption of filtered solutes and water
  - Tubular secretion of organic and nonorganic ions

### History

- General: malaise and growth failure
- Gastrointestinal (GI): feeding difficulties, vomiting, anorexia, and GI bleeding at times
- Asymptomatic in many cases
- Neonatal history
  - The most common prenatal diagnosis is hydronephrosis.
  - Edematous/hypertrophied placenta (>25% of birth weight) suggests congenital nephrotic syndrome.
  - Maternal infection. Congenital TORCH infections can present as neonatal nephrotic syndrome and seeding of renal parenchyma with infections (e.g., cytomegalovirus); maternal sepsis can cause hypoperfusion and injury to the infant's kidneys.
  - Perinatal asphyxia with macroscopic hematuria in neonatal period might suggest renal venous thrombosis in the same child with hematuria when older.
- Family history: inherited renal conditions such as cystic kidney diseases (ARPKD, ADPKD, nephronophthisis), thin basement membrane disease, Alport syndrome, and some nephrotic syndromes because of inherited mutations
- Past medical history: recurrent gross hematuria suggestive of IgA nephropathy
- Dietary history

### Physical Examination

Look for the following aspects of the physical examination to assist with diagnosing renal disease.
- Growth and nutrition
- Hydration status (edema or dehydration)
- Circulation, including four extremity pulses, precordium, lungs (pulmonary edema), and abdominal palpation
- Careful physical examination
  - Concentrate on the abdomen in newborns because many renal diseases are associated with other congenital defects (GI [imperforate anus]; VACTERL association; single umbilical artery; WAGR syndrome, with Denys-Drash syndrome with or without nephrotic syndrome, gonadal dysgenesis, and Wilms tumor).
  - Palpate for renal masses (enlarged kidney in renal vein thrombosis, renal tumors, and cystic kidney [e.g., multicystic dysplastic kidney]).

### Urinalysis

The following is a list of urinalysis findings that suggest or confirm renal disease.
- Abnormalities of appearance

**359**

| TABLE 22-1 | Laboratory Differentiation of Oliguria | |
| --- | --- | --- |
| Test | Prerenal oliguria* | Intrinsic renal oliguria* |
| Specific gravity | >1.020 (>1.015) | <1.010 (<1.010) |
| Urine osmolality (mosmol/kg) | >500 (>400) | <350 (<400) |
| Urine/plasma osmolality | >1.3 (>2.0) | <1.3 (<1.0) |
| Urine sodium (mEq/L) | <20 (<30) | >40 (>70) |
| FE$_{Na}$ | <1 (<2.5) | >3 (>10) |
| Urine/plasma urea | >8 (>30) | <3 (<6) |
| FE$_{Urea}$ | >70 | <30 |
| Urine/plasma creatinine | >40 (>30) | <20 (<10) |
| FE$_{\beta2\ microglobulin}$ | <0.4 | >0.5 |

*Indices for neonates who are >32 weeks are given in parentheses.
*FE*, fractional excretion

- Hematuria (confirm with urinalysis and microscopic examination; brown color could be because of hemoglobin, myoglobin, porphyria, beet root, or certain food colorings)
  - Cloudy or otherwise suggestive of infection or crystalluria
  - Stone or gravel (in the United States, most stones are a result of calcium)
- Abnormalities of urine volume
  - Anuria: complete cessation of urine output
  - Oliguria: insufficient urine for homeostasis (usually <500 mL/24 hours for adults or 1 mL/kg/hr in infants). See Table 22-1 for laboratory values that indicate a prerenal or renal cause.
  - Polyuria: increased fluid intake, failure of antidiuretic hormone (ADH) release, resistance to ADH, and osmotic diuresis

- Abnormalities of urination
  - Incontinence/enuresis
  - Poor urinary stream
  - Frequency/dysuria

- Blood: tests for heme moiety (hemoglobin and myoglobin). If positive, it is necessary to confirm red blood cell morphology by microscopic examination.
- Protein: standard Clinistix detects albumin; less sensitive for free light-chain proteins (Bence Jones) or low-molecular-weight "tubular" proteins
- Glucose: standard Clinistix detects glucose alone; to test for other sugars, a Clinitest is necessary
- Nitrite: 90% of common urinary pathogens are nitrite-forming bacteria
- Urinary concentration: tested by specific gravity, but osmolality is more accurate with large molecules such as glucose
- Urine bilirubin: elevated in any disease that causes increased conjugated bilirubin in the bloodstream (negative in hemolytic disease)
- Urine urobilinogen: increased in conditions that increase the production of bilirubin or decrease the liver's ability to remove reabsorbed urobilinogen from the portal circulation (positive in both liver disease and hemolytic disease)
- Microscopic examination
  - In healthy children, 1–2 red blood cells (RBCs)/high-power field (HPF) or 1–2 white blood cells (WBCs)/HPF is normal.
  - Casts: precipitation of debris in renal tubules
    - Hyaline casts: fever following exercise, dehydration, diuretic use, congestive heart failure, nephrotic syndrome
    - Waxy casts: indicative of many chronic renal diseases; not diagnostic
    - Red cell casts: hematuria of glomerular origin suggestive of glomerulonephritis
    - Fatty casts (Maltese-cross structures): commonly seen in nephrotic syndrome

- Crystals
  - Calcium oxalate: hypercalciuria (envelope or dumbbell shape of crystals)
  - Uric acid crystals: hyperuricosuria (appear as rhombic plates or rosettes)
  - Hexagonal (benzene ring structure) cystine crystals: cystinuria
  - Ammonium magnesium phosphate crystals: only form in alkaline pH; seen with urease-splitting organisms (coffin-lid appearance of crystals)
- Fine, needlelike crystals: tyrosinemia

## Calculating Creatinine Clearance

- Schwartz formula: used to calculate the glomerular filtration rate (GFR) mL/min/1.73 m$^2$

$$GFR = \frac{k \times L}{P_{Cr}}$$

- L = length in cm
- k = constant of proportionality
  - Full-term newborn through first year: 0.45
  - Children up to 13 years: 0.55
  - Adolescent males (13–21 years): 0.7
  - Adolescent females (13–21 years): 0.57
  - $P_{Cr}$ = plasma creatinine

- Blood urea nitrogen (BUN): not an accurate predictor of renal function
  - Factors that increase serum BUN: GI hemorrhage, dehydration, increased protein intake, and increased protein catabolism (systemic infection, burns, glucocorticoid therapy, early phase of starvation)
  - Factors that decrease serum BUN: decreased protein intake, advanced starvation, and liver disease
- Calculation of GFR using U × V/P
  - To standardize: Creatinine clearance

$$(mL/min/1.73\ M^2) = \frac{U_{Cr}\ (mg/dL) \times V\ (mL) \times 1.73}{P_{Cr}\ (mg/dL) \times 1440 \times SA\ (m^2)}$$

  - $U_{Cr}$ = urinary concentration of creatinine
  - V = urine volume in 24 hours
  - $P_{Cr}$ = plasma concentration of creatinine
  - SA = body surface area
  - If a child >3 years of age has <15 mg/kg/day of creatinine in a 24-hour urine collection, it probably means that the collection did not actually occur over 24 hours or that not all the urine has been collected.

- For normal values of GFR, see Table 22-2.
- Renal function can be categorized as glomerular, tubular, or hormonal (Table 22-3).

# ACUTE RENAL FAILURE

- Defined as an increase in creatinine of 0.5 mg/dL over the baseline

## Etiology

- Acute tubular necrosis (ATN): 45% (ischemia or nephrotoxins)
- Prerenal: 21% (heart failure, sepsis, or volume depletion)
- Acute on chronic: 13% (mostly because of ATN and prerenal diseases, such as acute nephrotoxin-induced injury with preexisting renal condition such as congestive heart failure)
- Urinary tract obstruction: 10%
- Glomerulonephritis or vasculitis: 4%
- Acute interstitial nephritis: 2%

| TABLE 22-2 | Normal Glomerular Filtration Rate (GFR) By Age |
|---|---|

| Age | GFR (mL/min/1.73 M$^2$) |
|---|---|
| Birth | 20.8 |
| 1 wk | 46.6 |
| 3–5 wk | 60.1 |
| 6–9 wk | 67.5 |
| 3–6 mo | 73.8 |
| 6 mo to 1 yr | 93.7 |
| 1–2 yr | 99.1 |
| 2–5 yr | 126.5 |
| 5–15 yr | 116.7 |

## Laboratory Studies

- Serum BUN/creatinine ratio (use with caution in children)
  - Prerenal >20:1
  - Other causes of high BUN: GI bleed, steroids, and tetracycline
  - Other causes of low creatinine: reduced muscle mass in chronically ill children
- Urinalysis
  - Prerenal: possibly hyaline casts
  - Intrinsic renal disease: brown granular casts, RBC casts, WBC casts, renal epithelial cells, and RBCs and WBCs
- Urine sodium concentration
  - Prerenal: <20 mEq/L
  - Intrinsic disease: >40 mEq/L
- Fractional excretion of Na ($FE_{Na}$) = ($U_{Na} \cdot Cr$)/($P_{Na} \cdot U_{Cr}$) × 100
  - Prerenal: <1 %
  - ATN: >2 %
  - Unequivocal if 1%–2%
  - Not useful if patients are taking diuretics

| TABLE 22-3 | Summary of Diagnostic Renal Evaluation by Function |
|---|---|

| Glomerular function | Tubular function | Hormonal function |
|---|---|---|
| Blood urea nitrogen | Water metabolism<br>• Urine specific gravity<br>• Urine osmolality<br>• Maximal urine concentrating ability | Erythropoietin<br>• Hematocrit<br>• Reticulocyte |
| Serum creatinine and inulin clearance Iothalamate glomerular filtration rate study | Acid-base metabolism<br>• Urine pH<br>• Urine titratable acid excretion<br>• Urine ammonium excretion<br>• Urine-blood $Pco_2$<br>• Fractional excretion of bicarbonate at normal serum bicarbonate level | Vitamin D<br>• Serum 1,25-$(OH)_2D_3$ concentration<br>• Serum calcium concentration |

- Fractional excretion (FE) of urea = $(U_{urea} \cdot P_{Cr})/(P_{urea} \cdot U_{Cr}) \times 100$
  - Prerenal: $<35\%$
  - Intrinsic: $>60\%-65\%$

- Urine osmolality
  - Prerenal: $>500$ milliosmol
  - Intrinsic: $<450$ milliosmol

- Urine-to-plasma creatinine concentration
  - Prerenal: $>40$
  - Intrinsic: $<20$

# METABOLIC ACIDOSIS

- Increased anion gap
  - Causes that result in an increase in unmeasured anions include diabetic ketoacidosis; lactic acidosis; uremia; and ingestion of salicylates, ethylene glycol, and methanol.
  - Severe diarrhea can also cause an increased anion gap acidosis in children and infants.

- Normal anion gap
  - GI bicarbonate loss (diarrhea, intestinal/pancreatic fistulas, resins)
  - Renal tubular acidosis (RTA)
  - Type I: defective proton ($H^+$) secretion
  - Type II: defective $HCO_3$ absorption
  - Type IV: hypoaldosteronism

- Tests for diagnosis of RTA (Table 22-4)
  - Urine pH
    - pH: $<5.5$ proximal type I and type IV
    - pH: $>5.5$ distal type I
  - Urine ammonia levels: low in distal type I
  - Urine anion gap
    - Negative in proximal type I
    - Positive in distal type I and type IV

### TABLE 22-4 Types of Renal Tubular Acidosis

|  | Distal type 1 | Proximal type II | Type IV |
|---|---|---|---|
| Urine anion gap | Positive | Negative | Positive |
| Urine ammonia | Low | Appropriately high | Low |
| Plasma potassium | Low | Low | High |
| Urine pH (when acidotic) | >6 | <6 | <6 |
| Defect | Abnormal $H^+$ pump | Abnormal $HCO_3$ transport | Low distal sodium transport, low aldosterone |
| Treatment | Bicarbonate | Investigate and treat underlying disease | Fludrocortisone (Florinef), surgery |
| Examples | Amphotericin, nephrocalcinosis | Fanconi syndrome (e.g., cystinosis), heavy metal poisoning, drugs (e.g., ifosfamide), primary hyperparathyroidism | Obstructive uropathy, chronic dehydration |

# PROTEINURIA

## Definition and Epidemiology

- Normal protein excretion: $<4$ mg/m$^2$/hr
  - Severe proteinuria: $>1$ g/day
  - Nephrotic range proteinuria: $>40$ mg/m$^2$/hr
  - Protein excretion highest in infants (immaturity of renal function); decreases slowly until reaches adult levels in late adolescence
  - Asymptomatic proteinuria: range, 0.6%–6.3% m$^2$/hr; usually transient and intermittent, with 10% having proteinuria after 6–12 months

## History

- History of the present illness
  - Age of onset (the younger the age, the more likely a significant cause is found)
  - Associated symptoms
    - Urethral dysuria: inflammation/irritation around urethra or bladder
    - Suprapubic tenderness: bladder
    - Flank/unilateral back pain: kidney
    - Dysuria, frequency, incontinence, foul smelling urine, or purulent urethral discharge: urethritis
    - Hemoptysis: Goodpasture syndrome, Wegener granulomatosis, or tuberculosis
    - Lower extremity bruising, arthritis, abdominal pain, or testicular swelling/discomfort: Henoch-Schönlein purpura (HSP)
    - Bloody diarrhea: hemolytic-uremic syndrome (HUS)
    - Arthritis, Raynaud phenomenon, alopecia, photosensitivity, weight loss, or malar rash: systemic lupus erythematosus (SLE) or other rheumatologic disorder
- Past medical history
  - Recurrent pyelonephritis/unexplained fever in infancy: scarred kidney
  - Recent streptococcal infection: poststreptococcal acute glomerulonephritis
  - History of hepatitis or tuberculosis
  - Recent viral infection: postinfectious glomerulonephritis
  - Presence of hematuria and symptoms of upper respiratory infection: IgA nephropathy, hereditary nephritis, thin membrane disease, or membranoproliferative glomerulonephritis
  - Right-sided congestive heart failure or pericarditis: renal vein congestion syndrome
  - Infant of diabetic mother, nephrotic syndrome, severe dehydration: renal vein thrombosis
  - Congenital heart disease: proliferative glomerulonephritis associated with subacute bacterial endocarditis
  - Travel history
  - Drug use
- Family history: deafness or visual disorders suggestive of hereditary nephritis

## Physical Examination

- Weight, height, occipitofrontal circumference (growth failure)
- Blood pressure and heart rate
- Edema (periorbital, presacral, genital, ankle)
- Polythelia, preauricular sinus, single umbilical artery, low-set/malformed ear: may point to congenital urinary problem (hydronephrosis, cystic/dysplastic kidneys)
- Large bladder: urethral obstruction

## Laboratory Studies

- First-morning urinalysis and another urinalysis later in the day (to rule out orthostatic proteinuria; need multiple samples)

- Microscopic examination: looking at color, stones, WBCs, eosinophils, WBC casts, RBC casts, dysmorphic RBCs, lipid bodies/casts
- Quantitative protein excretion measurement (or urine protein/creatinine ratio)
  - Protein excretion >1 g/24 hr implies glomerular dysfunction; <1 g/24 hr implies tubular dysfunction
- Urine protein/creatinine ratio
  - Total urine protein (g/m$^2$/day) = 0.63 × (U$_{Pr}$/U$_{Cr}$)
  - Adults and children >2 years: U$_{Pr}$/U$_{Cr}$ <0.2
  - Children 6 months–2 years: U$_{Pr}$/U$_{Cr}$ <0.5
  - Nephrotic range proteinuria: U$_{Pr}$/U$_{Cr}$ >3
  - Not valid in severe malnutrition and significant reductions of GFR
- Dipstick: proteinuria defined as 1+ or more
  - False-positive result: concentrated urine (specific gravity >1.030), alkaline urine, heavy mucus/blood/pus/semen/vaginal secretions
  - False-negative result: dilute urine (specific gravity <1.010), acidic urine, other proteins besides albumin (dipsticks are preferential to albumin)
- Sulfosalicylic acid turbidimetry: add 3 drops of 20% sulfosalicylic acid to 5 mL urine to cause precipitation of proteins in acid environment; note turbidity by inspection
  - Advantage: not limited to albumin
  - Disadvantage: needs urine with specific gravity >1.015
  - False-positive results: radiographic contrast, high doses of penicillin, cephalosporin, or sulfonamides
- Timed urine collection over 12 or 24 hours: difficult to obtain
- Complete blood count (CBC), basic metabolic panel, erythrocyte sedimentation rate
- Other laboratory tests, depending on differential diagnosis (C3 if suspecting glomerulonephritis, antistreptolysin O (ASO)/DNAse B if recent streptococcal infection, dsDNA if SLE is suspected)

## Imaging

- Ultrasound of urinary tract with Doppler of renal veins to rule out anatomical abnormalities
- Voiding cystourethrogram if the patient has small or scarred kidneys or a history of pyelonephritis
- Dimercaptosuccinic acid (DMSA) scan if the patient has renal scarring

## Indications for Renal Biopsy

- Definitive criteria: symptoms accompanied by (1) hematuria, (2) hypertension, (3) persistently low complement, (4) persistently depressed GFR, (5) signs or symptoms of collagen vascular disease, (6) chronic renal failure, (7) family history of chronic renal failure, (8) proteinuria >1 g/m$^2$/day, (9) nephrotic syndrome presenting in patients <1 year of age or >13 years of age, and (10) nephrotic syndrome unresponsive to a 4-week course of prednisone
- Debatable criteria: proteinuria with a later stage of onset, not responsive to therapy, or proteinuria lasting from 6 months to 1 year

## Differential Diagnosis

- Functional (or transient) proteinuria (cold exposure, CHF, epinephrine, fever, seizures, abdominal surgery, extreme exercise)
- Overflow proteinuria (excessive albumin transfusion, intravascular hemolysis, rhabdomyolysis)
- Orthostatic proteinuria
- Glomerular disease: nephrotic syndrome, glomerulonephritis (see below for specific discussions)
- Interstitial nephritis
  - Primary/isolated: infection, drug exposure, immunologic disease, idiopathic
  - Associated with glomerulonephritis and nephrotic syndrome

- Associated with structural renal disease: vesicoureteric reflux, obstruction, cystic disease
- Hereditary/metabolic: idiopathic familial interstitial nephritis, cystinosis, Wilson syndrome, sickle cell disease, hypercalcemia, hyperuricemia, Lesch-Nyhan syndrome, hyperoxaluria, hypokalemia
- Neoplastic disease
- Associated with chronic progressive renal disease of any etiology
- Other conditions: allograft rejection, heavy metals, radiation, Balkan nephropathy, idiopathic

- Renal tubular disorders
  - Fanconi syndrome (e.g., cystinosis, Dent disease, galactosemia, hereditary fructose intolerance, Lowe syndrome)
  - Tubular toxins: medications (aminoglycosides, penicillin), primary renal tubular disorders (isolated tubular proteinuria, polymyxins, cephalosporin, phenacetin, naproxen, allopurinol, phenindione), heavy metals
  - Ischemic tubular injury
- Other conditions: reflux nephropathy, polycystic kidney disease, renal transplant rejection

## Treatment

- Treat the cause if known.

# NEPHROTIC SYNDROME

## Definition and Epidemiology

- Nephrotic syndrome is a clinical state characterized by:
  - Massive proteinuria ( >40 mg/m$^2$/hr)
  - Hypoalbuminemia (albumin <2.5 g/dL)
  - Edema
  - Hypercholesterolemia

- It is a functional state associated with many glomerular diseases.
- For information about its incidence, see Table 22-5.

## Classification

- Congenital nephrotic syndrome (Finnish type, diffuse mesangial sclerosis, secondary to congenital infection)
- Primary or idiopathic nephrotic syndrome (minimal change disease and primary focal segmental sclerosis without any identifiable cause)
- Secondary nephrotic syndrome: SLE, HSP, acute glomerulonephritis, HUS, bacterial endocarditis, bee stings, drugs, sickle cell anemias, diabetic nephropathy, chronic nephritis

**TABLE 22-5** Incidence of Nephrotic Syndrome

| Types of primary nephrotic syndrome | Age 1–12 yr | Age 13–19 yr |
|---|---|---|
| Minimal change nephrotic syndrome | 76% | 43% |
| Focal segmental glomerulosclerosis | 7% | 13% |
| Membranoproliferative glomerulonephropathy | 7% | 14% |
| Membranous nephropathy | 2% | 22% |
| Others | 8% | 8% |

**TABLE 22-6**

| Complications | Cause |
|---|---|
| Infection: peritonitis (*Streptococcus pneumoniae* and *Escherichia coli*) | Edema<br>Low serum IgG<br>Low factor B<br>Decreased mesenteric blood flow |
| Thromboembolus: generally venous | Loss of antithrombin III in urine<br>High fibrinogen<br>High blood viscosity<br>Decreased renal blood flow |
| Hyperlipidemia | Increased very low density lipoproteins produced by liver.<br>Urinary loss of high-density lipoprotein and lipoproteins |
| Hypocalcemia | Artifactual hypocalcemia secondary to hypoalbuminemia and true hypocalcemia from urinary loss of vitamin D. |
| Copper, zinc, and iron deficiencies | Loss of carrier proteins |
| Artifactual hypothyroidism | Loss of thyroxine binding globulin |

## Treatment (Primary or Idiopathic)

- Prednisone 60 mg/m$^2$/day in divided doses for 6 weeks, followed by 40 mg/m$^2$/day in a single dose every other day for 6 weeks
- Relapse: defined as proteinuria of >2+ for 3 consecutive days
  - Treat with 60 mg/m$^2$/day in divided doses until resolved for 3 days, followed by tapering.
  - If >4 relapses/year, consider chlorambucil or cyclophosphamide with tapered prednisone every other day.

- Additional measures
  - Adequate protein in diet for endogenous synthesis of albumin
  - Restricted salt in diet
  - Fluid restriction: 600–800 mL

## Complications (Table 22-6)

## Indications for Renal Biopsy

- Steroid-resistant nephrotic syndrome
- Steroid-responsive nephrotic syndrome with frequent relapses
- Low serum complement (low C3) at presentation
- Patients <1 year of age (risk of congenital nephrotic syndrome)
- Evidence of renal insufficiency with high creatinine at presentation
- SLE with proteinuria or nephrotic syndrome

# HEMATURIA

## Definition and Epidemiology

- Defined as >5 RBCs/HPF
- Isolated hematuria: hematuria without proteinuria (hematuria associated with persistent proteinuria (>1+) should be referred to pediatric nephrologist)
- Prevalence: 1.5% in pediatrics (0.5%–1% have microhematuria lasting >1 month). The condition is mostly transient or intermittent.

## Etiology

- The differential diagnosis is obtained by determining the source of bleeding.
  - Glomerular: postinfectious glomerulonephritis (most common and may last up to a year), IgA nephropathy, lupus nephritis, nephritis of anaphylactoid purpura, Alport syndrome, benign familiar hematuria, focal segmental glomerulosclerosis, minimal change nephritic syndrome, membranoproliferative glomerulonephritis, or membranous nephropathy
  - Nonglomerular
    - Tubulointerstitial: infectious, metabolic, allergic vasculitis, drug- or poison-induced, or ATN
    - Vascular: renal venous thrombosis, sickle cell nephropathy, or malformations
    - Proliferative: Wilms tumor, renal cell carcinoma, polycystic kidney disease, or simple cyst
  - Renal pelvic and ureteral: kidney stones, trauma, vascular malformations, papillary necrosis, hydronephrosis, infections, or vasculitis
  - Bladder: infection/inflammation, kidney stones, drugs (cyclophosphamide), trauma, tumors, or vascular malformations
  - Urethral: infection/inflammation or trauma
  - Undefined: hypercalciuria or exercise-induced disease

## History

- Characteristics of hematuria: timing, onset, and duration
- Associated signs and symptoms: concurrent illnesses, joint pain, dysuria, edema, flank pain, rash, abdominal pain, vigorous exercise, or drug ingestion
- Past medical history: cystic kidney disease, sickle cell disease, skin and throat infections, SLE, malignancy, and neonatal course
- Family history: cystic kidney disease, deafness, hematuria, renal failure, sickle cell disease/trait, and/or nephrolithiasis

## Physical Examination

- Check for ear abnormalities and evaluate hearing (Alport syndrome).
- Palpate abdomen for masses (polycystic kidney disease, Wilms tumor) and costovertebral/flank tenderness.
- Check external genitalia for trauma.
- Check for edema (periorbital or pedal) and skin lesions (malar rash, purpuric lesions in HSP, impetigo).

## Laboratory Studies and Imaging

- A workup for hematuria is necessary if microscopic hematuria persists for >1 month.
- Urinalysis
  - Repeat urinalysis 2–3 times at intervals of a few days is necessary.
  - Many conditions can cause discolored urine, whether heme positive or negative. Heme-negative causes include beets, blackberries, ibuprofen, iron sorbitol, methyldopa, metronidazole, nitrofurantoin, rifampin, and sulfasalazine.
  - Dipsticks detect heme moiety, so results are positive for hemoglobinuria or myoglobinuria with or without true hematuria. If dipstick is positive for heme, this must be followed with a microscopic examination to determine presence of true hematuria.
  - Urinalysis can provide a hint to the location of the bleeding; glomerular hematuria requires more extensive evaluation (renal ultrasound; CBC; complement levels; antinuclear antibody (ANA), antineutrophilic cytoplasmic antibody (ANCA), and ASO titers; hepatitis B screen; and possibly renal biopsy). See Table 22-7 for more information.
- Urine culture
- Sickle cell "prep" for African-American patients (sickle cell trait can cause hematuria)
- Urine calcium and urine calcium/creatinine ratio (idiopathic hypercalciuria defined as ratio >0.20, urine calcium >20 mg/dL, or 24-hour urine calcium excretion >4 mg/kg/day)

| TABLE 22-7 Characteristics of Glomerular Versus Nonglomerular Bleeding | |
|---|---|
| Glomerular | Nonglomerular |
| Brown or "tea" colored urine | Red or pink urine |
| RBC casts, cellular casts, tubular cells | Blood clots |
| Dysmorphic RBCs | Isomorphic RBCs |
| >2+ proteinuria | No proteinuria |
| RBC, red blood cell. | |

- Electrolytes, BUN, creatinine
- Renal ultrasound
- Complement (C3)

## Treatment

- Therapy depends on cause.
  - For hypercalciuria, increase fluids, sodium or potassium citrate, and thiazides.
  - For postinfectious glomerulonephritis, use salt restriction, diuretics if needed, and close follow-up.
  - For SLE, use steroids with or without other immunosuppressants and close follow-up.
  - For Alport syndrome, use dialysis or transplant.
- If the workup points to isolated hematuria without serious pathologic cause, follow up every 6 months to a year without further workup. Follow growth pattern, blood pressure, and urinalysis. See "Glomerulonephritis" section.

## GLOMERULONEPHRITIS

- This glomerular disease with inflammation of glomerular tuft is characterized by hematuria (RBCs and RBC casts), proteinuria in the subnephrotic range (severe cases or some glomerulonephritis may show a nephrotic range), oliguria and edema, azotemia, and hypertension.
- The differential diagnosis of glomerulonephritis is presented in Table 22-8.

### Diagnosis

- Biopsy
  - Persistently low C3 (membranoproliferative glomerulonephritis) or low C4 (SLE)
  - Positive ANA
  - Normal complements with progressive disease or persistent symptoms
  - Nephrotic syndrome at presentation
  - Progressive azotemia (rapidly progressive glomerulonephritis)
- Outcome depends on:
  - Histology of glomerulus
  - Tubulointerstitial inflammation/scarring
  - Renal function at diagnosis
  - Hypertension
  - Degree of proteinuria

### Treatment

- Immunosuppressive therapy, depending on the type of glomerulonephritis

**TABLE 22-8** Differential Diagnosis of Glomerulonephritis

| Cause of glomerulonephritis (GN) | Serologic findings | Biopsy findings | Management |
|---|---|---|---|
| Acute poststreptococcal GN | Low C3 | EM: subepithelial "humps" IM: positive deposits along capillary loops and mesangium | Conservative; treat hypertension and persistent streptococcal infection |
| IgA nephropathy | None | EM and IM: mesangial deposits + IgA | Nonnephrotic range proteinuria: ACE I NS: Prednisone |
| Thin basement membrane disease | None | EM measurement of GBM <300 nm | Proteinuria: ACE inhibitor |
| Hereditary nephritis | None | EM: splitting of lamina densa and lucent areas in GBM | Proteinuria: ACE inhibitor |
| Henoch-Schönlein purpura | None | IM and EM: mesangial deposits- + IgA | Nonnephrotic range proteinuria: ACE inhibitor; Nephrotic syndrome or RPGN: Prednisone |
| Membranoproliferative GN | Low C3 +/−C4 | IM: positive mesangial and capillary deposits EM: subendothelial deposits in types 1 and 3; GBM deposits in type 2 | Immunosuppressive therapy based on biopsy findings |
| Systemic lupus erythematosus GN | Low C3 +/−C4 | IM: positive mesangial and capillary deposits EM: subendothelial or subepithelial deposits | Immunosuppressive therapy based on biopsy findings |
| Vasculitis | + ANCA | ± Immune mesangial deposition | Immunosuppressive therapy based on biopsy findings |
| RPGN | Varies based on underlying pathology | >50% of glomeruli with crescents | Aggressive immunosuppressive therapy |

*ACE,* Angiotensin-converting enzyme.
*C,* Complement.
*IM,* Immunofluorescence microscopy.
*EM,* Electron microscopy.
*RPGN,* rapidly progressive glomerular nephritis.
*GBM,* glomerular basement membrane.

# HYPERTENSION

## Definitions

- Hypertension: defined as blood pressure ≥95th percentile on three separate occasions. (See Appendix F for tables of normal blood pressure by age and height.)
- Stages of hypertension
  - Normal: systolic and diastolic blood pressure <90th percentile for sex and age (normotensive)
  - Prehypertension hypertension: systolic and diastolic blood pressure ≥90th percentile but <95th percentile or blood pressure exceeding 120/80 mm Hg even if <90th percentile
  - Stage 1 hypertension: systolic and/or diastolic blood pressure between the 95th and 5 mm Hg above the 99th percentile
  - Stage 2 hypertension: systolic and/or diastolic blood pressure ≥99th percentile plus 5 mm of Hg.

## Epidemiology

- Screening: annual blood pressure measurements starting at 3 years of age
- Prevalence: 0.8%–5% in pediatrics overall
- Symptoms in only half of severely hypertensive patients
  - In the first year of life, patients may present with failure to thrive, irritability, feeding problems, cyanosis, respiratory distress, heart failure, or seizures.
  - The condition is often silent after 1 year of age.

## Etiology

- Hypertension can be divided into transient (usually more drug-induced, acute renal injury with recovery, hypervolemia from volume overload, after surgeries such as renal transplants, genitourinary or orthopedic surgery, Guillain-Barré syndrome, increased intracranial pressure, and lead poisoning). The sustained type may represent:
  - Primary/essential hypertension (12%–18%)
  - Renal disease: chronic pyelonephritis/reflux nephropathy, chronic glomerulonephritides, chronic renal failure, HUS, polycystic kidney disease, or Wilms tumor
  - Renal vascular disease: fibromuscular dysplasia, congenital renal arterial stenosis, neurofibromatosis, or renal transplant arterial stenosis (including calcineurin induced)
  - Cardiovascular conditions: coarctation of the aorta or Takayasu arteritis
  - Endocrine conditions: catecholamine-secreting tumors (pheochromocytoma or neuroblastoma) or enzymatic defects in adrenal steroid synthesis
  - Other conditions: sickle cell anemia, Williams syndrome, idiopathic arterial calcification of infancy, obesity, closure of abdominal wall defects in neonates
- Age often helps determine the cause (Table 22-9).

## History

- Family history of hypertension or neonatal history (umbilical artery catheter in infancy)
- Abdominal pain, dysuria, frequency, nocturia, or enuresis: may suggest underlying renal disease
- Joint pain/swelling or edema: connective tissues disease and/or nephritis
- Weight loss, failure to gain weight, sweating, flushing, fevers, or palpitations: may suggest pheochromocytoma, hyperthyroidism
- Muscle cramps, weakness, or constipation: hypokalemia or hyperaldosteronism
- Age of onset of menarche and sexual development: hydroxylase deficiencies
- Medication use (over-the-counter drugs, oral contraceptive pills, illegal drugs): drug induction

| TABLE 22-9 | Differential Diagnosis of Hypertension |
|---|---|
| Age group | Causes |
| Neonates | Renal artery thrombosis, renal artery stenosis, congenital renal malformations, coarctation of the aorta, bronchopulmonary dysplasia, patent ductus arteriosus, intraventricular hemorrhage |
| Infancy–10 yr | Renal parenchymal disease, coarctation of the aorta<br>Less common: renal artery stenosis, hypercalcemia, neurofibromatosis, pheochromocytoma, mineralocorticoid excess, hyperthyroidism, transient hypertension status-post genitourinary surgery or immobilization, primary hypertension |
| Adolescence | Primary hypertension, renal parenchymal disease<br>Less common: same as for Infancy–10 yr |

## Physical Examination

- General
  - Examine the skin for pallor, flushing, increased sweating, and pale mucous membranes.
  - Note edema, cushingoid features, dysmorphic features (Turner or Williams syndrome), thyroid enlargement, and birthmarks, such as café-au-lait spots or neurofibromas.
- Cardiovascular
  - Note femoral pulses if absent or delayed or if there is a discrepancy between upper and lower extremity pulses. Obtain four extremity blood pressures.
  - Examine heart size, rate, rhythm, murmurs, work of breathing, hepatomegaly, and bruits over major vessels.
- Abdomen
  - Palpate for masses (unilateral or bilateral) or epigastric bruits.
- Neurologic
  - Examine fundi and note neurologic deficits.

## Laboratory Studies and Imaging

- Suspected essential hypertension: CBC, urinalysis, BUN, creatinine, uric acid, fasting cholesterol, triglycerides, high-density lipoprotein cholesterol, low-density lipoprotein cholesterol, and echocardiogram
- Suspected secondary etiology
  - Tailor depending on suspected cause.
  - Starting studies include CBC, urinalysis (and culture for suspected renal pathology), electrolytes with BUN, creatinine, and uric acid, as well as an echocardiogram.
  - Other studies to consider, depending on suspected etiology: renal ultrasound and radionuclide studies, abdominal computed tomography (looking at kidneys and adrenals), urine and plasma catecholamines, plasma renin and aldosterone, thyroid and thyroid-stimulating hormone, and adrenal hormones if hydroxylase or other enzyme defects suspected

## Treatment

- General counseling about cardiovascular risk factors (obesity, exercise, smoking) is necessary. Treatment, especially of primary hypertension, should begin with nonpharmacologic therapy and lifestyle modification (weight loss, dietary modifications, and exercise); this should continue whether or not medications are needed.

- Pharmacologic therapy is indicated for patients with symptomatic hypertension, severe hypertension (defined as 99th percentile and above), end-organ damage secondary to hypertension, or hypertensive refractory to nonpharmacologic treatment.
  - The "stepped care" approach is useful. Begin one medication at a low dose and increase until blood pressure is controlled, the maximum dose is reached, or side effects occur. Failing adequate control, switch to or add a second agent and proceed as above. Consult a specialist before adding a third medication.
  - The same classes of antihypertensives (including diuretics, β-blockers, angiotensin-converting enzyme inhibitors, and calcium channel antagonists) are used in children as in adults, but there is less information about efficacy and long-term safety in children.
- If weight is a factor:
  - In obese patients or those with weight >90% for age and with blood pressure in the high normal range, start with nonpharmacologic treatment such as weight loss with salt restriction. If blood pressure is high normal and weight is >90th percentile from obesity, suggest weight loss and continue to monitor blood pressure regularly.
  - If weight is acceptable, then monitor blood pressure every 6 months.

## Suggested Readings

Kher K, Makker S. Clinical Pediatric Nephrology. New York: McGraw-Hill, 1992.

Barratt T, Avner E, Harmon W. Pediatric Nephrology. Baltimore: Lippincott Williams & Wilkins, 1999:317–329.

Fernandes E, McCrindle BW. Diagnosis and treatment of hypertension in children and adolescents. Can J Cardiol 2000;16(6):801–811.

Flynn JT. Neonatal hypertension: diagnosis and management. Pediatr Nephrol 2000:14:332–341.

Roy S. Proteinuria. Pediatr Ann May 1997;25(5):277–282.

Leung AKC, Robson WL. Evaluating the child with proteinuria. J Royal Society Promotion Health March 2000;120(1):16–22.

Loghman-Adham M. Evaluating proteinuria in children. Am Fam Physician 1998;58(5): 1145–1152, 1158–1159.

Roy S III. Hematuria. Pediatr Rev 1998;19(6):209–212.

Cruz CC, Spitzer A. When you find protein or blood in the urine. Contemp Pediatr 1998;15(9):89–109.

# RHEUMATOLOGIC DISEASES

**23**

*Megan A. Cooper and Andrew J. White*

■ Pediatric rheumatology is a broad field that deals with disorders of the joints, connective tissues, muscles, and vasculature, as well as autoimmune and autoinflammatory disorders.

## APPROACH TO THE CHILD WITH JOINT PAIN AND/OR SWELLING

■ Joint pain is a common complaint in children.
■ It is generally transient, secondary to trauma and/or increased activity.

### Etiology and Differential Diagnosis

■ It is important to determine if the pain is secondary to joint, muscular, ligament, or bone, or if it is referred pain.
■ Joint pain (arthralgia) should be distinguished from arthritis, which has objective physical examination findings of effusion, warmth, and/or erythema.
■ Joint pain may be because of various conditions depending on the number and kind of joints involved.
  ■ Single joint (monoarticular):
    • Infectious: septic joint, osteomyelitis, Lyme arthritis, or gonococcal infection
    • Fracture
    • Hemarthrosis (primarily seen in sickle cell disease)
    • Malignancy: primary bone tumor or leukemia
    • Inflammatory: juvenile rheumatoid arthritis (JRA) or other inflammatory arthritis (e.g., psoriatic arthritis, spondyloarthropathies, sarcoidosis)
  ■ Multiple joints (polyarticular)
    • Inflammatory: JRA, juvenile ankylosing spondylitis, psoriatic arthritis, Henoch-Schönlein purpura (HSP), systemic lupus erythematosus (SLE), serum sicknesslike reaction, sarcoidosis, inflammatory bowel disease (IBD)–associated arthritis, or Kawasaki disease
    • Malignancy: leukemia
    • Infectious: Lyme arthritis or *Neisseria gonorrhoeae*
    • Reactive arthritis: *Salmonella, Shigella, Yersinia, Campylobacter,* or *Chlamydia*
    • Rickets
  ■ Hip involvement (rare as the sole presentation of an inflammatory arthritis in children)
    • Avascular necrosis: Legg-Calve-Perthes disease, sickle cell disease, or chronic steroid use
    • Slipped capital femoral epiphysis (SCFE)
    • Transient synovitis (formerly known as toxic synovitis)
    • Septic joint
    • Lyme arthritis

### Laboratory Studies

*Initial Evaluation*
■ Blood cultures: any time there is fever and new-onset joint pain
■ Complete blood count (CBC):
  ■ Elevated white blood cells (WBCs): infection, inflammatory arthritis, malignancies

**TABLE 23-1** | Properties of Synovial Joint Fluid

| | Normal | Reactive arthritis | Inflammatory (e.g., JRA) | Infectious |
|---|---|---|---|---|
| Color | Variable | Yellow | Yellow | Variable |
| Clarity | Clear | Clear to cloudy | Clear to cloudy | Cloudy, turbid |
| White blood cell count (per mm$^3$) | <200 | 5,000–10,000 | 5,000–>100,000 | >50,000 |
| % neutrophils | <25% | >50% | >50% | >75% |
| Culture | Negative | Negative | Negative | Positive |

*JRA*, juvenile rheumatoid arthritis.

- Cytopenias: SLE
- Microcytic anemia: IBD, systemic JRA
- Erythrocyte sedimentation rate (ESR) and C-reactive protein (CRP): elevated in infectious and inflammatory conditions; these are both nonspecific but can be useful for tracking established disease activity
- Renal function panel: SLE, vasculitis (e.g., HSP, ANCA-positive vasculitis, Goodpasture syndrome)
- Antinuclear antibody (ANA): if there is clinical concern for SLE

### Joint Fluid Analysis (Table 23-1)

- For isolated effusions with fever, joint aspiration is necessary to exclude a septic joint and should be done quickly and before initiation of antibiotics if the patient is stable.
- Do not consider a rheumatologic etiology or initiate steroids in a child with fever and joint effusion before conducting a thorough investigation for a septic joint or osteomyelitis.

### Imaging

- Plain film radiographs of involved joints may show evidence of trauma, arthritis, and bony abnormalities.
- In cases where there is a history of trauma or concern for septic joint and/or osteomyelitis, a computed tomography or magnetic resonance imaging scan can be useful.

### Treatment

- A patient who presents with joint pain and fever must be presumed to have a septic joint or osteomyelitis until proven otherwise.
- A potentially septic joint or osteomyelitis is an emergency that requires prompt recognition, involvement of orthopedic surgery, radiologic imaging, and initiation of intravenous (IV) antibiotics once blood and synovial fluid (if appropriate) cultures are obtained.
- Drugs frequently used in rheumatology are described in Table 23-2.

## JUVENILE RHEUMATOID ARTHRITIS

- JRA is thought to be an autoimmune disease, but its exact etiology is unknown.
- This disease may be classified into three subsets: pauciarticular, polyarticular, and systemic (Table 23-3).

**TABLE 23-2** Common Drugs Used in Rheumatology[*]

| Drug | Mechanism/actions | Dosage | Major side effects |
|---|---|---|---|
| **NSAIDs** | | | |
| Naproxen | Anti-inflammatory | 20 mg/kg/day PO div. q12h | Easy bleeding and bruising |
| Ibuprofen | Cyclooxygenase enzyme inhibition | 10 mg/kg/dose PO q 6h | Gastrointestinal: gastritis, bleeding |
| Aspirin | | 75–90 mg/kg/day PO div. q.i.d | Reye syndrome (aspirin) |
| | | | Nephrotoxicity |
| **Corticosteroids** | | | |
| Prednisone (PO) | Anti-inflammatory | Varies, 0.5–2 mg/kg/d PO | Cushing syndrome, growth delay, |
| Methylprednisolone (IV) | Immunosuppressive (T cell) | Pulse dose: 30 mg/kg/d IV, max 1 g/day | osteoporosis, avascular necrosis |
| **Immunosuppressives** | | | |
| Methotrexate | Inhibits purine synthesis | 5–15 mg/m² once weekly PO or SC | Hepatotoxicity |
| | | | Cytopenias |
| **Cytotoxic Agents** | | | |
| Cyclophosphamide | Alkylating agent | Varies, pulse therapy monthly | Cystitis |
| | Causes lymphopenia | is 500–1,000 mg/m² IV | Increased risk of infection |
| | | | Risk of infertility with high total dose |
| Cyclosporine | Thought to inhibit T-cell activation | Not standardized | Nephrotoxicity |
| **Biologic Agents** | | | Hepatotoxicity |
| Rituximab | Anti-CD20 mAb (anti-B cell) | Pediatric dosing not standardized, given | Infusion reactions |
| | | as an IV infusion | Increased risk of infection including |
| | | | re-activation of JC virus |
| Intravenous immune globulin | Pooled human immunoglobulin | Up to 2 g/kg IV | Infusion reactions |
| | | | Aseptic meningitis |
| Anakinra | Soluble IL-1Ra (anti-IL-1) | Pediatric dosing not standardized, SC daily | Local injection site reactions |
| **Anti-TNF-α Agents** | | | **For all Anti-TNF-α agents:** |
| Etanercept (Enbrel) | Soluble TNF-α receptor | 0.4 mg/kg SC twice weekly | Infusion/injection site reactions |
| Infliximab (Remicade) | Anti-TNF-α chimeric mAb | 3–10 mg/kg IV q 4–8 weeks | Reactivation of tuberculosis |
| Adalimumab (Humira) | Humanized anti-TNF-α mAb | SC; dosing in pediatrics not standardized | Possible increased risk of malignancy |

[*]These medications are each used in a variety of rheumatologic diseases; many are investigational and all should be given in consultation with a pediatric rheumatologist.
Abbreviations: *NSAID*, nonsteroidal anti-inflammatory drug; *TNF*, tumor necrosis factor; *SC*, subcutaneous.

**TABLE 23-3  Classification of Juvenile Rheumatoid Arthritis (JRA)**

| | Pauciarticular (oligoarthritis) | Polyarticular | Systemic |
|---|---|---|---|
| **Diagnostic criteria** | | | |
| Number of joints | ≤4 | ≥5 | Any number, usually >5 |
| Length of arthritis | 6 wk | 6 wk | 6 weeks |
| Other | | | Daily fever >39°C for at least 2 weeks |
| **Gender** | Female > Male | Female > Male | Male=Female |
| **Peak Age** | 2–4 yr | 1–4 yr and 6–12 yr | None |
| Extra-articular manifestations | Systemic symptoms rare | Fatigue | Ill appearance |
| | Uveitis (15%–20%) | Poor growth | Erythematous macular rash |
| | | Low-grade fever | Cardiac disease |
| | | Uveitis (5%–10%) | Lymphadenopathy and splenomegaly |
| | | | Pulmonary disease |
| | | | Uveitis is rare |
| **Laboratory Findings** | 65%–85% ANA+ | ~50% ANA+ | ↑ WBC, platelets |
| | ↑ ESR, CRP | ↑ ESR, CRP | ↓ hemoglobin |
| | | ↑ WBC, platelets | ↑ ESR, CRP |
| | | 5% RF+ | Usually ANA and RF negative |
| **Prognosis** | Excellent overall | Can be chronic | Guarded initially |
| | ↑ uveitis with ANA+ | RF+ more severe | ~50% fully recover |

Adapted from Cassidy JT, et al. A study of classification criteria for a diagnosis of juvenile rheumatoid arthritis. Arthritis Rheum 1986, 29:274–281. Cassidy JT, Petty RE, Laxer RM, et al. Textbook of Pediatric Rheumatology, 5th Ed. Philadelphia: Elsevier Inc, 2005.

Abbreviations: ANA, antinuclear antibody; CRP, C-reactive protein; ESR, erythrocyte sedimentation rate; RF, rheumatoid factor; WBC, white blood cell.

## Diagnosis

- JRA is a diagnosis of exclusion (see Table 23-3).
- Diagnosis requires arthritis in one or more joint for at least 6 weeks, age of onset <16 years, and exclusion of other causes of joint inflammation.
- Laboratory values are of little use in diagnosis but can help to exclude other diagnoses, and are for prognosis (e.g., increased risk of uveitis with a positive ANA) and for tracking disease activity (ESR and CRP).
- Other classifications systems are sometimes used for juvenile arthritis. These are juvenile idiopathic arthritis (JIA), which is becoming the preferred term worldwide, and juvenile chronic arthritis (JCA). The terms JRA, JIA, and JCA may be used interchangeably as long as the subsets of diseases are kept in mind.

## Treatment

- Pharmacologic therapy
  - Anti-inflammatory agents
    - Nonsteroidal anti-inflammatory drugs (NSAIDs): naproxen 20 mg/kg/day divided q12h or ibuprofen 40 mg/kg/day divided q6h. Patients need to take this on a scheduled basis for initial therapy.
    - Aspirin: largely replaced by the use of NSAIDs
    - Corticosteroids: used for flares unresponsiveness to NSAIDs or severe systemic manifestations; can be given orally or as an intra-articular injection
  - Disease-modifying agents
    - Methotrexate: need to monitor liver function and blood counts
    - Antitumor necrosis factor (TNF)-α agents: etanercept, infliximab, adalimumab
  - See Table 23-2 for dosages and further information.
- Therapy for systemic JRA
  - Initial treatment often is instituted during hospitalization until systemic symptoms are under control.
  - NSAIDs are useful to control pain and swelling.
  - The early use of IV steroids and methotrexate should be strongly considered.
  - Early use of biologic agents (anti-TNF-α agents and anti-interleukin 1 [anakinra]) may be beneficial in some patients after evaluation by a pediatric rheumatologist.
- Other monitoring/therapies
  - Ophthalmology examinations for uveitis are necessary every 3–6 months for pauciarticular and polyarticular JRA and yearly for systemic JRA.
  - Physical therapy, occupational therapy, and psychological support can be important for long-term outcome. However, with improving therapies, fewer physical disabilities related to JRA now occur.

## Complications

- Most complications/emergencies are related to therapy for JRA, including infections associated with immunosuppressive therapy (corticosteroids and anti-TNF-α agents) or gastrointestinal bleeding related to NSAID use.
- Children with systemic JRA are often very ill and present with multiple extra-articular manifestations as described in Table 23-3.
- Macrophage activation syndrome is a rare life-threatening complication associated with systemic JRA and other autoimmune disorders. This syndrome is characterized by overwhelming systemic inflammation, disseminated intravascular coagulation, hepatic failure, and cytopenias; it is often fatal and swift recognition and treatment in consultation with a pediatric rheumatologist and/or pediatric hematologist is necessary.

# SYSTEMIC LUPUS ERYTHEMATOSUS

## Definition and Epidemiology

■ Systemic lupus erythematosus (SLE) is an autoimmune inflammatory disorder characterized by immune complex deposition in multiple organs.
■ It more commonly affects females.
■ It can develop at any age, but rarely occurs in children <5 years of age.

## Diagnosis and Laboratory Studies

■ SLE is a clinical diagnosis that requires the presence of at least four or more clinical and/or laboratory criteria (Table 23-4; think **MD SOAP BRAIN**)
■ In addition to the laboratory criteria listed in Table 23-4 that are used for diagnosis, the following can be used as markers of disease activity and for therapeutic monitoring in SLE.
   ▪ C3 and C4. Low levels indicate increased disease activity.
   ▪ CBC. Patients often have cytopenias.
   ▪ dsDNA. Titers are often elevated and may be reflective of disease activity.
   ▪ Kidney function. As many as 75% of children with SLE have lupus nephritis.
   ▪ Antiphospholipid antibodies (may also be present in patients without SLE or other autoimmune disease). Patients are at increased risk for thrombotic events. Diagnosis of antiphospholipid syndrome is made based on a history of thrombosis or pregnancy loss or prematurity plus persistent anticardiolipin antibody or lupus anticoagulant positivity 12 weeks apart.

 **TABLE 23-4**    Diagnostic Criteria for Systemic Lupus Erythematous

1. Malar rash: spares nasolabial folds and eyelids
2. Discoid rash: usually on scalp or limbs
3. Serositis: pleuritis or pericarditis
4. Oral or nasal mucocutaneous ulcers: usually painless
5. Arthritis: two or more peripheral joints, nonerosive
6. Photosensitivity: by history or examination
7. Blood: Cytopenias (one of the following):
   • Hemolytic anemia
   • Leukopenia (<4,000/mm$^3$) on two or more occasions
   • Lymphopenia (<1,500/mm$^3$) on two or more occasions
   • Thrombocytopenia (<100,000/mm$^3$)
8. Renal Disorder:
   • Proteinuria >0.5g/day, **or**
   • Cellular casts
9. ANA: positive in the absence of medications known to cause drug-associated lupus
10. Immunologic (one of the following):
   • Anti-dsDNA antibodies
   • Anti-Sm nuclear antigen
   • Antiphospholipid antibodies: anticardiolipin antibodies, lupus anticoagulant, or false positive serologic test for syphilis for at least 6 mo
11. Neurologic (one of the following):
   • Seizure
   • Psychosis

Adapted from Tan E, et al. The 1982 revised criteria for the classification of systemic lupus erythematosus. Arthritis Rheum 1982;25:1271–1277. Hochberg MC. Updating the American College of Rheumatology revised criteria for the classification of systemic lupus erythematosus. Arthritis Rheum 1997;40:1725.

## Treatment

- Goal: to control the immune system
- Pharmacologic therapies (for more information on specific agents, see Table 23-2)
  - NSAIDs (use with caution if patients have renal disease)
  - Corticosteroids
    - Oral prednisone, 0.5–2 mg/kg/day taper until improvement of laboratory markers of disease control; may require long-term use
    - Pulse dosing of IV steroids
  - Immunosuppressive/cytotoxic agents: cyclophosphamide, mycophenolate, azathioprine, and cyclosporine
  - Biologic modifiers: rituximab (monoclonal anti-CD20 antibody)
  - Anticoagulation: should be considered if patients have high titer antiphospholipid antibodies and a history of thrombosis, the optimal treatment is not standardized

## Complications

- Patients with SLE can present with a variety of emergent conditions, including cardiac tamponade; coronary artery disease; Libman-Sacks endocarditis; pleural effusions; pulmonary hemorrhage; renal failure; and thrombosis with stroke related to antiphospholipid syndrome.
- Immunosuppressive therapy makes these patients susceptible to infection.

# NEONATAL LUPUS

- This condition is seen in newborns as a result of transplacental passage of maternal autoantibodies (anti-Ro and anti-La). This is not a systemic disease, and symptoms are generally limited to the skin and heart.
- The majority of mothers of these infants do not have SLE or a connective tissue disorder.
- Clinical manifestations include rash, congenital heart block, liver disease, and cytopenias.
- Treatment is supportive until maternal antibodies are gone (generally by 6–8 months of age).
- If present, congenital heart block is usually permanent and may require a pacemaker.
- Infants do not appear to have an increased risk of developing SLE later in life.

# JUVENILE DERMATOMYOSITIS

## Definition and Epidemiology

- Juvenile dermatomyositis is an autoimmune disorder characterized by inflammation of the muscle and skin resulting in proximal muscle weakness and characteristic skin lesions. The mechanism appears to be related to a vasculopathy.
- Before therapy with corticosteroids, one-third of patients died, but now survival is >95%.
- The peak age of onset is 5–14 years.
- The condition is seen more commonly in girls.

## Clinical Presentation

- Patients may present acutely with inability to walk because of muscle weakness; look for Gower sign on physical examination.
- Characteristic rashes include a heliotropic rash with purplish discoloration of upper eyelids and periorbital edema, as well as Gottron papules (shiny, scaly, erythematous dermatitis over the dorsum of the metacarpophalangeal and proximal interphalangeal joints).

■ Other common findings include fever, fatigue, and weight loss; dysphagia; arthralgias and arthritis; subcutaneous calcinosis, sometimes resulting in ulcerations; nail bed telangiectasias, which are nearly pathognomonic; and vasculitis that affects visceral organs (GI bleeding) and skin.

## Treatment

■ Pharmacologic therapy. For more information on specific agents, see Table 23-2.
  ■ Corticosteroids: IV pulse or oral 2 mg/kg/day until symptoms improve (strength, muscle enzymes); then taper. However, these drugs may be required for years.
  ■ Immunosuppressives/cytotoxic agents: methotrexate, hydroxychloroquine, cyclophosphamide, cyclosporine, and azathioprine have been used
  ■ Biologic modifiers: IVIG and rituximab (experimental) have been used with some success

## Complications

■ Prompt recognition of symptoms and treatment advances have significantly reduced the morbidity and mortality of this disease.
■ However, patients are still at risk for cardiorespiratory failure because of muscle weakness; aspiration pneumonias; and organ damage such as gastrointestinal hemorrhage related to vasculitis.

# HENOCH-SCHÖNLEIN PURPURA

## Definition and Epidemiology

■ HSP is characterized by a purpuric rash with normal platelets, abdominal pain, and glomerulonephritis.
■ It is a common vasculitis in children, usually occurring between the ages of 3 and 15 years.
■ It is more frequent in winter months.
■ It often follows a viral upper respiratory infection.

## Clinical Presentation and Diagnosis

■ If other causes of purpura are excluded (e.g., infection, thrombocytopenia, DIC, and other vasculitides), HSP can be diagnosed if at least two of the following are present (adapted from American College of Rheumatology criteria):
  ■ Age <20 years
  ■ Purpuric rash without thrombocytopenia, usually in dependent areas such as legs and buttocks
  ■ Abdominal pain or bloody diarrhea indicating bowel wall ischemia
  ■ Biopsy (e.g., skin, kidney) showing granulocytes in the walls of blood vessels
■ Other common findings include arthritis and arthralgias in large joints; glomerulonephritis, which occurs in one third of cases and usually resolves but can result in renal failure (kidney biopsy may be required); orchitis and testicular torsion; and scalp edema.

## Treatment

■ Treatment is generally supportive and symptomatic.
■ Corticosteroids may be effective, and short-term therapy may help with arthritis, orchitis, and gastrointestinal hemorrhage.
■ Treatment of gastrointestinal hemorrhage and renal complications is necessary.

## Results

■ Most patients recover in 2–4 weeks, and the course of HSP is usually benign. One third of children experience recurrence with rash and abdominal pain, usually shortly after the initial episode.
■ <5% of patients with renal disease progress to renal failure and may require transplantation.

# RHEUMATIC FEVER

## Etiology and Epidemiology

- This multisystem inflammatory process follows pharyngitis with group A β-hemolytic *Streptococcus* infection. It does not occur after cutaneous group A *Streptococcus* infections.
- It is thought to be caused by autoreactive antibodies directed against antigens from the *Streptococcus* bacteria that mimic host antigens.
- Peak age of incidence is 6–15 years.

## Laboratory Studies and Imaging

- Throat culture or rapid streptococcal test
- Streptococcal antibody titers
- Echocardiogram for all patients with suspected cardiac disease

## Diagnostic Criteria

- Diagnosis of initial episode of rheumatic fever is based on the Jones criteria (Table 23-5). Evidence of prior streptococcal infection with two major criteria or one major and two minor criteria is necessary.
- Patients with a history of rheumatic fever are at increased risk for recurrence of subsequent streptococcal infections and do not have to meet the Jones criteria for diagnosis of an acute exacerbation.

## Treatment

- Therapy consists of antibiotic therapy and supportive care as well as prophylaxis against recurrent infection.

**TABLE 23-5** **The Jones Criteria for Rheumatic Fever**

**Evidence of prior *Streptococcus* infection**
1. Positive throat culture or rapid streptococcal test
2. Elevated or rising streptococcal antibody titers (ASO and/or DNAse)

**Major criteria:**
Joints: polyarthritis, generally migratory affecting knees, elbows, and wrists
♥, Carditis: valvular disease; pericarditis
Nodules-Subcutaneous: painless, over extensor joint surfaces
Erythema marginatum: serpiginous erythematous rash with clear center
Sydenham chorea: sudden rapid movements of trunk and/or extremities

**Minor criteria**
1. Fever
2. Arthralgia
3. Prolonged PR interval
4. Elevated erythrocyte sedimentation rate or C-reactive protein

Adapted from Guidelines for the diagnosis of rheumatic fever. Jones Criteria, 1992 update. Special Writing Group of the Committee on Rheumatic Fever, Endocarditis, and Kawasaki Disease of the Council on Cardiovascular Disease in the Young of the American Heart Association. JAMA 1992;268: 2069–2073.

- Initial treatment is aimed at eliminating the streptococcal infection, even if cultures at the time of diagnosis are negative. **One** of the following is appropriate:
  - Benzathine penicillin: 0.6 (<27 kg) or 1.2 (>27 kg) million international units IM once
  - Penicillin VK: 25–50 mg/kg/day (<27 kg) divided t.i.d.-q.i.d. (max dose 3 g/day) or 500 mg (>27 kg) b.i.d.-t.i.d. for 10 days
  - Erythromycin: 20–40 mg/kg/day (maximum 1 g/day) PO b.i.d.-q.i.d. for 10 days
  - Oral cephalosporin for 10 days
- Carditis. If there is evidence of carditis, initial treatment includes aspirin 80–100 mg/kg/day div. q.i.d. and cardiology consultation.
  - Rheumatic heart disease can progress to acute congestive heart failure, and patients with carditis should be monitored closely for cardiovascular compromise.
  - Corticosteroids are sometimes used for severe carditis and congestive heart failure.
- Aspirin or NSAIDs can help with arthritis.
- Prophylaxis for rheumatic heart disease
  - Prophylaxis is important for the prevention of recurrent infection and rheumatic heart disease and should be continued for a minimum of 5 years (American Heart Association [AHA] guidelines).
    - If heart disease does not develop, consider discontinuation at age 21 or 5 years (whichever is longer).
    - However, if there is evidence of carditis, patients may require prophylaxis for life.
  - **One** of the following agents should be used:
    - Benzathine penicillin 1.2 million IM every 3–4 weeks
    - Penicillin VK 250 mg PO b.i.d.
    - Erythromycin 250 mg PO b.i.d.
    - Sulfadiazine 0.5 g (<27 kg) or 1 g (>27 kg) PO daily

# KAWASAKI DISEASE

- The cause of this acute vasculitis is unknown, but an infectious etiology is suspected.

## Clinical Presentation and Diagnosis

- Kawasaki is a clinical diagnosis. In the absence of another disease process, clinical features as described by the American Academy of Pediatrics (AAP) and the AHA include:
  - Fever (usually >39°C) for ≥5 days and at least four of the following:
    - Bilateral conjunctivitis (bulbar), nonexudative
    - Mucositis: erythema of the lips, cracked lips, strawberry tongue, or oropharyngeal erythema
    - Cervical lymphadenopathy, >1.5 cm; typically unilateral and solitary
    - Polymorphic erythematous rash
    - Changes in extremities: swelling, erythema, or periungual peeling
  - Exceptions
    - If there are coronary artery abnormalities, Kawasaki disease can be diagnosed with less than four of the above criteria.
    - Even with a positive viral culture, Kawasaki disease should still be considered if the patient is not improving.
  - Other associated symptoms
    - Central nervous system: irritability, lethargy, aseptic meningitis, and hearing loss
    - Cardiovascular: coronary artery abnormalities, aneurysms of other medium-sized vessels, pericarditis, congestive heart failure, and valvular abnormalities
    - Gastrointestinal: abdominal pain, diarrhea, vomiting, hepatic dysfunction, and gallbladder hydrops
    - Genitourinary: urethritis and perineal desquamating rash
    - Musculoskeletal: arthritis and arthralgias

## Incomplete Kawasaki Disease

- This should be considered in children with unexplained fever for >5 days who meet only 2 or 3 of the additional clinical criteria.
- Guidelines suggested by the AAP and AHA include:
  - Treat and obtain an echocardiogram for patients with fever ≥5 days plus two to three clinical criteria, if CRP ≥3.0 mg/dL, or if ESR ≥40 mm/hr **and** patients have three or more additional laboratory criteria:
    - Albumin ≤3.0 g/dL
    - Elevated alanine aminotransferase
    - Anemia
    - Thrombocytosis ≥450,000/mm$^3$
    - WBC count ≥15,000 mm$^3$
    - Sterile pyuria (≥10 WBC/HPF)
  - If the patient does not have three additional laboratory criteria, obtain an echocardiogram if clinically indicated and treat if there are cardiac findings.
- Incomplete Kawasaki disease is more common in infants, and echocardiography should be considered with fever for ≥7 days in infants ≤6 months of age regardless of lack of other clinical criteria.

## Laboratory Studies and Imaging

- No laboratory studies are diagnostic. Common abnormalities include an elevated ESR and CRP, sterile pyuria, hypoalbuminemia, anemia, thrombocytosis (usually after 7 days), and cerebrospinal fluid pleocytosis.
- It is essential to assess cardiac function and coronary arteries with an echocardiogram if Kawasaki disease is diagnosed or suspected. Repeat echocardiograms should be performed after treatment at routine intervals depending on the degree of initial cardiac involvement.

## Treatment

- Therapy should be initiated before day no. 10 of fever and preferably within the first 7 days.
  - Standard therapy is aspirin and IVIG.
  - Treatment within the first 10 days of illness reduces the risk of coronary aneurysms, which decreases from approximately 20%–5%.
- Pharmacologic therapy includes:
  - Aspirin:
    - Start with high-dose aspirin 80–100 mg/kg/day divided 4 times daily.
    - Practice guidelines vary. It may be possible to switch to low-dose aspirin (3–5 mg/kg/day) anywhere from 48 hours after resolution of fever to 14 days after the beginning of illness; or after thrombocytosis resolves.
    - Continue low-dose aspirin for at least 6–8 weeks and longer if there is cardiac involvement.
  - IVIG
    - Start with 2 g/kg in a single infusion.
    - Give a second dose if the fever continues ≥36 hours after treatment.
  - Anticoagulation
    - This is necessary for patients with large coronary aneurysms or coronary artery thrombosis.
    - Aspirin, clopidogrel, dipyridamole, warfarin, and/or low-molecular-weight heparin can be used.

## Complications

- For patients without cardiac involvement, the outcome is excellent.
- For patients with cardiac involvement:
  - The highest risk for myocardial infarction is in the first year after diagnosis.
  - Approximately 50% of coronary lesions resolve after 1–2 years. Coronary or other medium-sized vessel aneurysms may rupture.

■ Reactions to IVIG (e.g., anaphylaxis with IgA deficiency) may occur.
■ Consultation with appropriate subspecialties (rheumatology, infectious diseases, and/or cardiology) may be prudent.

### Suggested Readings

Cassidy JT, Petty RE, Laxer RM, et al. Textbook of Pediatric Rheumatology, 5th Ed. Philadelphia: Elsevier Inc, 2005.

Dajani A, Taubert K, Ferrieri P, et al. Treatment of acute streptococcal pharyngitis and prevention of rheumatic fever: a statement for health professionals. Committee on Rheumatic Fever, Endocarditis, and Kawasaki Disease of the Council on Cardiovascular Disease in the Young, the American Heart Association. Pediatrics 1995;96:758–764.

Mills JA, Michel BA, Bloch DA, et al. The American College of Rheumatology 1990 criteria for the classification of Henoch-Schönlein purpura. Arthritis Rheum 1990;33: 1114–1121.

Newburger JW, Takahashi M, Gerber MA, et al. Diagnosis, treatment and long-term management of Kawasaki disease: a statement for health professionals. Committee on Rheumatic Fever, Endocarditis, and Kawasaki Disease, Council on Cardiovascular Disease in the Young, American Heart Association. Pediatrics 2004;114:1708–1733.

Special Writing Group of the Committee on Rheumatic Fever, Endocarditis, and Kawasaki Disease of the Council on Cardiovascular Disease in the Young of the American Heart Association. Guidelines for the diagnosis of rheumatic fever. JAMA 1992;268: 2069–2073.

Tan EM, Cohen AS, Fries JF, et al. The 1982 revised criteria for the classification of systemic lupus erythematosus. Arthritis Rheum 1982;25:1271–1277.

### Rheumatology Web Sites

The American College of Rheumatology, http://www.rheumatology.org/.
The Arthritis Foundation, http://www.arthritis.org/default.asp.
Pediatric Rheumatology European Section, http://www.pres.org.uk/.

# SEDATION
## 24
### Lynne M. Strauser Sterni, Douglas W. Carlson, Jennifer W. Cole, and Robert M. Kennedy

- Goals of sedation include alleviation of procedure-related pain and anxiety, immobility when necessary to complete the procedure, and maintenance of patient safety with limitation of sedation-related complications.
- There is an increased need for procedural sedation in pediatrics.
    - Many procedures and imaging studies require patient cooperation with little to no movement, and others require pain control and the need for reduced anxiety and relaxation.
    - Because of developmental status and age-related behaviors in children, completing these procedures often requires sedation.
- Sedative medications should never be prescribed and administered at home, either before or after the procedure. This is associated with increased risks of respiratory depression and death. It is strongly discouraged by the American Academy of Pediatrics (AAP).
- Although many institutions have sedation protocols in place, the safest alternative is a designated pediatric sedation service or unit run by experienced sedation providers trained in airway management and sedation techniques.
    - Sedations in the emergency department setting are considered "urgent" and should be performed by emergency department providers with training in airway and sedation skills.
    - Both emergency departments and sedation units should have accessibility to extra personnel in case of adverse events and backup by anesthesiologists if needed.
- During procedural sedation, from the time a sedative drug is administered until the child awakens, continuous monitoring by both electronic monitors and medical providers trained in pediatric advanced life support is necessary.
    - Pediatric-sized airway equipment should be readily available, as well as an oxygen source and emergency medications.
    - Sedation personnel should observe the airway, respiratory and cardiac status, and vital signs.
        - They are responsible for managing any sedation-related complications that may arise.
        - They should not be performing any significant role in the procedure itself, so as not to be distracted from the airway and observation of the patient.
- When patients who are considered at high risk for sedation complications are encountered, this chapter suggests reasons for involvement of anesthetic care.
- This chapter is meant to serve as a reference for physicians trained in sedation. It should not be considered all-inclusive of the subject or a substitute for formal sedation training before participating in sedation-related patient care.

## DEFINITIONS

- The term "conscious sedation" is no longer used by the authors.
- The following are definitions from American Society of Anesthesiologists (ASA), AAP, and Joint Commission (formerly the Joint Commission on Accreditation of Healthcare Organizations [JCAHO]) guidelines:
    - Minimal sedation: drug-induced state during which patients respond normally to verbal commands. Although cognitive function and coordination may be impaired, ventilatory and cardiovascular functions are unaffected.

- Moderate sedation/analgesia: a drug-induced depression of consciousness during which patients respond purposefully to verbal commands, either alone or accompanied by light to moderate tactile stimulation. No interventions are required to maintain a patent airway, and spontaneous ventilation is adequate. Cardiovascular function is usually maintained.
- Deep sedation/analgesia: a drug-induced depression of consciousness during which patients cannot be easily aroused or respond purposefully following repeated or painful stimulation. The ability to maintain ventilatory function independently may be impaired. Patients may require assistance in maintaining a patent airway and spontaneous ventilation may be inadequate. Cardiovascular function is usually maintained.

## STAGES OF SEDATION AND RECOVERY

- **Presedation:** physical examination and evaluation, sedation plan, and informed consent; gathering of equipment, medications, and obtaining intravenous (IV) access.
- **Sedation**
  - Induction: administration of sedation/analgesia (higher risk of apnea or laryngospasm at this phase). The provider should not leave the patient's bedside from this point on.
  - Maintenance: maintaining a preplanned depth of sedation
    - This may require additional doses or titration of medications, keeping in mind the length of the procedure (avoid prolonging sedation) and the type of agent needed (analgesia versus anxiolytic/hypnotic).
    - A sedation score should be recorded every 15 minutes during the sedation until the patient is ready for discharge or transfer. At St. Louis Children's Hospital, the authors use the following scoring system:
      0 = awake and alert
      1 = minimally sedated: tired/sleepy, appropriate response to verbal conversation and/or sound
      2 = moderately sedated: somnolent/sleeping, easily aroused with light tactile stimulation or a simple verbal command
      3 = deeply sedated: deep sleep, arousable with purposeful response to significant physical stimulation
      4 = unarousable or nonpurposeful response to significant physical stimulation
      The University of Michigan Sedation Scale or a similar system can also be used.
  - Emergence: recovering from effects of sedation. The patient should be fully monitored with the provider or **credentialed** nurse at bedside (higher risk of laryngospasm at this phase as well).
- **Recovery**
  - Phase I (deep sedation with recovery score $\geq 3$; see Table 24-1 for Aldrete recovery scoring system). Continuous monitoring and recording of vital signs every 5 minutes is necessary.
    - Sedation, pain, oxygen saturation, end-tidal $CO_2$ ($ETCO_2$), and recovery scores are documented every 15 minutes.
    - The transition to phase II recovery begins when the level of consciousness is consistent with moderate sedation (sedation score is 2); the patient is clinically stable and vital signs are at baseline ($+/- 20\%$); supplemental $O_2$, airway, ventilation, and cardiovascular support are not required; and the recovery score is 8 and pain score is 6 or less.
  - Phase II (minimal to moderate sedation with sedation score $\leq 2$): recovery provider must be immediately available.
    - Vital signs and sedation score are recorded every 15 minutes until conclusion of phase II recovery.
    - Pain and recovery scores are documented at end of phase II recovery.
    - Noninvasive blood pressure monitoring and electrocardiogram may be waived if they are disruptive to patient and recovery care, provided the vital signs are stable.

| TABLE 24-1 Aldrete Scoring System for Recovery from Sedation* | |
|---|---|
| **Condition** | **Score** |
| **Activity** | |
| Able to move four extremities voluntarily or on command | 2 |
| Able to move two extremities voluntarily or on command | 1 |
| Able to move zero extremities voluntarily or on command | 0 |
| **Respirations** | |
| Able to deep breathe and cough freely | 2 |
| Dyspnea or limited breathing | 1 |
| Apneic | 0 |
| **Circulation** | |
| Blood pressure +/− 20% of presedation level | 2 |
| Blood pressure +/− 20%–50% of presedation level | 1 |
| Blood pressure =/− 50% or more of presedation level | 0 |
| **Consciousness** | |
| Fully awake | 2 |
| Arousable with verbal stimulation | 1 |
| Not responding | 0 |
| **Color** | |
| Pink | 2 |
| Pale, dusky, blotchy, jaundiced | 1 |
| Cyanotic | 0 |
| *Need score of 9 for discharge or 8 for admission | |

- Phase II recovery concludes with discharge once standard discharge criteria are met by the patient, and care can be transferred to responsible parent/legal guardian/inpatient care team.

## Discharge/Transfer Criteria

■ It is suggested that all eight of the following criteria be met before discharge or transfer to another unit following sedation:
  ■ Vital signs at baseline +/− 20%
  ■ No respiratory distress
  ■ $SpO_2$ at baseline (+/−3%) or ≥95% on room air
  ■ Motor function baseline or sits/stands with minimal assistance
  ■ Fluids/hydration normal and no emesis/nausea
  ■ Aldrete recovery score ≥9 for discharge, ≥8 for admission to a hospital floor, where monitoring is not one-to-one (see Table 24-1)
  ■ Pain score ≤4 for discharge or ≤6 for admission (or pain score reduced 50% post-procedure)
  ■ Sedation score ≤1 for discharge or ≤2 for admission; no reversal given for 2 hours

■ It is important to stress to parents at discharge that after sedation, children should not climb, bathe, or swim alone; be left alone in a car seat; or participate in activities requiring physical coordination for 24 hours.

## PRESEDATION EVALUATION

■ The goal is to identify the difficult airway and prevent sedation complications.

## History

■ The history and physical examination should determine the risks versus benefits of sedation. Any problems should be discussed with an attending physician experienced in sedation or anesthesia. These include concerns regarding the history and physical examination; any patients ASA classes III, IV, or V (see later discussion for ASA classification system); or any unstable patients.

■ Importance of past medical history:
  ▪ Congenital heart disease: history of arrhythmias, most recent echocardiography report, past surgical interventions, current medications, or blood pressure issues. Address endocarditis prophylaxis if warranted.
  ▪ Respiratory issues: history of wheezing, upper respiratory infection (URI), pneumonia, any respiratory medications/inhalers, history of croup, respiratory syncytial virus, prematurity or prolonged intubation, chronic enlarged tonsils, obstructive sleep apnea, or any potential airway masses/tumors/hemangiomas
  ▪ Gastrointestinal issues: history of gastroesophageal reflux disease and controller medications, frequent vomiting, delayed gastric emptying, melena or known gastrointestinal blood loss (check hemoglobin and/or hematocrit)
  ▪ Seizure disorder: last seizure, frequency, seizure characteristics, rescue treatment, and maintenance therapy
  ▪ Neuromuscular disease: involvement of respiratory musculature, potential $K^+$ imbalance, or history of respiratory disease/infections
  ▪ Renal disease: potential electrolyte disturbances, decreased renal function with pharmacologic consequences, hypoalbuminemia from renal losses, hypertension issues, IV fluid needs/limitations, history of oliguria or anuria, and intermittent catheterization with possible latex sensitivity
  ▪ Liver disease: decreased tidal volumes because of hepatomegaly and drug clearance/drug metabolism changes because of hepatic dysfunction
  ▪ Hematology/oncology issues
    • Most recent complete blood count/electrolytes, last chemotherapy regimen, and any central lines
    • Porphyria: avoid barbiturates
  ▪ Endocrine disease: current blood glucose level needed recent electrolytes
  ▪ Genetic disease
    • Many syndromes are associated with cardiac, renal, and metabolic derangements as well as craniofacial/airway abnormalities.
    • Be familiar with details of syndrome.

■ Drug allergies affecting sedation
  ▪ Latex allergy
  ▪ Personal or family history of computed tomography contrast allergy or allergy to shellfish (iodine)

■ Importance of past sedation/anesthesia records
  ▪ **Sedation/anesthesia records should be reviewed** as available to assess size of endotracheal tubes and laryngoscope blades needed, any difficulty with mask ventilation or intubation, and any adverse reactions or outcomes
  ▪ History of postoperative nausea or vomiting
  ▪ Sedative agents used in past (if known) and any complications/parental concerns
  ▪ Family history of adverse reactions or events with sedation or anesthesia particularly addressing malignant hyperthermia (relevant if using succinylcholine)

## Classification Systems

### Mallampati Classification System

■ During presedation evaluation, each patient should be assigned a Mallampati score, with the understanding that each classification is associated with anticipation of an increasingly difficult airway. There are four classes (Figure 24-1). Class 4 is considered the most difficult.

■ Mallampati scoring should be done during the physical examination in conjunction with determination of neck mobility, ability to open mouth without temporomandibular

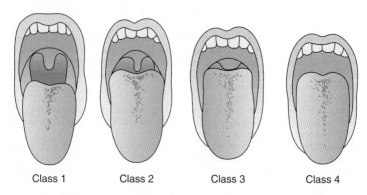

Class 1          Class 2          Class 3          Class 4

**Figure 24-1.** Mallampati classification system for use during presedation evaluation. From Mallampati S, Gatt S, Gugino L, et al. A clinical sign to predict difficult tracheal intubation: a prospective study. Can Anaesth Soc J 1985;32(4):429–434.

joint or jaw pathology, dentition status, mouth and tongue size, and cricoid-mandible distance.
- This helps give the sedation provider an idea of degree of difficulty in managing the airway if mask ventilation or intubation should become necessary.

### ASA Physical Status Classification
- During presedation evaluation, each patient should also be assigned an ASA score to determine the appropriate physical status of the patient before sedation. There are five classes.
  - Class I: normal healthy patient with no chronic medical conditions
  - Class II: patient with a mild to moderate but well-controlled medical condition
  - Class III: patient with severe systemic disease
  - Class IV: patient with severe systemic disease that is life-threatening
  - Class V: moribund patient with little chance of survival; surgery is last effort to save life
- Patients with class III, IV, or V status require specially trained and experienced sedation physicians; patients with class IV or V status warrant consultation with anesthesiology.

## High-Risk Problems
- Medical conditions
  - ASA classes III, IV, or V
  - Pulmonary airway obstruction (tonsils/adenoids): loud snoring, obstructive sleep apnea
  - Poorly controlled asthma
  - Morbid obesity (>2 times ideal body weight)
  - Cardiovascular conditions (cyanosis, congestive heart failure, history of congenital heart disease)
  - Prematurity with residual pulmonary, cardiovascular, gastrointestinal, or neurologic problems
  - Neurologic conditions: poorly controlled seizures or central apnea
  - Gastrointestinal conditions: uncontrolled gastroesophageal reflux, poor gastrointestinal motility
  - Age <3 months
  - Pregnancy or suspected pregnancy
  - Current URI or wheezing
  - Neuromuscular disease

- Procedures requiring deep sedation in patients with a full stomach
- Conditions that put patients at risk for failed sedation
  - Severe developmental delay
  - Difficulties with control
  - History of failed sedation, oversedation, or paradoxical response to sedatives (hyperactive)

## Screening for Acute Illness

- Patients also should be screened for acute illnesses that may increase their risk for sedation-related adverse effects.
  - When acute illness is detected, the sedation provider must weigh the increased risk of sedation against the need for the diagnostic or therapeutic procedure.
  - If the procedure is considered elective, the following guidelines are suggested:
- Indications for cancellation or delay of elective sedations include:
  - Illness and fever >100.4°F (38°C) within 24 hours
  - Active childhood infections (i.e., varicella, measles, mumps)
  - Active vomiting within 12 hours of sedation
  - Any respiratory infection with wheezing **not** ameliorated by a bronchodilator
- Rescheduling recommendations include:
  - Asthma without underlying infection: 7 days
  - Asthma with infectious component: 3 weeks
  - URI with cough/congestion: 3 weeks
    - URI symptoms may increase the risk of laryngospasm, bronchospasm, and hypoxia during sedation.
    - Mild URI symptoms alone (nonpurulent rhinitis, afebrile status, cough that clears) may not be an indication to cancel or delay a procedure; management should reflect anticipation of above potential complications.
    - Severe URI (febrile, purulent discharge, wet cough) should prompt consideration of cancellation; discuss with advanced sedation provider to review the risks versus the urgency of the procedure.
  - Fever: back to baseline >24 hours and acting well
  - Emesis: resolved for 24 hours and tolerating clear liquids, normal urine production and hydration
  - Croup: 3 weeks, with presedation visit to primary care physician
  - Pneumonia: 4 weeks
  - Influenza: 3 weeks
  - Respiratory syncytial virus: 6 weeks, with presedation visit to primary care physician
  - Children with known infection (e.g., otitis/tonsillitis) >24 hours without fever on therapy, if any

# PEDIATRIC AIRWAY AND POSITIONING

## Anatomy

- The larynx is at the level of C3-C6 and serves as the area of phonation. It also protects the lower airways from the contents of the oropharynx.
- The larynx is made of distinct cartilages: thyroid, cricoid, arytenoids, corniculates, and epiglottis.
- The vocal cords lie beneath the overhang of the epiglottis, at the level of the thyroid cartilage.
- The opening between the true vocal cords is the glottic opening, where intubation tubes are passed. This is the narrowest part of the airway in children >10 years of age. In children <10 years of age, the airway is narrowest at the level of the cricoid ring, just below the vocal cords.
- Laryngeal innervation is supplied by two branches of the vagus nerve: the superior and recurrent laryngeal nerves.

- The trachea begins at the level of C6, branching to the right and left mainstem bronchi at T5.
- Receptors sensitive to mechanical and chemical stimuli lie in the trachea, and are involved in regulating rate and depth of breathing, as well as causing cough and bronchoconstriction reflexive actions.
- Positioning of the pediatric airway is complicated by a large occiput size in relation to body size, a large tongue in relation to mouth size, and vocal cords which are more angled anteriorly in comparison to adults. The larynx is more cephalad than in adults, with narrowing below the vocal cords.

### Positioning Techniques

- Place towel roll underneath shoulders (if infant or toddler) or head to align airway, to achieve "sniffing" position.
- Avoid head flexion or extreme head extension.
- Adult-sized patients may require roll underneath head instead of shoulders to align airway.
- Obese patients may require several folded towels placed under shoulder blades for airway positioning.

### Identifying the Potential Difficult Airway

- Head: prominent occiput or misshapen skull
- Back: moderate to severe scoliosis or kyphosis
- Neck: short neck, fat neck, poor cervical mobility, neck masses, and cervical collar or traction in place
- Face: craniofacial abnormalities such as small mouth opening, jaw abnormalities, large tongue, narrow palate (associated with difficult airways), cleft palate, or micrognathia
- Airway: history of snoring, stridor, hoarseness, drooling, enlarged tonsils, or leaning forward to open airway
- Past medical history: history of prolonged intubation, airway tumors/hemangiomas/inflammation, obesity, or hypothyroidism
- Syndromes: craniofacial syndromes such as Crouzon, Apert, Goldenhar, or Pierre-Robin syndromes; Down, Turner, or Hurler/Hunter syndromes.

## AIRWAY EQUIPMENT, MEDICATIONS, AND PERSONNEL

### Equipment

#### At Bedside or Immediately Available

- Endotracheal tubes (ETTs): Three (estimated size for age, plus one size above and below)
  - Remember that ETTs should be uncuffed if children are <5 years of age.
  - To determine ETT size, use the following formula:

$$\text{Uncuffed tubes: } \frac{16 + \text{age}}{4} \qquad \text{Cuffed tubes: } \frac{\text{age} + 3}{4}$$

- Laryngeal mask airway (LMA)
  - The LMA should be appropriate for patient weight.

- Oral and nasopharyngeal airways
- Laryngoscope plus curved and straight blades (make sure light works)
- Rolled towel for positioning
- Stylet
- Clean extra syringes and needles to draw additional medications

#### In Room

- Suction unit, turned on
- Anesthesia bag (continuous positive airway pressure [CPAP] bag) with appropriate mask size assembled and attached to 10 L oxygen
- Nasal cannula +/− ETCO$_2$ with **full** oxygen tank to accompany patient during transport

- Continuous cardiorespiratory monitoring (transport monitor if needed)
- Second IV setup readily available in case of loss of IV access

## Medications (Immediately Available)

- Emergency medications
  - Succinylcholine (20 mg/mL), drawn in 5-mL syringe
  - Atropine (2 mL; 0.4 mg/mL)
  - Epinephrine (**diluted to 10 µg/mL**); take 1 ampule of epinephrine (1 ampule = 1 mg/mL) and dilute this in 100 mL of normal saline to yield (10 **µg**/mL)
- Sedation medications (see Tables 24-2 and 24-3 for sedation medications and dosing). The drugs in listed in Tables 24-4 and 24-5 may also be useful. Attendants should:
  - Be ready with extra doses as anticipated.
  - Have normal saline, with 10-mL syringes, available for flushing medications.
  - Know medication doses for reversal (i.e., flumazenil or naloxone).

## Personnel Required

- The AAP recommends that one nurse, one sedationist/anesthesiologist, and one proceduralist (if one is warranted) are necessary.
- Monitoring sedation and vital signs should be the only job for the sedationist during moderate to deep sedation.
- Following sedation, the patient should continue to be monitored, with vital signs recorded every 5 minutes, until the patient has reached baseline mental status. A designated recovery area should be staffed and equipped appropriately in case of airway compromise during recovery.
- Propofol sedation is performed only by credentialed sedationists/anesthesiologists at the authors' institution.

# RECOGNIZING INEFFECTIVE VENTILATION

- Understand that supplemental oxygen use often masks early hypoxemia and delays recognition of ineffective breathing. It is preferred that $ETCO_2$ be used when supplemental oxygen is used to prevent adverse events. If $ETCO_2$ is not used, then strong consideration should be given to having the patient breathe room air so that ineffective ventilation causing a fall in pulse oximetry is recognized early.
- Signs of ineffective ventilation include:
  - Color. Watch for paleness/cyanosis.
  - Chest wall movement. A chest rise should be visible at all times; remove burdensome clothing.
  - Watch for abdominal breathing. No "see-saw" retractions should occur; this is a sign of upper airway obstruction.
  - Snoring/upper airway sounds. Recognize that this is a sign of upper airway obstruction and requires either airway repositioning, placement of oral or nasal airway, or possible need for more definitive airway (i.e., LMA or ETT).
  - Pulse oximetry with audible tone (volume can be turned up on the monitors). This allows early detection of ineffective respiration.
  - End-tidal capnography. This should read 30–50 mm Hg unless metabolic derangement is present. $ETCO_2$ is more sensitive than pulse oximetry and is the earliest warning sign of apnea/obstruction.
    - Decreased $ETCO_2$ indicates poor ventilation and obstruction versus apnea.
    - Increased $ETCO_2$ indicates poor ventilation and possibly inadequate respiratory rate.

# SEDATION CHECKLIST

- Verify patient information, name, medical record, and procedure to be performed with the family/guardian/patient and the medical team.

- Complete sedation record to document:
  - History of the present illness: diagnosis, reason for sedation
  - Past medical history
  - Past sedation/anesthesia history/records
  - Drug allergies/sensitivities
  - Review of systems
  - Laboratory tests
  - Baseline vital signs
  - Physical examination
  - NPO status (Table 24-6)
  - ASA classification
  - Mallampati classification
  - Obtaining of informed consent
- Develop and document assessment and plan for performing sedation. Inform parents and assisting team members of plan.
- Perform checklist for preparation before performing sedation. (Think **SOAP ME.)**
  **S**uction: size-appropriate Yankauer catheter with power "on" and tested
  **O**xygen: nasal cannula, CPAP bag available and hooked up, and oxygen tank with adequate supply and/or functioning wall supply
  **A**irway: size-appropriate nasopharyngeal and oropharyngeal airways, ETTs, and LMA. Check laryngoscope blades to be sure these are functional, and have stylets available.
  **P**harmacy: intubation medications, emergency medications, with known doses/concentrations. Have normal saline flush available.
  **M**onitors: pulse oximetry, noninvasive blood pressure, $ETCO_2$ as appropriate, and ECG monitoring on patient. Have stethoscope available.
  **E**quipment: any anticipated special equipment. Have crash cart/airway cart available and nearby.
- Have anesthesia and CODE team contact numbers ready and available should assistance be needed.
- Ensure appropriately staffed and equipped recovery area for postsedation monitoring.
- Have responsible attending physician in room or immediately available and aware that sedation is about to begin.
- Have IV line in place, patent, and running well; check flow before giving medications.
- Preoxygenate as appropriate (if $ETCO_2$ will be used).
- If all checklist items have been completed, the patient is ready for sedation. **Before starting sedation, be sure to double-check the dose for age and weight as well as for maximum doses allowed.** Be sure to note times of medications and any premedications given. Vital signs are recorded every 5 minutes in sedation record.
- Document any sedation-related complications: any airway repositioning or nasopharyngeal/oral airways, need for larger than usual drug dosing to achieve sedation, any signs of airway obstruction (snoring, desaturation, poor chest rise) or difficult intubations/multiple attempts. This is valuable information for the next sedationist/anesthesiologist.

## ADVERSE EVENTS DURING SEDATION

### Upper Airway Obstruction/Laryngospasm

- Reposition using chin lift or jaw thrust.
- Consider oral airway placement **unless laryngospasm is obvious.**
- Oxygen with CPAP by anesthesia bag. Hold continuous pressure at 15–20 mm Hg.
- If no response, give succinylcholine 0.25–0.5 mg/kg plus continuous hand bagging. **Call for help.**
- Wait 30–60 seconds.
- If still the child cannot be oxygenated, proceed to intubation. Use cricoid pressure during intubation to try to lessen the risk of aspiration after bag-mask ventilation.
- Once the airway is stabilized, consider nasogastric tube placement for gastric decompression.

**TABLE 24-2** Common Sedation and Analgesic Medications

| Drug | Onset | Route | Dosing | Contraindications | Duration of action | Comments |
|------|-------|-------|--------|-------------------|--------------------|----------|
| **Sedative/Hypnotics** | | | | | | |
| Propofol | 15–30 sec | IV | For use only by propofol credentialed/anesthesia approved attending physicians | Egg allergy (relative) History of difficult airway; if cardiac, renal, or pulmonary disease, discuss with anesthesia | 3–5 min if no infusion | Can cause profound respiratory depression, apnea, and hypotension |
| Midazolam | 2–3 min | IV | 6 mo–6 yr: 0.05 mg/kg (anxiolysis) and 0.1 mg/kg (sedation); may titrate doses at 0.05 mg/kg to maximum of 0.6 mg/kg 6–12 yr: 0.025–0.05 mg/kg initially (anxiolysis) and 0.05–0.1 mg/kg (sedation); maximum single dose of 2.5 mg, to a maximum of 0.4 mg/kg | History of paradoxical reaction | 45–60 min IV 60–90 min PO | Can cause respiratory depression, bradycardia, and hypotension. Serum levels increased with cimetidine, erythromycin, clarithromycin, and antifungals. Anxiolytic doses should not exceed 2–4 mg total; sedation doses should not exceed 10 mg total. |
| | 20–30 min | PO | 0.5–0.75 mg/kg once only | | | |
| Pentobarbital | 3–5 min | IV | 1st dose 2.5mg/kg; may repeat 1.25 mg/kg three times to max of 7.5mg/kg OR 200 mg total | History of paradoxical reaction; porphyria. Apnea when used with other agents. | 15–45 min IV 60–240 min PO | May cause arrhythmias or respiratory depression. |
| | 15–60 min | PO/PR | (<4yr) 3–6mg/kg to max 100 mg total (>4yr) 1.5–3mg/kg to max 100 mg total | Not recommended in congestive heart failure, hypotension, or liver failure. | | |

*(continued)*

395

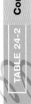

**TABLE 24-2** Common Sedation and Analgesic Medications *(Continued)*

| Drug | Onset | Route | Dosing | Contraindications | Duration of action | Comments |
|---|---|---|---|---|---|---|
| Chloral Hydrate | 15–30 min | PO | (6 m–12 m) 75 mg/kg, 2nd dose 25 mg/kg to max of 2 g (>1yr) 75–100 mg/kg, 2nd dose 25 mg/kg to max 2 g | History of paradoxical reaction. Effects unreliable >3yr. Avoid with renal, hepatic, or cardiac disease. Can potentiate warfarin. | 60–120 min | Can cause myocardial depression, hypotension, or gastrointestinal irritation. |
| **Analgesics** | | | | | | |
| Fentanyl | 2–3 min | IV | 0.5–1 µg/kg. Administer over 30–60 min; may repeat q2–3 min to desired effect, with a maximum dose of 100 µg in 30-min span. Consult experienced sedation attending if larger dose is required in larger patients. | Apnea when used with other agents, especially benzodiazepines (midazolam). Adjust dose in renal failure. Use with caution in bradycardia, hypotension, or respiratory depression. | 30–60 min | Rapid infusion may cause chest wall rigidity or respiratory depression. |
| Ketamine | 1 min | IV | 0.25–0.5 mg/kg to repeat as needed every 10 min | Contraindicated in patient with increased intracranial pressure, seizure disorder, recent craniotomy, hypertension, aneurysm, thyrotoxicosis, or psychotic disorder. | Dissociation: 15–30 min Recovery: 90–150 min | Consider glycopyrrolate 5 µg/kg IV (max 0.2 mg) once for secretions; especially if multiple doses of ketamine are anticipated or if intraoral procedure is being done (e.g., peritonsillar abscess, dental). |

| Drug | Onset | Route | Dose | Cautions | Duration | Adverse Effects |
|---|---|---|---|---|---|---|
| Nitrous Oxide | 2–5 min | mask | 50%–70% mixed with $O_2$: Suggest 50/50 mix blend with oxygen and titrate from 30% to 50% nitrous slowly over 2 min. | Can cause hypertension, tachycardia, nystagmus, nausea and vomiting, salivation, and emergent reaction. Laryngospasm can occur. Associated with pneumothorax, intestinal obstruction, recent ear/eye/sinus/cranial surgery, increased intracranial pressure, cystic fibrosis, emphysema, craniofacial or sinus injury, 1st trimester pregnancy, or ethanol/drug intoxication. | <5 min | Adverse effects include nausea and vomiting, diaphoresis, and hallucinations. Long-term use is associated with megaloblastic anemia, myeloneuropathy, and impaired fetal development. Works best with distraction in children >2 years of age; must tolerate mask. |
| Morphine | 5–10 min | IV | 0.1–0.15 mg/kg q 10–20 min, max dose 15 mg. Peak effect at 20 min. | Can cause histamine release with itching, bronchospasm. Use with caution in patients with hypotension, cardiac disease, and respiratory depression. | 180–300 min | Adverse effects include nausea and vomiting, itching, central nervous system or respiratory depression, miosis, biliary spasm, increased intracranial pressure, and hypotension/bradycardia. Use naloxone for reversal. |
| Oxycodone | 30–60 min | PO | 0.1–0.3 mg/kg for hospital dosing; home use is limited to 0.05–0.15 mg/kg/dose—max dose 15 mg. | Use with caution in patients with renal failure, shock/hypotension, cardiac disease, and respiratory depression. | 120–180 min | |

**TABLE 24-3** Chloral Hydrate and Pentobarbital Dosing Protocols

| Chloral hydrate sedation protocol | 3 mo | 4–6 mo | 6–18 mo | 18–36 mo | >36 mo |
|---|---|---|---|---|---|
| 25 mg/kg PO/PR; additional 25 mg/kg after 30 min if needed. | X | | | | |
| 50 mg/kg PO/PR; additional 25 mg/kg after 30 min if needed. | | X | | | |
| 75 mg/kg PO/PR; additional 37.5 mg/kg after 30 min if needed. | | | X | | |
| 100 mg/kg PO/PR; additional 25 mg/kg after 30 min if needed. | | | | X | X |

Maximum total dose of chloral hydrate: 2,000 mg or 125 mg/kg PO/PR

| Pentobarbital sedation protocol | <6 mo | 6–18 mo | 18–36 mo | >36 mo |
|---|---|---|---|---|
| IV: 2.5 mg/kg, followed by 1.25 mg/kg as needed × 2. May give additional 1.25 mg/kg × 2 if needed. | | X | X | X |
| IM: 5 mg/kg; additional 2 mg/kg IM after 15 min as needed | | X | X | X |

Maximum total dose of pentobarbital: 200 mg IV/IM
May give midazolam 0.05 mg/kg IV as needed for agitation associated with pentobarbital.
From St. Louis Children's Hospital.

## Apnea With or Without Hypoxia

- Reposition using chin lift or jaw thrust.
- Administer 100% oxygen.
- Decrease or discontinue infusion rate of sedative, if applicable.
- Give a sternal rub to stimulate.
- Bag with anesthesia bag or bag-valve-mask.
- Consider flumazenil or naloxone as appropriate:
  - Flumazenil: 0.01 mg/kg IV (maximum dose 0.2 mg) over 15 seconds; may repeat this dose 4 times to a maximum of 1 mg
  - Naloxone: 0.01–0.02 mg/kg IV, may repeat every 2–3 minutes as needed; may need 0.1 mg/kg IV for true emergencies when unable to perform bag-mask ventilation

- Perform intubation if necessary, and call appropriate back-up.

**TABLE 24-4** Antinausea Agents*

| Antinausea medications | Class | Route | Dose |
|---|---|---|---|
| Ondansetron (Zofran) | Antiserotonin | IV/PO | 0.15 mg/kg q8h |
| Metoclopramide (Reglan) | Benzamides | IV/PO | 0.05–0.1 mg/kg q6h (max 10 mg) |
| Diphenhydramine (Benadryl) | Antihistamine | PO/IV | 0.5–1 mg/kg q4–6h (max 50 mg) |
| Promethazine (Phenergan) | Antihistamine | IV | 0.25–0.5 mg/kg q6h |

*Some sedation procedures may be complicated by postprocedure nausea and vomiting. Medications can be given to help counteract these side effects and decrease complications. Using two agents from *different* classes may be necessary if the patient is not responding to a single drug. Be aware that antihistamines may worsen postsedation drowsiness.

| TABLE 24-5 | Emergency Drugs* |
| --- | --- |

| Drug | Dose |
| --- | --- |
| Atropine | 0.02 mg/kg/dose IV q 3–5 min (0.1 mg minimum dose)<br>Maximum 1 mg total dose for child<br>Maximum 2 mg total dose for adolescent |
| Epinephrine | 0.01 mg/kg/dose (or 0.1 mL/kg of 1:10,000) IV/IO q 3–5 min |
| Flumazenil | 0.01 mg/kg IV (max dose 0.5 mg) q 1–2 min to maximum of 3 mg<br>Monitor for resedation; use with caution in patients on benzodiazepine therapy for seizures because flumazenil may induce seizure |
| Naloxone | 0.00 –0.002 mg/kg (1–2 μg/kg) titrated to effect<br>Maximum of 2 mg<br>Monitor for resedation |
| Rocuronium | 0.6 mg/kg/dose for paralysis for intubation |
| Succinylcholine | 1–2 mg/kg/dose IV/IO (maximum 80 mg) for paralysis for intubation<br>0.1–0.5 mg/kg/dose for laryngospasm<br>Contraindicated in children with burns >48 hours old, neuromuscular disease, hyperkalemia, muscular dystrophy, suspected increased intracranial pressure, or prolonged immobilization; these patients should be discussed with anesthesia before any sedation and may require anesthesia level care. |

*Drug math:
1:100,000 = 10 μg/mL = 0.01 mg/mL
1:10,000 = 100 μg/mL = 0.1 mg/mL
1:1,000 = 1,000 μg/mL = 1 mg/mL

## Hypotension

- Hypotension is a decrease in systolic blood pressure by >20%.
- To increase blood pressure:
  - Consider etiologies; perform a physical examination.
    - Sedation medication possibly causing hypotension
    - Allergic reaction: see protocol
    - Cardiac rhythm disturbance
    - Shock or poor perfusion
  - Increase IV fluid rate, or administer normal saline bolus of 10–20 mL/kg if no contraindications (cardiac, renal, or pulmonary disease).

| TABLE 24-6 | Nothing-by-Mouth (NPO) Guidelines for Elective Sedation* |
| --- | --- |

| | Age | Time |
| --- | --- | --- |
| Clear Liquids | All ages | 3 hr |
| Breast Milk/Formula/Solids | 0–6 mo | 4 hr |
| Breast Milk/Formula/Solids | >6 mo | 6 hr |

*These guidelines are strictly adhered to for all elective sedations, and any NPO violations are rescheduled or delayed until criteria are met. Refer to the Chapter 4, Emergencies for recommendations regarding urgent/emergent sedation in the emergency department setting.
Clear liquids: Water, sugar water, Kool-aid, Pedialyte, soda, apple or grape juice without pulp, Gatorade.
Solids: All food, cow milk, unstrained fruit juices, tube feedings, candy, and gum.
*Source:* St. Louis Children's Hospital.

- Change blood pressure cuff cycling rate to every 1–3 minutes until blood pressure is stabilized.
- Consider decreasing infusion rate of sedation agent (as applicable).
- If no response, turn off infusion and allow recovery.

## Allergic Reaction

- Place patient in Trendelenburg position and call for help.
- Administer 100% oxygen and establish IV access.
- Give epinephrine 0.01 mL/kg (1:1,000) IM/SQ; OR give 10 μg/kg (0.01 mg/kg) epinephrine (1:10,000) IV; may repeat every 15 minutes as needed.
- Give 20-mg/kg IV bolus of normal saline; repeat as necessary.
- If respiratory state compromised, it may be necessary to give nebulized albuterol (2.5 or 5 mg in 3 mL normal saline) or intubate if severe respiratory involvement.
- As soon as possible, administer:
  - H-1 receptor antagonist (diphenhydramine 1 mg/kg IM/IV/PO [maximum dose 50 mg])
  - H-2 receptor antagonist (e.g., cetirizine: 6 months to 5 years 2.5 mg PO; 6 years to adult 5–10 mg PO)
  - Corticosteroids (methylprednisolone 2 mg/kg IV bolus or prednisone 2 mg/kg PO once)
- Observe for 6–24 hours to watch for late-phase rebound symptoms.

## Aspiration

- Turn head/body to side and suction immediately; interrupt procedure as needed.
- Turn off infusion medication (if applicable) and allow for recovery.
- Administer oxygen as needed; if ongoing emesis or continued desaturation may need definitive airway (ETT).
- Obtain chest radiograph to evaluate for signs of aspiration if clinically indicated (new cough, tachypnea, new oxygen requirement, lung auscultation findings)
- Admit for overnight hospitalization for observation if any new oxygen requirement present.
- Contact physician who ordered study.

### Suggested Readings

Cote CJ, Tordres ID, Ryan JF, et al., eds. A Practice of Anesthesia for Infants and Children, 3rd Ed. Philadelphia: WB Saunders, 2001.

American Society of Anesthesiology. Practice guidelines for sedation and analgesia by non-anesthesiologists. Anesthesiology 2002, 96(4):1004–1017.

Kennedy B. St Louis Children's Hospital sedation curriculum, revised 2007.

Motoyama EK, Davis PJ. Smith's Anesthesia for Infants and Children, 7th Ed. Philadelphia: Mosby, 2006.

Miller RD. Miller's Anesthesia. 6th Ed. New York: Churchill Livingstone, 2005.

Gregory GA. Pediatric Anesthesia, New York: Churchill Livingstone, 2002.

Shankar V, Deshpande JK. Procedural sedation in the pediatric patient. Anesthesiol Clin North Am 2005;23(4):635–654.

Doyle L, Colletti JE. Pediatric sedation and analgesia. Pediatr Clin North Am 2006; 53(2):279–292.

American Society of Anesthesiologists. Continuum of depth of sedation: definition of general anesthesia and levels of sedation/analgesia. Available at http://www.asahq.org/standards/20.htm. Accessed February 13, 2001.

Joint Commission on Accreditation of Healthcare Organizations. Standards and intents for sedation and anesthesia care. In: Revisions to anesthesia care standards, comprehensive accreditation manual for hospitals, Oakbrook Terrace, Ill. Joint Commission on Accreditation of Healthcare Organizations: 2001. Available at http://www.jcaho.org/standard/aneshap.html. Accessed February 13, 2001.

American Academy of Pediatrics. December 2006 Guidelines for monitoring and management of pediatric patients during and after sedation. Pediatrics 2006;118(6): 2587–2602.

Malviya S, Voepel-Lewis T, Tait AR, et al. Depth of sedation in children undergoing computed tomography: validity and reliability of the University of Michigan Sedation Scale (UMSS). Br J Anaesth 2002;88:241–245.

**Kristina N. Bryowsky**

$\mathcal{T}$his list is by no means comprehensive. Classes of medications that change frequently (i.e., human immunodeficiency virus medications) or that should be administered only with the aid of a specialist (i.e., antiarrhythmics) have not been included. This list represents the most common medications prescribed by general pediatricians as well as pediatricians-in-training. Because of the incomplete data on pediatric dosing, many drug dosages will be modified after the publication of this text. **The specific concentrations of medications administered by injection are NOT listed in the formulary because these are prepared for each individual patient by the physician's pharmacy.**

The authors recommend that the reader check product information and published literature for changes in dosing, especially for newer medications. For dosing information about anesthetics and sedatives, see Chapter 24, Sedation.

A day refers to a 24-hour period. Other abbreviations: *sol*, solution; *supp*, suppository; *tab*, tablet; *cap*, capsule; *susp*, suspension; *oint*, ointment; *SR*, sustained release; *ER*, extended release; *MDI*, metered dose inhaler; *DPI*, dry powder inhalation; *max*, maximum; *prn*, as needed; *R*, adjust in renal failure; *INR*, international normalized ratio; *PMA*, post menstrual age = gestational age + postnatal age; *AAP*, American Academy of Pediatrics; *MAOI*, monoamine oxidase inhibitor; *JRA*, juvenile rheumatoid arthritis; *GI*, gastrointestinal; *TB*, tuberculosis; *CMV*, cytomegalovirus; *PCP*, *Pneumocystis jiroveci* (formerly *carinii*) pneumonia.

| Name | Oral or Topical forms | Dosage | Comments |
|------|----------------------|--------|----------|
| acetaminophen (Tylenol) | Drops: 80 mg/0.8 mL<br>Susp: 160 mg/5 mL<br>Elixir: 120 mg, 160 mg/5 mL<br>Cap: 500, 650 mg<br>Gelcap: 500 mg<br>Chewable tab: 80, 160 mg<br>Supp: 80, 120, 325, 650 mg | Neonate dosing: 15 mg/kg/dose PO/PR q6–12h (lower interval for PMA <32 wk)<br>Children: 10–15 mg/kg/dose PO/PR q4–6h; max: 4 g/day | — |
| acetaminophen/ codeine (Tylenol #2, #3, #4) | Tab: all with 300 mg of acetaminophen<br>Tylenol #2: 15 mg codeine<br>Tylenol #3: 30 mg codeine<br>Tylenol #4: 60 mg codeine<br>Elixir: 12 mg codeine/120 mg acetaminophen in 5 mL | Based on the codeine component: 0.5–1 mg/kg/dose q4–6h prn<br>3–6 yr old: 5 mL t.i.d.-q.i.d. prn<br>7–12 yr old: 10 mL t.i.d.-q.i.d. prn<br>>12 yr old: 15 mL q4h prn | Respiratory depression may occur |
| acetazolamide (Diamox) | Tab: 125, 250 mg<br>Susp: 25, 30, 50 mg/mL<br>Cap, SR: 500 mg | Diuretic: 5 mg/kg/dose PO/IV q.d.-q.o.d.<br>Glaucoma: 20–40 mg/kg/day IM/IV q6h (max: 1 g/day) or 8–30 mg/kg/day PO q6–8h<br>Seizures: 8–30 mg/kg/day PO q6–12h<br>Urine alkalinization: 5 mg/kg/dose PO b.i.d.-t.i.d. | R |

*(continued)*

| Name | Oral or Topical forms | Dosage | Comments |
|------|----------------------|--------|----------|
| | | Hydrocephalus: initial: 20 mg/kg/day PO/IV q8h, titrate to 100 mg/kg/day; max: 2 g/day | |
| acyclovir (Zovirax) | Cap: 200 mg<br>Tab: 400, 800 mg<br>Susp: 200 mg/5 mL | Neonates: 20 mg/kg IV q8h Immunocompetent patients:<br>Mucocutaneous HSV: Initial infection: IV 15 mg/kg/day q8h × 5–7 day or PO 1,200 mg/day q8h × 7–10 day<br>Recurrence: PO 1,200 mg/day q8h<br>Suppressive: PO 800–1,000 mg/day 2–5×/day for up to 1 yr<br>Max: 80 mg/kg/day q6–8h<br>Zoster: IV 30 mg/kg/day q8h × 7–10 day or if >12 yr old: PO 4,000 mg/day 5 times/day × 5–7 day<br>Varicella: IV 30 mg/kg/day div. q8h × 7–10 day or PO 80 mg/kg/day q.i.d. × 5 day. Max: 3,200 mg/day Immunocompromised patients: dosing is different; consult AAP Red Book or Physicians' Desk Reference | R<br>Adequate hydration and slow IV administration are necessary to prevent crystallization in renal tubules. |
| adapalene (Differin) | Cream, gel, solution: 0.1% | Apply to affected area q.h.s. | — |
| albendazole (Albenza) | Tab: 200 mg | >6 yr old: 15 mg/kg/day PO b.i.d. with meals; use for 28 day, stop for 14 day then repeat for a total of 3 cycles; max: 800 mg/day<br>Neurocysticercosis: 15 mg/kg/day PO b.i.d.; max: 800 mg<br>Cutaneous larva migrans: 400 mg PO × 3 day<br>Roundworm, hookworm, whipworm: 400 mg × 1 PO<br>Pinworms: 400 mg PO × 1, repeat in 2 wk | — |
| albuterol (Ventolin, Proventil, salbutamol) | MDI: 90 μg/actuation<br>Nebulizer sol: 0.083%, 0.5% | MDI: 1–2 puff q4–6h<br>Nebulization:<br><1 yr old: 0.05–0.15 mg/kg/dose q4–6 h<br>1–5 yr old: 1.25–2.5 mg/dose q4–6h<br>5–12 yr old: 2.5 mg/dose q4–6h | Nebulization may be given more frequently if necessary<br>Always use MDI with spacer; it enhances efficacy |

| Name | Oral or Topical forms | Dosage | Comments |
|------|----------------------|--------|----------|
| | | >12 yr old: 2.5–5 mg/dose q6h | Side effects: palpitations, tremor, insomnia, nervousness, nausea and headache |
| alprostadil (PGE1) | | 0.0125–0.1 μg/kg/min | Possible apnea, pyrexia, hypotension |
| alteplase (t-PA) (Cathflo Activase) | 2-mg vial | For use in occluded IV catheters: <10 kg: 0.5 mg to each lumen; ≥10 kg: 1–2 mg to each lumen; instill into catheter over 1–2 min and leave in place for 2–4 hours before blood withdrawal; may be repeated ×1 | Do not infuse into patient |
| amantadine (Symmetrel) | Tab: 100 mg Susp: 50 mg/5 mL | Influenza A prophylaxis and treatment: 1–9 yr old: 5 mg/kg/day PO q.d.-b.i.d.; max: 150 mg/day >9 yr old: 5 mg/kg/day PO q.d.-b.i.d.; max: 200 mg/day | R Possible dizziness, depression, and anxiety Initiate therapy within 2 day of onset of symptoms. |
| amikacin (Amikin) | | Neonates: 0–4 wk, <1,200 g: 7.5 mg/kg/dose q18–24h Postnatal age ≤7 day: 1,200–2,000 g: 7.5 mg/kg/dose q12h >2,000 g: 7.5–10 mg/kg/dose q12h Postnatal age >7 day: 1,200–2,000 g: 7.5–10 mg/kg/dose q8–12h >2,000 g: 10 mg/kg/dose q8h Infants/children: 15–22.5 mg/kg/day q8h IV/IM | R Check peak and trough with third dose |
| amitriptyline (Elavil) | Tab: 10, 25, 50, 75, 100, 150 mg | Depression: Children, PO: start with 1 mg/kg/day t.i.d. for 3 day then increase to 1.5 mg/kg/day; may increase up to a max of 5 mg/kg/day. Adolescents, PO: start with 10 mg t.i.d. with 20 mg q.h.s.; increase to a max of 200 mg/day Chronic pain: start with 0.1 mg/kg/dose q.h.s. PO and increase over 2–3 wk to 0.5–2 mg/kg/dose q.h.s. | Contraindicated in narrow-angle glaucoma, seizures, severe cardiac disorders, and MAOIs. Antidepressants may worsen depression and increase suicidal ideation in children and young adults. Avoid abrupt discontinuation. |

*(continued)*

| Name | Oral or Topical forms | Dosage | Comments |
|---|---|---|---|
| amlodipine (Norvasc) | Tab: 2.5, 5, 10 mg<br>Susp: 1 mg/mL | Start with 0.1 mg/kg/dose PO q.d.-b.i.d. and titrate up q5–7 day to a max of 0.6 mg/kg/day or 20 mg/day | — |
| amoxicillin (Amoxil) | Cap: 250, 500 mg<br>Chewable tab: 125, 200, 250, 400 mg<br>Susp: 50 mg/mL, 125, 200, 250, 400 mg/5 mL<br>Tab: 500, 875 mg | Standard dose: 25–50 mg/kg/day b.i.d.-t.i.d. PO<br>High dose: 80–90 mg/kg/day b.i.d. PO; max: 2–3 g/day<br>Recurrent otitis media prophylaxis: 20 mg/kg/dose q.h.s. PO | R |
| amoxicillin clavulanate (Augmentin) | Chewable tab: 125/31.25 mg, 200/28.5 mg, 250/62.5 mg, 400/57 mg<br>Tab: 250/125, 500/125, 875/125 mg,<br>Augmentin ES: 600/42.9 mg/5 mL<br>Susp (per 5 mL): 125/31.25 mg, 200/28.5 mg, 250/62.5 mg, 400/57 mg | Dosage based on amoxicillin component:<br><3 mo: 30 mg/kg/day b.i.d. PO >3 mo: 20–40 mg/kg/day t.i.d. PO or 25–45 mg/kg/day b.i.d. PO<br>Augmentin ES:<br>>3 mo and >40 kg: 90 mg/kg/day b.i.d. PO<br>Max: 2 g/day | R |
| amphotericin B lipid formulations (Amphotec, Abelcet) | | 5 mg/kg/dose IV q24h, run over 2 hrs<br>Check basic metabolic panel and Mg 2×/wk | Possible hypokalemia, hypomagnesemia, renal tubular acidosis<br>Possible fever, chills, hypotension with infusion; give meperidine for chills<br>Premedicate with acetaminophen and diphenhydramine |
| ampicillin (Principen) | Cap: 250, 500 mg<br>Susp: 125, 250 mg/5 mL | Neonates: 100 mg/kg/dose IV q12h If ampicillin interval is not q12h, use 50 mg/kg/dose with interval from below:<br>PMA (wk) Age (day) Interval<br><29    0–28    q12h<br>          >28    q8h<br>30–36  0–14    q12h<br>          >14    q8h<br>37–44  0–7     q12h<br>          >7     q8h<br>>45    All     q6h<br>Children:<br>Mild-moderate infections: IM/IV: 100–200 mg/kg/day q6h; PO: 50–100 mg/kg/day q6h; max PO: 2–3 g/day<br>Severe infections: 200–400 mg/kg/day q4–6h IM/IV; max IV/IM dose: 12 g/day | R |

| Name | Oral or Topical forms | Dosage | Comments |
|---|---|---|---|
| ampicillin sulbactam (Unasyn) | | Dose base on ampicillin component<br>Neonate: 100 mg/kg/dose IV q12h; if ampicillin interval is not q12h, use 50 mg/kg/dose with interval from below:<br>PMA (wk)Age (day) Interval<br><29   0–28   q12h<br>       >28   q8h<br>30–36  0–14   q12h<br>       >14   q8h<br>37–44  0–7    q12h<br>       >7    q8h<br>>45   All    q6h<br>>1 mo. infant:<br>   mild/moderate infection: 100–150 mg/kg/day q6h IM/IV<br>Severe infection: 200–300 mg/kg/day q6h IM/IV<br>Children:<br>Mild/moderate infection: 100–200 mg/kg/day q6h IM/IV<br>Severe infection: 200–400 mg/kg/day q4–6h IM/IV<br>Max: 8 g/day | R |
| aspirin (Ecotrin, Bayer) | Tab: 325, 500 mg<br>Enteric-coated tab: 81, 165, 325, 500, 650 mg<br>Buffered tab: 325, 500 mg<br>Chewable tab: 81 mg<br>Supp: 60, 120, 125, 200, 300, 325, 600, 650 mg | Anti-inflammatory: 60–90 mg/kg/day PO q6–8h<br>Kawasaki disease: 80–100 mg/kg/day PO q.i.d. during febrile phase then 3–5 mg/kg/day every AM when defervesces; give until erythrocyte sedimentation rate and platelet count are normal | R<br>Do not use if <16 yr old in patient with flu or varicella because of risk of Reye syndrome |
| atenolol (Tenormin) | Tab: 25, 50, 100 mg<br>Susp: 2 mg/mL | 0.5–1 mg/kg/day PO; max: 2 mg/kg/day | R<br>Contraindicated in pulmonary edema and cardiogenic shock |
| atomoxetine (Strattera) | Tab: 10, 18, 25, 40, 60, 80, 100 mg | <70 kg×: start with 0.5 mg/kg PO every AM × 3 day; then titrate up prn to max of 1.4 mg/kg/day.<br>>70 kg: start with 40 mg PO every AM × 3 day; then titrate up prn to max of 100 mg/day. | Avoid use with MAOIs.<br>May have increased risk of suicidal ideation.<br>Consider dose adjustment with hepatic impairment. |
| azathioprine (Imuran) | Susp: 50 mg/mL<br>Tab: 50 mg | Initial: 2–5 mg/kg/day IV/PO q.d.<br>Maintenance: 1–3 mg/kg/day IV/PO q.d.<br>Max: 3 mg/kg/day | R<br>Hematologic toxicities |

*(continued)*

| Name | Oral or Topical forms | Dosage | Comments |
|------|----------------------|--------|----------|
| azithromycin (Zithromax) | Tab: 250, 600 mg Susp: 100, 200 mg/5 mL | Otitis media or pneumonia: 10 mg/kg PO day 1 (max 500 mg) then 5 mg/kg/day PO (max 250 mg) q.d. × 4 more day. Pharyngitis: 12 mg/kg/day PO q.d. × 5 day (max: 500 mg/day) | — |
| aztreonam (Azactam) | | Children: 90–120 mg/kg/day IV/IM q6–8h Cystic fibrosis: 150–200 mg/kg/day IV/IM q6–8h Max: 8 g/day. | R |
| bacitracin | Oint: 500 U/g | Apply small amount to affected area q.d.-t.i.d. | — |
| bacitracin/ polymyxin (Polysporin) | Oint: 500 U/10,000 U/g | Apply small amount to affected area q.d.-t.i.d. | — |
| bacitracin/neomycin/ polymyxin (Neosporin) | Oint: 400 U/3.5 mg/5,000 U/g | Apply small amount to affected area q.d.-t.i.d. | — |
| baclofen (Lioresal) | Tab: 10, 20 mg Susp: 5, 10 mg/mL | >2 yr old: 10–15 mg/day PO q8h Titrate dose q3d by increments of 5–15 mg/day to max of 40 mg/day if <8 yr old and max of 60 mg/day if >8 yr old | R Possible drowsiness Do not abruptly withdraw |
| benzathine penicillin G (Bicillin L-A) | | Group A streptococcus: 25,000–50,000 U/kg/dose IM × 1; max: 1.2 million U/dose Rheumatic fever prophylaxis: 25,000–50,000 U/kg/dose IM q3–4wk; max: 1.2 million U/dose | Provides sustained levels for 2–4 wk Do not give IV |
| benzocaine/ antipyrine (Auralgan) | Sol: 1.4%/5.4% | Fill ear canal, place cotton in external ear; may repeat q1–2h prn | — |
| benzoyl peroxide | Gel, wash, cream, lotion 2.5%, 5%, 10% | Apply to affected area q.d.-b.i.d. | — |
| bisacodyl (Correctol, Dulcolax) | Tab: 5 mg Supp: 5, 10 mg Enema: 10 mg/30 mL | PO: 0.3 mg/kg/day; max: 15 mg/day. PR: <2 yr old: 5 mg q.d. 2–11 yr old: 5–10 mg q.d. >11 yr old: 10 mg q.d. | — |
| budesonide (Pulmicort Turbuhaler, Pulmicort Respules) | DPI: 200 μg/actuation Respules: 0.25 mg/2 mL, 0.5 mg/2 mL | DPI: 200 μg b.i.d. and titrate up to max of 400 μg b.i.d. Respules: 250 μg b.i.d. and titrate up to a max of 1 mg/day. | Rinse mouth after use |

| Name | Oral or Topical forms | Dosage | Comments |
|------|----------------------|--------|----------|
| budesonide (Rhinocort) | Nasal aerosol or spray: 32 μg/actuation | >6 yr old: initial: 2 sprays each nostril every AM and q.h.s.; then reduce gradually to lowest effective dose | — |
| bumetanide (Bumex) | Tab: 0.5, 1, 2 mg | Neonates: 0.05–0.1 mg/kg IV >6 mo: 0.015–0.1 mg/kg/ dose PO/IV/IM q24–48; max: 10 mg/day | — |
| calamine | Lotion: 8% | Apply a thin layer to affected area q.d.-q.i.d. | — |
| calcitriol (vitamin D, Rocaltrol) | Cap: 0.25, 0.5 μg Sol: 1 μg/mL | Renal failure: PO: 0.01–0.05 μg/kg/day q.d.; titrate in 0.005–0.01 μg/kg/day in 1–2 month increments; max: 0.5 μg/day IV: 0.01–0.05 μg/kg/dose 3×/week. Hypoparathyroidism: <1 yr old: 0.04–0.08 μg/kg q.d. PO 1–5 yr old: 0.25–0.75 μg/kg q.d. PO >6 yr old: 0.5–2 μg q.d. PO Vitamin D–dependent rickets: 1 μg q.d. PO Vitamin D–resistant rickets: initial 0.015–0.02 μg/kg PO q.d.; maintenance 0.03–0.06 μg/kg/day q.d.; max: 2 μg q.d. | — |
| captopril (Capoten) | Tab: 12.5, 25, 50, 100 mg Susp: 1 mg/mL | Infants: Initially: 0.15 mg–0.3 mg/kg/dose PO; titrate upward if needed to max of 6 mg/kg/day q.d.-q.i.d. Children: Initially: 0.3–0.5 mg/kg/dose PO q8h; titrate upward to max of 6 mg/kg/day b.i.d.-q.i.d. | R May cause cough. |
| carbamazepine (Tegretol, Carbatrol) | Tab: 200 mg Chewable tab: 100 mg Tab (ER): 100, 200, 400 mg Cap (ER): 100, 200, 300 mg Susp: 100 mg/5 mL | <6 yr old: 10–20 mg/kg/day PO b.i.d.; increase q 5–7 day up to 35 mg/ kg/day b.i.d.-t.i.d. PO. 6–12 yr old: 100 mg PO b.i.d.; increase 100 mg/ day at 1-week intervals; max: 1,000 mg/day or 35 mg/kg/day >12 yr old: initial: 200 mg PO b.i.d., increase 200 mg/day at 1-week intervals b.i.d.-t.i.d.; max: 1,200 mg/day. | R Should not be taken with cloza- pine because of increased risk of bone marrow suppression, agranulocytosis Many drug interactions |

*(continued)*

| Name | Oral or Topical forms | Dosage | Comments |
|---|---|---|---|
| carbamide perox-ide (Debrox) | Sol: 6.5% | 1–5 drops b.i.d. for up to 4 day | — |
| caspofungin (Cancidas) | | 2–11 yr old. IV load 70 mg/m² (max 70 mg) on day 1 then 50 mg/m²/day (max: 50 mg) q24 <br> >12 yr old.: IV load 70 mg on day 1 then 50 mg q24 | Adjust for hepatic dysfunction |
| cefaclor (Ceclor) | Cap: 250, 500 mg <br> Susp: 125, 187, 250, 375 mg/5 mL | 20–40 mg/kg/day PO q8h; max: 2 g/day. | R |
| cefazolin (Ancef) | | Neonate dosing: 25 mg/kg/dose IV at the following intervals: <br> EGA (wk) Age (day) Interval <br> <29    0–28    q12h <br>             >28    q8h <br> 30–36   0–14   q12h <br>             >14    q8h <br> 37–44   0–7    q12h <br>             >7     q8h <br> >45    All     q6h <br> >1 mo.: 50–100 mg/kg/day q8h IV/IM; max: 6 g/day | R <br> Does not penetrate well into central nervous system |
| cefdinir (Omnicef) | Cap: 300 mg <br> Susp: 125 mg/5 mL | 6 mo–12 yr old: 14 mg/kg/day PO q12h; max: 600 mg/day <br> >12 yr old 600 mg/day PO q12h | R |
| cefepime (Maxipime) | | >2 mo: 100 mg/kg/day q12h IV/IM <br> Meningitis, fever and neu-tropenia, cystic fibrosis: 150 mg/kg/day q8h IV/IM; max 6 g/day | R |
| cefixime (Suprax) | Tab: 200, 400 mg <br> Susp: 100 mg/5 mL | 8 mg/kg/day q12–24h; max: 400 mg/day | R |
| cefotaxime (Claforan) | | Neonatal dosing: 50 mg/kg/dose IV at the following intervals: <br> PMA (wk) Age (day) Interval <br> <29    0–28    q12h <br>             >28    q8h <br> 30–36   0–14   q12h <br>             >14    q8h <br> 37–44   0–7    q12h <br>             >7     q8h <br> >45    All     q6h <br> <50 kg: 100–200 mg/kg/day q6–8h IV/IM; max: 12 g/day <br> >50 kg: 1–2 g/dose q6–8h IV/IM; max: 12 g/day | R |
| cefoxitin (Mefoxin) | | Neonates: 90–100 mg/kg/day IM,IV q8h <br> Infants and children: 80–160 mg/kg/day IM/IV q4–8h; max: 12 g/day | R |

| Name | Oral or Topical forms | Dosage | Comments |
|------|----------------------|--------|----------|
| cefprozil (Cefzil) | Tab: 250, 500 mg<br>Susp: 125, 250 mg/5 mL | Otitis media: 6 mo–12 yr old: 30 mg/kg/day PO q12h<br>Pharyngitis: 2–12 yr old: 15 mg/kg/day PO q12h<br>Acute sinusitis: 6 mo–12 yr old: 15–30 mg/kg/day PO q12–24h<br>Skin infection: >2 yr old: 20 mg/kg/day PO q24h<br>Max: 1 g/day | R |
| ceftazidime (Fortaz) | | 90–150 mg/kg/day q8h IV/IM<br>Meningitis or cystic fibrosis: 150 mg/kg/day IV/IM q8h; max: 6 g/day | R |
| ceftriaxone (Rocephin) | | Neonate gonococcal ophthalmia: 25–50 mg/kg/dose IM/IV × 1; max: 125 mg/dose<br>Child: 50–75 mg/kg/dose q12–24h IM/IV<br>Meningitis: 100 mg/kg/day IM/IV q12h; max: 4 g/day<br>Otitis media: 50 mg/kg IM × 1; max: 1 g | May cause hyperbilirubinemia in neonates; use with caution<br>Do not administer with calcium-containing solutions in newborns because of risk of precipitation of calcium-ceftriaxone salt; fatal reactions have occurred. |
| cefuroxime (Ceftin) | Tab: 125, 250, 500 mg<br>Susp: 125, 250 mg/5 mL | Neonates: 25–50 mg/kg/dose IV q12h (term infants >30 day: use q8h dosing)<br>Children: IM/IV: 75–150 mg/kg/day q8h; max: 6 g/day; PO<br>Pharyngitis: susp: 20 mg/kg/day q12h; max: 500 mg/day<br>Otitis media: susp: 30 mg/kg/day q12h; max: 1 g/day | R<br>Tablets and suspension are not bioequivalent; cannot substitute on a mg/mg basis. |
| cephalexin (Keflex) | Cap: 250, 500 mg<br>Susp: 125, 250 mg/5 mL<br>Tab: 250 mg, 500 mg | 25–100 mg/kg/day PO q6h; max 4 g/day | R |
| cetirizine (Zyrtec) | Syrup: 5 mg/5 mL<br>Tab: 5, 10 mg<br>ER tab with pseudoephedrine: 5 mg/120 mg | 2–5 yr old: 2.5 mg PO q.d.<br>>5 yr old: 5–10 mg PO q.d.<br>ER tab >11 yr old: 1 tab b.i.d. | R |
| chlorhexidine gluconate (Peridex) | 0.12% | Immunocompetent: 15 mL b.i.d.<br>Immunocompromised: 10–15 mL b.i.d.-t.i.d. | — |
| chlorothiazide (Diuril) | Tab: 250, 500 mg<br>Susp: 250 mg/5 mL | <6 mo: 20–40 mg/kg/day IV, PO divided q12h or lower doses of 2–8 mg/kg/dose IV divided q12h | R<br>May cause hypercalcemia, alkalosis, |

*(continued)*

| Name | Oral or Topical forms | Dosage | Comments |
|---|---|---|---|
| | | PO: 20 mg/kg/day b.i.d.; max: 1 g/day<br>IV: 4 mg/kg/day q.d.-b.i.d.; max: 500 mg/day. | hypokalemia, hypomagnesemia |
| chlorpheniramine (Chlor-Trimeton) | Tab: 4 mg<br>ER tab: 8, 12 mg<br>Chewable tab: 2 mg<br>Syrup: 2 mg/5 mL | 2–6 yr old: 1 mg/dose PO q4–6h; max: 6 mg/day<br>6–12 yr old: 2 mg/dose PO q4–6h; max: 12 mg/day.<br>>12 yr old: 4 mg/dose q4–6h PO; max: 24 mg/day.<br>ER, 6–12 yr old: 8 mg/dose PO q12h, >12 yr old: 8–12 mg PO q12h<br>IV/SC/IM: 5–20 mg × 1; max: 40 mg/day | — |
| ciprofloxacin (Cipro) | Tab: 100, 250, 500, 750 mg<br>Susp: 250, 500 mg/5 mL | Children:<br>PO: 20–30 mg/kg/day q12h; max: 1.5 g/day<br>IV: 10–20 mg/kg/day q12h; max: 800 mg/day.<br>Cystic fibrosis:<br>PO: 40 mg/kg/day q12h; max: 2 g/day<br>IV: 30 mg/kg/day q8h; max: 1.2 g/day. | R |
| ciprofloxacin/hydrocortisone (Cipro HC Otic) | Susp: 0.2%/1% | >1 yr old: instill 3 drops into affected ear(s) b.i.d. for 7 day. | — |
| clarithromycin (Biaxin) | Tab: 250, 500 mg<br>Susp: 125, 250 mg/5 mL | 15 mg/kg/day PO q12h.<br>Max.: 1 g/day | R<br>Can prolong QT interval. |
| clindamycin (Cleocin T) | Gel, lotion, solution: 1%, 2% | >12 yr old: Apply to area b.i.d. | — |
| clindamycin (Cleocin) | Cap: 75, 150, 300 mg<br>Susp: 75 mg/5 mL | Neonates: 5–7.5 mg/kg/dose IV at the following intervals:<br>PMA (wk) Age (Day) Interval<br><29  0–28  q12h<br>     >28  q8h<br>30–36  0–14  q12h<br>     >14  q8h<br>37–44  0–7  q8h<br>     >7  q6h<br>>45  All  q6h<br>Children:<br>PO: 10–30 mg/kg/day q6–8h (max: 1.8 g/day)<br>IM/IV: 25–40 mg/kg/day q6–8h (max: 4.8 g/day) | May cause pseudomembranous colitis<br>Poor tasting suspension |
| clonazepam (Klonopin) | Tab: 0.5, 1, 2 mg<br>Wafer: 0.125, 0.25, 0.5, 1, 2 mg<br>Susp: 100 μg/mL | <10 yr old or <30 kg: initial: 0.01–0.03 mg/kg/day PO b.i.d. or t.i.d., increase 0.25–0.5 mg/day q3 day up to max of 0.1–0.2 mg/kg/day. | Contraindicated in severe liver disease, acute narrow-angle glaucoma<br>Do not discontinue abruptly |

| Name | Oral or Topical forms | Dosage | Comments |
|------|----------------------|--------|----------|
| | | >10 yr old or >30 kg: initial: 1.5 mg/day PO t.i.d.; increase 0.5–1 mg/day q3d; max: 20 mg/day | Steady state achieved after 5–8 day of therapy with same dose |
| clonidine (Catapres) | Tab: 0.1, 0.2, 0.3 mg<br>Patch: 0.1, 0.2, 0.3 mg | 5–7 μg/kg/day PO q6–12h; titrate up q5–7d to 5–25 μg/kg/day PO q6h; max: 0.9 mg/day | — |
| clotrimazole (Mycelex, Lotrimin) | Cream: 1%<br>Vaginal supp: 200 mg<br>Vaginal cream: 1%, 2%<br>PO troche 10 mg | Vaginal candidiasis: 100 mg/dose q.h.s. × 7 day or 200 mg/dose q.h.s. × 3<br>Thrush: >3 yr old: Dissolve one troche 5×/day × 14 day<br>Topical: Apply b.i.d. | — |
| codeine | Tab: 15, 30, 60 mg<br>Sol: 15 mg/5 mL | >6 yr old: 1–1.5 mg/kg/day PO in doses q4–6h prn; max: 120 mg/day. | R |
| cromolyn sodium (Opticrom) | Ophthalmologic sol: 4% | 1–2 drops each eye 4–6 times/day | |
| cyproheptadine (Periactin) | Tab: 4 mg<br>Syrup: 2 mg/5 mL | 0.25–0.5 mg/kg/day PO q8–12h<br>Max in 2–6 yr old: 12 mg/day<br>Max in 7–14 yr old: 16 mg/day<br>Max in adults: 0.5 mg/kg/day | Contraindicated in neonates<br>Contraindicated in asthma, glaucoma |
| desmopressin (DDAVP) | Tab: 0.1, 0.2 mg<br>Nasal sol: 100 μg/mL, 1,500 μg/mL<br>Nasal spray: 10 μg/mL (may be compounded by hospital pharmacy), 100 μg/mL | Diabetes insipidus:<br>PO: Start with 0.05 mg/dose q.d.-b.i.d. and titrate to effect.<br>Intranasal: 5–30 μg/day q.d.-b.i.d.; max: 40 μg/day<br>IV/SC: 2–4 μg/day b.i.d.<br>Hemophilia A and von Willebrand's disease:<br>Intranasal: <50 kg: 150 μg, >50 kg: 300 μg,<br>IV 0.2–0.4 μg/kg/dose over 15–30 min<br>Nocturnal enuresis:<br>PO: 0.2 mg q.h.s. titrated to max of 0.6 mg<br>Intranasal: 20 μg q.h.s. to max of 40 μg | — |
| dexamethasone (Decadron) | Tab: 0.25, 0.5, 0.75, 1, 1.5, 2, 4, 6 mg<br>Elixir: 0.5 mg/5 mL<br>Oral sol: 1 mg/mL | Physiologic replacement: 0.03–0.15 mg/kg/day q6–12h IV/IM/PO<br>Cerebral edema: loading dose: 1–2 mg/kg/dose IV/IM × 1 then maintenance: 1–1.5 mg/kg/day q4–6h; max: 16 mg/day<br>Airway edema: 0.5–2 mg/kg/day IV/IM/PO q6h | Contraindicated in active, untreated infections<br>May cause hyperglycemia, mood changes, osteopenia<br>Taper if given for more than 7 day |

*(continued)*

| Name | Oral or Topical forms | Dosage | Comments |
|------|----------------------|--------|----------|
| | | Croup: 0.6 mg/kg/dose PO/IV/IM × 1<br>Antiemetic: initial: 10 mg/m²/dose IV (max: 20 mg), then 5 mg/m²/dose q6h IV<br>Anti-inflammatory: 0.08–0.3 mg/kg/day PO/IV/IM q6–12h<br>Spinal cord compression: 2 mg/kg/day IV q6h | |
| dextroamphetamine (Dexedrine) | Tab: 5, 10 mg<br>Tab (SR): 5, 10, 15 mg | 3–5 yr old: 2.5 mg/day PO every AM, increase by 2.5 mg/day every week to a max of 40 mg/day q.d.-t.i.d.<br>>5 yr old: 5 mg/day PO, increase by 5 mg/day every week to max of 40 mg/day q.d.-t.i.d. | Controlled II substance.<br>Use has been associated with serious cardiovascular events.<br>Potential for drug dependency.<br>Avoid use with MAOIs.<br>Use with caution in patients with hypertension or cardiovascular disease. |
| dextroamphetamine/racemic amphetamine (Adderall) | Tab: 5, 7.5, 10, 12.5, 15, 20, 30 mg<br>Susp: 1 mg/mL<br>Tab (ER): 5, 10, 15, 20, 25, 30 mg | 3–5 yr old: 2.5 mg/day PO every AM, increase by 2.5 mg/day every week to max of 40 mg/day q.d.-t.i.d.<br>>5 yr old: 5 mg/day PO, increase by 5 mg/day every week to max of 40 mg/day q.d.-t.i.d. | Use with caution in patients with hypertension or cardiovascular disease.<br>Controlled II substance.<br>Use has been associated with serious cardiovascular events<br>Potential for drug dependency.<br>Avoid use with MAOIs. |
| dextromethorphan (Delsym) | Delsym (SR): 30 mg/5 mL | 6 yr old: 2.5–7.5 mg PO q4–8h; SR: 15 mg/dose PO b.i.d.<br>7–12 yr old: 5–10 mg PO q4h or 15 mg PO q6–8h, SR: 30 mg/dose PO b.i.d.<br>>12 yr old: 10–30 mg PO q4–8h; SR: 60 mg/dose PO b.i.d. | Cough medicine is not recommended for children under the age of 6. |
| diazepam (Valium, Diastat) | Tab: 2, 5, 10 mg<br>Sol: 1, 5 mg/mL<br>Rectal gel: 2.5, 5, 10, 20 mg | Conscious sedation for procedures: PO 0.2–0.3 mg/kg (max 10 mg) 45–60 min before procedure<br>Status epilepticus: 0.2–0.5 mg/kg IV; see algorithm in Appendix G; Diastat: 1–5 yr old, 0.5 mg/kg | May cause hypotension, respiratory depression<br>Do not use with protease inhibitors. |

| Name | Oral or Topical forms | Dosage | Comments |
|---|---|---|---|
| | | 6–11 yr old, 0.3 mg/kg<br>12+ yr old, 0.2 mg/kg<br>Muscle relaxant: IV/IM:<br>0.04–0.3 mg/kg/dose<br>q2–4 h (max: 0.6 mg/kg<br>in 8 hr); PO: 0.12–0.8<br>mg/kg/day q6–8h | |
| diazoxide<br>(Proglycem) | Cap: 50 mg<br>Susp: 50 mg/mL | Hyperinsulinemic hypo-<br>glycemia:<br>Infants: 8–15 mg/kg/day PO<br>q8–12h<br>Children: 3–8 mg/kg/day PO<br>q8–12h | May cause hypona-<br>tremia, ketoaci-<br>dosis, hyper-<br>uricemia. |
| dicloxacillin<br>(Dynapen) | Cap: 125, 250, 500 mg | <40 kg: 25–50 mg/kg/day<br>PO q6h; max: 2 g/day<br>>40 kg: 125–500 mg/dose<br>PO q6h; max: 2 g/day | — |
| digoxin (Lanoxin) | Cap: 50, 100, 200 µg<br>Tab: 125, 250, 500 µg<br>Elixir: 50 µg/mL | 1 mo–2 yr old:<br>Initial: 35–60 µg/kg PO or<br>30–50 µg/kg IV/IM<br>Maintenance: 10–15 µg/<br>kg/day PO or 7.5–12<br>µg/kg/day IV/IM<br>2–5 yr old:<br>Initial: 30–40 µg/kg PO or<br>25–35 µg/kg IV/IM.<br>Maintenance: 7.5 µg/kg/<br>day PO or 6–9 µg/kg/ day<br>IV/IM.<br>5–10 yr old:<br>Initial: 20–35 µg/kg PO or<br>15–30 µg/kg IV/IM.<br>Maintenance: 5–10 µg/kg/<br>day PO or 4–8 µg/kg/ day<br>IV/IM.<br>>10 yr old:<br>Initial: 10–15 µg/kg PO or<br>8–12 µg/kg IV/IM.<br>Maintenance: 2.5–5 µg/kg/<br>day PO or 2–3 µg/kg/ day<br>IV/IM. | R<br>Give one half of<br>total initial dose<br>then give one<br>quarter of the<br>remaining dose<br>in each of the<br>subsequent two<br>doses at 6–12 hr<br>intervals. Obtain<br>electrocardio-<br>gram 6 hr after<br>each dose to<br>assess toxicity.<br>Toxic conditions:<br>bradycardia,<br>heart block, ven-<br>tricular arrhyth-<br>mias, vertigo,<br>hyperkalemia,<br>abdominal pain |
| digoxin immune<br>Fab (Digibind) | | To determine dose, calculate<br>the total body load (TBL)<br>of digoxin:<br>TBL (in mg) = serum<br>digoxin level (in ng/mL) ×<br>5.6 × body weight (in<br>kg) by 1,000. Dose of<br>digoxin immune Fab (in<br>mg) IV = TBL × 76 | — |
| dihydrotachysterol<br>(vitamin D) | Sol: 0.2 mg/mL<br>Cap: 0.125 mg<br>Tab: 0.125, 0.2, 0.4 mg | Hypoparathyroidism:<br>infants/young children:<br>initial 1–5 mg/day PO ×<br>4 day then 0.5–1.5<br>mg/day PO.<br>Older children: initial: 0.75–2.5<br>mg/day PO × 4 day then<br>0.2–1.5 mg/day PO | Use caution in<br>patients with<br>renal stones,<br>renal failure, and<br>heart disease. |

*(continued)*

| Name | Oral or Topical forms | Dosage | Comments |
|---|---|---|---|
| | | Nutritional rickets: 0.5 mg × 1 PO or 13–50 µg/day PO q.d. until healing Renal osteodystrophy: 0.1–0.5 mg/day PO | |
| diltiazem (Cardizem) | Cap, ER: 60, 90, 120, 180, 240, 300 mg Cap, SR: 60, 90, 120 mg Tab: 30, 60, 90, 120 mg Elixir: 12 mg/mL | Initial: 1.5–2 mg/kg/day PO t.i.d.-q.i.d.; max: 3.5 mg/kg/day | — |
| diphenhydramine (Benadryl) | Elixir, syrup, liquid: 12.5 mg/5 mL Cap/tab: 25, 50 mg Chewable tab: 12.5 mg | 5 mg/kg/day q6h PO/IV/IM; max: 300 mg/day For anaphylaxis: 1–2 mg/kg IV slowly | R |
| docusate sodium (Colace) | Cap: 50, 100, 240, 250 mg Tab: 100 mg Syrup: 16.7, 20 mg/5 mL Liquid: 10 mg/mL | 5 mg/kg/day PO q.d.-q.i.d.; max: 400 mg/day | — |
| dornase alfa (Pulmozyme) | Nebulizer sol: 1 mg/mL | >5 yr old: 2.5 mg q.d.-b.i.d. | Do not mix with other nebulized drugs |
| doxycycline (Vibramycin) | Cap or tab: 20, 50, 100 mg Susp: 25 mg/5 mL Syrup: 50 mg/5 mL | 2–4 mg/kg/day PO/IV q12–24h; max: 200 mg/day. | Use with caution in children <8 yr old because of risk of tooth enamel hypoplasia and discoloration |
| enalapril (Vasotec) enalaprilat (IV) | Tab: 2.5, 5, 10, 20 mg Susp: 1 mg/mL | Infants and children: PO: 0.1 mg/kg/day q.d.-b.i.d., titrate up as needed over 2 wk to max of 0.5 mg/kg/day. IV: 5–10 µg/kg/dose q8–24h | R |
| enoxaparin (Lovenox) | 30 mg/0.3 mL | Deep vein thrombosis (DVT): <2 mo: 1.5 mg/kg/dose q12h SC >2 mo.: 1 mg/kg/dose q12h SC DVT prophylaxis: <2 mo.: 0.75 mg/kg/dose q12h SC >2 mo.: 0.5 mg/kg/dose q12h SC | R Check factor Xa level 4 hr after dose |
| epinephrine (EpiPen, EpiPen Jr.) | EpiPen: 0.3 mg EpiPen Jr.: 0.15 mg. | <30 kg: 0.15 mg/dose IM ≥30 kg: 0.3 mg/dose IM | To be used only in severe hypersensitivity reactions |
| epinephrine racemic (AsthmaNefrin, MicroNefrin) | Nebulizer sol: 2.25% | Nebulizer: 0.5 mL/dose diluted in 3 mL normal saline over 15 min | — |
| erythromycin | Oint, gel, solution: 2% | Apply to affected area b.i.d. | — |

| Name | Oral or Topical forms | Dosage | Comments |
|------|----------------------|--------|----------|
| erythromycin (Ilotycin) | Ophthalmologic oint: 0.5% | Apply 0.5 inch ribbon to affected eye b.i.d.-q.i.d. | — |
| erythromycin preparations (E-mycin) | Base: Cap, enteric 250 mg Tab, enteric: 250, 333, 500 mg Ethyl succinate (EES): Chewable tab: 200 mg Susp: 200, 400 mg/5 mL Drops: 100 mg/2.5 mL Tab: 400 mg Others: Chewable tab: 125, 250 mg Tab: 500 mg Cap: 125, 250 mg | Chlamydia conjunctivitis and pneumonia: 50 mg/kg/day PO q6h × 14 day. Pertussis: estolate salt: 50 mg/kg/day PO q6h × 14 day Other infections: base, estolate, and ethylsuccinate: 30–50 mg/kg/day PO q6–8h; max: 2 g/day as base or 3.2 g/day as ethylsuccinate | R Many drug interactions. |
| erythropoietin (Epogen) | | Anemia in cancer or renal failure: SC/IV: Initial dose of 50–100 U/kg/dose 3 × week; increase dose if hematocrit does not rise by 5–6% after 8 wk. | Iron supplementation recommended before and during therapy |
| etanercept (Enbrel) | 25 mg/mL 50 mg/mL Injection: 50 mg/mL | 4–17 yr old: 0.4 mg/kg/dose SC 2×/wk 72–96h apart; max: 25 mg/dose | Contraindicated in serious infections. Do not administer live vaccines concurrently Onset of action: 1–4 wk |
| ethambutol (Myambutol) | Tab: 100, 400 mg | TB: 15–25 mg/kg/dose PO q.d. or 50 mg/kg/dose PO twice weekly; max: 2.5 g/day Non-TB mycobacterial infection: 15–25 mg/kg/day; max: 1 g/day | R Possible reversible optic neuritis |
| famotidine (Pepcid) | Liquid: 40 mg/5 mL Tab: 10, 20, 40 mg Gel cap: 10 mg Disintegrating oral tab: 20, 40 m Chewable tab: 10 mg | Neonates: 1 mg/kg/dose IV, PO q24h Children: IV/PO: 0.5–1 mg/kg/day b.i.d.; max: 80 mg/day. | R |
| fexofenadine (Allegra) | Tab: 30, 60, 180 mg Cap: 60 mg ER tab with pseudoephedrine: 60 mg/120 mg | 6–11 yr old: 30 mg PO b.i.d. >11 yr old: 60 mg PO b.i.d. or 180 mg PO q.d.; ER: >11 yr old: 1 tab PO b.i.d. | R |
| filgrastim (G-CSF, Neupogen) | | IV/SC: 5–10 μg/kg/dose q24h × 14 day or until absolute neutrophil count >10,000/mm$^3$ May increase dose by 5 μg/kg/day if desired effect not achieved within 7 day. | Use with caution in myeloid malignancies |
| fluconazole (Diflucan) | Tab: 50, 100, 150, 200 mg Susp: 10, 40 mg/mL | Neonates: load of 12 mg/kg, then maintenance of 6 mg/ | R Do not use |

*(continued)*

| Name | Oral or Topical forms | Dosage | Comments |
|---|---|---|---|
| | | kg/dose IV, PO q24h; prophylaxis: 3 mg/kg/dose IV q24h<br>Children: load of 10 mg/kg IV/PO, then maintenance of (24h after load) 3–6 mg/kg q.d. IV/PO; max: 12 mg/kg/day<br>Vaginal candidiasis: 150 mg PO× 1 | concurrently with terfenadine, astemizole |
| fludrocortisone (Florinef) | Tab: 0.1 mg | 0.05–0.2 PO mg q.d. | Contraindicated in congestive heart failure and fungal infections |
| fluoxetine (Prozac) | Liquid: 20 mg/5 mL<br>Cap: 10, 20, 40 mg<br>Delayed release (weekly): 90 mg<br>Tab: 10, 20 mg | Depression: >5 yr old: 5–10 mg PO q.d.; max: 20 mg/day; adolescent max: 60 mg/day.<br>Bulimia: 60 mg every AM PO. | Avoid use with MAOIs.<br>Avoid abrupt discontinuation.<br>Divide doses >20 mg/24h q.d. or b.i.d.<br>Antidepressants may worsen depression and increase suicidal ideation in children and young adults.<br>Consider dose adjustment with hepatic impairment. |
| fluticasone (Flonase) | Nasal spray: 50 μg/actuation | >4 yr old: 1 spray per nostril q.d.; can increase to 2 sprays per nostril every day when symptomatic | — |
| fluticasone (Flovent, Flovent Rotadisk) | DPI: 50,100, 250 μg/dose<br>MDI: 44, 110, 220 μg/dose | MDI: 88 μg b.i.d. and titrate up to max of 440 μg b.i.d.<br>DPI: 50 μg b.i.d. and titrate up to max of 500 μg b.i.d. | May cause dysphonia, oral thrush.<br>Has less effect on suppressing linear growth compared with beclomethasone |
| fluticasone/salmeterol (Advair Diskus) | DPI 100/50, 250/50, 500/50 μg/μg/dose | 100/50 μg 1 puff b.i.d.; may titrate up to effect. | May cause dysphonia, oral thrush<br>Has less effect on suppressing linear growth compared with beclomethasone<br>Rinse mouth after use |
| foscarnet (Foscavir) | | CMV retinitis:<br>Induction: 60 mg/kg IV q8h<br>Maintenance: 90–120 mg/kg/day IV | R<br>Nephrotoxicity, electrolyte imbalances |

| Name | Oral or Topical forms | Dosage | Comments |
|------|----------------------|--------|----------|
| | | Acyclovir-resistant herpes simplex virus: 40 mg/kg/dose IV q8h or 40–60 mg/kg/dose q12h for up to 3 wk or until lesions heal | |
| fosphenytoin (Cerebyx) | | Status epilepticus: see algorithm in Appendix G Status epilepticus: 10–20 mg/kg IV Nonemergent loading dose: 10–20 mg phenytoin equivalent (PE)/kg IV/IM. Initial maintenance dose: 4–6 mg PE/kg/day IV/IM | R Possible signs of overdose: slurred speech, dizziness, ataxia, rash, nystagmus, tinnitus, diplopia, vomiting Many drug interactions Therapeutic levels: 10–20 mg/L Consider dosage adjustment in hepatic impairment or hypoalbuminemia |
| furosemide (Lasix) | Tab: 20, 40, 80 mg Sol: 10 mg/mL, 40 mg/5 mL | Neonates: 1 mg/kg/dose IV, 2 mg/kg/dose PO, interval varies PO: 1–6 mg/kg/day q6–12h. IV/IM: 1–2 mg/kg/dose q6–12h. Max: 6 mg/kg/dose | R Contraindicated in anuria and hepatic coma Possible hypokalemia, alkalosis, hyperuricemia, hypercalciuria |
| gabapentin (Neurontin) | Cap: 100, 300, 400 mg Tab: 600, 800 mg Sol: 250 mg/5 mL | 3–12 yr old: day 1: 10–15 mg/kg/day PO t.i.d., increase to the following over 3 day: 3–4 yr old: 40 mg/kg/day PO t.i.d. >5 yr old: 25–35 mg/kg/day PO t.i.d.; max: 50 mg/kg/day | R Do not withdraw abruptly. |
| ganciclovir (Cytovene) | Cap: 250 mg | Congenital CMV: 6 mg/kg IV q12h CMV infection or CMV prevention in transplant: >3 mo Induction: 5 mg/kg/dose IV q12h Maintenance: 5 mg/kg/dose IV q.d. or 6 mg/kg/dose IV q.d. for 5 day/week; oral maintenance: 30 mg/kg/dose q8h; max: 1,000 mg t.i.d. | R Common side effects: neutropenia, thrombocytopenia |
| gentamicin (Garamycin) | | Neonates: PMA (wk) Age (day) Dose ≤28 0–30 3 mg/kg q24h | R Everyday dosing not appropriate in weight >20% |

*(continued)*

| Name | Oral or Topical forms | Dosage | Comments |
|---|---|---|---|
| | | >30   5 mg/kg q24h<br>29–32  0–21  3 mg/kg q24h<br>      21–45  5 mg/kg q24h<br>      45–60  4 mg/kg q12h<br>      >60  4 mg/kg q12h[1] or 2.5 mg/kg q8h[2]<br>33–34  0–14  3 mg/kg q24h<br>      14–45  5 mg/kg q24h<br>      >45  4 mg/kg q12h[1] or 2.5 mg/kg q8h[2]<br>≥35  0–30  5 mg/kg q24h<br>      >30  4 mg/kg q12h[1] or 2.5 mg/kg q8h[2]<br>Monitoring peak 6–15 $\mu$g/mL, trough ≤1.5 $\mu$g/mL, (2.5 mg/kg/dose: peak 6–10, trough <2). Check levels with 4th dose if patient is being evaluated for sepsis, and 3rd when treating a known infection.<br>[1]Preferred for all patients, including those with renal and cardiac dysfunction<br>[2]If using 2.5 mg/kg/dose in renal or cardiac dysfunction, use q12–24h<br><br>1 mo–18 yr old: 2.5 mg/kg/dose IV q8 up to a max of 150 mg IV q8 | ideal body weight, ascites, >20% burns, altered renal function, endocarditis, tularemia, meningitis, osteomyelitis, or hemodynamic instability<br>Dosing may need to be adjusted in patients with cystic fibrosis<br>Check peak and trough |
| glucagon (Glucagon) | 1 mg = 1 unit | <20 kg: 0.5 mg/dose (or 0.02–0.03 mg/kg/dose) IM every 20 min prn, >20 kg: 1 mg/dose IM every 20 min prn | — |
| glycerin | Rectal sol: 4 mL per application<br>Supp: infant/child, adult | Neonate: 0.5 mL/kg/dose of rectal sol as enema<br><6 yr old: 1 infant supp prn<br>≥6 yr old: 1 adult supp | — |
| griseofulvin microsize | Microsize: tab: 250, 500 mg; cap: 125, 250 mg; susp: 125 mg/5 mL | Microsize: >2 yr old: 10–20 mg/kg/day PO q.d.-b.i.d.; max: 1 g/day | Contraindicated in hepatic disease |

| Name | Oral or Topical forms | Dosage | Comments |
|------|----------------------|--------|----------|
| | Ultramicrosize: tab: 125, 165, 250, 330 mg | Ultramicrosize: >2 yr old: 5–10 mg/kg/day PO q.d.-b.i.d.; max dose: 750 mg/day | |
| guaifenesin (Hytuss, Robitussin) | Tab: 100 mg<br>Syrup: 100 mg/5 mL | Cough medicine is not recommended for children under the age of 6.<br>6–11 yr old: 100–200 mg PO q4h; max: 1.2 g/day<br>>11 yr old: 200–400 mg PO q4h; max 2.4 g/day | — |
| haloperidol (Haldol) | Tab: 0.5, 1, 2, 5, 10, 20 mg<br>Sol: 2 mg/mL | 3–12 yr old: PO initial dose of 0.25–0.5 mg/day b.i.d.-t.i.d. and increase by 0.25–0.5 mg/day q5–7 day prn to max of 0.15 mg/kg/day.<br>>12 yr old: 0.5–5 mg b.i.d.-t.i.d.; max: 30 mg/day<br>IM: 6–12 yr old: 1–3 mg/dose q4–8h; max: 0.15 mg/kg/day<br>Acute agitation, >12 yr old: 2–5 mg/dose IM, repeat in 1h prn<br>Psychosis: 2–5 mg/dose q4–8h IM prn or 1–15 mg/day b.i.d.-t.i.d. PO<br>Max: 30 mg/day. | Use with caution in patients with cardiac disease (risk of hypotension) or epilepsy (lowers seizure threshold) IM form comes in immediate and long-acting forms. Contraindicated with narrow-angle glaucoma, bone marrow suppression, and severe cardiac and hepatic disease. Increased risk of QT prolongation and torsades de pointes. May cause extrapyramidal symptoms |
| heparin (Hepalean) | | Anticoagulation: 50–100 units/kg IV bolus and then maintenance: 10–25 unit/kg/hr IV. Adjust dose q4h based on activated partial thromboplastin time (aPTT): if <50: give 50 units/kg bolus and increase rate by 10%, if 50–59: increase rate by 10%, if 60–85: keep rate the same, if 86–95: decrease rate by 10%, if 96–120: hold infusion for 30 min then resume with rate decreased by 10%, if >120: hold infusion for 60 min then resume with rate decreased by 15%. Remeasure aPTT 4h after each change. | Check PTT q6h while adjusting dose and then every day while on steady dose. |
| hydrochlorothiazide (HCTZ, HydroDIURIL) | Cap: 12.5 mg<br>Tab: 25, 50, 100 mg<br>Sol: 50 mg/5 mL | <6 mo: 2–4 mg/kg/day b.i.d. PO; max: 37.5 mg/day<br>>6 mo: 2 mg/kg/day b.i.d. PO; max: 100 mg/day | R<br>May cause hypercalcemia, alkalosis, hypokalemia, hypomagnesemia |

*(continued)*

| Name | Oral or Topical forms | Dosage | Comments |
|------|----------------------|--------|----------|
| hydrocortisone (Cortef) | Tab: 5, 10, 20 mg<br>Susp: 10 mg/5 mL | Acute adrenal insufficiency: 1–2 mg/kg/dose IV bolus, then 25–250 mg/day IM/IV q6–8h<br>Congenital adrenal hyperplasia: initial: 10–20 mg/m$^2$/day PO t.i.d.; maintenance: 2.5–10 mg/day PO t.i.d.<br>Physiologic replacement: PO: 0.5–0.75 mg/kg/day q8h; IM: 0.25–0.35 mg/kg/day q.d.<br>Status asthmaticus: 8 mg/kg/day IV q6h<br>Anti-inflammatory/immunosuppressive: PO: 2.5–10 mg/kg/24h q6–8h; IM/IV: 1–5 mg/kg/24h q12–24h | Contraindicated in active, untreated infections<br>May cause hyperglycemia, mood changes, osteopenia<br>Taper if given for more than 7 day. |
| hydrocortisone/polymyxin/neomycin (Cortisporin Otic) | Sol, susp: 10 mg/10,000 U, 5 mg/mL | 3 drops into affected ear t.i.d.-q.i.d. | — |
| hydroxychloroquine sulfate (Plaquenil) | Tab: 200 mg | JRA: 3–5 mg/kg/day PO q.d.-b.i.d.; max: 400 mg/day. | R<br>Bone marrow suppression, retinal toxicity |
| ibuprofen (Motrin, Advil, NeoProfen) | Susp: 100 mg/5 mL<br>Drops: 40 mg/mL<br>Chewable tab: 50, 100 mg<br>Cap: 100, 200 mg<br>Tab: 100, 200, 300, 400, 600, 800 mg | Analgesic, antipyretic: 4–10 mg/kg/dose PO q6–8h; max 40 mg/kg/day or 2,400 mg/day<br>Closure of ductus: 10 mg/kg IV ×1, then 5 mg/kg IV q24h × 2 doses | R<br>Contraindicated with GI bleeding and ulcer disease; inhibits platelet aggregation<br>Monitor urine output and platelet count during therapy; do not give subsequent doses if either falls too low. |
| imiquimod (Aldara) | Cream: 5% | Apply 3 X/wk; leave on skin 6–10 h and then wash off. Use for up to 16 wk | — |
| indomethacin (Indocin) | Cap: 25, 50 mg<br>Cap, ER: 75 mg<br>Supp: 50 mg<br>Susp: 25 mg/5 mL | Anti-inflammatory: ≥2 yr old: 1–2 mg/kg/day PO b.i.d.-q.i.d.; max: 150–200 mg/day or 4 mg/kg/day<br>Closure of ductus: 0.1–0.2 mg/kg/dose IV q12–24h × 3 total doses | R<br>Contraindicated in bleeding, necrotizing enterocolitis, coagulopathies<br>Monitor urine output and platelet count during therapy; do not give subsequent doses if either falls too low. |

| Name | Oral or Topical forms | Dosage | Comments |
|------|----------------------|--------|----------|
| ipratropium bromide (Atrovent) | Nebulizer sol: 0.02% (500 µg/2.5 mL) MDI: 17 µg/actuation | Acute asthma exacerbations: 250–500 µg/dose neb q6h 4–8 puffs prn Maintenance dose: 250–500 µg/dose neb q6h 1–2 puffs (<12 yr old) or 2–3 puffs (≥12 yr) q6h | More effective in first 24 hr of reactive airway disease management May combine with albuterol |
| isoniazid (INH) | Tab: 50, 100, 300 mg Syrup: 50 mg/5 mL | Prophylaxis: 10 mg/kg PO q.d.; max: 300 mg; after 1 mo. of q.d., may change to 20–40 mg/kg (max 900 mg) per dose PO, twice a week Treatment: 10–15 mg/kg (max dose 300 mg) PO q.d. or 20–30 mg/kg PO (max 900 mg) per dose twice a week with rifampin | Supplemental pyridoxine recommended. |
| isotretinoin (Accutane) | Cap: 10, 20, 40 mg | 0.5–2 mg/kg/day PO b.i.d. for 15–20 wk. | Known teratogen; contraindicated in pregnancy May cause hyperlipidemia, pseudotumor cerebri, elevated transaminases |
| ivermectin (Stromectol) | Tab: 3, 6 mg | >15 kg: Strongyloidiasis, scabies: 200 µg/kg PO × 1 dose Onchocerciasis: 150 µg/kg PO × 1 dose | — |
| ketoconazole (Nizoral) | Tab: 200 mg Susp: 100 mg/5 mL Cream: 2% Shampoo: 2% | PO: >2 yr old: 3.3–6.6 mg/kg q.d.; max: 800 mg/day b.i.d. Topical: 1–2 applications/day Shampoo: twice weekly for 4 wk | Do not use concurrently with cisapride, terfenadine, astemizole Monitor liver function tests in long-term use |
| ketorolac (Toradol) | Tab: 10 mg | IM/IV: 0.5 mg/kg/dose q6h; max: 30 mg q6h or 120 mg/day PO: >50 kg: 10 mg prn q6h; max: 40 mg/day | R Do not exceed 5 day of therapy. |
| lactulose (Cephulac) | Syrup: 10 g/15 mL | Constipation: 7.5 mL/day PO; may increase to max of 60 mL/day. Hepatic encephalopathy: infants; 2.5–10 mL/day PO t.i.d.-q.i.d.; children: 40–90 mL/day PO t.i.d.-q.i.d. | Contraindicated in galactosemia |
| lansoprazole (Prevacid) | Cap: 15, 30 mg Granules for susp: 15 mg, 30 mg/packet | Neonates: 1.5 mg/kg/dose PO q24h (max for <10 kg: 7.5 mg PO q24h) | — |

*(continued)*

| Name | Oral or Topical forms | Dosage | Comments |
|------|----------------------|--------|----------|
| | | 10–20 kg: 15 mg PO q.d.<br>>20 kg: 15–30 mg PO q.d. | |
| levalbuterol<br>(Xopenex) | Nebulizer sol: 0.36, 0.73,<br>1.25 mg/3 mL<br>MDI: 45 μg/actuation | <6 yr old: 0.16–1.25 mg<br>inhalation t.i.d.<br>6–11 yr old: 0.31–0.63 mg<br>inhaled t.i.d. prn<br>>12 yr old: 0.63–1.25 mg<br>inhaled t.i.d. | — |
| levofloxacin<br>(Levaquin) | Tab: 250, 500 mg | 5–10 mg/kg/dose PO/IV<br>q.d.; max: 500 mg. | R |
| levothyroxine<br>(Synthroid) | Tab: 25, 50, 75, 88, 100,<br>112, 125, 137, 150, 175,<br>200 , 300 μg<br>Susp: 25 μg/mL | PO:<br>0–6 mo.: 8–10 μg/kg/dose<br>q.d.<br>6–12 mo.: 6–8 μg/kg/dose<br>q.d.<br>1–5 yr old: 5–6 μg/kg/ dose<br>q.d.<br>6–12 yr old: 4–5 μg/kg/<br>dose q.d.<br>>12 yr old: 2–3 μg/kg/<br>dose q.d.<br>IM/IV: 50–75% of PO dose | Contraindicated in<br>acute myocardial<br>infarction,<br>thyrotoxicosis,<br>uncorrected<br>adrenal<br>insufficiency. |
| lidocaine/prilocaine<br>(EMLA) | Cream: 2.5%/2.5% | Total max dose: <5 kg: 1 g<br>(10 cm$^2$), 5–10 kg: 2 g<br>(20 cm$^2$), 10–20 kg: 10 g<br>(100 cm$^2$), >20 kg: 20 g<br>(200 cm$^2$) | Do not use on<br>mucous<br>membranes<br>or eyes. |
| linezolid (Zyvox) | Susp: 100 mg/5 mL<br>Tab: 400, 600 mg | 10 mg/kg/dose IV/PO q8–12h;<br>max: 600 mg/dose | Bacteriostatic |
| loratadine<br>(Claritin) | Tab: 10 mg<br>RediTab: 10 mg<br>Syrup: 1 mg/mL<br>ER tab with<br>pseudoephedrine: 12 hr:<br>5 mg/120 mg; 24 hr:<br>10 mg/240 mg | 2–5 yr old: 5 mg PO q.d.<br>>5 yr old: 10 mg PO q.d.<br>ER >11 yr old: 1 tab PO<br>b.i.d. for 12 h and 1 tab<br>q.d. for 24 h | R |
| lorazepam (Ativan) | Tab: 0.5, 1, 2 mg<br>Sol: 2 mg/mL | Status epilepticus: see<br>algorithm in Appendix G;<br>0.1 mg/kg/dose IV, max<br>dose 4 mg | Contraindicated in<br>narrow-angle<br>glaucoma and<br>severe hypoten-<br>sion. May cause<br>respiratory<br>depression. |
| mannitol | | Cerebral edema: 0.25 g/kg/<br>dose IV over 20–30 min;<br>may increase to 1 g/kg/<br>dose if needed. | R<br>Contraindicated in<br>severe renal dis-<br>ease, active<br>intracranial bleed,<br>dehydration, pul-<br>monary edema |
| mebendazole<br>(Vermox) | Chewable tab: 100 mg | Pinworm: 1 tab PO × 1 dose<br>Whipworm, common<br>roundworm, hookworm:<br>1 tab b.i.d. PO × 3 day | — |

| Name | Oral or Topical forms | Dosage | Comments |
|------|----------------------|--------|----------|
| meclizine (Antivert) | Tab: 12.5, 25, 50 mg<br>Chewable tab: 25 mg | >12 yr old: 25–100 PO mg/day | — |
| meropenem (Merrem IV) | | Neonates:<br>Sepsis: 20 mg/kg/dose IV q8–12h<br>Meningitis: 40 mg/kg/dose IV q8h<br>Mild to moderate infection (>3 mo): 20 mg/kg/dose IV q8h; max: 3 g/day.<br>Severe infections (including meningitis): 40 mg/kg/dose IV q8h; max: 6 g/day | R |
| mesalamine (Asacol, Rowasa, Pentasa) | Caps, controlled release: (Pentasa): 250 mg<br>Tab, delayed release (Asacol): 400 mg<br>Supp (Rowasa): 500 mg | Cap: 50 mg/kg/day q6–12h PO<br>Tab: 50 mg/kg/day q8–12h PO; max: 4 g/day<br>Supp (adolescents): 500 mg b.i.d. PR × 3–6 wk | R<br>Do not use in children with flulike symptoms. Contraindicated in active peptic ulcer disease, severe renal failure. |
| metformin (Glucophage) | Tab: 500, 850, 1,000 mg<br>Tab ER: 500 mg | 10–16 yr old: initial dose of 500 mg b.i.d. PO; increase every week to max of 2,000 mg/day<br>>17 yr old: same dosing except max is 2,500 mg/day | R<br>Contraindicated in renal impairment, congestive heart failure, metabolic acidosis<br>Possibly fatal lactic acidosis |
| methimazole (Tapazole) | Tab: 5, 10 mg | Initial: 0.4–0.7 mg/kg/day PO q8h; then maintenance: 1/3–2/3 of initial dose q8h; max: 30 mg/day | — |
| methotrexate (Rheumatrex) | Tab: 2.5, 5, 7.5, 15 mg | JRA: 5–15 mg/m$^2$/wk PO/SQ/IM as a single dose or in 3 doses given 12h apart | R<br>Hepatic toxicity<br>Give folate replacement while on therapy |
| methylphenidate (Ritalin, others) | Tab (Ritalin): 5, 10, 20 mg<br>Tab (ER)<br>  Metadate ER: 10, 20 mg<br>  Concerta: 18, 27, 36, 54 mg<br>Cap (ER)<br>  Metadate CD: 10, 20, 30, 40, 50, 60 mg<br>  Ritalin LA: 10, 20, 30, 40 mg<br>Tab (SR): Ritalin SR, 20 mg<br>Chewable tab: 2.5, 5, 10 mg<br>Patch: 10, 15, 20, 30 mg<br>Sol: 1 mg/mL, 2 mg/mL | >5 yr old: initial 0.3 mg/kg/dose given before breakfast and lunch; increase by 0.1 mg/kg/dose PO every week until 0.3–1 mg/kg/day reached; max: 2 mg/kg/day or 60 mg/day<br>Once-daily dosing (Concerta): start with 18 mg PO every AM; increase every week at 18 mg increments to max of 54 mg/day. | Controlled II substance.<br>Use has been associated with serious cardiovascular events.<br>Contraindicated in glaucoma, anxiety disorders, motor tics, Tourette syndrome.<br>Avoid use with MAOIs.<br>Potential for drug dependency. |
| methylprednisolone (Solu-Medrol, Medrol) | Tab: 2, 8, 16 mg | Anti-inflammatory/ immunosuppressive: 0.5–1.7 mg/kg/day PO/IV/IM q6–12h | Contraindicated in active, untreated infections |

*(continued)*

| Name | Oral or Topical forms | Dosage | Comments |
|---|---|---|---|
| | | Status asthmaticus: 2 mg/kg/day IM/IV q6h<br>Acute spinal cord injury: 30 mg/kg IV over 15 min followed in 45 min by a continuous infusion of 5.4 mg/kg/hr × 23h | May cause hyperglycemia, mood changes, osteopenia<br>Taper if given for more than 7 day |
| metoclopramide (Reglan, others) | Tab: 5, 10 mg<br>Syrup: 5 mg/5 mL | Gastroesophageal reflux (PO, IV, IM) (infant/child): 0.4–0.8 mg/kg/day t.i.d.-q.i.d.<br>Antiemetic (PO, IV): 1–2 mg/kg/dose q2–4h (pretreat with diphenhydramine to reduce extrapyramidal symptoms)<br>Postoperative nausea/vomiting (IV) (child): 0.1–0.2 mg/kg/dose q6–8h prn | — |
| metolazone (Zaroxolyn) | Tab: 2.5, 5, 10 mg<br>Susp: 1 mg/mL | 0.2–0.4 mg/kg/day PO q.d.-b.i.d. | Contraindicated in patients with anuria or hepatic coma<br>May cause electrolyte imbalances, hyperglycemia, marrow suppression |
| metronidazole (Flagyl) | Tab: 250, 500 mg<br>Tab, ER: 750 mg<br>Cap: 375 mg<br>Susp: 20, 50 mg/mL<br>Gel, topical: 0.75%<br>Cream, topical: 0.75%<br>Gel, vaginal: 0.75% | Neonates: anaerobic infections:<br>PO, IV: 0–4 wk, <1,200 g: 7.5 mg/kg q48h<br>Postnatal ≤7 day: 1,200–2,000 g: 7.5 mg/kg/day given q24h<br>>2,000 g: 15 mg/kg/day divided q12h<br>Postnatal age >7 day: 1,200–2,000 g: 15 mg/kg/day divided q12h<br>>2,000 g: 30 mg/kg/day divided q12h<br>Infants and children:<br>Amebiasis: 35–50 mg/kg/day PO t.i.d.; max: 750 mg/dose<br>*Clostridium difficile*, anaerobic infection: 30 mg/kg/day IV/PO q6h; max: 4 g/day<br>Bacterial vaginosis: 500 mg b.i.d. PO × 7 day or 2 g PO × 1 dose or 5 g vaginal gel q.d.-b.i.d. ×5 day<br>Giardiasis: 15 mg/kg/day PO t.i.d. × 5 d; max: 250 mg PO t.i.d. | Patients should avoid alcohol while taking. |

| Name | Oral or Topical forms | Dosage | Comments |
|---|---|---|---|
| | | Trichomoniasis: 15 mg/kg/day PO t.i.d. × 7 d (max: 250–375 mg PO t.i.d.) or 2 g PO × 1 | |
| miconazole (Monistat) | Cream, lotion, oint, sol: 2%, vaginal supp: 100, 200 mg | Tinea cruris or corporis or candidiasis: apply b.i.d. Tinea versicolor: apply q.d. Vaginal: 1 applicator full of cream or 100 mg supp. q.h.s. × 7 day | — |
| mineral oil | Rectal liquid: 133 mL | 5–11 yr old: 30–60 mL PR × 1 >11 yr old: 60–150 mL PR × 1 | Use as laxative, should not exceed 1 wk |
| minocycline (Minocin) | Cap: 50, 75, 100 mg Tab: 50, 100 mg Susp: 50 mg/5 mL | 8–12 yr old: 4 mg/kg/dose × 1 PO/IV then 2 mg/kg/dose q12h PO/IV; max: 200 mg/day >12 yr old: 200 mg/dose × 1 PO/IV then 100 mg q12h PO/IV Acne: 50 mg PO q.d.-t.i.d. | Use with caution in children <8 yr old because of risk of tooth enamel hypoplasia and discoloration |
| montelukast (Singulair) | Chewable tab: 4, 5 mg Tab: 10 mg | 2–5 yr old: 4 mg PO q.h.s. 6–14 yr old: 5 mg PO q.h.s. >15 yr old: 10 mg PO q.h.s. | Contraindicated in phenylketonuria Adjust dose with phenobarbital and rifampin. |
| morphine | Tab: 10, 15, 30 mg Controlled release tab (MS Contin): 15, 30, 60, 100, 200 mg Sol: 10 mg/5 mL, 20 mg/5 mL Concentrated oral sol: 20 mg/mL | Neonates: 0.05 mg/kg IV, IM, SQ q4–8h prn (max: 0.1 mg/kg) Infants/children: 0.2–0.5 mg/kg/dose PO q4–6h prn; 0.1–0.2 mg/kg/dose IV, IM, SQ q2–4h prn Continuous IV infusion: Neonates: 10–20 μg/kg/hr Infant/child: 10–40 μg/kg/hr (postoperatively); 40–70 μg/kg/hr (sickle cell/cancer) | Respiratory depression may occur Controlled release product: not intended for prn use; for mild pain, immediate postoperative pain, or pain that is not expected to persist for extended period |
| mupirocin (Bactroban) | Cream, oint: 2% | Apply b.i.d.-t.i.d. Intranasal: b.i.d.-q.i.d. × 5–14 day | Avoid contact with eyes. |
| nafcillin (Nallpen) | Tab: 500 mg Cap: 250 mg | Neonates: IM, IV: 0–4 wk, <1,200 g: 50 mg/kg/day in divided doses q12h ≤7 day: 1,200–2,000 g: 50 mg/kg/day in divided doses q12h >2,000 g: 75 mg/kg/day in divided doses q8h >7 day 1,200–2,000 g: 75 mg/kg/day in divided doses q8h >2,000 g: 100 mg/kg/day in divided doses q6h | R |

*(continued)*

| Name | Oral or Topical forms | Dosage | Comments |
|------|----------------------|--------|----------|
| | | Children:<br>PO: 50–100 mg/kg/day q6h,<br>IM/IV: mild to moderate<br>infections: 50–100<br>mg/kg/day q6h.<br>Severe infection: 100–200<br>mg/kg/day q4–6h<br>Max: 12 g/day | |
| naproxen/naproxen sodium (Naprosyn, Aleve, Anaprox) | Tab (naproxen): 250, 375, 500 mg, Tab (naproxen sodium):<br>Anaprox: 275 mg (250 mg base), 550 mg (500 mg base)<br>Aleve: 220 mg (200 mg base)<br>Susp (naproxen): 125 mg/5 mL | >2 yr old:<br>Analgesic: 5–7 mg/kg/dose PO q8–12h<br>JRA: 10–20 mg/kg/day PO q12h; max: 1,000 mg/day | R<br>Possible GI bleeding, easy bruising, thrombocytopenia |
| neomycin/baci-tracin/polymyxin B (Neosporin) | Ophthalmologic oint: 3.5 mg/400 U/10,000 U/g | Apply small amount to conjunctiva q.d.-q.i.d. | — |
| neomycin/ polymyxin/ hydrocortisone (Cortisporin) | Cream: 5 mg/10,000 U/5 mg/g<br>Oint (also has 400 U of bacitracin): 5 mg/5,000 U/10 mg/g | Apply thin layer to affected area b.i.d.-q.i.d. | — |
| nifedipine (Procardia) | Cap: 10, 20 mg<br>Tab (ER or SR): 30, 60, 90 mg | Hypertension: 0.25–0.5 mg/kg/dose q4–6h prn PO/SL; max: 10 mg/dose or 3 mg/kg/day<br>Hypertrophic cardiomyopathy: 0.5–0.9 mg/kg/day q6–8h PO/SL | — |
| nitrofurantoin (Furadantin) | Caps: 25, 50, 100 mg<br>Susp: 25 mg/5 mL | >1 mo: 5–7 mg/kg/day PO q6h; max: 400 mg/day<br>Upper respiratory tract infection prophylaxis: 1–2 mg/kg/dose PO q.h.s. PO; max: 100 mg/day. | R |
| nitroprusside sodium (Nipride) | | IV, continuous infusion: start at 0.3–0.5 $\mu$g/kg/min, titrate to effect; usual dose is 3–4 $\mu$g/kg/min; max: 10 $\mu$g/kg/min | R<br>Contraindicated in patients with decreased cerebral perfusion<br>Converted to cyanide, which may produce metabolic acidosis and methemoglobinemia |
| nortriptyline (Pamelor) | Cap: 10, 25, 50, 75 mg<br>Sol: 10 mg/5 mL | Depression:<br>Avoid use in pediatric patients<br>6–12 yr old: 1–3 mg/kg/day t.i.d.-q.i.d. PO<br>>12 yr old: 1–3 mg/kg/day t.i.d.-q.i.d. PO; max: 150 mg/day. | Contraindicated in angle-closure glaucoma and with MAOIs. Antidepressants may worsen and |

| Name | Oral or Topical forms | Dosage | Comments |
|------|----------------------|--------|----------|
| | | | increase suicidal ideation in children and young adults |
| nystatin | Tab: 500,000 units<br>Troche: 200,000 units<br>Susp: 100,000 units /mL<br>Cream/oint: 100,000 units/g<br>Topical powder: 100,000 U/g, Vaginal tab: 100,000 units | PO:<br>Preterm infants: 0.5 mL to each side of mouth q.i.d.<br>Term infants: 1 mL to each side of mouth q.i.d.<br>Children: Susp: 4–6 mL swish and swallow q.i.d. or troche: 200,000–400,000 U 4–5 ×/day<br>Vaginal: 1 tab q.h.s. × 14 day<br>Topical: Apply b.i.d.-q.i.d. | — |
| octreotide (Sandostatin) | | IV/SC: 1–10 $\mu$g/kg/day q12–24h; max: 1,500 $\mu$g/day.<br>Continuous infusion: 1 $\mu$g/kg/hr | R |
| olopatadine (Patanol) | Ophthalmologic sol: 0.1% | 1–2 drops in affected eyes b.i.d. | Do not use while wearing contact lenses. |
| omeprazole (Prilosec) | Cap: 10, 20, 40 mg | Start with 0.6–0.7 mg/kg/dose PO q.d.; increase to 0.6–0.7 mg/kg/dose PO b.i.d. | — |
| ondansetron (Zofran) | Tab: 4, 8 mg<br>Tab, orally disintegrating: 4, 8 mg<br>Sol: 4 mg/5 mL | Prevention of nausea/vomiting associated with chemotherapy (give 30 min before) or radiation (give 1–2 hour before)<br>Oral:<br>Based on body surface area:<br><0.3 m$^2$: 1 mg t.i.d.<br>0.3–0.6 m$^2$: 2 mg t.i.d.<br>0.6–1 m$^2$: 3 mg t.i.d.<br>>1 m$^2$: 4 mg t.i.d.<br>Based on age:<br>4–11 yr old: 4 mg t.i.d.<br>>11 yr old: 8 mg t.i.d. or 24 mg q.d.<br>IV:<br>6 mo–18 yr old: 0.15 mg/kg/dose 30 min before, then 4 and 8 hr after chemotherapy, then q4h prn.<br>Prevention of postoperative nausea/vomiting (administered immediately before anesthesia or postoperatively if symptomatic) | Additional postoperative doses for controlling nausea/vomiting may not provide any benefits |

*(continued)*

| Name | Oral or Topical forms | Dosage | Comments |
|------|----------------------|--------|----------|
| | | ≥2 yr, <40 kg: 0.1 mg/kg IV, IM<br>>40 kg: 4 mg IV, IM | |
| oseltamivir (Tamiflu) | Cap: 75 mg<br>Susp: 12 mg/mL | Treatment of influenza (all for 5 day): 1–12 yr old based on weight:<br><15 kg: 30 mg PO b.i.d.<br>15–23 kg: 45 mg PO b.i.d.<br>23–40 kg: 60 mg PO b.i.d.<br>>40 kg: 75 mg PO b.i.d.<br>>12 yr old: 75 mg PO b.i.d. | R<br>Initiate therapy within 2 day of onset of symptoms. |
| oxacillin (Bactocill) | Cap: 250, 500 mg | Neonates: IM, IV:<br>0–4 wk, <1,200 g: 50 mg/kg/day in divided doses q12h<br>≤7 day:<br>1,200–2,000 g: 50 mg/kg/day in divided doses q12h<br>>2,000 g: 75 mg/kg/day in divided doses q8h<br>>7 day<br>1,200–2,000 g: 75 mg/kg/day in divided doses q8h<br>>2,000 g: 100 mg/kg/day in divided doses q6h<br>Children:<br>PO: 50–100 mg/kg/day q6h,<br>IM/IV: mild to moderate infections: 50–100 mg/kg/day q6h.<br>Severe infection: 100–200 mg/kg/day q4–6h<br>Max: 12 g/day | R |
| oxycodone | Tab: 5, 15, 30 mg<br>Cap: 5 mg<br>Sol: 5 mg/5 mL<br>Controlled release tab (OxyContin): 10, 20, 40, 60, 80, 160 mg | Children: 0.05–0.15 mg/kg/dose PO q4–6h prn (up to 5 mg/dose) | Respiratory depression may occur<br>Controlled release product: not intended for prn use; or for mild pain, immediate postoperative pain, or pain that is not expected to persist for an extended period |
| oxycodone/acetaminophen (Percocet, Roxicet) | Tab: 5 mg/325 mg (most common)<br>Other forms: 2.5 mg/325 mg, 7.5 mg/325 or 500 mg, 10 mg/325 or 650 mg<br>Sol (Roxicet): 5 mg/325 mg in 5 mL | Based on amount of oxycodone and acetaminophen | Respiratory depression may occur |
| oxymetazoline (Afrin) | Nasal drops: 0.025%, 0.05%<br>Nasal spray: 0.05% | 2–5 yr old: 2–3 drops of 0.025% solution in each nostril b.i.d.<br>>5 yr old: 2–3 sprays or 2–3 drops of 0.05% solution in each nostril b.i.d. | Do not exceed 3 day of therapy because rebound nasal congestion may occur. |

| Name | Oral or Topical forms | Dosage | Comments |
|---|---|---|---|
| palivizumab (Synagis) | 50 or 100 mg vials | Respiratory syncytial virus (RSV) prophylaxis: 15 mg/kg IM every month during RSV season | — |
| pamidronate (Aredia) | | Hypercalcemia: Mild: 0.5–1 mg/kg/dose IV × 1; may repeat in 7 day. Severe: 1.5–2 mg/kg/dose; may repeat in 7 day | R Maintain adequate hydration and urinary output during treatment. Infuse over 2–24 hr Because of increased risk of nephrotoxicity, doses should not exceed 90 mg. |
| paroxetine (Paxil) | Tab: 10, 20, 30, 40 mg Tab (controlled release): 12.5, 25, 37.5 mg Susp: 10 mg/5 mL | Depression: avoid in pediatric patients; in adults, start with 10 mg PO q.d. and adjust upward as needed q7d after 4 wk of initial therapy to max of 50 mg/day. Obsessive-compulsive disorder: start with 10 mg PO q.d. and adjust upward 10 mg/day q2wk to a max of 60 mg/day. Panic disorder: start with 10 mg PO q.d. and adjust upward by 10 mg/day every week to a max of 60 mg/day. Social/generalized anxiety disorder: 20 mg PO every AM | R Avoid use with MAOIs. Avoid abrupt discontinuation. Antidepressants may worsen depression and increase suicidal ideation in children and young adults. Consider dose adjustment with hepatic impairment. |
| penicillin G (aqueous crystalline) | | Neonates: Meningitis 75,000–100,000 units/kg/dose IV Sepsis: 25,000–50,000 units/kg/dose IV Group B streptococcal infections: Bacteremia: 200,000 units/kg/day Meningitis: 450,000 units/kg/day Intervals: PMA (wk)Age (day) Interval <29 0–28 q12h >28 q8h 30–36 0–14 q12h >14 q8h 37–44 0–7 q12h >7 q8h >45 All q6h | — |
| penicillin G procaine | | Newborns: 50,000 units/ kg/day IM q.d. (congenital syphilis) | Provides sustained levels for 2–4 day |

*(continued)*

| Name | Oral or Topical forms | Dosage | Comments |
|---|---|---|---|
| | | Children: 25,000–50,000 U/kg/day q12–24h IM. Max: 4.8 million U/day. | Do not give IV. |
| penicillin V potassium | Tab: 125, 250, 500 mg Susp: 125, 250 mg/mL | 25–50 mg/kg/day q6–8h PO; max 3 g/day. Acute group A streptococcus: 250 mg PO b.i.d.-t.i.d. × 10 day Rheumatic fever/pneumo-coccal prophylaxis: <5 yr old: 125 mg PO b.i.d.; >5 yr old: 250 mg PO b.i.d. | R |
| pentamidine (Pentam, NebuPent) | | PCP: 4 mg/kg/day IM/IV q.d. × 14–21 day Trypanosomiasis: 4 mg/kg/day IM q.d. × 10 day Visceral leishmaniasis: 2–4 mg/kg/dose IM q24h or q48h for 15 doses Cutaneous leishmaniasis: 2–3 mg/kg/dose IM q24h or q48h × 4–7 doses Prophylaxis (PCP): IM/IV: 4 mg/kg/dose q2–4wk (≥5 yr old: 300 mg nebulized in 6 mL water every month) | R |
| permethrin (Elimite, Nix) | Cream: 5% Rinse: 1% | Head lice: saturate hair and scalp with 1% rinse after shampooing and towel drying hair; leave on 10 min; rinse; may repeat in 7–10 day Scabies: apply 5% cream from neck to toes; wash off with water in 8–14 hr; may repeat in 7 day | — |
| phenobarbital (Luminal) | Tab: 15, 30, 60, 100 mg Elixir: 20 mg/5 mL | Status epilepticus: see algorithm in Appendix G; 10–20 mg/kg IV Maintenance: Infants: 5–6 mg/kg/day PO q.d.-b.i.d. 1–5 yr old: 6–8 mg/kg/day PO q.d.-b.i.d. 5–12 yr old: 4–6 mg/kg/day PO q.d.-b.i.d. >12 yr old: 1–3 mg/kg/day PO q.d.-b.i.d. | R Contraindicated in porphyria, severe respiratory disease May cause respiratory depression or hypotension. Many drug interactions Therapeutic levels: 15–40 mg/L. Consider dosage adjustment with hepatic impair-ment |
| phenylephrine (Neo-Synephrine) | Nasal drops: 0.125, 0.16, 0.25, 0.5% Nasal spray: 0.25, 0.5, 1% | >6 mo: 1–2 drops of 0.16% solution q3h prn <6 yr old: 2–3 drops of 0.125% solution q4h prn | Do not exceed 3 day of therapy because rebound nasal |

| Name | Oral or Topical forms | Dosage | Comments |
|---|---|---|---|
| | | 6–12 yr old: 2–3 drops of 0.125% or 1–2 sprays of 0.25% solution q4h prn<br>>12 yr old: 2–3 drops or 1–2 sprays of 0.25% or 0.5% solution q4h prn | congestion may occur. |
| phenytoin (Dilantin) | Chewable tab: 50 mg<br>Prompt cap: 100 mg<br>Cap (ER): 30, 100 mg<br>Susp: 125 mg/5 mL | Status epilepticus: see algorithm in Appendix G; 10–20 mg/kg IV<br>Epilepsy: start with 5 mg/kg/day PO/IV q8–12h; usual dose range:<br>neonates: 5–8 mg/kg/day<br>6 mo–3 yr old: 8–10 mg/kg/day<br>4–6 yr old: 7.5–9 mg/kg/day<br>7–9 yr old: 7–8 mg/kg/day<br>>9 yr old: 6–7 mg/kg/day | R<br>Contraindicated in heart block or sinus bradycardia.<br>May cause gingival hyperplasia, hirsutism, dermatitis, ataxia, lupus-like syndrome, liver damage.<br>Many drug interactions<br>Therapeutic levels: 10–20 mg/L<br>Consider dose adjustment with hepatic impairment. |
| phytonadione (vitamin K) | Tab: 5 mg<br>Susp: 1 mg/mL | Neonatal hemorrhagic disease: Prophylaxis: 0.5–1 mg IM × 1, Treatment: 1–2 mg/day IM/SC<br>Vitamin K deficiency: PO: 2.5–5 mg/day IM/SC: 1–2 mg/dose × 1<br>Adults: PO 2.5–25 mg/24 hr SQ, IM, IV 10 mg | Monitor prothrombin/partial thromboplastin time.<br>SC route is preferred; IM/IV should be restricted to situations when SC route is not feasible.<br>IV dosing may cause flushing, dizziness, hypotension, cardiac arrest |
| pimecrolimus (Elidel) | Cream: 1% | Apply a thin layer to affected areas b.i.d. | May use on face. Do not place over areas of infected skin. |
| piperacillin (Pipracil) | | Neonates: IM, IV<br>≤7 day: 150 mg/kg/day q8h<br>>7 day: 200 mg/kg/day q6h<br>Infants and children: 200–300 mg/kg/day IM/IV q4–6h; max: 24 g/day<br>Cystic fibrosis: 350–600 mg/kg/day IM/IV q4–6h; max: 24 g/day | R |
| piperacillin/tazobactam (Zosyn) | | Dosages based on piperacillin component. | R |

*(continued)*

| Name | Oral or Topical forms | Dosage | Comments |
|---|---|---|---|
| | | <6 mo: 150–300 mg/kg/day IV q6–8h >6 mo: 200–400 mg/kg/day IV q6–8h. Cystic fibrosis dosing same as piperacillin | |
| podofilox (Condylox) | Sol: 0.5% Gel: 0.5% | Apply b.i.d. for 3 day, then wait 4 day; continue to reapply for 3 day, wait for 4 day, for a maximum of 4 one-week cycles | — |
| polyethylene glycol (GoLYTELY, MiraLAX) | Powder for PO solution | Bowel cleansing (GoLYTELY): 25–40 mL/kg/hr PO until rectal effluent is tan/clear. Constipation (MiraLAX): 8.5–17 g PO q.d. | Bowel cleansing contraindicated in toxic megacolon, gastric retention, colitis, bowel perforation Use with caution in patients with altered mental status or impaired gag |
| prednisolone (Pediapred, Prelone, Orapred) | Tab: 5 mg Syrup: 15 mg/5 mL (Prelone, Orapred), 5 mg/5 mL (Pediapred) | Anti-inflammatory/ immunosuppressive: 0.5–2 mg/kg/day PO q.d.-b.i.d. Acute asthma: 2 mg/kg/day PO q.d.-b.i.d.; max: 80 mg/day Nephrotic syndrome: start at 2 mg/kg/day PO q.d.-b.i.d.; max: 80 mg/day | Contraindicated in active, untreated infections May cause hyperglycemia, mood changes, osteopenia Taper if given for more than 7 day |
| prednisone | Tab: 1, 2.5, 5, 10, 20, 50 mg Syrup: 5 mg/mL | Anti-inflammatory/ immunosuppressive: 0.5–2 mg/kg/day PO q.d.-b.i.d. Acute asthma: 2 mg/kg/day PO q.d.-b.i.d. Nephrotic syndrome: start at 2 mg/kg/day PO q.d.-t.i.d. Max: 80 mg/day | Contraindicated in active, untreated infections May cause hyperglycemia, mood changes, osteopenia Taper if given for more than 7 day |
| promethazine (Phenergan) | Tab: 12.5, 25, 50 mg Syrup: 6.25 mg/5 mL Supp: 12.5, 25, 50 mg | >2 yr old: 0.1 mg/kg/dose PO q6h and 0.5 mg/kg/ dose q.h.s. PO prn | Use with extreme caution in children and avoid use in children <2 yr old due to potential for severe and potentially fatal respiratory depression |
| propranolol (Inderal) | Cap, ER: 60, 80, 120, 160 mg Sol: 20, 40 mg/5 mL Tab: 10, 20, 40, 60, 80 mg | Neonates: PO: Initial dose 0.25 mg/kg/dose q6–8h; | R Contraindicated in asthma, heart |

| Name | Oral or Topical forms | Dosage | Comments |
|------|----------------------|--------|----------|
| | | increase slowly as needed to maximum of 5 mg/kg/day<br>IV: Initial: 0.01 mg/kg slow IV push over 10 minutes; may repeat q6–8h as needed; increase slowly to maximum of 0.15 mg/kg/dose q6–8h.<br>Arrhythmias (infants and children)<br>PO: Initial: 0.5–1 mg/kg/day in divided doses q6–8h; titrate dosage upward q3–5d; usual dose: 2–4 mg/kg/day; higher doses may be needed; do not exceed 16 mg/kg/day or 60 mg/day<br>IV: 0.01–0.1 mg/kg slow IV over 10 minutes; max: 1 mg (infants); 3 mg (children)<br>Hypertension (children): PO: initial: 0.5–1 mg/kg/day q6–12h; increase q3–5d prn to max of 8 mg/kg/day.<br>Migraine prophylaxis: <35 kg: 10–20 mg PO t.i.d., >35 kg: 20–40 mg PO t.i.d.<br>Tetralogy spells (infants and children):<br>PO; usual 1–2 mg/kg/dose q6h; may initiate at half the usual dose; may increase by 1 mg/kg/day q24h to max of 5 mg/kg/day<br>IV: 0.15–0.25 mg/kg/dose slow IV. May repeat in 15 min × 1.<br>Thyrotoxicosis:<br>Neonates: PO: 2 mg/kg/day in divided doses q6–12h; occasionally higher doses may be required<br>Adolescents and adults: 10–40 mg/dose PO q6h. | failure, and heart block |
| propylthiouracil (PTU) | Tab: 50 mg<br>Susp: 5 mg/mL | Neonates: 5–10 mg/kg/day in divided doses q8h<br>Children: initial: 5–7 mg/kg/day PO q8h, then maintenance after 2 mo. ⅓ to ⅔ of initial dose; max: 300 mg/day | R |
| protamine | | IV: 1 mg protamine neutralizes 115 units porcine intestinal heparin or | — |

*(continued)*

| Name | Oral or Topical forms | Dosage | Comments |
|---|---|---|---|
| | | 90 units of beef lung heparin or 100 mg SC low-molecular-weight heparin Max: 50 mg | |
| pyrantel (Pin-X) | Susp: 50 mg/mL Liquid: 50, 144 mg/mL Cap: 180 mg | Roundworm: 11 mg/kg/dose PO × 1 Pinworm: 11 mg/kg/dose PO × 1 dose, repeat 2 wk later Hookworm: 11 mg/kg/dose PO q.d. × 3 day; max: 1 g/dose | — |
| pyridostigmine (Mestinon) | Syrup: 60 mg/5 mL Tab: 60 mg Tab (SR): 180 mg | Myasthenia gravis: Neonates: PO: 5 mg q4–6h Children: PO: 7 mg/kg/day in 5–6 divided doses. Neonates and children IM/IV: 0.05–0.15 mg/kg/dose q4–6h; max IM/IV dose: 10 mg/dose | R Contraindicated in mechanical intestinal or urinary obstruction |
| ranitidine (Zantac) | Tab: 75, 150, 300 mg Effervescent tab: 150 mg Liquid: 15 mg/mL (syrup and solution) Cap: 150, 300 mg Sol: 5, 10 mg/mL | Ulcer: PO, treatment: 2–4 mg/kg/day q12h; max. 300 mg/day; maintenance: 2–4 mg/day q12h; max: 150 mg/day IV: 2–4 mg/kg/day q6–8h; max: 150 mg/day. Gastroesophageal reflux disease/erosive esophagitis: PO: 5–10 mg/kg/day q12h; max: 300 mg/day. IV: 2–4 mg/kg/day q6–8h; max: 150 mg/day. | R |
| rifampin (Rimactane, Rifadin) | Cap: 150, 300 mg Susp: 10, 15 mg/mL | TB: twice weekly therapy may be used after 1–2 mo of daily therapy; 10–20 mg/kg/day IV/PO q12–24 h then 10–20 mg/kg/day PO twice weekly; max: 600 mg/day *Neisseria meningitidis* prophylaxis: 0–1 mo: 10 mg/kg/day PO q12h × 2 day >1 mo: 20 mg/kg/day PO q12h × 2; max: 600 mg/day Synergy for *Staphylococcus aureus*: neonates: 5–20 mg/kg/day IV, PO q12h | R Causes orange discoloration of bodily fluids Many drug interactions Give 1 hr before or 2 hr after meals |
| rimantadine (Flumadine) | Tab: 100 mg Syrup: 50 mg/5 mL | Influenza A prophylaxis: <10 yr old: 5 mg/kg/day PO q.d.; max: 150 mg/day. >10 yr old: 100 mg PO b.i.d. | R Initiate therapy within 2 day of onset of symptoms. |

| Name | Oral or Topical forms | Dosage | Comments |
|---|---|---|---|
| | | Treatment: <10 yr old or <40 kg: 5 mg/kg/day PO q.d.-b.i.d. × 5–7 day; max: 150 mg/day >10 yr old and >40 kg: 100 mg PO b.i.d. × 5–7 day | |
| salmeterol (Serevent) | MDI: 25 $\mu$g/actuation DPI: 50 $\mu$g/dose | >4 yr old: 42 $\mu$g b.i.d. DPI or 50 $\mu$g b.i.d. MDI | — |
| selenium sulfate (Selsun) | Shampoo: 1%, 2.5% | Dandruff: massage 5–10 mL into wet scalp, leave on 5–10 min then rinse off. Tinea versicolor: 2.5% lotion in a thin layer covering body from face to knees, leave on 30 min then rinse. Apply daily for 7 day then every month for 3 months. | — |
| senna (Senokot) | Granules: 326 mg/5 mL Rectal: 652 mg Syrup: 218 mg/5 mL Tab: 187, 217, 374, 600 mg Liquid: 33.3 mg/mL | PO: 10–20 mg/kg/dose PO q.h.s. with max by age: 1 mo–1 yr old: 218 mg/day; 1–5 yr old: 436 mg/day; 5–15 yr old: 872 mg/day. PR: >27 kg: 326 mg q.h.s. | — |
| sertraline (Zoloft) | Tab: 25, 50, 100 mg Sol: 20 mg/mL | Depression or obsessive-compulsive disorder: 6–12 yr old: not approved by Food and Drug Administration; start with 12.5 mg PO q.d. and increase by 25 mg q3–4d up to a max of 200 mg/day >12 yr old: Start at 50 mg PO q.d. and increase by 50 mg every week to max of 200 mg/day. | Avoid use with MAOIs. Antidepressants may worsen depression and increase suicidal ideation in children and young adults. Consider dose adjustment with hepatic impairment. Avoid abrupt discontinuation. |
| silver sulfadiazine (Silvadene) | Cream: 1% | Apply q.d.-b.i.d. to thickness of ¹⁄₁₆ inch | Contraindicated in infants <2 mo old May cause bone marrow suppression, interstitial nephritis |
| sirolimus (Rapamune) | Tab: 1, 2 mg Sol: 1 mg/mL | Children ≥13 yr old and <40 kg: 3 mg/m$^2$ PO × 1 immediately after transplant; maintenance dose: 1 mg/m$^2$/day q12h or q.d. | Tablets and oral solution are not bioequivalent because of differences in absorption; |

*(continued)*

| Name | Oral or Topical forms | Dosage | Comments |
|------|----------------------|--------|----------|
| | | Intestinal transplant (adults): 2–3 mg/m$^2$; maintenance dose 1 mg/m$^2$ q.d. to achieve troughs 8–10 ng/mL | however, clinical equivalence has been demonstrated at the 2-mg dose level. Target serum trough concentration: 6–15 ng/mL |
| sodium phosphate (Fleet enema) | Enema: 6 g Na phosphate and 16 g Na biphosphate/ 100 mL, Pediatric size: 67.5 mL, adult: 133 mL | 2–12 yr old: 67.5 mL PR × 1 >12 yr old: 133 mL PR × 1 | R Contraindicated in patients with severe renal failure, megacolon, bowel obstruction, congestive heart failure May cause hyperphosphatemia, hypernatremia, hypocalcemia, hypotension, dehydration, acidosis |
| spironolactone (Aldactone) | Tab: 25, 50, 100 mg Susp: 1, 2, 5, 25 mg/mL | Diuretic: Neonates: PO: 1–3 mg/kg/day q12–24h Children: 1–3.3 mg/kg/day PO q.d.-q.i.d. Max: 200 mg/day Primary aldosteronism: 125–375 mg/m$^2$/day PO hr b.i.d.-q.i.d.; max: 400 mg q.d. | R Contraindicated in acute renal failure Possible hyperkalemia |
| sulfasalazine (Azulfidine, Azulfidine EN-tabs, Salazopyrin EN-tabs) | Tab: 500 mg | JRA: >6 yr old: start with 10 mg/kg/day b.i.d. PO and increase by 10 mg/kg/day q7d until maintenance of 30–50 mg/kg/day b.i.d.; max: 2 g/day. | R Contraindicated in sulfa allergy, porphyria, GI obstruction May cause orange-yellow discoloration of skin and mucous membranes |
| sulfasalazine (Azulfidine, Azulfidine EN-tabs, Salazopyrin EN-tabs) | Tab: 500 mg | Ulcerative colitis (>6 yr old); initial dosing: Moderate to severe: 50–75 mg/kg/day q4–6h PO; max: 6 g/day Mild: 40–50 mg/kg/day PO q6 Maintenance: 30–50 mg/kg/day PO q4–8h PO; max: 2 g/day | R Contraindicated in sulfa allergy, porphyria, GI obstruction May cause orange-yellow discoloration of skin and mucous membranes |

| Name | Oral or Topical forms | Dosage | Comments |
|---|---|---|---|
| sumatriptan (Imitrex) | Tab: 25, 50, 100 mg<br>Susp: 5 mg/mL<br>Nasal spray: 5 mg, 20 mg/ 100 microliters<br>Unit use syringe: 8 mg/mL, 12 mg/mL syringe (0.5 mL) | PO: 25 mg with onset of headache; may give 25–100 mg more if no relief after 2 hr up to a max of 200 mg/day<br>SC: 6 mg × 1 with onset of headache; may give additional dose if no relief up to max of 12 mg/day<br>Nasal: 5–20 mg/dose with onset of headache; may give up to 40 mg/day if no response in 2 hr; may repeat dose up to max of 40 mg/day. | R<br>Contraindicated with ergotamines, ischemic heart disease, or peripheral vascular syndromes<br>Flushing and dizziness may occur |
| tacrolimus (Protopic) | Oint: 0.03%, 0.1% | >2 yr old: Apply 0.03% oint to affected areas b.i.d. Continue for 1 wk after resolution of symptoms. | — |
| tazarotene (Tazorac) | Gel: 0.05%, 0.1% | Apply to affected area every PM. | — |
| terbutaline (Brethine, Bricanyl) | | Continuous infusion: 2–10 $\mu$g/kg IV loading dose followed by 0.1–0.4 $\mu$g/kg/min; titrate in increments of 0.1–0.2 $\mu$g/kg/min every 30 min; max: 10 $\mu$g/kg/min | — |
| testosterone | | IM (cypionate or enanthate ester): Initiation of pubertal growth: 40–50 mg/m$^2$/dose monthly until growth rate falls to prepubertal levels. Terminal growth phase: 100 mg/m$^2$/dose monthly until growth ceases<br>Maintenance virilizing dose: 100 mg/m$^2$/dose twice monthly<br>Delayed puberty: 40–50 mg/m$^2$/dose monthly for 6 mo | Contraindicated in severe renal, cardiac, or hepatic disease |
| tetracycline (e.g., Achromycin, Sumycin) | Tab: 250, 500 mg<br>Cap: 250, 500 mg<br>Susp: 125 mg/5 mL | >8 yr old: 25–50 mg/kg/day PO q6h; max: 3 g/day. | R<br>Use with caution in children <8 yr old because of tooth enamel hypoplasia and discoloration. |
| ticarcillin/ clavulanate (Timentin) | | Neonates: 75–100 mg/kg/dose IV to max of 300 mg/kg/day; for intervals, see the following: | R |

*(continued)*

| Name | Oral or Topical forms | Dosage | Comments |
|------|----------------------|--------|----------|
| | | PMA (wk) Age (day) Interval<br><29    0–28   q12h<br>           >28   q8h<br>30–36  0–14   q12h<br>           >14   q8h<br>37–44  0–7    q12h<br>           >7    q8h<br>>45    All    q6h<br>Children: 200–300 mg/kg/day IM/IV q4–6h; max: 24 g/day.<br>Cystic fibrosis: 300–600 mg/kg/day IM/IV; max: 24 g/day. | |
| tobramycin (Nebcin, TOBI) | | Neonates:<br>PMA (wk) Age (day) Dose<br>≤28 0–30 3 mg/kg q24h<br>     >30 5 mg/kg q24h<br>29– 0–21 3 mg/kg q24h<br>32  21–45 5 mg/kg q24h<br>   45–60 4 mg/kg q12h<br>     >60 4 mg/kg q12h[1]<br>     or 2.5 mg/kg  q8h[2]<br>33– 0–14 3 mg/kg q24h<br>34  14–45 5 mg/kg q24h<br>     >45 4 mg/kg q12h[1]<br>     or 2.5 mg/kg  q8h[2]<br>≥35 0–30 5 mg/kg q24h<br>     >30 4 mg/kg q12h[1]<br>     or 2.5 mg/kg  q8h[2]<br>Monitoring peak 6–15 μg/mL, trough ≤1.5 μg/mL, (2.5 mg/kg/dose: peak 6–10, trough <2), Check levels with 4th dose when evaluating a patient for sepsis, and 3rd when treating a known infection.<br>[1]Preferred for all patients, including those with renal and cardiac dysfunction<br>[2]If using 2.5 mg/kg/dose in renal or cardiac dysfunction, use q12–24h<br>1 mo–18 yr old: 2.5 mg/kg/dose IV q8 up to a max of 150 mg IV q8 | R<br>Everyday dosing not appropriate in weight >20% ideal body weight, ascites, >20% burns, altered renal function, endocarditis, tularemia, meningitis, osteomyelitis, or hemodynamic instability. Dosing may need to be adjusted in patients with cystic fibrosis. Check peak and trough. |
| tobramycin (Tobrex) | Ophthalmologic oint: 0.3%<br>Ophthalmologic sol: 0.3% | Apply thin ribbon of ointment to affected eye b.i.d.-t.i.d. or 1–2 drops of solution to affected eye q4h | — |
| tretinoin (Retin-A) | Cream: 0.025%, 0.05%, 0.1%<br>Gel: 0.01%, 0.025%, 0.1%<br>Liquid: 0.05% | Apply to affected area q.h.s. | Avoid excessive sun exposure while using |

| Name | Oral or Topical forms | Dosage | Comments |
|---|---|---|---|
| trimethoprim/ sulfamethox-azole; TMP (Bactrim) | Tab: Double-strength: 160–800 mg Single-strength: 80–400 mg Susp: 40–200 mg/5 mL | Doses based on TMP component: Minor infections: 8–10 mg/kg/day PO/IV b.i.d.; max: 320 mg/day Urinary tract infection prophylaxis: 2–4 mg/kg/day PO q.d. PCP treatment: 20 mg/kg/day PO/IV q6–8h PCP prophylaxis: 5–10 mg/kg/day PO/IV b.i.d. or 150 mg/m²/day b.i.d. × 3 consecutive day/wk | R May cause kernicterus in newborns. |
| ursodiol (Actigall) | Susp: 60 mg/mL Cap: 300 mg Tab: 250 mg | 10–15 mg/kg PO q.d. Max: 30 mg/kg/day t.i.d. | Contraindicated in renal stones |
| valproic acid (Depakene, Depakote) | Cap: 250 mg Sprinkles: 125 mg Syrup: 250 mg/5 mL Tab delayed release: 125, 250, 500 Tab (ER): 250, 500 | Seizures: PO: Initial: 10–15 mg/kg/day q.d.-t.i.d.; increase 5–10 mg/kg/day weekly to max of 60 mg/kg/day Maintenance: 30–60 mg/kg/day b.i.d.-t.i.d. IV: same dose as PO but q6h. Migraine prophylaxis: 15–30 mg/kg/day PO b.i.d.; max: 1,000 mg/day. Status migrainosus: 15 mg/kg IV loading dose, max 1,000 mg, then 5–8 mg/kg/dose IV q8h max 750 mg | Contraindicated in hepatic disease May cause hepatic dysfunction, pan-creatitis, throm-bocytopenia, rash, platelet dysfunction, and hyperammone-mia Many drug interactions Therapeutic levels: 50–100 mg/L R Consider dose adjustment with hepatic impairment. |
| vancomycin (Vancocin) | Cap; 125, 250 g | Neonate: 15 mg/kg/dose PMA (wk) Age (day) Interval ≤29      0–14      q18h           >14       q12h 30–36   0–14      q12h           >14       q8h 37–44   0–7       q12h           >7        q8h >45 day  All       q8h Monitoring: trough 5–15 μg/mL, check with 4th dose (peak only necessary for meningitis, goal 30–40 μg/mL with trough:10–15 μg/mL) Children: central nervous system infection: 60 mg/kg/day IV q6h, other infections: 40 mg/kg/day IV q6–8h; max: 1 g/dose *Clostridium difficile* colitis: 40–50 mg/kg/day PO q6h; max: 500 mg/day | R Associated with "red man syndrome" Treat with diphen-hydramine and slower vancomycin infusion. Monitor drug levels. Infuse over 60 minutes; slow to 2 hr in "red man syndrome." |

*(continued)*

| Name | Oral or Topical forms | Dosage | Comments |
|------|----------------------|--------|----------|
| vasopressin (Pitressin) | | Diabetes insipidus:<br>Titrate dose to effect:<br>SC/IM: 2.5–10 units b.i.d.-q.i.d.<br>Continuous infusion: start at 0.5 milliunit/kg/hr, double dose every 30 min up to max of 10 milliunit/kg/hr<br>GI hemorrhage: start at 0.002–0.005 units/kg/min IV and titrate to max of 0.01 units/kg/min | Use with caution in vascular disease.<br>Do not abruptly stop infusion. |
| voriconazole (Vfend) | Tab: 50, 200 mg | IV:<br>2–11 yr old: 6 mg/kg q12h for 2 doses, then 4 mg/kg b.i.d.<br>≥12 yr old – adult: 6 mg/kg q12h for 2 doses, then 4 mg/kg b.i.d.<br>(candidemia: 3 mg/kg b.i.d.)<br>PO:<br>>12 yr old and ≥40 kg: 200 mg b.i.d.<br>>12 yr old and <40 kg: 100 mg b.i.d.<br>Limited info on oral use in children: may use 3–5 mg/kg/dose q12h in patients <25 kg | R for IV form only<br>Concurrent use of cyclosporine or tacrolimus results in increased concentrations of cyclosporine/tacrolimus; empirically decrease dose of cyclosporine/tacrolimus dose by 50% when initiating voriconazole<br>Coadministration with sirolimus is contraindicated. |
| warfarin (Coumadin) | Tab: 1, 2, 2.5, 3, 4, 5, 6, 7.5, 10 mg | Loading dose: baseline INR: 1–1.3: 0.1–0.2 mg/kg/dose PO q.d. × 2 day; max: 10 mg/dose<br>Maintenance: 0.05–0.34 mg/kg/day PO q.d.<br>Adjust to desired prothrombin time or INR. | R<br>Contraindicated in severe liver or kidney disease, uncontrolled bleeding, gastrointestinal ulcers, or malignant hypertension<br>Many drug interactions<br>Monitor INR 5–7 day after new dosage before readjustment. |

## Suggested Readings

Briggs GG, Freeman RK, Yaffe SJ, eds. Drugs in Pregnancy and Lactation, 8th Ed. Baltimore: Lippincott Williams & Wilkins, 2008.

Pickering LK, ed. Red Book: Report of the Committee on Infectious Diseases. 27th Ed. Elk Grove Village, Ill: American Academy of Pediatrics; 2006.

Taketomo CK, Hodding JH, Kraus DM, eds. Lexi Comp's Pediatric Dosage Handbook. 14th Ed. Hudson, Ohio: Lexi-Comp Inc, 2007–2008.

Young T, Mangum B. Neofax. 20th Ed. Montvale, NJ: Thomson Healthcare, 2007.

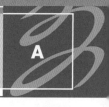

# CHILD AND ADOLESCENT IMMUNIZATION GUIDELINES, 2008

**A**

*For those who fall behind or start late, see the catch-up schedule*

| Vaccine ▼   Age ▶ | Birth | 1 month | 2 months | 4 months | 6 months | 12 months | 15 months | 18 months | 19–23 months | 2–3 years | 4–6 years |
|---|---|---|---|---|---|---|---|---|---|---|---|
| Hepatitis B[1] | HepB | HepB | *see footnote 1* | | HepB | | | | | | |
| Rotavirus[2] | | | Rota | Rota | Rota | | | | | | |
| Diphtheria, Tetanus, Pertussis[3] | | | DTaP | DTaP | DTaP | *see footnote 3* | DTaP | | | | DTaP |
| *Haemophilus influenzae* type b[4] | | | Hib | Hib | Hib[4] | Hib | | | | | |
| Pneumococcal[5] | | | PCV | PCV | PCV | PCV | | | | PPV | |
| Inactivated Poliovirus | | | IPV | IPV | | IPV | | | | | IPV |
| Influenza[6] | | | | | | Influenza (Yearly) | | | | | |
| Measles, Mumps, Rubella[7] | | | | | | MMR | | | | | MMR |
| Varicella[8] | | | | | | Varicella | | | | | Varicella |
| Hepatitis A[9] | | | | | | HepA (2 doses) | | | | HepA Series | |
| Meningococcal[10] | | | | | | | | | | MCV4 | |

Range of recommended ages

Certain high-risk groups

This schedule indicates the recommended ages for routine administration of currently licensed childhood vaccines, as of December 1, 2007, for children aged 0 through 6 years. Additional information is available at www.cdc.gov/vaccines/recs/schedules. Any dose not administered at the recommended age should be administered at any subsequent visit, when indicated and feasible. Additional vaccines may be licensed and recommended during the year. Licensed combination vaccines may be used whenever any components of the combination are indicated and other components of the vaccine are not contraindicated and if approved by the Food and Drug Administration for that dose of the series. Providers should consult the respective Advisory Committee on Immunization Practices statement for detailed recommendations, including for **high-risk conditions:** http://www.cdc.gov/vaccines/pubs/ACIP-list.htm. Clinically significant adverse events that follow immunization should be reported to the Vaccine Adverse Event Reporting System (VAERS). Guidance about how to obtain and complete a VAERS form is available at **www.vaers.hhs.gov** or by telephone, **800-822-7967.**

**1. Hepatitis B vaccine (HepB).** *(Minimum age: birth)*
**At birth:**
- Administer monovalent HepB to all newborns prior to hospital discharge.
- If mother is hepatitis B surface antigen (HBsAg) positive, administer HepB and 0.5 mL of hepatitis B immune globulin (HBIG) within 12 hours of birth.
- If mother's HBsAg status is unknown, administer HepB within 12 hours of birth. Determine the HBsAg status as soon as possible and if HBsAg positive, administer HBIG (no later than age 1 week).
- If mother is HBsAg negative, the birth dose can be delayed, in rare cases, with a provider's order and a copy of the mother's negative HBsAg laboratory report in the infant's medical record.

**After the birth dose:**
- The HepB series should be completed with either monovalent HepB or a combination vaccine containing HepB. The second dose should be administered at age 1–2 months. The final dose should be administered no earlier than age 24 weeks. Infants born to HBsAg-positive mothers should be tested for HBsAg and antibody to HBsAg after completion of at least 3 doses of a licensed HepB series, at age 9–18 months (generally at the next well-child visit).

**4-month dose:**
- It is permissible to administer 4 doses of HepB when combination vaccines are administered after the birth dose. If monovalent HepB is used for doses after the birth dose, a dose at age 4 months is not needed.

**2. Rotavirus vaccine (Rota).** *(Minimum age: 6 weeks)*
- Administer the first dose at age 6–12 weeks.
- Do not start the series later than age 12 weeks.
- Administer the final dose in the series by age 32 weeks. Do not administer any dose later than age 32 weeks.
- Data on safety and efficacy outside of these age ranges are insufficient.

**3. Diphtheria and tetanus toxoids and acellular pertussis vaccine (DTaP).** *(Minimum age: 6 weeks)*
- The fourth dose of DTaP may be administered as early as age 12 months, provided 6 months have elapsed since the third dose.
- Administer the final dose in the series at age 4–6 years.

**4. Haemophilus influenzae type b conjugate vaccine (Hib).** *(Minimum age: 6 weeks)*
- If PRP-OMP (PedvaxHIB® or ComVax® [Merck]) is administered at ages 2 and 4 months, a dose at age 6 months is not required.
- TriHIBit® (DTaP/Hib) combination products should not be used for primary immunization but can be used as boosters following any Hib vaccine in children age 12 months or older.

**5. Pneumococcal vaccine.** *(Minimum age: 6 weeks for pneumococcal conjugate vaccine [PCV]; 2 years for pneumococcal polysaccharide vaccine [PPV])*
- Administer one dose of PCV to all healthy children 24–59 months having any incomplete schedule.
- Administer PPV to children aged 2 years and older with underlying medical conditions.

**6. Influenza vaccine.** *(Minimum age: 6 months for trivalent inactivated influenza vaccine [TIV]; 2 years for live, attenuated influenza vaccine [LAIV])*
- Administer annually to children aged 6–59 months and to all eligible close contacts of children aged 0–59 months.
- Administer annually to children 5 years of age and older with certain risk factors, to other persons (including household members) in close contact with persons in groups at higher risk, and to any child whose parents request vaccination.
- For healthy persons (those who do not have underlying medical conditions that predispose them to influenza complications) ages 2–49 years, either LAIV or TIV may be used.
- Children receiving TIV should receive 0.25 mL if age 6–35 months or 0.5 mL if age 3 years or older.
- Administer 2 doses (separated by 4 weeks or longer) to children younger than 9 years who are receiving influenza vaccine for the first time or who were not vaccinated for the first time last season but only received one dose.

**7. Measles, mumps, and rubella vaccine (MMR).** *(Minimum age: 12 months)*
- Administer the second dose of MMR at age 4–6 years. MMR may be administered before age 4–6 years, provided 4 weeks or more have elapsed since the first dose.

**8. Varicella vaccine.** *(Minimum age: 12 months)*
- Administer second dose at age 4–6 years; may be administered 3 months or more after first dose.
- Do not repeat second dose if administered 28 days or more after first dose.

**9. Hepatitis A vaccine (HepA).** *(Minimum age: 12 months)*
- Administer to all children aged 1 year (i.e., aged 12–23 months). Administer the 2 doses in the series at least 6 months apart.
- Children not fully vaccinated by age 2 years can be vaccinated at subsequent visits.
- HepA is recommended for certain other groups of children, including in areas where vaccination programs target older children.

**10. Meningococcal vaccine.** *(Minimum age: 2 years for meningococcal conjugate vaccine (MCV4) and for meningococcal polysaccharide vaccine (MPSV4))*
- Administer MCV4 to children aged 2–10 years with terminal complement deficiencies or anatomic or functional asplenia and certain other high-risk groups. MPSV4 is also acceptable.
- Administer MCV4 to persons who received MPSV4 3 or more years previously and remain at increased risk for meningococcal disease.

The Recommended Immunization Schedules for Persons Aged 0–18 Years are approved by the Advisory Committee on Immunization Practices (www.cdc.gov/vaccines/recs/acip), the American Academy of Pediatrics (http://www.aap.org), and the American Academy of Family Physicians (http://www.aafp.org).

CS103164

**Figure A-1.** Recommended immunization schedule for persons aged 0–6 years. Source: Centers for Disease Control and Prevention, Morbidity & Mortality Weekly Report (MMWR); Jan. 11, 2008. The most current immunization guidelines can be fount at http://www.cdc.gov/vaccines/recs/schedules/child-schedule.htm

*For those who fall behind or start late, see the green bars and the catch-up schedule*

| Vaccine ▼        Age ▶ | 7–10 years | 11–12 years | 13–18 years |
|---|---|---|---|
| Diphtheria, Tetanus, Pertussis[1] | *see footnote 1* | Tdap | Tdap |
| Human Papillomavirus[2] | *see footnote 2* | HPV (3 doses) | HPV Series |
| Meningococcal[3] | MCV4 | MCV4 | MCV4 |
| Pneumococcal[4] | PPV | | |
| Influenza[5] | Influenza (Yearly) | | |
| Hepatitis A[6] | HepA Series | | |
| Hepatitis B[7] | HepB Series | | |
| Inactivated Poliovirus[8] | IPV Series | | |
| Measles, Mumps, Rubella[9] | MMR Series | | |
| Varicella[10] | Varicella Series | | |

Range of recommended ages

Catch-up immunization

Certain high-risk groups

This schedule indicates the recommended ages for routine administration of currently licensed childhood vaccines, as of December 1, 2007, for children aged 7–18 years. Additional information is available at www.cdc.gov/vaccines/recs/schedules. Any dose not administered at the recommended age should be administered at any subsequent visit, when indicated and feasible. Additional vaccines may be licensed and recommended during the year. Licensed combination vaccines may be used whenever any components of the combination are indicated and other components of the vaccine are not contraindicated and if approved by the Food and Drug Administration for that dose of the series. Providers should consult the respective Advisory Committee on Immunization Practices statement for detailed recommendations, including for **high risk conditions: http://www.cdc.gov/vaccines/pubs/ACIP-list.htm.** Clinically significant adverse events that follow immunization should be reported to the Vaccine Adverse Event Reporting System (VAERS). Guidance about how to obtain and complete a VAERS form is available at www.vaers.hhs.gov or by telephone, **800-822-7967.**

**1. Tetanus and diphtheria toxoids and acellular pertussis vaccine (Tdap).** *(Minimum age: 10 years for BOOSTRIX® and 11 years for ADACEL™)*
- Administer at age 11–12 years for those who have completed the recommended childhood DTP/DTaP vaccination series and have not received a tetanus and diphtheria toxoids (Td) booster dose.
- 13–18-year-olds who missed the 11–12 year Tdap or received Td only are encouraged to receive one dose of Tdap 5 years after the last Td/DTaP dose.

**2. Human papillomavirus vaccine (HPV).** *(Minimum age: 9 years)*
- Administer the first dose of the HPV vaccine series to females at age 11–12 years.
- Administer the second dose 2 months after the first dose and the third dose 6 months after the first dose.
- Administer the HPV vaccine series to females at age 13–18 years if not previously vaccinated.

**3. Meningococcal vaccine.**
- Administer MCV4 at age 11–12 years and at age 13–18 years if not previously vaccinated. MPSV4 is an acceptable alternative.
- Administer MCV4 to previously unvaccinated college freshmen living in dormitories.
- MCV4 is recommended for children aged 2–10 years with terminal complement deficiencies or anatomic or functional asplenia and certain other high-risk groups.
- Persons who received MPSV4 3 or more years previously and remain at increased risk for meningococcal disease should be vaccinated with MCV4.

**4. Pneumococcal polysaccharide vaccine (PPV).**
- Administer PPV to certain high-risk groups.

**5. Influenza vaccine.**
- Administer annually to all close contacts of children aged 0–59 months.
- Administer annually to persons with certain risk factors, health-care workers, and other persons (including household members) in close contact with persons in groups at higher risk.

- Administer 2 doses (separated by 4 weeks or longer) to children younger than 9 years who are receiving influenza vaccine for the first time or who were vaccinated for the first time last season but only received one dose.
- For healthy nonpregnant persons (those who do not have underlying medical conditions that predispose them to influenza complications) ages 2–49 years, either LAIV or TIV may be used.

**6. Hepatitis A vaccine (HepA).**
- Administer the 2 doses in the series at least 6 months apart.
- HepA is recommended for certain other groups of children, including in areas where vaccination programs target older children.

**7. Hepatitis B vaccine (HepB).**
- Administer the 3-dose series to those who were not previously vaccinated.
- A 2-dose series of Recombivax HB® is licensed for children aged 11–15 years.

**8. Inactivated poliovirus vaccine (IPV).**
- For children who received an all-IPV or all-oral poliovirus (OPV) series, a fourth dose is not necessary if the third dose was administered at age 4 years or older.
- If both OPV and IPV were administered as part of a series, a total of 4 doses should be administered, regardless of the child's current age.

**9. Measles, mumps, and rubella vaccine (MMR).**
- If not previously vaccinated, administer 2 doses of MMR during any visit, with 4 or more weeks between the doses.

**10. Varicella vaccine.**
- Administer 2 doses of varicella vaccine to persons younger than 13 years of age at least 3 months apart. Do not repeat the second dose if administered 28 or more days following the first dose.
- Administer 2 doses of varicella vaccine to persons aged 13 years or older at least 4 weeks apart.

The Recommended Immunization Schedules for Persons Aged 0–18 Years are approved by the Advisory Committee on Immunization Practices (www.cdc.gov/vaccines/recs/acip), the American Academy of Pediatrics (http://www.aap.org), and the American Academy of Family Physicians (http://www.aafp.org).

**Figure A-2.** Recommended immunization schedule for persons aged 7–18 years. Source: Centers for Disease Control and Prevention, Morbidity & Mortality Weekly Report (MMWR); Jan. 11, 2008; http://www.cdc.gov/vaccines/recs/schedules/child-schedule.htm

The table below provides catch-up schedules and minimum intervals between doses for children whose vaccinations have been delayed. A vaccine series does not need to be restarted, regardless of the time that has elapsed between doses. Use the section appropriate for the child's age.

| Vaccine | Minimum Age for Dose 1 | Minimum Interval Between Doses | | | |
|---|---|---|---|---|---|
| | | **Dose 1 to Dose 2** | **Dose 2 to Dose 3** | **Dose 3 to Dose 4** | **Dose 4 to Dose 5** |
| **CATCH-UP SCHEDULE FOR PERSONS AGED 4 MONTHS–6 YEARS** | | | | | |
| Hepatitis B[1] | Birth | 4 weeks | 8 weeks (and 16 weeks after first dose) | | |
| Rotavirus[2] | 6 wks | 4 weeks | 4 weeks | | |
| Diphtheria, Tetanus, Pertussis[3] | 6 wks | 4 weeks | 4 weeks | 6 months | 6 months[3] |
| Haemophilus influenzae type b[4] | 6 wks | 4 weeks if first dose administered at younger than 12 months of age<br>8 weeks (as final dose) if first dose administered at age 12-14 months<br>No further doses needed if first dose administered at 15 months of age or older | 4 weeks[4] if current age is younger than 12 months<br>8 weeks (as final dose)[4] if current age is 12 months or older and second dose administered at younger than 15 months of age<br>No further doses needed if previous dose administered at age 15 months or older | 8 weeks (as final dose) This dose only necessary for children aged 12 months-5 years who received 3 doses before age 12 months | |
| Pneumococcal[5] | 6 wks | 4 weeks if first dose administered at younger than 12 months of age<br>8 weeks (as final dose) if first dose administered at age 12 months or older or current age 24-59 months<br>No further doses needed for healthy children if first dose administered at age 24 months or older | 4 weeks if current age is younger than 12 months<br>8 weeks (as final dose) if current age is 12 months or older<br>No further doses needed for healthy children if previous dose administered at age 24 months or older | 8 weeks (as final dose) This dose only necessary for children aged 12 months-5 years who received 3 doses before age 12 months | |
| Inactivated Poliovirus[6] | 6 wks | 4 weeks | 4 weeks | 4 weeks[6] | |
| Measles, Mumps, Rubella[7] | 12 mos | 4 weeks | | | |
| Varicella[8] | 12 mos | 3 months | | | |
| Hepatitis A[9] | 12 mos | 6 months | | | |
| **CATCH-UP SCHEDULE FOR PERSONS AGED 7–18 YEARS** | | | | | |
| Tetanus, Diphtheria/ Tetanus, Diphtheria, Pertussis[10] | 7 yrs[10] | 4 weeks | 4 weeks if first dose administered at younger than 12 months of age<br>6 months if first dose administered at age 12 months or older | 6 months if first dose administered at younger than 12 months of age | |
| Human Papillomavirus[11] | 9 yrs | 4 weeks | 12 weeks (and 24 weeks after first dose) | | |
| Hepatitis A[9] | 12 mos | 6 months | | | |
| Hepatitis B[1] | Birth | 4 weeks | 8 weeks (and 16 weeks after first dose) | | |
| Inactivated Poliovirus[6] | 6 wks | 4 weeks | 4 weeks | 4 weeks[6] | |
| Measles, Mumps, Rubella[7] | 12 mos | 4 weeks | | | |
| Varicella[8] | 12 mos | 4 weeks if first dose administered at age 13 years or older<br>3 months if first dose administered at younger than 13 years of age | | | |

**1. Hepatitis B vaccine (HepB).**
- Administer the 3-dose series to those who were not previously vaccinated.
- A 2-dose series of Recombivax HB® is licensed for children aged 11–15 years.

**2. Rotavirus vaccine (Rota).**
- Do not start the series later than age 12 weeks.
- Administer the final dose in the series by age 32 weeks.
- Do not administer a dose later than age 32 weeks.
- Data on safety and efficacy outside of these age ranges are insufficient.

**3. Diphtheria and tetanus toxoids and acellular pertussis vaccine (DTaP).**
- The fifth dose is not necessary if the fourth dose was administered at age 4 years or older.
- DTaP is not indicated for persons aged 7 years or older.

**4. Haemophilus influenzae type b conjugate vaccine (Hib).**
- Vaccine is not generally recommended for children aged 5 years or older.
- If current age is younger than 12 months and the first 2 doses were PRP-OMP (PedvaxHIB® or ComVax® [Merck]), the third (and final) dose should be administered at age 12–15 months and at least 8 weeks after the second dose.
- If first dose was administered at age 7–11 months, administer 2 doses separated by 4 weeks plus a booster at age 12–15 months.

**5. Pneumococcal conjugate vaccine (PCV).**
- Administer one dose of PCV to all healthy children aged 24–59 months having any incomplete schedule.
- For children with underlying medical conditions, administer 2 doses of PCV at least 8 weeks apart if previously received less than 3 doses, or 1 dose of PCV if previously received 3 doses.

**6. Inactivated poliovirus vaccine (IPV).**
- For children who received an all-IPV or all-oral poliovirus (OPV) series, a fourth dose is not necessary if third dose was administered at age 4 years or older.

- If both OPV and IPV were administered as part of a series, a total of 4 doses should be administered, regardless of the child's current age.
- IPV is not routinely recommended for persons aged 18 years and older.

**7. Measles, mumps, and rubella vaccine (MMR).**
- The second dose of MMR is recommended routinely at age 4–6 years but may be administered earlier if desired.
- If not previously vaccinated, administer 2 doses of MMR during any visit with 4 or more weeks between the doses.

**8. Varicella vaccine.**
- The second dose of varicella vaccine is recommended routinely at age 4–6 years but may be administered earlier if desired.
- Do not repeat the second dose in persons younger than 13 years of age if administered 28 or more days after the first dose.

**9. Hepatitis A vaccine (HepA).**
- HepA is recommended for certain groups of children, including in areas where vaccination programs target older children. See MMWR 2006;55(No. RR-7):1–23.

**10. Tetanus and diphtheria toxoids (Td) and tetanus and diphtheria toxoids and acellular pertussis vaccine (Tdap).**
- Tdap should be substituted for a single dose of Td in the primary catch-up series or as a booster if age appropriate; use Td for other doses.
- A 5-year interval from the last Td dose is encouraged when Tdap is used as a booster dose. A booster (fourth) dose is needed if any of the previous doses were administered at younger than 12 months of age. Refer to ACIP recommendations for further information. See MMWR 2006;55(No. RR-3).

**11. Human papillomavirus vaccine (HPV).**
- Administer the HPV vaccine series to females at age 13–18 years if not previously vaccinated.

Information about reporting reactions after immunization is available online at http://www.vaers.hhs.gov or by telephone via the 24-hour national toll-free information line 800-822-7967. Suspected cases of vaccine-preventable diseases should be reported to the state or local health department. Additional information, including precautions and contraindications for immunization, is available from the National Center for Immunization and Respiratory Diseases at http://www.cdc.gov/vaccines or telephone, 800-CDC-INFO (800-232-4636).

**Figure A-3.** Catch-up immunization schedule for persons aged 4 months–18 years who start late or who are >1 month behind. Source: Centers for Disease Control and Prevention, Morbidity & Mortality Weekly Report (MMWR); Jan. 11, 2008; http://www.cdc.gov/vaccines/recs/schedules/child-schedule.htm

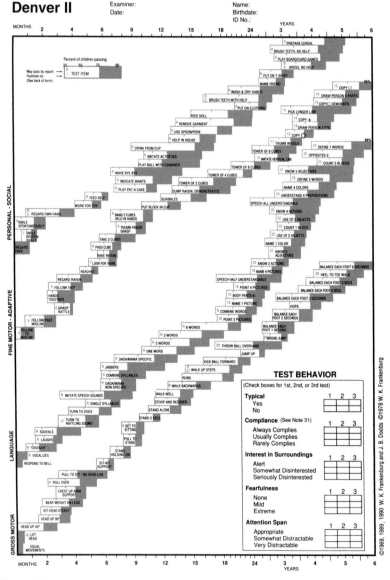

**Figure B-1.** Denver development assessment (Denver II). Reprinted with permission from William K. Frankenburg, MD.

# DIRECTIONS FOR ADMINISTRATION

1. Try to get child to smile by smiling, talking or waving. Do not touch him/her.
2. Child must stare at hand several seconds.
3. Parent may help guide toothbrush and put toothpaste on brush.
4. Child does not have to be able to tie shoes or button/zip in the back.
5. Move yarn slowly in an arc from one side to the other, about 8″ above child's face.
6. Pass if child grasps rattle when it is touched to the backs or tips of fingers.
7. Pass if child tries to see where yarn went. Yarn should be dropped quickly from sight from tester's hand without arm movement.
8. Child must transfer cube from hand to hand without help of body, mouth, or table.
9. Pass if child picks up raisin with any part of thumb and finger.
10. Line can vary only 30 degrees or less from tester's line. $\sqrt{}$
11. Make a fist with thumb pointing upward and wiggle only the thumb. Pass if child imitates and does not move any fingers other than the thumb.

         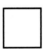

| 12. Pass any enclosed form. Fail continuous round motions. | 13. Which line is longer? (Not bigger.) Turn paper upside down and repeat. (pass 3 of 3 or 5 of 6) | 14. Pass any lines crossing near midpoint. | 15. Have child copy first. If failed, demonstrate. |

When giving items 12, 14, and 15, do not name the forms. Do not demonstrate 12 and 14.

16. When scoring, each pair (2 arms, 2 legs, etc.) counts as one part.
17. Place one cube in cup and shake gently near child's ear, but out of sight. Repeat for other ear.
18. Point to picture and have child name it. (No credit is given for sounds only.)
   If less than 4 pictures are named correctly, have child point to picture as each is named by tester.

19. Using doll, tell child: Show me the nose, eyes, ears, mouth, hands, feet, tummy, hair. Pass 6 of 8.
20. Using pictures, ask child: Which one flies?... says meow?... talks?... barks?... gallops? Pass 2 of 5, 4 of 5.
21. Ask child: What do you do when you are cold?... tired?... hungry? Pass 2 of 3, 3 of 3.
22. Ask child: What do you do with a cup? What is a chair used for? What is a pencil used for?
   Action words must be included in answers.
23. Pass if child correctly places and says how many blocks are on paper. (1, 5)
24. Tell child: Put block **on** table; **under** table; **in front of** me, **behind** me. Pass 4 of 4.
   (Do not help child by pointing, moving head or eyes.)
25. Ask child: What is a ball?... lake?... desk?... house?... banana?... curtain?... fence?... ceiling? Pass if defined in terms of use, shape, what it is made of, or general category (such as banana is fruit, not just yellow). Pass 5 of 8, 7 of 8.
26. Ask child: If a horse is big, a mouse is __? If fire is hot, ice is __? If the sun shines during the day, the moon shines during the __? Pass 2 of 3.
27. Child may use wall or rail only, not person. May not crawl.
28. Child must throw ball overhand 3 feet to within arm's reach of tester.
29. Child must perform standing broad jump over width of test sheet (8½ inches).
30. Tell child to walk forward, 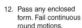 heel within 1 inch of toe. Tester may demonstrate.
   Child must walk 4 consecutive steps.
31. In the second year, half of normal children are noncompliant.

**OBSERVATIONS:**

**Figure B-2.** Questions to ask during administration of Denver Development Assessment. Reprinted with permission from William K. Frankenburg, MD.

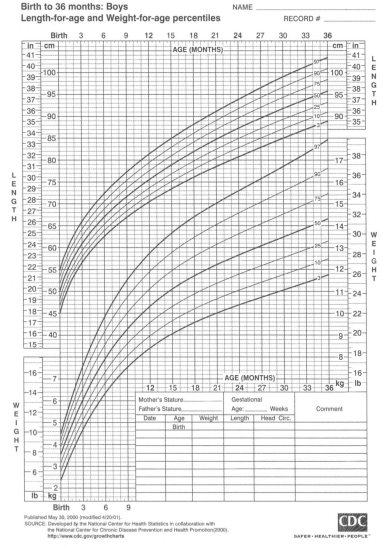

**Figure C-1.** Birth to 36 months: boys' length-for-age and weight-for-age percentiles. Source: National Center for Health Statistics in collaboration with the National Center for Chronic Disease Prevention and Health Promotion, May 30, 2000 (modified 4/20/01).

Birth to 36 months: Girls
Length-for-age and Weight-for-age percentiles

NAME _____

RECORD # _____

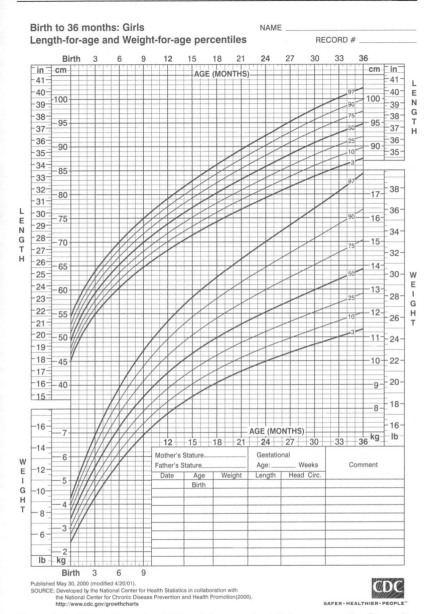

Published May 30, 2000 (modified 4/20/01).
SOURCE: Developed by the National Center for Health Statistics in collaboration with
the National Center for Chronic Disease Prevention and Health Promotion(2000).
http://www.cdc.gov/growthcharts

SAFER·HEALTHIER·PEOPLE™

**Figure C-2.** Birth to 36 months: girls' length-for-age and weight-for-age percentiles. Source: National Center for Health Statistics in collaboration with the National Center for Chronic Disease Prevention and Health Promotion, May 30, 2000 (modified 4/20/01).

Birth to 36 months: Boys
Head circumference-for-age and
Weight-for-length percentiles

NAME _____

RECORD # _____

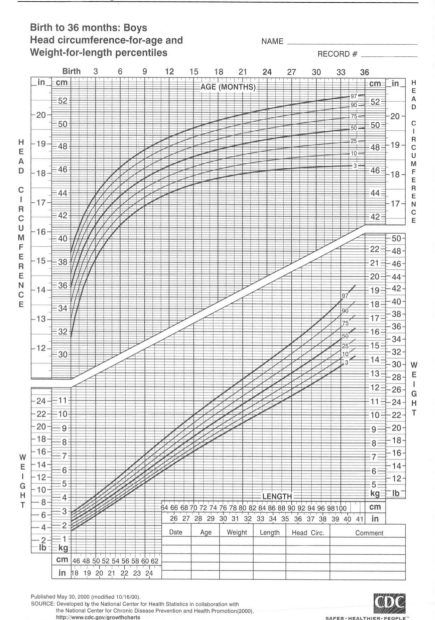

Published May 30, 2000 (modified 10/16/00).
SOURCE: Developed by the National Center for Health Statistics in collaboration with
the National Center for Chronic Disease Prevention and Health Promotion(2000).
http://www.cdc.gov/growthcharts

CDC
SAFER·HEALTHIER·PEOPLE™

**Figure C-3.** Birth to 36 months: boys' head circumference-for-age and weight-for-length percentiles. Source: National Center for Health Statistics in collaboration with the National Center for Chronic Disease Prevention and Health Promotion, May 30, 2000 (modified 4/20/01).

Birth to 36 months: Girls
Head circumference-for-age and
Weight-for-length percentiles

NAME _____

RECORD # _____

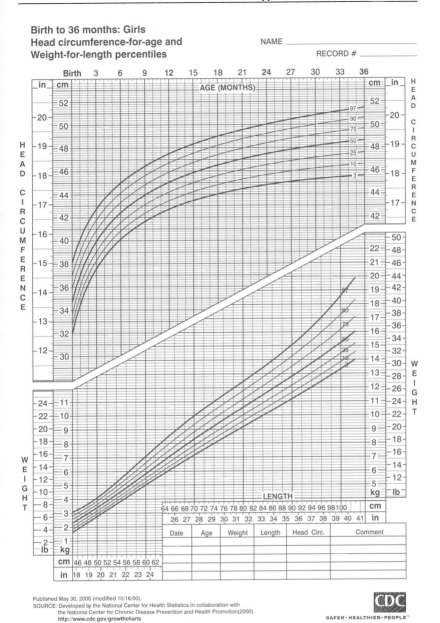

Published May 30, 2000 (modified 10/16/00).
SOURCE: Developed by the National Center for Health Statistics in collaboration with
the National Center for Chronic Disease Prevention and Health Promotion(2000).
http://www.cdc.gov/growthcharts

**Figure C-4.** Birth to 36 months: girls' head circumference-for-age and weight-for-length percentiles. Source: National Center for Health Statistics in collaboration with the National Center for Chronic Disease Prevention and Health Promotion, May 30, 2000 (modified 4/20/01).

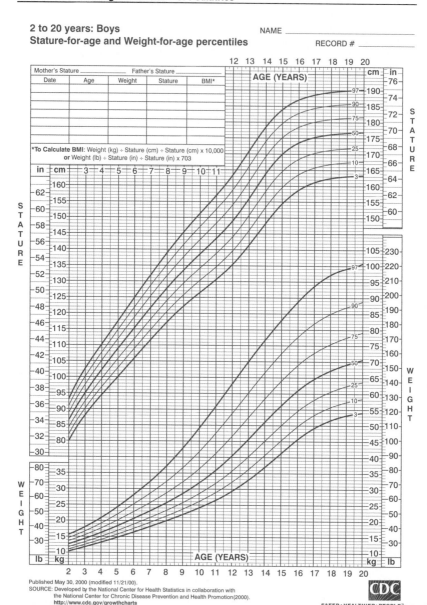

**Figure C-5.** 2 to 20 years: boys' stature-for-age and weight-for-age percentiles. Source: National Center for Health Statistics in collaboration with the National Center for Chronic Disease Prevention and Health Promotion, May 30, 2000 (modified 4/20/01).

## 2 to 20 years: Girls
## Stature-for-age and Weight-for-age percentiles

NAME _____

RECORD # _____

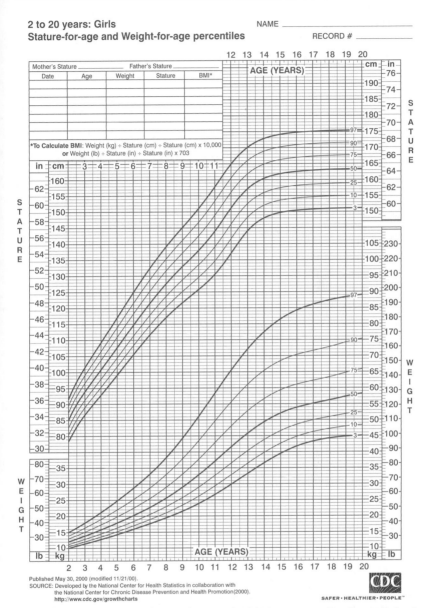

*To Calculate BMI: Weight (kg) ÷ Stature (cm) ÷ Stature (cm) x 10,000
or Weight (lb) ÷ Stature (in) ÷ Stature (in) x 703

Published May 30, 2000 (modified 11/21/00).
SOURCE: Developed by the National Center for Health Statistics in collaboration with
the National Center for Chronic Disease Prevention and Health Promotion(2000).
http://www.cdc.gov/growthcharts

SAFER·HEALTHIER·PEOPLE™

**Figure C-6.** 2 to 20 years: girls' stature-for-age and weight-for-age percentiles. Source: National Center for Health Statistics in collaboration with the National Center for Chronic Disease Prevention and Health Promotion, May 30, 2000 (modified 4/20/01).

**2 to 20 years: Boys**
**Body mass index-for-age percentiles**

NAME _____

RECORD # _____

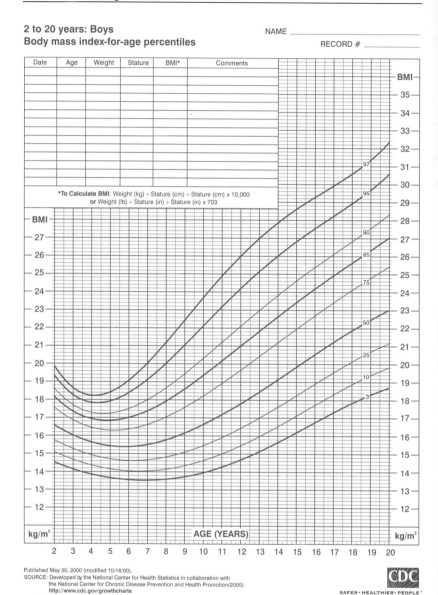

*To Calculate BMI: Weight (kg) ÷ Stature (cm) ÷ Stature (cm) x 10,000
or Weight (lb) ÷ Stature (in) ÷ Stature (in) x 703

Published May 30, 2000 (modified 10/16/00).
SOURCE: Developed by the National Center for Health Statistics in collaboration with
the National Center for Chronic Disease Prevention and Health Promotion(2000).
http://www.cdc.gov/growthcharts

**Figure C-7.** 2 to 20 years: boys' body mass index (BMI)-for-age percentiles. Source: National Center for Health Statistics in collaboration with the National Center for Chronic Disease Prevention and Health Promotion, May 30, 2000 (modified 4/20/01).

**2 to 20 years: Girls**
**Body mass index-for-age percentiles**

NAME _____

RECORD # _____

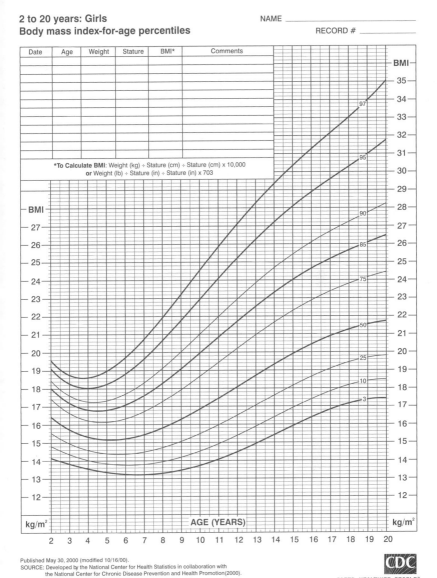

| Date | Age | Weight | Stature | BMI* | Comments |
|------|-----|--------|---------|------|----------|

*To Calculate BMI: Weight (kg) ÷ Stature (cm) ÷ Stature (cm) x 10,000
or Weight (lb) ÷ Stature (in) ÷ Stature (in) x 703

AGE (YEARS)

Published May 30, 2000 (modified 10/16/00).
SOURCE: Developed by the National Center for Health Statistics in collaboration with
the National Center for Chronic Disease Prevention and Health Promotion(2000).
http://www.cdc.gov/growthcharts

CDC
SAFER·HEALTHIER·PEOPLE™

**Figure C-8.** 2 to 20 years: girls' body mass index (BMI)-for-age percentiles. Source: National Center for Health Statistics in collaboration with the National Center for Chronic Disease Prevention and Health Promotion, May 30, 2000 (modified 4/20/01).

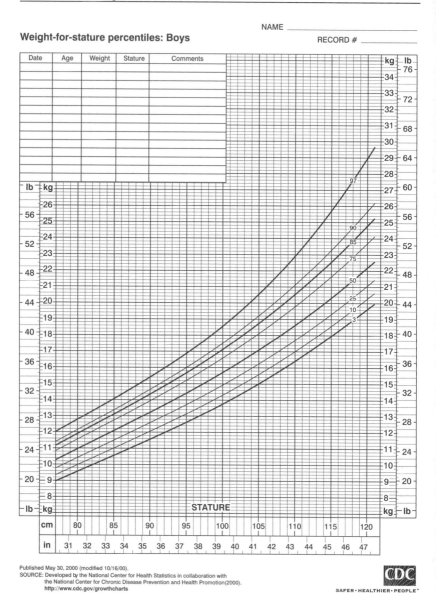

**Figure C-9.** Boys' weight-for-stature percentiles. Source: National Center for Health Statistics in collaboration with the National Center for Chronic Disease Prevention and Health Promotion, May 30, 2000 (modified 4/20/01).

## Weight-for-stature percentiles: Girls

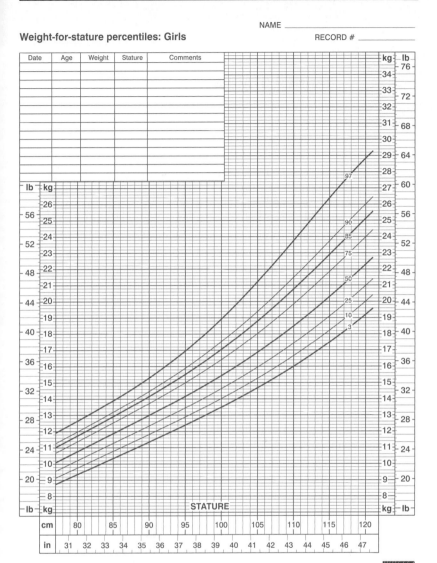

Published May 30, 2000 (modified 10/16/00).
SOURCE: Developed by the National Center for Health Statistics in collaboration with
the National Center for Chronic Disease Prevention and Health Promotion(2000).
http://www.cdc.gov/growthcharts

SAFER·HEALTHIER·PEOPLE™

**Figure C-10.** Girls' weight-for-stature percentiles. Source: National Center for Health Statistics in collaboration with the National Center for Chronic Disease Prevention and Health Promotion, May 30, 2000 (modified 4/20/01).

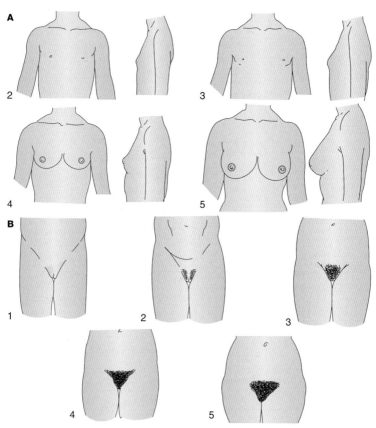

**Figure D-1.** Female Tanner stages. **(A)** Female breast development. Sex maturity rating 1 (not shown): prepubertal; elevation of papilla only. Sex maturity rating 2: breast buds appear; areola is slightly widened and projects as small mound. Sex maturity rating 3: enlargement of the entire breast with no protrusion of the papilla or the nipple. Sex maturity rating 4: enlargement of the breast and projection of areola and papilla as a secondary mound. Sex maturity rating 5: adult configuration of the breast with protrusion of the nipple; areola no longer projects separately from remainder of breast. **(B)** Female pubic hair development. Sex maturity rating 1: prepubertal; no pubic hair. Sex maturity rating 2: straight hair extends along the labia and, between rating 2 and 3, begins on the pubis. Sex maturity rating 3: Pubic hair increased in quantity, darker, and present in the typical female triangle but in smaller quantity. Sex maturity rating 4: pubic hair more dense, curled, and adult in distribution but less abundant. Sex maturity rating 5: abundant, adult-type pattern; hair may extend onto the medial part of the thighs. (Adapted from Tanner JM. Growth at Adolescence. 2nd Ed. Oxford: Blackwell,1962.) From Pillitteri A. Maternal and Child Nursing. 5th Ed. Philadelphia: Lippincott Williams & Wilkins, 2007.

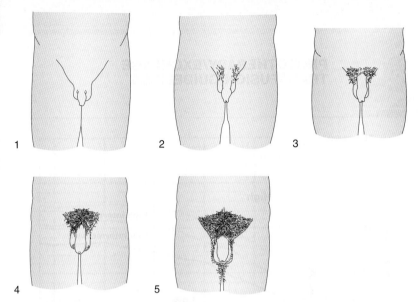

**Figure D-2.** Male Tanner stages. Male genital and pubic hair development. Ratings for pubic hair and for genital development can differ in a typical boy at any given time because pubic hair and genitalia do not necessarily develop at the same rate. Sex maturity rating 1: prepubertal; no pubic hair; genitalia unchanged from early childhood. Sex maturity rating 2: light, downy hair develops laterally and later becomes dark; penis and testes may be slightly larger; scrotum becoming more textured. Sex maturity rating 3: pubic hair has extended across the pubis; testes and scrotum are further enlarged; penis is larger, especially in length. Sex maturity rating 4: more abundant pubic hair with curling; genitalia resemble those of an adult; glans has become larger and broader; scrotum is darker. Sex maturity rating 5: adult quantity and pattern of pubic hair, with hair present along inner borders of thighs; testes and scrotum are adult in size. (Adapted from Tanner JM. Growth at Adolescence. 2nd Ed. Oxford: Blackwell,1962.) From Pillitteri A. Maternal and Child Nursing. 5th Ed. Philadelphia: Lippincott Williams & Wilkins, 2007.

# PHOTOTHERAPY/EXCHANGE TRANSFUSION GUIDELINES

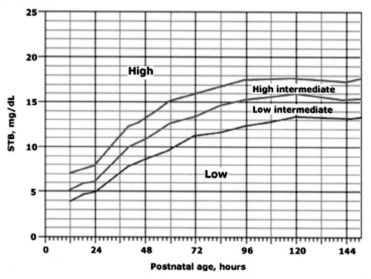

**Figure E-1.** Nomogram of hour specific serum total bilirubin. Source: Subcommittee on Hyperbilirubinemia. Management of hyperbilirubinemia in the newborn infant 35 or more weeks of gestation. Pediatrics 2004;114:297. ©2004 The American Academy of Pediatrics.

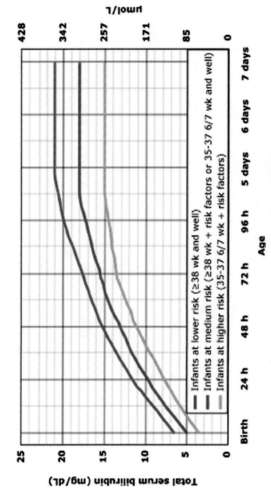

**Figure E-2.** Total serum bilirubin guideline for phototherapy. Source: Subcommittee on Hyperbilirubinemia. Management of hyperbilirubinemia in the newborn infant 35 or more weeks of gestation. Pediatrics 2004;114:297. ©2004 The American Academy of Pediatrics.

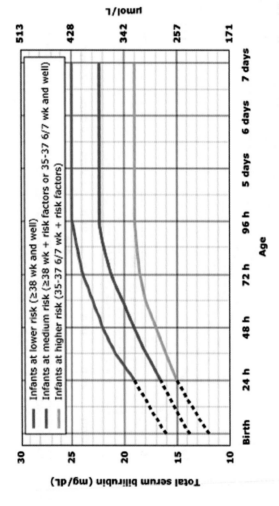

**Figure E-3.** Total serum bilirubin guideline for exchange transfusion. Source: Subcommittee on Hyperbilirubinemia. Management of hyperbilirubinemia in the newborn infant 35 or more weeks of gestation. Pediatrics 2004;114:297. ©2004 The American Academy of Pediatrics.

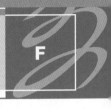

# HYPERTENSION IN CHILDREN AND ADOLESCENTS

**TABLE F-1  Blood Pressure Levels for Boys by Age and Height Percentile**

| Age, y | BP percentile | SBP, mm Hg | | | | | | | DBP, mm Hg | | | | | | |
| --- | --- | --- | --- | --- | --- | --- | --- | --- | --- | --- | --- | --- | --- | --- | --- |
| | | Percentile of height | | | | | | | Percentile of height | | | | | | |
| | | 5th | 10th | 25th | 50th | 75th | 90th | 95th | 5th | 10th | 25th | 50th | 75th | 90th | 95th |
| 1 | 50th | 80 | 81 | 83 | 85 | 87 | 88 | 89 | 34 | 35 | 36 | 37 | 38 | 39 | 39 |
| | 90th | 94 | 95 | 97 | 99 | 100 | 102 | 103 | 49 | 50 | 51 | 52 | 53 | 53 | 54 |
| | 95th | 98 | 99 | 101 | 103 | 104 | 106 | 106 | 54 | 54 | 55 | 56 | 57 | 58 | 58 |
| | 99th | 105 | 106 | 108 | 110 | 112 | 113 | 114 | 61 | 62 | 63 | 64 | 65 | 66 | 66 |
| 2 | 50th | 84 | 85 | 87 | 88 | 90 | 92 | 92 | 39 | 40 | 41 | 42 | 43 | 44 | 44 |
| | 90th | 97 | 99 | 100 | 102 | 104 | 105 | 106 | 54 | 55 | 56 | 57 | 58 | 58 | 59 |
| | 95th | 101 | 102 | 104 | 106 | 108 | 109 | 110 | 59 | 59 | 60 | 61 | 62 | 63 | 63 |
| | 99th | 109 | 110 | 111 | 113 | 115 | 117 | 117 | 66 | 67 | 68 | 69 | 70 | 71 | 71 |
| 3 | 50th | 86 | 87 | 89 | 91 | 93 | 94 | 95 | 44 | 44 | 45 | 46 | 47 | 48 | 48 |
| | 90th | 100 | 101 | 103 | 105 | 107 | 108 | 109 | 59 | 59 | 60 | 61 | 62 | 63 | 63 |
| | 95th | 104 | 105 | 107 | 109 | 110 | 112 | 113 | 63 | 63 | 64 | 65 | 66 | 67 | 67 |
| | 99th | 111 | 112 | 114 | 116 | 118 | 119 | 120 | 71 | 71 | 72 | 73 | 74 | 75 | 75 |
| 4 | 50th | 88 | 89 | 91 | 93 | 95 | 96 | 97 | 47 | 48 | 49 | 50 | 51 | 51 | 52 |
| | 90th | 102 | 103 | 105 | 107 | 109 | 110 | 111 | 62 | 63 | 64 | 65 | 66 | 66 | 67 |
| | 95th | 106 | 107 | 109 | 111 | 112 | 114 | 115 | 66 | 67 | 68 | 69 | 70 | 71 | 71 |
| | 99th | 113 | 114 | 116 | 118 | 120 | 121 | 122 | 74 | 75 | 76 | 77 | 78 | 78 | 79 |
| 5 | 50th | 90 | 91 | 93 | 95 | 96 | 98 | 98 | 50 | 51 | 52 | 53 | 54 | 55 | 55 |
| | 90th | 104 | 105 | 106 | 108 | 110 | 111 | 112 | 65 | 66 | 67 | 68 | 69 | 69 | 70 |
| | 95th | 108 | 109 | 110 | 112 | 114 | 115 | 116 | 69 | 70 | 71 | 72 | 73 | 74 | 74 |
| | 99th | 115 | 116 | 118 | 120 | 121 | 123 | 123 | 77 | 78 | 79 | 80 | 81 | 81 | 82 |
| 6 | 50th | 91 | 92 | 94 | 96 | 98 | 99 | 100 | 53 | 53 | 54 | 55 | 56 | 57 | 57 |
| | 90th | 105 | 106 | 108 | 110 | 111 | 113 | 113 | 68 | 68 | 69 | 70 | 71 | 72 | 72 |
| | 95th | 109 | 110 | 112 | 114 | 115 | 117 | 117 | 72 | 72 | 73 | 74 | 75 | 76 | 76 |
| | 99th | 116 | 117 | 119 | 121 | 123 | 124 | 125 | 80 | 80 | 81 | 82 | 83 | 84 | 84 |

| Age | BP Percentile | SBP | | | | | | | DBP | | | | | | |
|---|---|---|---|---|---|---|---|---|---|---|---|---|---|---|---|
| 7 | 50th | 92 | 94 | 95 | 97 | 99 | 100 | 101 | 55 | 55 | 56 | 57 | 58 | 59 | 59 |
|  | 90th | 106 | 107 | 109 | 111 | 113 | 114 | 115 | 70 | 70 | 71 | 72 | 73 | 74 | 74 |
|  | 95th | 110 | 111 | 113 | 115 | 117 | 118 | 119 | 74 | 74 | 75 | 76 | 77 | 78 | 78 |
|  | 99th | 117 | 118 | 120 | 122 | 124 | 125 | 126 | 82 | 82 | 83 | 84 | 85 | 86 | 86 |
| 8 | 50th | 94 | 95 | 97 | 99 | 100 | 102 | 102 | 56 | 56 | 57 | 58 | 59 | 60 | 61 |
|  | 90th | 107 | 109 | 110 | 112 | 114 | 115 | 116 | 71 | 71 | 72 | 73 | 74 | 75 | 76 |
|  | 95th | 111 | 112 | 114 | 116 | 118 | 119 | 120 | 75 | 75 | 76 | 77 | 79 | 79 | 80 |
|  | 99th | 119 | 120 | 122 | 123 | 125 | 127 | 127 | 83 | 83 | 84 | 85 | 87 | 87 | 88 |
| 9 | 50th | 95 | 96 | 98 | 100 | 102 | 103 | 104 | 57 | 57 | 58 | 59 | 60 | 61 | 62 |
|  | 90th | 109 | 110 | 112 | 114 | 115 | 117 | 118 | 72 | 72 | 73 | 74 | 76 | 76 | 77 |
|  | 95th | 113 | 114 | 116 | 118 | 119 | 121 | 121 | 76 | 76 | 77 | 78 | 80 | 81 | 81 |
|  | 99th | 120 | 121 | 123 | 125 | 127 | 128 | 129 | 84 | 84 | 85 | 86 | 88 | 88 | 89 |
| 10 | 50th | 97 | 98 | 100 | 102 | 103 | 105 | 106 | 58 | 58 | 59 | 60 | 61 | 61 | 62 |
|  | 90th | 111 | 112 | 114 | 115 | 117 | 119 | 119 | 73 | 73 | 73 | 74 | 75 | 76 | 77 |
|  | 95th | 115 | 116 | 117 | 119 | 121 | 122 | 123 | 77 | 77 | 77 | 78 | 79 | 80 | 81 |
|  | 99th | 122 | 123 | 125 | 127 | 128 | 130 | 130 | 85 | 85 | 85 | 86 | 87 | 88 | 89 |
| 11 | 50th | 99 | 100 | 102 | 104 | 105 | 107 | 107 | 59 | 59 | 59 | 60 | 61 | 62 | 63 |
|  | 90th | 113 | 114 | 115 | 117 | 119 | 120 | 121 | 74 | 74 | 74 | 75 | 76 | 77 | 78 |
|  | 95th | 117 | 118 | 119 | 121 | 123 | 124 | 125 | 78 | 78 | 78 | 79 | 80 | 81 | 82 |
|  | 99th | 124 | 125 | 127 | 129 | 130 | 132 | 132 | 86 | 86 | 86 | 87 | 88 | 89 | 90 |
| 12 | 50th | 101 | 102 | 104 | 106 | 108 | 109 | 110 | 59 | 60 | 60 | 61 | 62 | 63 | 63 |
|  | 90th | 115 | 116 | 118 | 120 | 121 | 123 | 123 | 74 | 75 | 75 | 76 | 77 | 78 | 79 |
|  | 95th | 119 | 120 | 122 | 123 | 125 | 127 | 127 | 78 | 79 | 80 | 80 | 81 | 82 | 82 |
|  | 99th | 126 | 127 | 129 | 131 | 133 | 134 | 135 | 86 | 87 | 88 | 88 | 89 | 90 | 90 |
| 13 | 50th | 104 | 105 | 106 | 108 | 110 | 111 | 112 | 60 | 60 | 61 | 62 | 63 | 64 | 64 |
|  | 90th | 117 | 118 | 120 | 122 | 124 | 125 | 126 | 75 | 75 | 76 | 77 | 78 | 79 | 79 |
|  | 95th | 121 | 122 | 124 | 126 | 128 | 129 | 130 | 79 | 79 | 80 | 81 | 82 | 83 | 83 |
|  | 99th | 128 | 130 | 131 | 133 | 135 | 136 | 137 | 87 | 87 | 88 | 89 | 90 | 91 | 91 |

*(continued)*

## TABLE F-1 Blood Pressure Levels for Boys by Age and Height Percentile

| Age, y | BP percentile | SBP, mm Hg Percentile of height | | | | | | | DBP, mm Hg Percentile of height | | | | | | |
|---|---|---|---|---|---|---|---|---|---|---|---|---|---|---|---|
| | | 5th | 10th | 25th | 50th | 75th | 90th | 95th | 5th | 10th | 25th | 50th | 75th | 90th | 95th |
| 14 | 50th | 106 | 107 | 109 | 111 | 113 | 114 | 115 | 60 | 61 | 62 | 63 | 64 | 65 | 65 |
| | 90th | 120 | 121 | 123 | 125 | 126 | 128 | 128 | 75 | 76 | 77 | 78 | 79 | 79 | 80 |
| | 95th | 124 | 125 | 127 | 128 | 130 | 132 | 132 | 80 | 80 | 81 | 82 | 83 | 84 | 84 |
| | 99th | 131 | 132 | 134 | 136 | 138 | 139 | 140 | 87 | 88 | 89 | 90 | 91 | 92 | 92 |
| 15 | 50th | 109 | 110 | 112 | 113 | 115 | 117 | 117 | 61 | 62 | 63 | 64 | 65 | 66 | 66 |
| | 90th | 122 | 124 | 125 | 127 | 129 | 130 | 131 | 76 | 77 | 78 | 79 | 80 | 80 | 81 |
| | 95th | 126 | 127 | 129 | 131 | 133 | 134 | 135 | 81 | 81 | 82 | 83 | 84 | 85 | 85 |
| | 99th | 134 | 135 | 136 | 138 | 140 | 142 | 142 | 88 | 89 | 90 | 91 | 92 | 93 | 93 |
| 16 | 50th | 111 | 112 | 114 | 116 | 118 | 119 | 120 | 63 | 63 | 64 | 65 | 66 | 67 | 67 |
| | 90th | 125 | 126 | 128 | 130 | 131 | 133 | 134 | 78 | 78 | 79 | 80 | 81 | 82 | 82 |
| | 95th | 129 | 130 | 132 | 134 | 135 | 137 | 137 | 82 | 83 | 83 | 84 | 85 | 86 | 87 |
| | 99th | 136 | 137 | 139 | 141 | 143 | 144 | 145 | 90 | 90 | 91 | 92 | 93 | 94 | 94 |
| 17 | 50th | 114 | 115 | 116 | 118 | 120 | 121 | 122 | 65 | 66 | 66 | 67 | 68 | 69 | 70 |
| | 90th | 127 | 128 | 130 | 132 | 134 | 135 | 136 | 80 | 80 | 81 | 82 | 83 | 84 | 84 |
| | 95th | 131 | 132 | 134 | 136 | 138 | 139 | 140 | 84 | 85 | 86 | 87 | 87 | 88 | 89 |
| | 99th | 139 | 140 | 141 | 143 | 145 | 146 | 147 | 92 | 93 | 93 | 94 | 95 | 96 | 97 |

The 90th percentile is 1.28 SD, the 95th percentile is 1.645 SD, and the 99th percentile is 2.326 SD over the mean.
For research purposes, the SDs in Table BI allow one to compute BP Z scores and percentiles for boys with height percentiles given in Table 3 (ie, the 5th, 10th, 25th, 50th, 75th, 90th, and 95th percentiles). These height percentiles must be converted to height Z scores given by: 5% = −1.645; 10% = −1.28; 25% = −0.68; 50% = 0; 75% = 0.68; 90% = 1.28; and 95% = 1.645, and then computed according to the methodology in steps 2 through 4 described in Appendix B. For children with height percentiles other than these, follow steps 1 through 4 as described in Appendix B.
From National High Blood Pressure Education Program Working Group on High Blood Pressure in Children and Adolescents: The Fourth Report on the Diagnosis, Evaluation, and Treatment of High Blood Pressure in Children and Adolescents. Pediatrics 2004;114(2);555–576. ©2004 The American Academy of Pediatrics.

**TABLE F-2  Blood Pressure Levels for Girls by Age and Height Percentile**

| Age, y | BP percentile | SBP, mm Hg | | | | | | | DBP, mm Hg | | | | | | |
| | | Percentile of height | | | | | | | Percentile of height | | | | | | |
| | | 5th | 10th | 25th | 50th | 75th | 90th | 95th | 5th | 10th | 25th | 50th | 75th | 90th | 95th |
|---|---|---|---|---|---|---|---|---|---|---|---|---|---|---|---|
| 1 | 50th | 83 | 84 | 85 | 86 | 88 | 89 | 90 | 38 | 39 | 39 | 40 | 41 | 41 | 42 |
| | 90th | 97 | 97 | 98 | 100 | 101 | 102 | 103 | 52 | 53 | 53 | 54 | 55 | 55 | 56 |
| | 95th | 100 | 101 | 102 | 104 | 105 | 106 | 107 | 56 | 57 | 57 | 58 | 59 | 59 | 60 |
| | 99th | 108 | 108 | 109 | 111 | 112 | 113 | 114 | 64 | 64 | 65 | 65 | 66 | 67 | 67 |
| 2 | 50th | 85 | 85 | 87 | 88 | 89 | 91 | 91 | 43 | 44 | 44 | 45 | 46 | 46 | 47 |
| | 90th | 98 | 99 | 100 | 101 | 103 | 104 | 105 | 57 | 58 | 58 | 59 | 60 | 61 | 61 |
| | 95th | 102 | 103 | 104 | 105 | 107 | 108 | 109 | 61 | 62 | 62 | 63 | 64 | 65 | 65 |
| | 99th | 109 | 110 | 111 | 112 | 114 | 115 | 116 | 69 | 69 | 70 | 70 | 71 | 72 | 72 |
| 3 | 50th | 86 | 87 | 88 | 89 | 91 | 92 | 93 | 47 | 48 | 48 | 49 | 50 | 50 | 51 |
| | 90th | 100 | 100 | 102 | 103 | 104 | 106 | 106 | 61 | 62 | 62 | 63 | 64 | 64 | 65 |
| | 95th | 104 | 104 | 105 | 107 | 108 | 109 | 110 | 65 | 66 | 66 | 67 | 68 | 68 | 69 |
| | 99th | 111 | 111 | 113 | 114 | 115 | 116 | 117 | 73 | 73 | 74 | 74 | 75 | 76 | 76 |
| 4 | 50th | 88 | 88 | 90 | 91 | 92 | 94 | 94 | 50 | 50 | 51 | 52 | 52 | 53 | 54 |
| | 90th | 101 | 102 | 103 | 104 | 106 | 107 | 108 | 64 | 64 | 65 | 66 | 67 | 67 | 68 |
| | 95th | 105 | 106 | 107 | 108 | 110 | 111 | 112 | 68 | 68 | 69 | 70 | 71 | 71 | 72 |
| | 99th | 112 | 113 | 114 | 115 | 117 | 118 | 119 | 76 | 76 | 76 | 77 | 78 | 79 | 79 |
| 5 | 50th | 89 | 90 | 91 | 93 | 94 | 95 | 96 | 52 | 53 | 53 | 54 | 55 | 55 | 56 |
| | 90th | 103 | 103 | 105 | 106 | 107 | 109 | 109 | 66 | 67 | 67 | 68 | 69 | 69 | 70 |
| | 95th | 107 | 107 | 108 | 110 | 111 | 112 | 113 | 70 | 71 | 71 | 72 | 73 | 73 | 74 |
| | 99th | 114 | 114 | 116 | 117 | 118 | 120 | 120 | 78 | 78 | 79 | 79 | 80 | 81 | 81 |
| 6 | 50th | 91 | 92 | 93 | 94 | 96 | 97 | 98 | 54 | 54 | 55 | 56 | 56 | 57 | 58 |
| | 90th | 104 | 105 | 106 | 108 | 109 | 110 | 111 | 68 | 68 | 69 | 70 | 70 | 71 | 72 |
| | 95th | 108 | 109 | 110 | 111 | 113 | 114 | 115 | 72 | 72 | 73 | 74 | 74 | 75 | 76 |
| | 99th | 115 | 116 | 117 | 119 | 120 | 121 | 122 | 80 | 80 | 80 | 81 | 82 | 83 | 83 |

*(continued)*

**TABLE F-2** 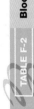 **Blood Pressure Levels for Girls by Age and Height Percentile (Continued)**

| Age, y | BP percentile | SBP, mm Hg | | | | | | | DBP, mm Hg | | | | | | |
|---|---|---|---|---|---|---|---|---|---|---|---|---|---|---|---|
| | | Percentile of height | | | | | | | Percentile of height | | | | | | |
| | | 5th | 10th | 25th | 50th | 75th | 90th | 95th | 5th | 10th | 25th | 50th | 75th | 90th | 95th |
| 7 | 50th | 93 | 93 | 95 | 96 | 97 | 99 | 99 | 55 | 56 | 56 | 57 | 58 | 58 | 59 |
| | 90th | 106 | 107 | 108 | 109 | 111 | 112 | 113 | 69 | 70 | 70 | 71 | 72 | 72 | 73 |
| | 95th | 110 | 111 | 112 | 113 | 115 | 116 | 116 | 73 | 74 | 74 | 75 | 76 | 76 | 77 |
| | 99th | 117 | 118 | 119 | 120 | 122 | 123 | 124 | 81 | 81 | 82 | 82 | 83 | 84 | 84 |
| 8 | 50th | 95 | 95 | 96 | 98 | 99 | 100 | 101 | 57 | 57 | 57 | 58 | 59 | 60 | 60 |
| | 90th | 108 | 109 | 110 | 111 | 113 | 114 | 114 | 71 | 71 | 71 | 72 | 73 | 74 | 74 |
| | 95th | 112 | 112 | 114 | 115 | 116 | 118 | 118 | 75 | 75 | 75 | 76 | 77 | 78 | 78 |
| | 99th | 119 | 120 | 121 | 122 | 123 | 125 | 125 | 82 | 82 | 83 | 83 | 84 | 85 | 86 |
| 9 | 50th | 96 | 97 | 98 | 100 | 101 | 102 | 103 | 58 | 58 | 58 | 59 | 60 | 61 | 61 |
| | 90th | 110 | 110 | 112 | 113 | 114 | 116 | 116 | 72 | 72 | 72 | 73 | 74 | 75 | 75 |
| | 95th | 114 | 114 | 115 | 117 | 118 | 119 | 120 | 76 | 76 | 76 | 77 | 78 | 79 | 79 |
| | 99th | 121 | 121 | 123 | 124 | 125 | 127 | 127 | 83 | 83 | 84 | 84 | 85 | 86 | 87 |
| 10 | 50th | 98 | 99 | 100 | 102 | 103 | 104 | 105 | 59 | 59 | 59 | 60 | 61 | 62 | 62 |
| | 90th | 112 | 112 | 114 | 115 | 116 | 118 | 118 | 73 | 73 | 73 | 74 | 75 | 76 | 76 |
| | 95th | 116 | 116 | 117 | 119 | 120 | 121 | 122 | 77 | 77 | 77 | 78 | 79 | 80 | 80 |
| | 99th | 123 | 123 | 125 | 126 | 127 | 129 | 129 | 84 | 84 | 85 | 86 | 86 | 88 | 88 |
| 11 | 50th | 100 | 101 | 102 | 103 | 105 | 106 | 107 | 60 | 60 | 60 | 61 | 62 | 63 | 63 |
| | 90th | 114 | 114 | 116 | 117 | 118 | 119 | 120 | 74 | 74 | 74 | 75 | 76 | 77 | 77 |
| | 95th | 118 | 118 | 119 | 121 | 122 | 123 | 124 | 78 | 78 | 78 | 79 | 80 | 81 | 81 |
| | 99th | 125 | 125 | 126 | 128 | 129 | 130 | 131 | 85 | 85 | 86 | 87 | 87 | 88 | 89 |
| 12 | 50th | 102 | 103 | 104 | 105 | 107 | 108 | 109 | 61 | 61 | 61 | 62 | 63 | 64 | 64 |
| | 90th | 116 | 116 | 117 | 119 | 120 | 121 | 122 | 75 | 75 | 75 | 76 | 77 | 78 | 78 |
| | 95th | 119 | 120 | 121 | 123 | 124 | 125 | 126 | 79 | 79 | 79 | 80 | 81 | 82 | 82 |
| | 99th | 127 | 127 | 128 | 130 | 131 | 132 | 133 | 86 | 86 | 87 | 88 | 88 | 89 | 90 |

| Age | BP % | SBP 5th | 10th | 25th | 50th | 75th | 90th | 95th | DBP 5th | 10th | 25th | 50th | 75th | 90th | 95th |
|-----|------|------|------|------|------|------|------|------|------|------|------|------|------|------|------|
| 13 | 50th | 104 | 105 | 106 | 107 | 109 | 110 | 110 | 62 | 62 | 62 | 63 | 64 | 65 | 65 |
|    | 90th | 117 | 118 | 119 | 121 | 122 | 123 | 124 | 76 | 76 | 76 | 77 | 78 | 79 | 79 |
|    | 95th | 121 | 122 | 123 | 124 | 126 | 127 | 128 | 80 | 80 | 80 | 81 | 82 | 83 | 83 |
|    | 99th | 128 | 129 | 130 | 132 | 133 | 134 | 135 | 87 | 87 | 88 | 89 | 89 | 90 | 91 |
| 14 | 50th | 106 | 106 | 107 | 109 | 110 | 111 | 112 | 63 | 63 | 63 | 64 | 65 | 66 | 66 |
|    | 90th | 119 | 120 | 121 | 122 | 124 | 125 | 125 | 77 | 77 | 77 | 78 | 79 | 80 | 80 |
|    | 95th | 123 | 123 | 125 | 126 | 127 | 129 | 129 | 81 | 81 | 81 | 82 | 83 | 84 | 84 |
|    | 99th | 130 | 131 | 132 | 133 | 135 | 136 | 136 | 88 | 88 | 89 | 90 | 90 | 91 | 92 |
| 15 | 50th | 107 | 108 | 109 | 110 | 111 | 113 | 113 | 64 | 64 | 64 | 65 | 66 | 67 | 67 |
|    | 90th | 120 | 121 | 122 | 123 | 125 | 126 | 127 | 78 | 78 | 78 | 79 | 80 | 81 | 81 |
|    | 95th | 124 | 125 | 126 | 127 | 129 | 130 | 131 | 82 | 82 | 82 | 83 | 84 | 85 | 85 |
|    | 99th | 131 | 132 | 133 | 134 | 136 | 137 | 138 | 89 | 89 | 90 | 91 | 91 | 92 | 93 |
| 16 | 50th | 108 | 108 | 110 | 111 | 112 | 114 | 114 | 64 | 64 | 65 | 66 | 66 | 67 | 68 |
|    | 90th | 121 | 122 | 123 | 124 | 126 | 127 | 128 | 78 | 78 | 79 | 80 | 81 | 81 | 82 |
|    | 95th | 125 | 126 | 127 | 128 | 130 | 131 | 132 | 82 | 82 | 83 | 84 | 85 | 85 | 86 |
|    | 99th | 132 | 133 | 134 | 135 | 137 | 138 | 139 | 89 | 90 | 90 | 91 | 92 | 93 | 93 |
| 17 | 50th | 108 | 109 | 110 | 111 | 113 | 114 | 115 | 64 | 65 | 65 | 66 | 67 | 67 | 68 |
|    | 90th | 122 | 122 | 123 | 125 | 126 | 127 | 128 | 78 | 79 | 79 | 80 | 81 | 81 | 82 |
|    | 95th | 125 | 126 | 127 | 129 | 130 | 131 | 132 | 82 | 83 | 83 | 84 | 85 | 85 | 86 |
|    | 99th | 133 | 133 | 134 | 136 | 137 | 138 | 139 | 90 | 90 | 91 | 91 | 92 | 93 | 93 |

*The 90th percentile is 1.28 SD, the 95th percentile is 1.645 SD, and the 99th percentile is 2.326 SD over the mean.

For research purposes, the SDs in Table B1 allow one to compute BP Z scores and percentiles for girls with height percentiles given in Table 4 (ie, the 5th, 10th, 25th, 50th, 75th, 90th, and 95th percentiles). These height percentiles must be converted to height Z scores given by: 5% = -1.645; 10% = -1.28; 25% = -0.68; 50% = 0; 75% = 0.68; 90% = 1.28; and 95% = 1.645 and then computed according to the methodology in steps 2 through 4 described in Appendix B. For children with height percentiles other than these, follow steps 1 through 4 as described in Appendix B.

From National High Blood Pressure Education Program Working Group on High Blood Pressure in Children and Adolescents: The Fourth Report on the Diagnosis, Evaluation, and Treatment of High Blood Pressure in Children and Adolescents. Pediatrics 2004;114(2):555-576. ©2004 The American Academy of Pediatrics.

**TABLE F-3** Classification of Hypertension in Children and Adolescents, with Measurement Frequency and Therapy Recommendations

| | SBP or DBP percentile* | Frequency of BP measurement | Therapeutic lifestyle changes | Pharmacologic therapy |
|---|---|---|---|---|
| Normal | <90th | Recheck at next scheduled physical examination | Encourage healthy diet, sleep, and physical activity | — |
| Prehypertension | 90th to <95th or if BP exceeds 120/80 even if <90th percentile up to <95th percentile† | Recheck in 6 mo | Weight-management counseling if overweight; introduce physical activity and diet management‡ | None unless compelling indications such as chronic kidney disease, diabetes mellitus, heart failure, or LVH exist |
| Stage 1 hypertension | >95th–99th percentile plus 5 mm Hg | Recheck in 1–2 wk or sooner if the patient is symptomatic; if persistently elevated on 2 additional occasions, evaluate or refer to source of care within 1 mo | Weight-management counseling if overweight; introduce physical activity and diet management‡ | Initiate therapy based on indications in Table 6 or if compelling indications (as shown above) exist |
| Stage 2 hypertension | >99th percentile plus 5 mm Hg | Evaluate or refer to source of care within 1 wk or immediately if the patient is symptomatic | Weight-management counseling if overweight; introduce physical activity and diet management‡ | Initiate therapy§ |

*For gender, age, and height measured on at least 3 separate occasions; if systolic and diastolic categories are different, categorize by the higher value.
† This occurs typically at 12 years old for SBP and at 16 years old for DBP.
‡ Parents and children trying to modify the eating plan to the Dietary Approaches to Stop Hypertension Study eating plan could benefit from consultation with a registered or licensed nutritionist to get them started.
§ More than 1 drug may be required.
From National High Blood Pressure Education Program Working Group on High Blood Pressure in Children and Adolescents: The Fourth Report on the Diagnosis, Evaluation, and Treatment of High Blood Pressure in Children and Adolescents. Pediatrics 2004;114(2):555–576. ©2004 The American Academy of Pediatrics.

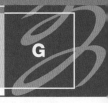

- Make yourself comfortable. This is the most important aspect of beginning a procedure.
  - If *you* are uncomfortable, the procedure will take longer, and is more likely to be unsuccessful.
- For all the procedures described below:
  - Wear a mask.
  - Wear a sterile gown and sterile gloves after scrubbing.
  - Prepare and drape the skin with povidone-iodine under aseptic precautions.

## UMBILICAL ARTERY CATHETERIZATION

### Indications

- Monitoring of arterial blood gases and blood pressure
- Administering total parenteral nutrition (TPN) or hypertonic solutions

### Complications

- Hemorrhage (from line displacement)
- Thrombosis
- Infection
- Ischemia/infarction of lower extremities, bowel, or kidney
- Arrhythmia
- Hypertension

### Line Placement and Catheter Length

- With a high line, place the tip of the catheter above the diaphragm, between T6 and T9 (above the renal and mesenteric arteries). This approach is less prone to complications.
- Use the formula to determine catheter length (high line):

$$\text{Catheter length (cm)} = (3 \times \text{birth weight (kg)} + 9)$$

### Procedure

- Determine the catheter length.
- Restrain infant. Using sterile technique, "prep" and drape umbilical cord and adjacent skin.
- Flush catheter with sterile saline (after attaching a three-way stopcock) before insertion to avoid air embolism
- Place sterile umbilical tape around base of cord. Cut through cord horizontally about 1.5–2.0 cm above the skin. Tighten umbilical tape to stop bleeding.
- Identify the one large, thin-walled vein and the two smaller, thicker-walled arteries. Use curved-tip forceps to gently open and dilate one of the arteries.
- Grasp catheter approximately 1 cm from the tip with toothless forceps and insert catheter into artery to the desired length. Feed catheter into artery using gentle pressure.
  - Do not force the catheter.
  - Forcing the catheter may create a false luminal tract.
- Secure catheter with a suture through the cord and around the catheter.

- Confirm catheter position with a radiograph. The catheter may be pulled back but not advanced once the sterile field is broken.

## UMBILICAL VEIN CATHETERIZATION

### Indications

- Administering crystalloids or colloids in the labor and delivery room to resuscitate neonates in shock
- Rapidly administering medications
- Administering hypertonic fluids or TPN

### Complications

- Hemorrhage from line displacement or vessel perforation
- Infection
- Air embolism
- Arrhythmia
- Portal vein thrombosis and portal hypertension (delayed complication)

### Line Placement and Catheter Length

- Place the catheter in the inferior vena cava above the level of the ductus venosus and the hepatic veins and below the level of the left atrium. Practically, this means at the level of the right dome of the diaphragm.
- Use the formula to determine catheter length:

  Catheter length (cm) = [0.5 × length of the umbilical artery catheter (cm)] + 1

### Procedure

- Follow procedure steps for umbilical artery catheter placement up to identifying the artery. In this case, identify the thin-walled vein and insert the catheter.
  - Gently advance catheter to desired distance.
  - Do not force the catheter because this may cause a false luminal tract.
- Secure catheter as in umbilical artery catheter placement.
- Confirm catheter placement with a radiograph.
- In the delivery room, where speed of placing the umbilical line is essential, insert the catheter to 5 cm in a term infant (or until you can first draw back blood easily); this is sufficient.

## LUMBAR PUNCTURE

### Indications

- Diagnosing meningitis (suspected sepsis in neonates, apnea and bradycardia, evaluation of neonates or children with positive blood cultures)
- Relieving increased intracranial pressure (ICP) in neonates with hydrocephalus (serial lumbar punctures)

### Contraindications

- Increased ICP
  - If signs or symptoms of increased ICP are present (papilledema, retinal hemorrhage, trauma with associated head injury), perform computed tomography (CT) before lumbar puncture.
  - Lumbar puncture should not be performed in very sick neonates who do not tolerate the required positioning.

- Bleeding diathesis
  - Platelet count $>50,000/mm^3$ is preferable.
  - Correction of clotting factor deficiencies before lumbar puncture prevents spinal cord hemorrhage and potential paralysis.
- Overlying skin infections, which may inoculate the cerebrospinal fluid (CSF).

## Complications

- Dry tap or traumatic tap (most common complication)
- Headache
- Acquired epidermal spinal cord tumor caused by implantation of epidermal material into spinal canal if no stylet used on skin entry
- Local back pain
- Infection
- Bleeding
- Herniations associated with increased ICP. Cerebellar tonsillar herniation is not a dreaded complication in neonates who have an open anterior fontanelle.

## Procedure

- Position the child either in the sitting position or in the lateral recumbent position with the hips, knees, and neck flexed. Monitor cardiorespiratory status for compromise.
- Locate either the L3-L4 or L4-L5 interspace by drawing an imaginary line between the two iliac crests.
- Clean the skin with povidone-iodine and drape the child in sterile fashion.
- Use a 20- to 22-gauge spinal needle of desired length.
- Anesthetize the overlying skin and subcutaneous tissue with 1% buffered lidocaine.
- Puncture midline just caudal to palpated spinous process, angling the needle slightly cephalad and toward the umbilicus. Advance the needle slowly; withdrawing the stylet every few millimeters to check for CSF flow.
- If resistance is met (i.e., you hit bone), withdraw the needle to the skin and redirect the angle of the needle.
- Send CSF for appropriate studies (tube 1 for culture and Gram's stain, tube 2 for glucose and protein, tube 3 for cell count and differential, and tube 4 for saved CSF or any additional specialized studies).The tube with the clearest CSF should be sent for cell count regardless of its number.
- To measure CSF pressure, patient must be lying straight (not curled up) on his or her side. Once free flow of CSF is established, attach the manometer and measure CSF pressure.

# CHEST TUBE PLACEMENT AND THORACENTESIS

## Indications

- Tension pneumothorax and pleural effusion

## Complications

- Pneumothorax or hemothorax
- Bleeding or infection
- Pulmonary contusion or laceration
- Puncture of diaphragm, liver, or spleen

## Procedure

### Needle Decompression

- For tension pneumothorax, decompress by inserting a 23-gauge butterfly or 22-gauge angiocatheter at the second intercostal space in the midclavicular line, taking aseptic precautions.

- Insert the needle or the angiocatheter attached to a three-way stopcock open to the syringe and aspirate as the needle is advanced. Stop advancing the needle as soon as air is aspirated in the syringe. Stop aspirating after the syringe is full of air and turn the stopcock off and empty the syringe.
- Turn the stopcock in line with the syringe and start aspirating again. Repeat until no air is aspirated.

## Chest Tube Placement

- Position child supine or with affected side up.
- Identify the entry point, which is the third to fifth intercostal space in the mid to anterior axillary line, usually at the level of the nipple. (Be careful to avoid breast tissue.)
- Locally anesthetize skin, subcutaneous tissue, chest wall muscles, and parietal pleura with lidocaine.
- Make an incision at the desired insertion point, and bluntly dissect through tissue layers until the superior portion of the rib is reached. (This avoids the neurovascular bundle on the inferior portion of each rib.)
- Push a Hemostat over the top of the rib, through the pleura, and into the pleural space. Enter the pleural space cautiously. Spread Hemostat to open, place chest tube in clamp, and guide into entry point.
- Insert the tube.
  - For a pneumothorax, insert the tube anteriorly toward the apex of the opposite lung.
  - For a pleural effusion, direct the tube inferiorly and posteriorly.
- Secure the tube with purse-string sutures.
- Attach the tube to the drainage system with –20 to –30 cm of water pressure.
- Apply a sterile occlusive dressing.
- Confirm position with a chest radiograph. A lateral chest radiograph is needed to confirm that the tip of the chest tube is in the anterior mediastinum especially if evacuating a pneumothorax.

## Thoracentesis

- Confirm fluid in pleural space with clinical examination, chest radiography, or sonography. Confirm that the volume of the fluid is large enough to be drained.
- Place child in sitting position leaning over a table if possible. Otherwise place child supine.
- Identify the point of entry in the seventh intercostal space and posterior axillary line.
- "Prep" and drape area under aseptic precautions.
- Anesthetize skin, subcutaneous tissue, chest wall muscles, and pleura with lidocaine.
- Advance an 18- to 22-gauge intravenous catheter or large-bore needle attached to a syringe and a stop cock and then "walk" the needle over the top of the rib into the pleural space while providing steady negative pressure.
- Aspirate fluid.
- After removing the needle or catheter, place an occlusive dressing and obtain a chest radiograph to rule out iotrogenic pneumothorax.

## SUTURING

### General Information

- Lacerations to be sutured should be <6 hours old (12 hours on the face).
- Usually, bite wounds should not be sutured.
- The longer sutures are left in place, the greater the potential for scarring and infection.

| TABLE G-1 | Suture Requirements for Lacerations by Location | |
| --- | --- | --- |
| Location | Suture (monofilament) | Removal (days) |
| Face | 6–0 | 3–5 |
| Scalp | 4–0 or 5–0, consider staples | 5–7 |
| Eyelid | 6–0 or 7–0 | 3–5 |
| Eyebrow | 5–0 or 6–0 | 3–5 |
| Trunk | 4–0 or 5–0 | 5–7 |
| Extremities | 4–0 or 5–0 | 7 |
| Joint surface | 4–0 | 10–14 |
| Hand | 5–0 | 7 |
| Sole of foot | 3–0 or 4–0 | 7–10 |

- Plastic surgery should be considered with any laceration involving the face, lips, hands, genitalia, mouth, or orbital area, including deep lacerations with nerve damage; stellate lacerations; flap lacerations; lacerations involving the vermilion border; lacerations with questionable tissue viability; and large, complex lacerations.

## Procedure

- Remove foreign bodies.
- Examine area for exposed nerves, tendons, and bone.
- Perform a neurovascular examination.
- Remember to ask about tetanus status and immunize if needed.
- Irrigate wound with copious amounts of sterile saline to clean area. (This is the most important step to prevent infection.)
- Apply anesthetic.
  - Injectable
    - No end-artery supply: 1% lidocaine with 1% epinephrine; maximum dose is 7 mg/kg
    - End-artery supply: 1% lidocaine without epinephrine; maximum dose is 3–5 mg/kg
  - Topical: lidocaine, epinephrine, tetracaine (LET), lidocaine (ELA-Max)
- Débride any necessary areas.
- Begin suturing (Table G-1).
- Apply antibiotic ointment and sterile dressing.

## APPLICATION OF SKIN ADHESIVES

- Appropriate uses: low-tension areas
- Inappropriate uses: high-tension areas, contaminated wounds, wounds across mucocutaneous junctions, animal or human bites, or wounds with evidence of infection

## Procedure

- Clean and dry area.
- Achieve hemostasis.
- Approximate wound edges.
- Squeeze adhesive onto wound edges then apply in a circular motion around wound.
- Apply at least three layers, allowing each layer to dry between applications.

## Postapplication

- Do not apply dressing. None is needed, and adhesive falls off in 5 to 10 days.
- Avoid topical ointments.
- Do not scrub or submerse area.

### Suggested Readings

Dieckman R, Fisher D, Selbst S. Pediatric Emergency and Critical Care Procedures. St. Louis: Mosby-Year Book, 1997.
The Cochrane Database of Systematic Reviews 2005 Issue 4, http://www.cochrane.org/reviews

Page numbers followed by f refer to figures; page numbers followed by t refer to tables.